HOSPITAL MEDICINE

HOSPITAL MEDICINE

SECRETS

Jeffrey J. Glasheen, MD
Assistant Professor of Medicine
Director, Hospital Medicine Program, University of Colorado Hospital
Director of Inpatient Medicine, University of Colorado Hospital
Associate Program Director, Internal Medicine Training Program
Program Director, Hospitalist Training Program
Department of Medicine
University of Colorado at Denver and Health Sciences Center
Denver, Colorado

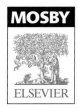

MOSBY

ELSEVIER

MOSBY
ELSEVIER

1600 John F. Kennedy Boulevard, Suite 1800
Philadelphia, PA 19103-2899

Hospital Medicine Secrets   ISBN-13: 978-0-323-04087-7
                                       ISBN-10: 0-323-04087-X

Library of Congress Cataloging-in-Publication Data

Hospital medicine secrets / [edited by] Jeffrey James Glasheen. – 1st ed.
    p. ; cm. – (Secrets series)
Includes bibliographical references and index.
ISBN 0-323-04087-X
    1. Clinical medicine–Examinations, questions, etc.   2. Hospital care–Examinations, questions, etc.   I. Glasheen, Jeffrey James.   II. Series.
    [DNLM: 1. Clinical Medicine–Examination Questions.   2. Hospitalization–Examination Questions.   WB 18.2 H828 2007]
    RC58.H67 2007
    616.0076–dc22

                                                            2006040956

Vice President, Medical Education: Linda Belfus
Developmental Editor: Stan Ward
Project Manager: Mary Stermel
Marketing Manager: Kate Rubin

Working together to grow
libraries in developing countries

www.elsevier.com | www.bookaid.org | www.sabre.org

ELSEVIER   BOOK AID International   Sabre Foundation

Printed in China.

Last digit is the print number: 9   8   7   6   5   4   3   2   1

ASSOCIATE EDITORS

Alpesh N. Amin, MD, MBA, FACP
Professor of Medicine, Executive Director, Hospitalist Program, and Vice Chair for Clinical Affairs and Quality, Department of Medicine; Associate Program Director, IM Residency, Medicine Clerkship Director, University of California at Irvine, Orange, California

Amir K. Jaffer, MD
Associate Professor of Medicine, Cleveland Clinic Lerner College of Medicine of Case Western Reserve University; Medical Director, IMPACT (Internal Medicine Preoperative Assessment Consultation and Treatment) Center; Medical Director, The Anticoagulation Clinic, Department of General Internal Medicine, Section of Hospital Medicine, Cleveland Clinic, Cleveland, Ohio

Sunil Kripalani, MD, MSc
Assistant Professor, Division of General Internal Medicine, Emory School of Medicine; Assistant Director for Research, Grady Hospitalist Program, Atlanta, Georgia

Joseph Ming Wah Li, MD
Director, Hospital Medicine Program, Department of Medicine, Beth Israel Deaconess Medical Center; Assistant Professor of Medicine, Harvard Medical School, Boston, Massachusetts

DEDICATION

To my parents, Jim and Cathy, for their unconditional, occasionally bordering on crazed, support of all that I have attempted. Without you I would not be where I am today. And to my love and inspiration, Hanna, without whom I would not be going where I will be tomorrow.

Jeffrey J. Glasheen

To my parents, my wife Hajra and my children Saniya and Salman, for their ongoing support of my career that has required so much time away from them.

Amir K. Jaffer

To my beautiful wife Sapna, for all her love and support, and to our daughter Sia, for always making me smile.

Sunil Kripalani

To my parents Navin and Harshila, my wife Sonali, my daughter Aanya, my sister Avani, and her husband Ashish for their endless support and love.

Alpesh N. Amin

Thank you to my wife Kelly, my daughters Grace and Hope, my parents, family, friends, colleagues, and mentor, Mark Aronson.

Joseph Ming Wah Li

CONTENTS

VI. GASTROENTEROLOGY

VII. NEPHROLOGY

VIII. INFECTIOUS DISEASE

IX. HEMATOLOGY AND ONCOLOGY

X. ENDOCRINOLOGY

XI. RHEUMATOLOGY

XII. DERMATOLOGY

XIII. ALLERGY

XIV. TOXICOLOGY

XV. GERIATRICS

XVI. PERIOPERATIVE AND CONSULTATIVE MEDICINE

XVII. PROCEDURES

XVIII. PALLIATIVE CARE MEDICINE AND END-OF-LIFE ISSUES

CONTRIBUTORS

Val Akopov, MD
Assistant Professor, Department of Medicine, Emory University School of Medicine; Director, Hospital Medicine Service, Emory Crawford Long Hospital, Atlanta, Georgia

Ashish Aneja, MBBS, MD
Associate Staff, Department of General Internal Medicine, Section of Hospital Medicine, Cleveland Clinic, Cleveland, Ohio

Julia Feliz Alvarado, MD
Assistant Professor of Medicine, University of Colorado School of Medicine, Denver, Colorado

Alpesh N. Amin, MD, MBA, FACP
Professor of Medicine, Executive Director, Hospitalist Program, and Vice Chair for Clinical Affairs and Quality, Department of Medicine; Associate Program Director, IM Residency, Medicine Clerkship Director, University of California at Irvine, Orange, California

Robin K. Avery, MD
Section Head, Transplant Infectious Disease, Department of Infectious Disease, Cleveland Clinic, Cleveland, Ohio

Vincent Barba, MD, FACP
Chief, Section of Hospital Medicine; Assistant Professor of Medicine, New Jersey Medical School, Newark, New Jersey

Preetha Basaviah, MD
Clinical Associate Professor of Medicine, Associate Course Director – Practice of Medicine, Stanford University School of Medicine, Stanford University, Stanford, California

Adrienne L. Bennett, MD, PhD
Associate Professor of Clinical Medicine, Director, Division of Hospital Medicine; Department of Internal Medicine, The Ohio State University Medical Center, Columbus, Ohio

Douglas Borg, MD
Clinical Instructor, Section of Hospital Medicine, Division of General Internal Medicine, University of Colorado at Denver and Health Sciences Center, Denver, Colorado

Sarah Bull, MD
Department of Medicine, Division of Endocrinology and Metabolism, University of Colorado Health Sciences Center, Aurora, Colorado

Gregory Busse, DO
Clinical Assistant Professor, University of Wisconsin Medical School, Madison, Wisconsin

Alex Carbo, MD
Hospitalist, Beth Israel Deaconess Medical Center; Instructor in Medicine, Harvard Medical School, Boston, Massachusetts

Jeffrey Carter, MD
Clinical Instructor, Section of Hospital Medicine, Division of General Internal Medicine, University of Colorado at Denver and Health Sciences Center, Denver, Colorado

Patrick S. Cawley, MD
Director, Hospitalist Program, Medical University of South Carolina, Charleston, South Carolina

Eugene S. Chu, MD
Director of Education, Director of Hospital Medicine, Denver Health and Hospital Authority, Assistant Professor of Medicine, University of Colorado at Denver and Health Sciences Center, Denver, Colorado

Barbara Cleary, MD
Hospitalist, Denver Health Medical Center; Assistant Professor, University of Colorado Health Sciences Center, Denver, Colorado

Scott E. Clemens, MD
Resident, University of Colorado School of Medicine, Denver, Colorado

Steven L. Cohn, MD, FACP
Chief, Division of General Internal Medicine; Director, Medical Consultation Service; Clinical Professor of Medicine, SUNY Downstate Medical Center, Brooklyn, New York

Natalie G. Correia, DO, MA
Senior Associate Director, Internal Medicine Residency, Advocate Lutheran General Hospital, Park Ridge, Illinois

Yvette M. Cua, MD
Assistant Professor of Medicine, Emory University School of Medicine, Atlanta, Georgia

Catherine Curley, MD, MS
Chief, Division of Hospital Medicine, Department of Medicine, MetroHealth Medical Center; Assistant Professor of Medicine, Case School of Medicine, Cleveland, Ohio

Amish Ajit Dangodara, MD
Associate Clinical Professor of Internal Medicine; Director, Inpatient Medical Consultation Service; Director, Preoperative Medicine Clinic; University of California at Irvine College of Medicine; Hospitalist Program, UCI Medical Center, Orange, California

Steven B. Deitelzweig, MD
Chairman, Hospital Medicine, Ochsner Clinic Foundation; Clinical Assistant Professor of Medicine, Tulane University Medical College, New Orleans, Louisiana

Robert Dexter, MD
Clinical Instructor, Section of Hospital Medicine, Division of General Internal Medicine, University of Colorado at Denver and Health Sciences Center, Denver, Colorado

Andrew H. Dombro, MD
Clinical Instructor, Section of Hospital Medicine, Division of General Internal Medicine, University of Colorado at Denver and Health Sciences Center, Denver, Colorado

Daniel D. Dressler, MD, MSc
Assistant Professor of Medicine, Director of Hospital Medicine, Emory University Hospital, Emory University School of Medicine, Atlanta, Georgia

Wassim H. Fares, MD
Assistant Professor of Medicine, Cleveland Clinic Lerner College of Medicine of Case Western Reserve University, Department of General Internal Medicine, Section of Hospital Medicine, Cleveland Clinic, Cleveland, Ohio

David Feinbloom, MD
Hospital Physician, Department of Medicine, Beth Israel Deaconess Medical Center; Instructor in Medicine, Harvard Medical School, Boston, Massachusetts

Kathleen Finn, MD, MPhil
Hospitalist, Medical Director of the General Medical Service, Brigham and Women's–Faulkner Hospitalist Program; Instructor in Medicine, Harvard Medical School, Boston, Massachusetts

Bradley Flansbaum, DO, MPH
Lennox Hill Hospital; Clinical Assistant Professor of Medicine; Chief, Hospitalist Services, New York University, New York, New York

Kevin Flemmons, MD
FirstHealth of the Carolinas Hospitalist Services, Pinehurst, North Carolina

Lorenzo Di Francesco, MD, FACP
Associate Professor of Medicine, Associate Program Director, GMH, J. Willis Hurst Internal Medicine Residency, Emory University School of Medicine, Altanta, Georgia

Adam L. Friedlander, MD
Fellow, Division of Pulmonary Sciences and Critical Care Medicine, Department of Medicine, University of Colorado at Denver and Health Sciences Center, Denver, Colorado

Joseph Michael Gergyes, MD
Assistant Professor, Department of Medicine, University of Wisconsin at Madison, Madison, Wisconsin

Jeffrey J. Glasheen, MD
Assistant Professor of Medicine, Director, Hospital Medicine Program, University of Colorado at Denver and Health Sciences Center, Denver, Colorado

Craig Gordon, MD
Hospitalist, Beth Israel Deaconess Medical Center; Instructor in Medicine, Harvard Medical School, Boston, Massachusetts

Barry S. Greenwald, PhD
Emeritus, Associate Professor of Psychology, University of Illinois at Chicago, Chicago, Illinois

Jeffrey L. Greenwald, MD
Assistant Professor of Medicine, Boston University School of Medicine, Boston, Massachusetts

Stephanie Grossman, MD
Assistant Professor of Medicine, Emory University School of Medicine; Co-Director, Palliative Care Consult Service, Emory Hospitals, Atlanta, Georgia

Ruben O. Halperin, MD, MPH
Physician, Core Faculty, Providence Ambulatory Care and Education Center (PACE); Providence Portland Medical Center, Portland, Oregon

Brian Harte, MD
Clinical Assistant Professor of Medicine, Cleveland Clinic Lerner College of Medicine at Case Western Reserve University; Associate Staff, Section of Hospital Medicine, Cleveland Clinic, Cleveland, Ohio

Anna Loa Helgason, MD, PhD
Instructor of Medicine, Harvard Medical School; Assistant Physician, Department of Medicine, Massachusetts General Hospital, Boston, Massachusetts

Benjamin A. Hohmuth, MD
Instructor, Harvard Medical School; Hospitalist, Harvard Vanguard Medical Associates; Brigham and Women's and Faulkner Hospitals, Boston, Massachusetts

Amir K. Jaffer, MD
Associate Professor of Medicine, Cleveland Clinic Lerner College of Medicine of Case Western Reserve University; Medical Director, IMPACT (Internal Medicine Preoperative Assessment Consultation and Treatment) Center; Medical Director, The Anticoagulation Clinic, Department of General Internal Medicine, Section of Hospital Medicine, Cleveland Clinic, Cleveland, Ohio

Daniel Johnson, MD
Chief, Palliative Care Department, Kaiser Permanente of Denver, Aurora, Colorado

James Joyner, MD
Hospitalist Program, University of California Irvine Medical Center, Orange, California

Nilesh Kalyanaraman, MD
Physician, Unity Health Care, Inc., Washington, DC

Ben Keidan, MD
Hospitalist, Department of Medicine, Beth Israel Deaconess Medical Center; Instructor of Medicine, Harvard Medical School, Boston, Massachusetts

Lisa S. Kettering, MD, FACP
Associate Director, In-Patient Services, Director, Evidence Based Medicine Curriculum, Department of Graduate Medical Education for Internal Medicine, Exempla-Saint Joseph Hospital; Assistant Clinical Professor, Department of Internal Medicine, University of Colorado School of Medicine, Denver, Colorado

Anna Kho, MD
Assistant Professor, Division of General Internal Medicine, Emory University School of Medicine, Atlanta, Georgia

Chong U. Kim, MD
Associate Professor of Medicine, University of California at Irvine College of Medicine; Hospitalist Program, UCI Medical Center, Orange, California

Jennifer Kleinbart, MD
Associate Professor of Medicine, Emory University School of Medicine; Associate Medical Director, Grady Health Outcomes Center, Atlanta, Georgia

Christin H. Ko, MD
Assistant Professor of Medicine, Emory University School of Medicine; Director, Hospital Medicine, Emory Dunwoody Medical Center; Associate Medical Director, Emory Healthcare Alliance, Atlanta, Georgia

Cynthia A. Korzelius, MD, MSc
Assistant Clinical Professor, Tufts University School of Medicine; Department of Internal Medicine, Newton Wellesley Hospital, Newton, Massachusetts

David Krakow, MD
Instructor in Medicine, Harvard Medical School; Beth Israel Deaconess Medical Center, Boston, Massachusetts

Susan Krekun, MD
Assistant Professor of Clinical Medicine, Division of General Internal Medicine, Hospital of the University of Pennsylvania, Philadelphia, Pennsylvania

Sunil Kripalani, MD, MSc
Assistant Professor of Medicine, Emory University School of Medicine; Assistant Director, Grady Hospitalist Program, Atlanta, Georgia

Ajay Kumar, MD, MRCP
Associate Staff, Department of General Internal Medicine, Section of Hospital Medicine, Cleveland Clinic, Cleveland, Ohio

Suzette LaRoche, MD
Assistant Professor of Neurology, Emory University School of Medicine, Atlanta, Georgia

Solomon Liao, MD
Associate Professor of Medicine, University of California at Irvine, Orange, California

Joseph Ming Wah Li, MD
Director, Hospital Medicine Program, Department of Medicine, Beth Israel Deaconess Medical Center; Assistant Professor of Medicine, Harvard Medical School, Boston, Massachusetts

Marina N. Magrey, MD
Fellow, Department of Rheumatology, Cleveland Clinic, Cleveland, Ohio

Melissa Mahoney, MD
Assistant Professor of Medicine, Emory University School of Medicine; Co-Director, Palliative Care Consult Service, Emory Hospitals, Atlanta, Georgia

Noble Maleque, MD
Instructor, Emory University School of Medicine, Atlanta, Georgia

Brian F. Mandell, MD, PhD, FACR
Professor and Vice Chairman of Medicine, Department of Rheumatic and Immunologic Diseases, Center for Vasculitis Care and Research, Cleveland Clinic, Cleveland, Ohio

Robert L. Matorin, MD, MS
Assistant Clinical Professor of Medicine, University of California at San Diego, San Diego, California

Melissa L.P. Mattison, MD
Instructor of Medicine, Harvard Medical School; Beth Israel Deaconess Medical Center, Boston, Massachusetts

Sylvia C.W. McKean, MD
Assistant Professor, Harvard Medical School; Medical Director, BWF Hospitalist Service, Brigham and Women's Hospital, Boston, Massachusetts

Margaret McLees, MD
Assistant Professor of Medicine, Section of Hospital Medicine, Division of General Internal Medicine, University of Colorado at Denver and Health Sciences Center, Denver, Colorado

Edward J. Merrens, MD
Assistant Professor, Dartmouth Medical School; Section Chief, Hospital Medicine, Department of Medicine, Dartmouth-Hitchcock Medical Center, Lebanon, New Hampshire

Jordan Messler, MD
Medical Director, Morton Plant Hospitalists, InCompass Health, Clearwater, Florida

Franklin A. Michota, MD, FACP
Head, Section of Hospital Medicine, Department of General Internal Medicine, Cleveland Clinic, Cleveland, Ohio

Gregory J. Misky, MD
Assistant Professor of Medicine, Section of Hospital Medicine, Division of General Internal Medicine, University of Colorado at Denver and Health Sciences Center, Denver, Colorado

Mandakolathur Murali, MD
Director, Clinical Immunology Laboratory, Division of Allergy, Immunology and Rheumatology, Massachusetts General Hospital; Harvard Medical School, Boston, Massachusetts

Jennifer S. Myers, MD
Assistant Professor of Clinical Medicine, Division of General Internal Medicine, Hospital of the University of Pennsylvania, Philadelphia, Pennsylvania

John Nelson, MD
Director, Hospitalist Practice, Overlake Hospital Medical Center, Bellevue, Washington

Mary H. Pak, MD
Clinical Associate Professor of Medicine, University of Wisconsin School of Medicine and Public Health, Madison, Wisconsin

Robert M. Palmer, MD, MPH
Head, Section of Geriatric Medicine, Department of General Internal Medicine, Cleveland Clinic, Cleveland, Ohio

James C. Pile, MD
Assistant Professor of Medicine, Case Medical School, Division of Hospital Medicine, Case Western Reserve University at MetroHealth Medical Center, Cleveland, Ohio

Michael J. Pistoria, DO, FACP
Associate Program Director, Internal Medicine Residency, Medical Director, Hospitalist Services, Lehigh Valley Hospital; Assistant Professor of Medicine, Pennsylvania State University College of Medicine, Allentown, Pennsylvania

Mark B. Reid, MD
Assistant Professor of Medicine, University of Colorado School of Medicine; Hospitalist, Denver Health Medical Center, Denver, Colorado

Daniel Robitshek, MD
Associate Professor of Clinical Medicine, University of California at Irvine; Department of Medicine, Hospitalist Program, UC Irvine Medical Center, Orange, California

David D.K. Rolston, MD, FACP
Staff Physician and Associate Program Director, Internal Medicine Residency Program, Cleveland Clinic, Cleveland, Ohio

James H. Roum, MD, PhD
Associate Clinical Professor of Medicine, Pulmonary and Critical Care Medicine, University of California at Irvine; Director, Medical Intensive Care, Hospitalist Program, University of California Irvine Medical Center, Orange, California

Bindu Sangani, MD, MPH
Staff Physician, Kaiser Permanente, Cleveland, Ohio

Gentian Scheer, MD
Clinical Instructor, Section of Hospital Medicine, Division of General Internal Medicine, University of Colorado at Denver and Health Sciences Center, Denver, Colorado

Hiren Shah, MD, MBA
Associate Director, Section of Hospital Medicine, Northwestern University; Feinberg School of Medicine, Chicago, Illinois

Bradley A. Sharpe, MD
Assistant Clinical Professor, Department of Medicine, University of California at San Francisco, San Francisco, California

Lisa Shieh, MD, PhD
Clinical Assistant Professor, Department of Medicine, Stanford University Medical Center, Stanford, California

Eric M. Siegal, MD
Regional Medical Director, Cogent Healthcare, Irvine, California

Vaishali Singh, MD, MPH, MBA
Department of Medicine, Section of Hospital Medicine, Cleveland Clinic, Cleveland, Ohio

Gerald W. Smetana, MD
Division of General Medicine and Primary Care, Beth Israel Deaconess Medical Center; Associate Professor of Medicine, Harvard Medical School, Boston, Massachusetts

Visalakshi Srinivasan, MD
Fellow, Section of Geriatric Medicine, Department of General Internal Medicine, Cleveland Clinic, Cleveland, Ohio

Sanjeev Suri, MD, MBA
Director of Clinical Operations, Section of Hospital Medicine, Department of General Internal Medicine, Cleveland, Ohio

Sheri Chernetsky Tejedor, MD
Assistant Professor of Medicine, Emory University School of Medicine, Atlanta, Georgia

Anjala Tess, MD
Hospitalist, Department of Medicine, Beth Israel Deaconess Medical Center; Instructor and Assistant Professor in Medicine, Harvard Medical School, Boston, Massachusetts

Alexandra Villa-Forte, MD, MPH
Director, Vasculitis Clinic, Department of Rheumatology, Universidade do Estado do Rio de Janeiro, Rio de Janeiro, Brazil

Michael D. Wang, MD
Assistant Clinical Professor, Department of Medicine, Hospitalist Program, Program in Geriatrics, University of California at Irvine, Orange, California

Martin C. Were, MD
Instructor, Emory University School of Medicine, Atlanta, Georgia

Chad T. Whelan, MD
Associate Professor of Medicine, University of Chicago, Chicago, Illinois

James H. Williams, Jr, MD
Adjunct Professor of Medicine, Pulmonary and Critical Care Hospitalist Physician Group; UC Irvine Medical Center, Orange, California

Mitchell J. Wilson, MD
Associate Professor of Medicine, Section Chief of Hospital Medicine, Medical Director, FirstHealth of the Carolinas Hospitalist Services, Division of General Medicine and Clinical Epidemiology, Department of Medicine, The University of North Carolina at Chapel Hill School of Medicine, Chapel Hill, North Carolina

Neil Winawer, MD
Director, Hospital Medicine Unit, Grady Memorial Hospital; Associate Professor of Medicine, Emory University School of Medicine, Atlanta, Georgia

Julius Yang, MD, PhD
Hospitalist, Department of Medicine, Beth Israel Deaconess Medical Center; Instructor in Medicine, Harvard Medical School, Boston, Massachusetts

Jeanie Youngwerth, MD
Associate Program Director, Colorado Palliative Medicine Fellowship; Clinical Instructor, Section of Hospital Medicine, Division of General Internal Medicine, University of Colorado at Denver and Health Sciences Center, Denver, Colorado

PREFACE

The field of hospital medicine has seen a meteoric rise in the number of practitioners in the past decade, fueling a new paradigm in the delivery of health care. With this growth has come the realization that hospitalists are more than just internists, family practitioners, and pediatricians who focus their clinical interest on the care of inpatients. It is now clear that hospitalists require an expert understanding of areas of health care that have traditionally stood outside the practice of most generalists—areas such as perioperative medicine, stroke management, inpatient orthopedics, and palliative care. Additionally, hospitalists are asked to lead change in hospitals, including leadership in the patient safety movement and systems and quality improvement. Unfortunately, the traditional educational venues have been slow to adapt to these rapid changes, leaving many practicing hospitalists feeling underprepared to deal with these expectations.

Hospital Medicine Secrets is intended to help fill this void. With sections devoted to quality improvement, patient safety, perioperative medicine, and palliative care, this book goes beyond the scope of most traditional organ-based texts. However, it does so while maintaining a strong backbone of clinical and procedural medicine, which remains the foundation of the practice of hospital medicine.

Inherent to the practice of inpatient medicine is the need to practice in teams. The ever more complicated world of hospital care demands that physicians, nurses, pharmacists, social workers, case managers, and other allied health professionals work in true collaboration to ensure the safe passage of patients throughout the hospital environment. As such, it is our intent that this book serve as a reference and learning tool for all providers who participate in the care of medical or surgical inpatients. To this end we created this book not only for the practicing hospitalist but also for students and practitioners of medicine, nursing and other allied health fields, to enhance their role in this evolving team.

Finally, I want to thank the host of contributors who gave of their time and energy so willingly. The handiwork of their passion, zeal, and work ethic is visible not only in the fabric of this book but also in the hospital medicine movement itself.

Jeffrey J. Glasheen, MD

TOP 100 SECRETS

These secrets are 100 of the top board alerts. They summarize the concepts, principles, and most salient details of hospital medicine.

1. Proper handwashing and gloving, contact precautions, and isolation all limit the spread of organisms. Routine hand decontamination is crucial, before and after each patient contact, either with an alcohol-based hand rub or at least 15 seconds of vigorous handwashing with soap and water.

2. The best approach to improve patient safety is one that focuses on training employees and fixing the system rather than blaming or punishing the individual.

3. Use of legible handwriting and universally accepted abbreviations only cuts down the chances of medication errors. Direct communication to the individual responsible for the actual administration of the medication further reduces the likelihood of medication errors.

4. In the stormy sea of litigation, documentation can be a life raft that keeps you afloat or an anchor that drags you down. If you would not want your note read in open court, rethink what you are writing.

5. Communicating expectations about hospital care and discharge is the best way to minimize the conflicts that arise during a hospitalization.

6. Develop a standard approach to communication with other professionals and patients, and follow this approach for every patient.

7. Medication reconciliation, the process of comparing a patient's list of discharge medicines with the list of medicines at the time of hospital admission, is not only a new JCAHO mandate but also a vital component of a safe handoff.

8. One in five adults aged 18–64 years is uninsured in America. The majority of them are employed.

9. Evidence-based medicine emphasizes the examination of evidence from clinical research and the integration of that evidence with clinical expertise and patient values.

10. In a ventilated patient, increasing the tidal volume, pressure support, or respiratory rate will tend to decrease the PCO_2, and increasing the FIO_2 or positive end-expiratory pressure will tend to increase the PaO_2.

11. The most important step in treating hypotension is to ensure the patient is adequately volume resuscitated. The ultimate goal for vasoactive agents is adequate tissue perfusion, not a prescribed blood pressure.

12. The hallmark of hypovolemic shock is a decreased pulmonary capillary wedge pressure (PCWP); the hallmark of cardiogenic shock is a decreased cardiac output; the hallmark of distributive

shock is a decreased systemic vascular resistance; and the hallmark of cardiac tamponade is an equalization of right atrial pressure, right ventricular diastolic pressure, and PCWP.

13. Brain death, the irreversible loss of function of both the cerebrum and the brain stem, is a prerequisite for donation of most solid organs (e.g., heart, lungs). Families must also consent for patients to become organ donors.

14. Patients presenting with acute, nonhemorrhagic stroke benefit most from intravenous thrombolytic therapy administered within 3 hours.

15. In all patients with new-onset seizures, a head computed tomography (CT) or magnetic resonance imaging scan should be performed at the time of presentation to exclude acute structural lesions. A lumbar puncture is indicated in patients with human immunodeficiency virus infection, fever, or otherwise high suspicion for infectious etiology.

16. In the evaluation of a patient for the cause of syncope, a good history and physical will often lead you to the answer. Routine diagnostic testing is not indicated; rather, testing should be targeted toward history and physical examination findings.

17. If a head CT scan is indicated before a lumbar puncture is performed in a patient with suspected bacterial meningitis, blood cultures should be drawn and dexamethasone (if indicated) and empiric antibiotics should be given before sending the patient for the head CT scan.

18. The risk of developing delirium can be lowered by identifying high-risk patients early in their hospitalization and implementing non-pharmacologic delirium prevention treatments.

19. Hypotension and tachycardia should be expected when patients with prolonged dyspnea are intubated because volume depletion is common, and positive pressure ventilation further impedes venous return to the chest.

20. All patients with community-acquired pneumonia should have a determination of their oxygenation within 24 hours of admission, blood cultures before antibiotics, appropriate antibiotics within 4 hours of admission, appropriate smoking counseling, and influenza and pneumococcal vaccinations (or documentation of prior immunization) before discharge.

21. Antibiotics are indicated in the treatment of chronic obstructive pulmonary disease (COPD) exacerbation when at least two of three cardinal symptoms are present: increased shortness of breath, increased sputum volume, and increased sputum purulence.

22. Respiratory drive is usually increased in acute asthma attacks, so the finding of an elevated or normal PCO_2 level indicates an episode of life-threatening severity.

23. Most pneumothoraces are due to COPD or *Pneumocystis jiroveci* infection in patients with acquired immunodeficiency syndrome.

24. Pleural effusions that layer >1.0 cm against the lateral chest wall on a decubitus radiograph are large enough to be tapped.

25. Acute vasoreactivity testing is essential in most forms of pulmonary arterial hypertension to determine responsiveness to calcium channel blockers, which imparts a simpler therapeutic course and an improved prognosis.

26. The five most important potentially life-threatening causes of chest pain are acute coronary syndromes, aortic dissection, pulmonary embolism, tension pneumothorax, and esophageal rupture.

27. The diagnosis of myocardial infarction is made in the presence of a typical rise and gradual fall (troponin) or more rapid rise and fall creatine kinase–myocardial bound (CK-MB) of cardiac enzymes along with one of the following: ischemic symptoms, development of pathologic Q waves on the electrocardiogram (ECG), ECG changes indicative of ischemia (ST segment elevation or depression), or coronary artery intervention (e.g., angioplasty).

28. Look for three key findings when evaluating a patient for acute aortic dissection: immediate onset of tearing or ripping chest/back pain, mediastinal/aortic widening on chest radiograph (>8 cm), and variable pulse pressure (20 mmHg). The absence of all three findings makes aortic dissection unlikely. The presence of any of these findings should prompt a further work-up.

29. No absolute blood pressure value defines hypertensive crises or differentiates hypertensive emergencies from hypertensive urgencies. All patients with systolic blood pressure >180 mmHg or diastolic blood pressure >120 mmHg should be screened, at least by history and physical examination, for evidence of acute/progressive end-organ damage indicating hypertensive emergency.

30. Unless contraindicated, all patients experiencing heart failure with systolic dysfunction, heart disease, or high risk for heart disease should take an angiotensin-converting enzyme inhibitor.

31. Acute pericarditis can present with ST elevation and mild troponin leak and must be excluded as a cause of chest pain before the initiation of anticoagulation because of the risk of conversion to hemorrhagic pericarditis.

32. The primary reason for anticoagulation in atrial fibrillation is stroke prevention. The risk for stroke is higher in persons with comorbid conditions, such as age greater than 65 years, ischemic heart disease, and congestive heart failure.

33. Sick sinus syndrome is the most common cause of symptomatic bradycardia.

34. Most patients with endocarditis have a murmur (85–95%), but only 5–10% have a new murmur or a change in an existing murmur.

35. A careful history and physical examination will provide a clue to the etiology of abdominal pain in most patients. Pain referred to the abdomen tends to be felt along dermatomal segments; it is sharp and associated with hyperalgesia. The finding of an "acute abdomen" does not necessarily imply the need for surgical intervention.

36. Antibiotics are the most common cause of diarrhea that develops in hospitalized patients.

37. Early assessment of upper versus lower source in the management of gastrointestinal bleed (GIB) is essential and can be accomplished through history and physical examination. Early endoscopy in cases of GIB provides diagnostic, prognostic, and therapeutic benefits.

38. Ulcerative colitis is usually confined to the colon and associated with continuous superficial inflammation and a high risk of malignant transformation; Crohn's disease is characterized by transmural skip lesions, fistulas, and noncaseating granulomas.

39. Alcoholic hepatitis can generally be differentiated from other liver diseases by the presence of modest transaminase elevation (< 500 IU/L) and an aspartate transaminase/alanine transaminase ratio >2.

40. Common precipitants of hepatic encephalopathy in patients with cirrhosis include constipation, high dietary protein intake, infections of any cause, gastrointestinal tract bleeding, metabolic alkalosis, hypokalemia, surgery, sedating medications, and lactulose noncompliance.

41. More than 80% of cases of acute pancreatitis are due to alcohol use or biliary disease, with most cases resolving with conservative therapy but some progressing to pseudocyst or abscess formation.

42. In gallstone pancreatitis, the patient may present primarily with symptoms of pancreatitis due to pancreatic ductal obstruction.

43. Carcinoma of the distal colon often presents with obstructive symptoms, whereas lesions involving the proximal colon more frequently present with anemia from chronic blood loss and only rarely obstruction.

44. Asymptomatic bacteriuria does not need to be treated except in pregnant women and in patients who have undergone urinary tract manipulation.

45. The most common cause of renal failure in hospitalized patients is intrinsic renal failure due to acute tubular necrosis.

46. In the treatment of hyponatremia, the serum sodium level should never be increased more than 12 mEq/day, and preferably less than 8 mEq/day, to lessen the risk of developing central pontine myelinolysis.

47. Decreased serum bicarbonate (HCO_3^-) may represent either an acidosis or compensation for respiratory alkalosis, thus interpretation of a patient's acid–base balance requires a blood gas analysis.

48. Patients with end-stage renal disease have a cardiac mortality rate 10–20 times higher than those without the disease.

49. When you give 1 L of normal saline or lactated Ringer's solution to a patient, only 200–300 mL of the fluid remains intravascularly.

50. Limiting oral calcium actually results in a *higher* likelihood of calcium stone formation because low-calcium diets stimulate intestinal oxalate absorption and hyperoxaluria.

51. The most common infectious sources of new fever in a hospitalized patient are urinary tract infections, pneumonia, and bloodstream infections.

52. Hospitalized patients become colonized with resistant bacteria after *transmission*, usually via the hands of hospital personnel, and *selection* via pressure with antibiotics that favor the growth of resistant bacteria.

53. Classic signs of inflammation (e.g., purulent sputum, peritoneal signs) are usually absent in neutropenic patients.

54. Steroids in relative adrenal insufficiency, activated protein C, early goal-directed therapy, intense glycemic control, and daily hemodialysis in acute renal failure have all been shown to significantly reduce mortality in sepsis.

55. *Sepsis* is defined as documented or suspected infection plus systemic inflammatory response syndrome (SIRS). SIRS includes temperature $<36°C$ or $>38.5°C$, tachycardia, tachypnea, and white blood cell count $<4000/\mu L$ or $>12,000/\mu L$.

56. Funguria usually represents colonization rather than true infection and should only be treated if a patient is symptomatic. Removal of a urinary catheter will often resolve the problem.

57. Prosthetic joint infections almost always require device removal and long-term antibiotic therapy.

58. Pulmonary embolism is one of the most common preventable causes of death in hospitalized patients. Aggressive identification and initiation of prophylaxis of at-risk medical and surgical patients is required to reduce this risk.

59. Hemolysis should be suspected in a patient with a rapid decline in hemoglobin and no identifiable bleeding and diagnosed with a high reticulocyte index, high lactate dehydrogenase and indirect bilirubin levels, and a low haptoglobin level.

60. Acute chest syndrome is the most common cause of death in patients with sickle cell disease. More than half of these patients initially present with an acute painful episode.

61. Immune-mediated heparin-induced thrombocytopenia (HIT) is the most serious cause of drug-induced thrombocytopenia and must be treated immediately.

62. The tumor lysis syndrome classically presents with hyperkalemia, hyperphosphatemia, hypocalcemia, hyperuricemia, and acute renal failure.

63. The therapeutic goals in the treatment of diabetic ketoacidosis and hyperglycemic hyperosmotic syndrome are similar and include volume resuscitation, electrolyte repletion, and correction of electrolyte and glucose abnormalities.

64. Patients receiving chronic steroids should always continue taking their steroids before and during surgery or illness. The need for supplemental steroids is determined by the degree of hypothalamic-pituitary-adrenal axis suppression and physiologic stress.

65. Gout and septic arthritis are the most common causes of acute arthritis that present in a hospitalized patient.

66. Although laboratory tests may support the diagnosis, there are no screening or diagnostic tests for vasculitis. When vasculitis is clinically suspected, biopsy or angiography may be indicated.

67. The incidence of community-acquired methicillin-resistant *Staphylococcus aureus* infections is rising sharply throughout the country.

68. Decubitus ulcers can occur with as little as 12 hours of direct pressure but are *very* slow to heal, causing a fourfold risk of prolonged hospitalization or death.

69. In patients with hereditary angioedema, standard treatment with antihistamines, steroids, and epinephrine has little or no effect because the reaction is not mediated by histamine.

70. Patients who are taking beta blockers and are experiencing anaphylaxis may not respond to epinephrine and may require intravenous glucagon instead.

71. In patients with a true immune-mediated reaction to penicillin, cephalosporins should not be used, or skin testing should be performed first. If the skin test result is negative or if the reaction history is consistent with a non–immune-mediated mechanism, use of a cephalosporin is probably safe.

72. Benzodiazepines are the only drugs that decrease both the signs and symptoms of alcohol withdrawal, as well as preventing withdrawal seizures and delirium tremens.

73. Empiric treatment for a patient with altered mental status may include thiamine, dextrose, naloxone, flumazenil, and/or activated charcoal.

74. Delirium, depression, and dementia (i.e., "the three Ds") are common and can be distinguished from one another based on clinical features.

75. Routine screening of all patients undergoing surgery with a panel of laboratory tests and imaging studies is not useful; an approach that targets individual findings on history and physical examination is more prudent and cost-effective.

76. Coronary revascularization is rarely indicated before noncardiac surgery to reduce the risk of cardiac complications and should only be performed in those patients who would derive a long-term mortality benefit from the procedure.

77. The absence of chest pain or dyspnea in a patient whose functional status is limited (e.g., due to claudication, arthritis, or sedentary lifestyle) does not rule out significant cardiac disease that may be unmasked by the stress of surgery.

78. Postoperative pulmonary complications are more common than postoperative cardiac complications after noncardiac surgery, but the use of routine spirometry, chest x-ray, and arterial blood gas is not warranted.

79. Beta blockers can attenuate perioperative risk in diabetic patients and should be used in diabetic patients undergoing major noncardiac surgery.

80. Maintain a high level of suspicion for, and give aggressive prophylaxis against, postoperative venous thromboembolism in patients undergoing major surgery.

81. Most fevers in the early postoperative period result from tissue trauma–related cytokine release.

82. Necessary radiologic studies should not be withheld just because a patient is pregnant. However, the amount of contrast and radiation should be limited, and all radioactive studies should be avoided.

83. In ventricular fibrillation/tachycardia arrest, the most critical intervention is early defibrillation. Guidelines state that defibrillation should be provided within 3 minutes of onset for an in-hospital arrest.

84. Causes of pulseless electrical activity/asystolic arrest can be remembered as the "6 Hs and 6 Ts": hypoxia, hypovolemia, H+ excess (acidosis), hyper-/hypokalemia, hypothermia, hypoglycemia, and thrombosis/coronary (myocardial infarction), thrombosis/pulmonary (pulmonary embolus), tension pneumothorax, tamponade (cardiac), tablets (overdose/ingestions), and trauma.

85. A positive deflection on an ECG tracing indicates that the electrical activity of the heart is moving toward that lead, whereas a negative deflection means that it is moving away from that lead.

86. A vertical line on the ECG tracing indicates the same point in time across all leads. By tracing a finding (such as a P wave) along its vertical line, it may make it easier to identify the same finding in other leads, where it may not be as obvious.

87. With every chest x-ray: (1) confirm administrative information; (2) assess the film type, penetration, positioning, and degree of inspiration; and (3) follow a systematic approach to interpretation.

88. The *silhouette sign,* an important feature for localizing abnormalities, refers to adjacent structures having nondiscrete borders.

89. Appropriate neuroimaging can decrease the risk of tonsillar herniation in patients at risk for a central nervous system mass lesion undergoing lumbar puncture.

90. A spun hematocrit test of grossly bloody pleural fluid assists in the diagnosis of hemothorax, in which the hematocrit level of the pleural fluid is more than 50% of the peripheral hematocrit level.

91. In patients with cirrhosis, a paracentesis should be performed to exclude spontaneous bacterial peritonitis for any change in clinical status such as fever, nausea, abdominal pain, or confusion.

92. Administration of intravenous fluids and blood products can be more rapidly achieved by large-bore peripheral venous catheters than by most central venous catheters.

93. If a patient has a chronic disease of any nature, a palliative care approach may be helpful in symptom management and addressing goals of care at any time in the illness, not only when the likelihood of death is within days.

94. Establishing the patients' goals for care is an essential step in creating a treatment plan for all patients, but especially for critically or terminally ill patients, in whom treatment choices may require trade-offs.

95. When discussing code status, establish an appropriate setting; ask the patient and family what they understand about the illness and resuscitation; find out what their expectations and wishes are; discuss the do-not-resuscitate (DNR) order; respond to emotions; and establish, document, and implement the plan.

96. Life experience and personal values help shape the way physicians view their patients and may lead to biases and difficulties communicating with patients if not acknowledged.

97. The key elements of discussing bad news with a patient are to think about what you want to say, explain the news simply, reassure the patient that you will continue to be there for him or her, and be silent and listen for the patient's reactions and questions.

98. Barriers to hospice care include misconceptions that patients must have less than a 6-month prognosis, must have decided against resuscitation, cannot get "aggressive treatment," and cannot come back to the hospital or emergency department.

99. Respiratory depression resulting from narcotics is rare in patients with pain. Pain is a potent stimulus to breathe.

100. Measurements of hypoxia and respiratory rate do not correlate with the sensation of dyspnea in advanced illness.

PREVENTION OF COMPLICATIONS IN THE HOSPITAL SETTING

Michael D. Wang, MD

1. **Define Iatrogenesis and primum non nocere.**

   Iatros is a Greek term indicating physicians, medicine, and treatment. *Iatrogenesis* denotes a negative response to a medical or surgical intervention. The concept of *primum non nocere*, first do no harm, beckons us to ensure that our attempts to help do not result in harm. The principle suggests that in situations of uncertainty about whether the benefits outweigh risks, inaction may be the ethically preferred choice.

2. **How can the hospital be a dangerous place?**

   The hospital concentrates ill, frail patients in a manner that almost encourages complications (Table 1-1). Nosocomial infections, immobilization and deconditioning, pressure ulcers, venous thromboembolism (VTE), contrast-induced nephropathy, falls, delirium, gastrointestinal stress ulcers, adverse drug events (ADEs), and medical errors all conspire to make the hospital a potentially dangerous place. Tightly packed patients with a variety of infections afford a microenvironment for cross-pollination by common staff. Patient mobility is limited, with the bed becoming the center of all care—meals in bed, television in bed, and a button to call for the nursing staff. Intravenous catheter pumps, continuous oxygen, bladder catheters, and sequential compression devices further tether patients to the bed. Tests often beget more tests and subsequent treatments that may cause adverse events, leading to more treatments. In the end, only attention to these issues and minimization of length of stay can help to reduce these complications.

TABLE 1-1. POTENTIAL CAUSES OF HARM IN HOSPITALIZED PATIENTS*

Malnutrition

Infection

Stress ulcers

Deconditioning (disability)

Encephalopathy (delirium)

Elixirs (polypharmacy)

Deep venous thrombosis

Sores (pressure ulcers)

*Mnemonic MISDEEDS can be used as a checklist of iatrogenic problems to anticipate upon admission.

---

3. **What are the risk factors for nosocomial infections?**

   Hospitalized patients are exposed to an astonishing array of bacteria via health care workers and other vectors. Host defenses are also often diminished with systemic factors, including acute illness, malnutrition, and medications (e.g., steroids, chemotherapy) that place patients at a higher risk of infection. Antibiotic use may alter the host's normal flora, leading to colonization with hospital-acquired bacteria. Additionally, the normally acidic pH of the gastric environment is often altered with antacid medications, leading to colonization of the upper gastrointestinal tract with hospital-acquired organisms. These organisms can then be aspirated, leading to hospital-acquired pneumonia. The presence of foreign bodies (e.g., intravenous and bladder catheters, nasogastric tubing, and intubation tubing) and impairment of reflexes (e.g., cough, sedation) also encourage infection.

4. **What preventive measures can be used to minimize nosocomial infections?**
Proper handwashing and gloving, contact precautions, and isolation all limit the spread of organisms. Routine hand decontamination is crucial, before and after each patient contact, either with an alcohol-based hand rub or at least 15–30 seconds of vigorous handwashing with soap and water. If urinary catheters and central venous catheters are required, proper aseptic technique for their placement and minimization of their duration are important. The minimization of antibiotics to type and duration indicated, and use of narrow-spectrum antibiotics, will minimize resistance and nosocomial infections. (See Chapter 55 for more details.)

5. **Why is deconditioning important? How can it be minimized?**
Deconditioning can prolong the problem of immobility. Strength can diminish by as much as 5% per day. Although this has minimal significance in younger patients with high reserve, it can often be disabling in older, frail patients. Admission to the hospital setting is strongly correlated with new-onset, sometimes persistent, functional decline in older adults. Functional decline has been associated with increased risk of fall, death, rehospitalization, and institutionalization. Two percent of patients fall during hospitalization, but as many as 15% of older patients will fall in the posthospitalization period. Deconditioning likely plays a role in these outcomes. Early mobilization and minimization of tethers that discourage mobility are worthy goals. Minimize the use of bed rest orders and ambulate the patient frequently. After discharge, home visits by physical and occupational therapists, assessments for home environmental hazards, home modifications, and assistive devices may be helpful.

6. **Why is it important to prevent pressure ulcers?**
Pressure ulcers, formerly known as decubitus ulcers, are a common complication in bedridden patients. They can lead to soft tissue infections and osteomyelitis. They can also serve as a reservoir for resistant organisms that may become pathogens if spread elsewhere. Pressure ulcer risk increases with prolonged operating room times, suggesting that ulcers may develop within 1 day of prolonged immobility.

7. **Describe the locations, staging, and prevention of pressure ulcers.**
Any bony protrusion exposed to gravity-induced pressure is at risk for pressure sores. Common locations for pressure ulcers in patients in bed include the sacrococcygeal area, greater trochanter, back, occiput, and heels. In patients with contractures, the lateral hips and medial and lateral aspects of the knees and ankles may be more exposed. These locations represent important places to screen on routine examination of bed-bound patients. The staging of pressure ulcers is summarized in Table 1-2.
  Preventive techniques include patient mobilization and repositioning every 2 hours, minimization of shear injury by use of draw sheets, and avoiding prolonged 60-degree head-up bed positions. In high-risk patients, special mattresses to disburse gravitational pressures over a larger surface area are helpful. Malnutrition is a strong risk factor for the development of pressure ulcers. Whether supplementation beyond adequate nutrition can accelerate wound healing is controversial. The data supporting the use of vitamin C, zinc sulfate, and increased protein intake is limited and inconclusive. (See Chapter 67 for more details.)

TABLE 1-2.	STAGING OF PRESSURE ULCERS
Stage I	Skin still intact, but there is nonblanching erythema.
Stage II	Superficial or partial-thickness necrosis. May include presence of bullae, dermal necrosis (black-colored), and shallow ulcer formation.
Stage III	Deep necrosis and ulcer formation with full-thickness skin loss extending down to, but not through, the fascia.
Stage IV	Full-thickness necrosis and ulceration with involvement of muscle and/or bone. Generally quite large and deep with ill-defined borders.

8. **Name risk factors for VTE.**
   Increasing age, prolonged immobility, previous deep venous thrombosis or pulmonary embolism, malignancy, major surgery, trauma, obesity, varicose veins, cardiac or pulmonary dysfunction, indwelling central venous catheters, inflammatory bowel disease, nephrotic syndrome, and pregnancy or estrogen use all increase the risk for VTE. (See Chapter 57 for more details.)

9. **How can VTE be prevented in the hospital?**
   Mobilization, graduated compression stockings, intermittent leg compression, and prophylactic anticoagulation. Anticoagulation methods include subcutaneous unfractionated heparin, low-molecular-weight heparins, fondaparinux, and oral warfarin (Table 1-3).

TABLE 1-3.	PROPHYLACTIC ANTICOAGULANT MEDICATIONS AND DOSING	
Medication	**Dosing (SQ)**	**Interval**
Heparin	5000 Units	b.i.d. to t.i.d.
Enoxaparin	30 mg	b.i.d.
	40 mg	Daily
Dalteparin	2500–5000 International Units	Daily
Fondaparinux	2.5 mg	Daily
Warfarin	Individualized	Daily

10. **How can the risk of renal insufficiency be minimized in a patient undergoing an intravenous contrast procedure?**
    Minimize risk of contrast by hydrating adequately, withholding nephrotoxins (e.g., nonsteroidal anti-inflammatory drugs [NSAIDs], diuretics), and adjusting medications affected by renal function (e.g., holding metformin in diabetics). If risk is higher (e.g., baseline renal insufficiency, diabetes, unavoidable nephrotoxins), ameliorate effects of contrast by administering *N*-acetylcysteine, 600 mg bid, two doses before and two doses after contrast. Bicarbonate infusions may also be helpful. Adjust type or volume of contrast to minimize risk. If risks are very high, delay the exposure until the risk is lower, or find an alternative, non-contrast procedure.

11. **How can delirium be prevented in elderly patients?**

    Delirium occurs in 10–25% of hospitalized elderly patients and is associated with increased length of stay, cost of care, and mortality. Factors associated with delirium included medical illness, anticholinergic or psychoactive medications, malnutrition, and restraining devices. Attention to medications, mobility, nutrition, and sensory deficits will go a long way toward avoidance of this difficult complication. (See Chapter 18 for more details.)

12. **Who should receive prophylaxis against gastrointestinal stress ulcers?**

    Stress ulcers develop as the protective mucosal barriers are diminished or overcome in the context of acute medical illness. They result from a combination of factors such as decreased mucosal blood flow (e.g., hypotension), decreased prostaglandin synthesis, and increased barrier disruption (e.g., steroids, NSAIDs). The incidence of stress ulcers increase with the severity of illness and length of hospitalization but appear most commonly in mechanically ventilated patients, those with coagulopathies, and patients with burns. Only 0.1% of patients without the first two factors will develop clinically important gastrointestinal tract bleeding such that prophylaxis can normally be safely withheld in these patients. Potential medications include sucralfate, H2 blockers, and proton pump inhibitors. Sucralfate does not affect the pH of the stomach but can impair absorption of a variety of medications and may not be as effective. The use of acid-reducing medications can impair the absorption of select medications (e.g., ferrous sulfate, itraconazole) and diminish the stomach's natural defense mechanism from exogenous bacteria. Drugs used for prevention are summarized in Table 1-4.

TABLE 1-4. STRESS ULCER PROPHYLAXIS		
Medication	**Dosing**	**Interval**
Sucralfate	1 gm PO/PNG	qid
Famotidine	20 mg IV	q12h
Ranitidine	50 mg IV	q8h
Omeprazole	20–40 mg PO/PNG	Daily
Lansoprazole	15–30 mg PO/PNG	Daily
Rabeprazole	20 mg PO/PNG	Daily
Esomeprazole	20–40 mg PO/PNG	Daily

13. **What is an ADE? How serious are ADEs?**

    An *adverse drug event* is defined as any toxic physical or psychological reaction to a medication. Studies have shown that ADEs occur in 4–20% of hospitalized patients. Twenty to thirty percent of all ADEs are categorized as "serious" (i.e., causing or prolonging hospitalization or death). They also may add to increased cost and length of stay. (See Chapter 3 for more details.)

14. **Why are elderly patients at higher risk for ADEs?**

    Older adults more commonly have impaired renal and hepatic function, thereby altering drug metabolism and elimination. They generally are taking more medications and have more comorbidities. The risk of ADEs appears to increase with increasing comorbidity and use of scheduled medications (i.e., five or more scheduled medications).

KEY POINTS: PREVENTION OF COMPLICATIONS

1. Proper handwashing and gloving, contact precautions, limitation of broad-spectrum antibiotics, and isolation of patients with resistant organisms all limit the spread of organisms.

2. Methods to minimize deconditioning include early mobilization, minimizing tethers (e.g., oxygen administration, intravenous lines, bedrails, bladder catheters), avoiding bed rest orders, and initiating early physical and occupational therapy.

3. Pressure ulcers are a common complication in bedridden patients that can lead to soft tissue infections and osteomyelitis as well as serve as a reservoir for resistant organisms that may become pathogens if spread elsewhere.

4. Hospital-acquired VTE is a leading cause of morbidity and mortality in hospitalized patients; all medical and surgical patients should be considered for mechanical or chemoprophylactic therapy.

5. Delirium occurs in 10–25% of hospitalized elderly patients and is associated with increased length of stay, cost of care, and mortality.

6. The primary indications for stress ulcer prophylaxis are mechanical ventilation and coagulopathy. Patients without these indications most often do not require prophylaxis.

---

15. **What is a transition in care? When do transitions in care occur?**
    A transition in care is simply a transfer of care between one team of caregivers and another. They commonly occur in a large hospital setting and include admission to the hospital, transfers between floors, transfers between services, transfers to and from the operating room/recovery room, cross coverage, change of rotation, and discharge from the hospital. (See Chapter 8 for more details.)

16. **How can medication errors in transition be prevented?**
    One study suggests a 20% incidence of ADEs due to medication changes in patients transferring from and back to a nursing facility. Most changes occurred in the hospital setting, but many of the reactions did not occur until after discharge. This suggests a need for increased vigilance over medications in transitions of care and the discharge planning process. Medications should be reconciled with every transition of care. This involves reviewing the medication list, determining which were actually taken and ascertaining why others were not. Reconciling medications at the time of discharge is especially important—some drugs are temporarily discontinued during hospitalization, whereas others are altered in dose or frequency, and still others are brand new. Explicit communication of the plan for discontinuation of temporary medications, anticipation of monitoring requirements for ADEs (e.g., laboratory and orthostatic monitoring), and streamlining medications all can contribute to posthospital success. (See Chapter 2 for more details.)

17. **What preventive medicine should be accomplished in the hospital setting?**
    The hospital setting is often the opportune time to intervene on chronic health issues. Initiating statin therapy in patients with unstable angina has some proof of benefit and is suggestive that other primary and secondary preventive measures started in the hospital may have merit. Examples of other opportunities include angiotensin-converting enzyme inhibitors in patients

with diabetes, congestive heart failure (CHF) with systolic dysfunction, or proteinuria; aspirin in patients with cerebrovascular or cardiac disease; and echocardiography to evaluate ejection fraction in patients with CHF. When appropriate, patients should receive cessation counseling for tobacco, alcohol, and illicit drug use. Pneumococcal, influenza, and tetanus vaccinations should be administered at the time of discharge, if indicated, according to the established guidelines. Arranging for primary care follow-up for patients with chronic diseases or requiring further health screening is also important.

WEBSITES

1. National Pressure Ulcer Advisory Panel
   http://www.npuap.org/

2. Centers for Disease Control and Prevention, Infection Control in Healthcare Settings
   http://www.cdc.gov/ncidod/dhqp/index.html

3. Food and Drug Administration Center for Drug Evaluation and Research
   http://www.fda.gov/cder/drug/drugReactions/default.htm

4. Agency for Healthcare Research and Quality
   http://www.ahcpr.gov/qual/errorsix.htm

BIBLIOGRAPHY

1. Boyce JM, Pittet D: Guideline for hand hygiene in healthcare settings. MMWR 51:1–44, 2002.
2. Cook DJ, Fuller HD, Guyatt GH: Risk factors for gastrointestinal bleeding in critically ill patients. Canadian Critical Care Trials Group. N Engl J Med 330:377–381, 1994.
3. Geerts WH, Heit JA, Clagett GP, et al: Prevention of venous thromboembolism. Chest 119 (Suppl 1):132s–175s, 2001.
4. Gill TM, Allore HG, Holford TR, et al: Hospitalization, restricted activity, and the development of disability among older persons. JAMA 292:2115–2124, 2004.
5. Kohn L, Corrigan J, Donaldson M (eds): To Err is Human: Building a Safer Health System. Washington, DC, National Academy Press, 2000, pp 1–68.
6. Langer G, Schloemer G, Knerr A, et al: Nutritional interventions for preventing and treating pressure ulcers. Cochrane Database Syst Rev 4:CD003216, 2003.
7. Lazarou J, Pomeranz BH, Corey PN: Incidence of adverse drug reactions in hospitalized patients: A meta-analysis of prospective studies. JAMA 279:1200–1205, 1998.
8. Mandell LA, Bartlett JG, Dowell SF, et al: Update of Practice Guidelines for the Management of Community-acquired Pneumonia in Immunocompetent Adults. Clin Infect Dis 37:1405–1433, 2003.

CHAPTER 2

PATIENT SAFETY AND QUALITY IN THE HOSPITAL

Anjala Tess, MD

1. **What is patient safety?**
   Patient safety is the field of health care practice and study that focuses on preventing harm to patients. An estimated 44,000–98,000 patients die each year due to medical errors at an estimated cost to society of $37.6–$50 billion. These estimates are based on population studies of hospitalized patients and place medical errors as the eighth leading cause of death in the United States.

2. **Who is responsible for patient safety?**
   Every member of the health care team is responsible for patient safety, from the care providers (i.e., physicians and trainees, nursing staff, pharmacists, and ancillary staff) to the hospital administration. Patients themselves can promote safe care by voicing concerns when they arise.

3. **How are adverse events, near misses, and medical errors defined?**
   An *adverse event* is any harm to a patient from medical care and could be the result of an error; these events may be preventable or not. A *near miss* is an event or situation that could have resulted in harm but did not. *Medical errors* include both near misses and preventable adverse events.

4. **How does the systems approach to medical error differ from the approach that focuses on the individual?**
   A systems approach accepts that humans are prone to make mistakes and focuses on identifying flaws in the system rather than blaming the individual (Fig. 2-1). *Active failures* are actions that eventually result in an error (e.g., writing an illegible prescription). *Latent conditions* are system design flaws that allow errors to occur. (e.g., no process to clarify clinician's order when writing is illegible.)

5. **What are the different types of human errors?**
   - **Errors of commission:** Carrying out an action that is incorrect (e.g., ordering penicillin for a patient with a known penicillin allergy).
   - **Errors of omission:** Not carrying out a necessary action that results in error (e.g., not asking the patient about drug allergies before ordering antibiotics).
   - **Slips:** The intention is correct but the action is incorrect (e.g., intending to write "200 pounds" but instead writing "200 kilograms").
   - **Mistakes:** The intention is incorrect due to lack of information or flawed judgment, resulting in an incorrect action (e.g., writing "200 kilograms" because you believe the patient weighs 200 kilograms when he actually weighs 200 pounds).

6. **List three factors that increase the likelihood that a human being will make an error.**
   Distraction, fatigue, and physical environments that impede natural workflow all increase the risk that errors will occur.

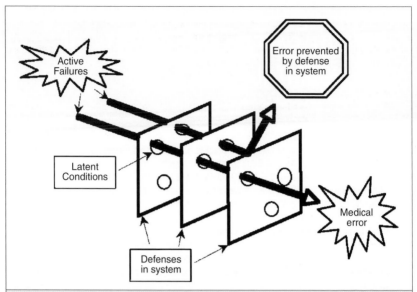

Figure 2-1. The "Swiss cheese model": the slices of cheese are potential defenses against an error except where the holes (latent conditions) of the system allow the error to pass through. (Adapted from Reason J: Human error: Models and management. BMJ 320:768–770, 2000.)

7. **List examples of errors that happen in the hospital setting.**
   See Table 2-1.

TABLE 2-1. EXAMPLES OF MEDICAL ERRORS IN HOSPITALIZED PATIENTS

Diagnostic error	A delay in diagnosis, failure to act on known information
Treatment error	Medication error, delay in treatment, inappropriate treatment for given condition, wrong site/wrong procedure or wrong patient/wrong procedure
Prevention error	Lack of appropriate prophylaxis, inadequate monitoring
Communication error	Failure in handoff between providers, poor teamwork

8. **What tools are available to document, study, and prevent errors?**
   - **Incident reporting systems:** These collect adverse events to identify cases to pinpoint breakdowns in the system of health care delivery. All frontline providers and patients can report incidents as they occur.
   - **Root cause analysis (RCA):** This allows for retrospective examination of an incident with the goal of identifying the active and latent failures of the system (root causes).
   - **Failure modes and effects analysis (FMEA):** This requires a prospective look at a process to identify weaknesses in the system before an incident occurs.

9. **What general barriers prevent hospitals from eliminating all medical errors?**
    - Every medical system that requires human interaction is prone to error.
    - Flaws in systems are often not recognized until adverse events occur.
    - Reluctance to report errors may exist because of fear, lack of training in identifying flaws, and lack of support for those who make mistakes.

10. **What is a culture of safety?**
    A culture of safety is one that promotes and facilitates safer care within a hospital. All health care providers, including the hospital administration, can endorse this culture and allow it to guide hospital policies and processes. Examples include training employees and not blaming them for error, emphasizing nonpunitive reporting with the aim of safer process design, and focusing on interventions to reduce error.

11. **List four strategies to improve teamwork among health care providers.**
    - Clarification of roles and encouraging team members to monitor each other
    - Assertiveness training to promote communication between members and team leader
    - Training in briefing techniques to improve communication during handoffs
    - Development of a shared mental model and common goals among team members

12. **What are adverse drug events (ADEs)? How frequently do they occur?**
    An ADE has occurred when harm befalls a patient due to a medication. ADEs can be preventable or unpreventable. A potential ADE occurs when an error happens but no harm befalls the patient. It is either intercepted or has no bad outcome. One study of more than 4000 inpatient admissions revealed 6.5 ADEs and 5.5 potential adverse drug events for every 100 admissions. Of the life-threatening and serious ADEs, 42% were preventable.

    Bates DW, Cullen DJ, Laird N, et al: Incidence of adverse drug events and potential adverse drug events: Implications for prevention. ADE Prevention Study Group. JAMA 274:29–34, 1995.

13. **List patient-, medication-, and prescriber-related risk factors for ADEs.**
    See Table 2-2.

TABLE 2-2. MEDICATION ERRORS IN THE HOSPITAL: RISK FACTORS		
Patient Factors	**Medication Factors**	**Prescriber Factors**
Extremes of age	Multiple medications	Writing illegibly
Need for urgent or critical care	Multiple drug allergies	Miscalculating doses
High-risk surgeries: vascular, neurosurgical, cardiothoracic	High-risk medications: anticoagulants, insulin, narcotics, sedatives, chemotherapy	Giving verbal orders
	Look-alike, sound-alike medications	Using ambiguous abbreviations

14. **List strategies to prevent medication errors.**
    - Prioritization of medication safety by all patients, providers, and hospitals
    - Encouragement of reporting and analysis of ADEs

- Close attention to high-risk factors to minimize risk
- Establish systems to create and maintain accurate medication lists
- Discuss medication risks/benefits and encourage reporting of side effects
- Use of real-time computer order entry for medication ordering

15. **What is the incidence and impact of falls in the hospital?**

Falls in the hospital are among the most common adverse events experienced by elderly hospitalized patients. One study reported an overall fall rate of 3.38 falls per 1000 patient-days (range across all hospital specialties, 0.83–6.12 falls per 1000 hospital days). Patients on neurology and medicine services had the highest rate of falls (6.12 falls/1000 patient days). Forty-two percent of falls resulted in some injury, with 8% causing moderate to severe injuries (e.g., fractures, subdural hematomas, lacerations, and death). Another study showed a 71% increase in length of stay and an increase of $4223 in hospital charges for patients who have fallen.

Bates DW, Pruess K, Souney P, et al: Serious falls in hospitalized patients: Correlated and resource utilization. Am J Med 99:137–143, 1995.

Hitcho EB, Krauss MJ, Birge S, et al: Characteristics and circumstances of falls in a hospital setting. J Gen Intern Med 19:732–739, 2004

16. **List hospital and patient risk factors for falls in elderly patients.**

See Table 2-3.

TABLE 2-3. RISK FACTORS FOR FALLS IN ELDERLY HOSPITALIZED PATIENTS	
Hospital Factors	**Patient Factors**
Unfamiliar environment	Age > 65 years
Poor lighting	History of previous falls
Equipment in room contributing to trip or fall	More than four medications (especially hypnotics, benzodiazepines, opioids)
	Unstable gait
	Postural hypotension
	Poor visual acuity
	Agitation or delirium
	Need for frequent toileting

17. **List strategies to prevent falls in the hospital.**
- Use "fall risk" identifying bracelets.
- Avoid sedation and unnecessary medications.
- Use physical restraints only if needed.
- Use bed alarms and make call alarms available.
- Maintain patient's mobility.
- Minimize environmental hazards.

18. **List three procedure-related errors and specific strategies to prevent them.**

See Table 2-4.

TABLE 2-4.   PROCEDURE-RELATED ERRORS AND PREVENTIVE STRATEGIES

Preventable Procedural Error	Strategy
Wrong patient, wrong procedure	Use of two patient identifiers (date of birth, name, identification number) to confirm patient identity
Wrong site, wrong procedure	Use of a preprocedure "time-out" to confirm type and site of a procedure
	Marking the site of the procedure before patient enters the operating room or procedure suite
Leaving foreign body in patient	Use of procedural checklist and equipment count

KEY POINTS: PATIENT SAFETY

1. No system that relies on human performance will ever be perfect.

2. Patient safety is the responsibility of everyone in the hospital from frontline providers to the CEO.

3. Near misses and adverse events can be studied to understand health care system flaws and improve them.

4. By understanding risk factors and preventive strategies for falls, ADEs, and procedural errors, hospital workers can play an active role in improving patient care.

19.   **How do hospitals monitor the quality of the care they provide?**
- Use of patient safety indicators to compare with regional or national benchmarks. Examples include rates of aspiration pneumonia, aspirin use in myocardial infarction, postoperative thrombosis or embolism, readmission for patients with congestive heart failure or pneumonia, and wound dehiscence. Some agencies require reporting of these patient safety measures to determine whether care is safe at a given hospital. For example, the Joint Commission for the Accreditation of Healthcare Organizations (JCAHO) is a not-for-profit organization that focuses on patient safety to evaluate and accredit more than 15,000 health care organizations and programs in the United States. *JCAHO core measures* are standard performance measures that all hospitals are expected to collect and report to JCAHO. Examples of current JCAHO core measures are listed in Table 2-5.
- Proactively studying institutional processes and systems to improve overall care. Examples: maintaining training for specific protocols such as conscious sedation; monitoring patient waiting times in the emergency room.
- Use of tools with a peer-review process to study individual incidents or trends as they occur. (See question 8.)

20.   **How does the Institute of Medicine define the six dimensions of health care quality?**
The Institute of Medicine reports that health care should strive to be safe, effective, patient centered, timely, efficient, and equitable.

21.   **What is rapid cycle improvement?**
Rapid cycle improvement is a methodology wherein a process or system goes through a series of small changes to improve its overall outcome. Rather than focusing on collecting large

TABLE 2-5. JCAHO CORE MEASURES FOR HOSPITALS

Condition	Core Measures
Acute myocardial infarction (AMI)	AMI-1 Aspirin at arrival
	AMI-2 Aspirin prescribed at discharge
	AMI-3 ACE inhibitor for left ventricular systolic dysfunction
	AMI-4 Adult smoking cessation advice/counseling
	AMI-5 Beta blocker prescribed at discharge
	AMI-6 Beta blocker at arrival
	AMI-7 Time to thrombolysis
	AMI-8 Time to percutaneous transluminal coronary angioplasty
	AMI-9 Inpatient mortality
Heart failure (HF)	HF-1 Discharge instructions
	HF-2 Left ventricular function assessment
	HF-3 ACE inhibitor for left ventricular systolic dysfunction
	HF-4 Adult smoking cessation advice/counseling
Community-acquired pneumonia (CAP)	CAP-1 Oxygenation assessment
	CAP-2 Pneumococcal screening and/or vaccination
	CAP-3 Blood cultures
	CAP-4a Adult smoking cessation advice/counseling
	CAP-4b Pediatric smoking cessation advice/counseling
	CAP-5 Antibiotic timing
Pregnancy-related conditions (PR)	PR-1 Vaginal birth after cesarean section
	PR-2 Inpatient neonatal mortality
	PR-3 Third- or fourth-degree laceration
Surgical infection prevention (SIP)	SIP-1 Prophylactic antibiotic received within 1 hour prior to surgical incision
	SIP-2 Prophylactic antibiotic selection for surgical patients
	SIP-3 Prophylactic antibiotics discontinued within 24 hours after surgery end time

amounts of data, hypotheses are tested and relatively small amounts of data are quickly collected to make improvements. By using the *Plan-Do-Study-Act cycle* (Fig. 2-2), small changes to an existing system can be designed and then tested. Results of the test can be used to design future changes to the system.

KEY POINTS: HEALTH CARE QUALITY

1. Health care should strive to be safe, effective, patient centered, timely, efficient, and equitable.

2. Patient safety benchmarks such as JCAHO measures and tools such as the *Plan-Do-Study-Act* cycle can be used to improve the quality of care we deliver as clinicians.

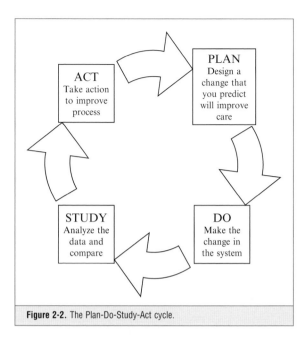

Figure 2-2. The Plan-Do-Study-Act cycle.

22. What is risk management in health care?

The field of measuring and assessing risk associated with health care and its consequences for patients and the hospital. Hospital risk managers can help support staff and provide guidance in improving patient safety, reducing medical errors, disclosing errors to patients, and documenting events in specific cases.

WEBSITES

1. Institute for Healthcare Improvement
   http://www.ihi.org

2. National Patient Safety Foundation
   http://www.npsf.org

3. Joint Commission for the Accreditation of Healthcare Organizations
   http://www.jcaho.org

4. The Leapfrog Group for Patient Safety
   http://www.leapfroggroup.org

5. Risk Management Foundation, Harvard Medical Institutions
   http://www.rmf.harvard.edu

BIBLIOGRAPHY

1. Bates DW, Cullen DJ, Laird N, et al: Incidence of adverse drug events and potential adverse drug events: Implications for prevention. ADE Prevention Study Group. JAMA 274:2934, 1995.

2. Bates DW, Pruess K, Souney P, et al: Serious falls in hospitalized patients: Correlated and resource utilization. Am J Med 99:137–143, 1995.

3. Hitcho EB, Krauss MJ, Birge S, et al: Characteristics and circumstances of falls in a hospital setting. J Gen Intern Med 19:732–739, 2004.

4. Kohn L, Corrigan J, Donaldson M (eds): To Err is Human: Building a Safer Health System. Washington, DC, National Academy Press, 2000, pp 1–68.

5. Leape L: The preventability of medical injury. In Bogner M (ed): Human Error in Medicine, 2nd ed. Hillsdale, NJ, L. Erlbaum Associates, 1994, pp 13–25.

6. Moray N: Error reduction as a systems problem. In Bogner M (ed): Human Error in Medicine, 2nd ed. Hillsdale, NJ, L. Erlbaum Associates, 1994, pp 67–91.

7. Reason J: Human error: Models and management. BMJ 320:768–770, 2000.

8. Reason J: Foreword. In Bogner M (ed): Human Error in Medicine, 2nd ed. Hillsdale, NJ, L. Erlbaum Associates, 1994, pp vii–xv.

CHAPTER 3

SAFE AND APPROPRIATE MEDICATION USE

Sanjeev Suri, MD, MBA, and Sunil Kripalani, MD, MSc

1. **What are iatrogenic injuries?**

   Iatrogenic injuries are those that are caused by medications and medical interventions. The Harvard Medical Practice Study was a landmark report describing how often medical errors occur in hospitalized patients. By reviewing records from 51 hospitals in New York State, the authors found that iatrogenic injuries occurred in 4% of the admissions with a mortality rate of 14%. Extrapolating these data to the entire nation would result in nearly 180,000 deaths per year or the equivalent of three jumbo jet crashes every 2 days. Most of these iatrogenic injuries were caused by medication errors.

2. **What is an adverse drug event (ADE)?**

   Adverse drug event refers to an injury related to the use of a medicine. This includes both the inappropriate use of a medication as well as an unintended consequence from the appropriate use of a medication. ADEs may be further subclassified as *preventable* (i.e., those from inappropriate use of medications) and *unpreventable* ADEs (i.e., those related to appropriate use of medications). *Potential* ADEs involve the possibility of an ADE that did not transpire because the medication error was intercepted before its administration, or cases in which the patient did not have an adverse event despite a medication error.

3. **What is the incidence of ADEs for hospitalized patients?**

   Studies have shown that ADEs occur in 4–20% of hospitalized patients. Of these ADEs, nearly half have been thought to be "serious" or "life threatening" and 28% to be preventable. Physicians are responsible for over half of these ADEs, with the remainder attributed to nursing, pharmacy, and clerical staff.

4. **What are the consequences of ADEs?**

   ADEs are associated with tangible economic costs such as additional medical costs, loss of economic productivity, and malpractice costs, as well as intangible economic costs related to the loss of the patient's quality of life. ADEs have been associated with an additional $2600 of hospital costs per event. This amounts to several million dollars per hospital per year, and approximately $4 billion annually throughout the United States. These costs do not include the impact of lost economic productivity and the impact on quality of life.

5. **What are the causes of ADEs?**

   Medication order fulfillment is a complex process involving multiple personnel in discrete stages. Medication errors may occur at any stage of the prescription-fulfillment process from the physician ordering the medication, to the unit clerk putting the order in the hospital computer system, to the pharmacy preparing the medication, to the nursing staff administering the medication (Table 3-1). For hospitalized patients, over 50% of errors occur in the ordering stage and approximately one-third at the administration stage. The probability of an ADE occurring is directly related to the number of prescriptions written, the severity of patient illness, and any metabolic derangements in the patient.

TABLE 3-1.   CAUSES OF MEDICATION ERRORS IN HOSPITALIZED PATIENTS AND PREVENTIVE MEASURES

Cause of Error	Definition	Level of Error	Examples	Possible Preventive Measures
Inadequate drug information	Inadequate knowledge of the indications for use, dosage, route of administration, and drug interactions	MD RN	Furosemide prescribed to patient with allergy to sulfa antibiotics; extended release formulation of ampicillin/sulbactam prescribed to a hemodialysis patient	CPOE; electronic drug database; continuing education; standardized formularies; pharmacists on physician rounds
Lack of patient information	Incomplete knowledge of patient's medical condition	MD RN Pharmacy	Ampicillin ordered for a patient with penicillin allergy; acetaminophen ordered for patient with severe liver failure	Cross-checking of information by computer software or by another individual at the time of drug ordering, dispensing, and/or administration; use of electronic drug databases
Rule violations	Failure to follow well-established procedures	MD RN Pharmacy	Incomplete medication order written; inappropriate drug preparation by pharmacy	Cross-checking of information at multiple levels as stated above
Transcription errors	Errors while putting orders in the computer system	Clerical staff RN Management systems	Errors of omission or commission such as dropped orders, missed orders, duplicate orders	Seamless electronic ordering and dispensing technology with multiple built-in checks; vigilance on part of MD, RN, and pharmacy
Faulty administration	Failure to give the appropriate medication in the appropriate manner to the patient	RN Pharmacy Management systems	Wrong drug or dose dispensed to a patient due to confusing nomenclature/drug package; delayed administrations of drug; heparin intravenously administered instead of subcutaneously as ordered	Cross-checking of patient and drug information; automated drug dispensing; administrative measures to reduce workload; improving system-wide operational efficiency

TABLE 3-1.   CAUSES OF MEDICATION ERRORS IN HOSPITALIZED PATIENTS AND PREVENTIVE MEASURES—CONT'D

Cause of Error	Definition	Level of Error	Examples	Possible Preventive Measures
Inadequate monitoring	Failure to adjust dose of medication based on continual monitoring of various patient parameters	MD RN	Failure to adjust medications such as vancomycin based on serum drug level; failure to monitor renal function and electrolytes for a patient taking amphotericin	Use of electronic drug databases; CPOE with built-in reminders for monitoring patient parameters; education and training; standard operating procedures for administration of medications that require intensive monitoring
Human errors		MD RN Pharmacy	Errors in dose calculation; inappropriate placement of a decimal resulting in 2.05 units instead of 20.5 units; medication given to wrong patient	Education and training; regular reminders about similar-sounding medications; CPOE with error-checking facility for dosing, allergy, etc.; automated medication dispensing; use of bar codes for patient identity; avoidance of abbreviations; encouragement of legible orders
Inadequate communication	Failure among various providers to communicate patient's medication regimens	MD RN Pharmacy	Miscommunication by physicians after transfer of a patient between services or hospitals; different consult services ordering drugs with potential interactions	Avoiding polypharmacy; use of legible writing; provider-to-provider communication encouraged; use of EMR for secure communication of patient's medical information

MD = physician, RN = nurse, CPOE = computerized physician order entry, EMR = electronic medical records.

6. **What are the common types of prescription errors made by ordering physicians?**

   Some of the common types of prescription errors seen are wrong drug for the indication, wrong dose for the disease being treated or for the patient's metabolic characteristics, wrong duration of treatment, inappropriate frequency of drug administration, and inappropriate route of administration.

7. **What are some of the common classes of medications associated with hospital ADEs?**

   Medications commonly involved in ADEs include antibiotics, antineoplastic agents, cardiovascular medications, anticoagulants, hypoglycemic agents, narcotics, and central nervous system depressants, including sedatives and antipsychotics. Central nervous system medications are the most common cause of preventable ADEs.

8. **What are computerized physician order entry (CPOE) and clinical decision support systems (CDSS)? How effective are they in reducing ADEs?**

   CPOE is software that helps automate the medication-ordering process to ensure standardized and complete orders. CDSS is software that provides advice regarding various aspects of the medication-ordering process such as dose, route of administration, drug interactions, and potential allergic reactions. Studies have shown that CPOE use markedly reduces serious medication errors and may improve prescribing behaviors. The data on CDSS are less encouraging, with some studies failing to show any benefit of the technology in reducing medication errors. Not enough data are available to comment on the effectiveness of either of these in reducing overall ADEs, and concerns have been raised that the use of these technologies will result in different types of ADEs. These relate to incorrect default doses and routes of administration and over-reliance on computerized advice resulting in neglect of human clinical judgment. These systems cannot eliminate all human errors and require extensive upfront and ongoing capital investments with no clear cost-effectiveness analysis available so far.

9. **What are some of the commonly used abbreviations that may cause medication errors?**

   See Table 3-2.

TABLE 3-2. UNDESIRABLE ABBREVIATIONS AND SUGGESTED ALTERNATIVES	
Undesirable Abbreviation	**Recommended Alternative**
qd; qod	Daily; every other day
U	Unit
IU	International unit
x3d	For three days or three doses
MS, MSO_4, $MgSO_4$	Morphine sulfate, magnesium sulfate
.5 mg	0.5 mg (place a "0" before a decimal)
1.0 mg	1 mg (avoid trailing zeros after decimal)
µg	Microgram
$Dram_3$, grain, minim	Use metric system

10. **What are Beers criteria?**

    Elderly patients have a high incidence of ADEs due to polypharmacy, altered metabolism, and a higher likelihood of being institutionalized. An estimated 350,000 ADEs occur annually in long-term care residents, and more than half of these are preventable. Beers criteria are a set of standards defining potentially inappropriate medication use in the elderly. These criteria have been useful in reducing medication errors. They cover medications that should generally be avoided in patients older than 65 years and medications that should not be used in older patients with specific medical conditions. Examples of some of the medications that should be avoided in the elderly patients and the adverse events they can cause are as follows:

- **Anticholinergics:** Urinary retention, cardiac dysrhythmias, dry mouth
- **Tricyclic antidepressants** (e.g., amitriptyline): Anticholinergic side effects
- **Sedative antihistamines** (e.g., diphenhydramine): Anticholinergic properties
- **Long-acting benzodiazepines** (e.g., chlordiazepoxide): Prolonged sedation and potential for falls
- **First- and second-generation antipsychotics:** Anticholinergic and extrapyramidal effects
- **Barbiturates:** Respiratory depression, potential for falls and risk of habituation

11. **Name several factors that need to be considered when prescribing medications.**
   Apart from selecting the proper drug class, physicians should consider the cost of therapy and the convenience of dosing. These factors influence patients' adherence to a medication regimen, which in turn influences the effectiveness of the treatment. It does little good to prescribe a medication if the patient cannot afford it or is unable to take it.

12. **How do brand-name and generic drugs compare?**
   Brand-name medications often cost $50–$150 per month. For patients taking multiple medications, costs can quickly reach several thousand dollars each year. Generic medications, by contrast, usually cost 30–60% less than the brand-name equivalent. Generic drugs are available once the patent on the branded medication has expired, which is usually 7–20 years after the drug's introduction. Generic medications are reviewed and approved by the U.S. Food and Drug Administration before being allowed on the market. Strict regulations ensure that generic drugs offer the same chemical structure, dosing, efficacy, and safety as their brand-name counterparts.

13. **Are new medications better than old ones?**
   New medications are heavily advertised in the medical and commercial media and aggressively marketed by pharmaceutical sales forces. Although these advertisements may imply that new drugs are more effective than their older counterparts, this is not always the case. In fact, with the exception of a few ground-breaking products, the older and more established drugs should be preferred due to their lower cost and more established safety profile.

14. **How common is patient nonadherence to medical therapy?**
   On average, fewer than 50% of patients take their medications as directed. A survey conducted by the Boston Consulting Group in 2003 found that during a 12-month period, 30% of patients took prescription medications less often than prescribed, 26% delayed filling a prescription, 21% stopped taking a prescription sooner than prescribed, 18% never filled a prescription, and 14% took smaller doses than prescribed.

   Alastair F, Thomas G, Deborah L, et al: The hidden epidemic: Finding a cure for unfilled prescriptions and missed doses. December 2003:1–8. Available at http://www.bcg.com/publications/publications_splash.jsp.

15. **What are the consequences of nonadherence?**
   Poor adherence to medical therapy leads to reduced drug effectiveness. In other words, the full effect of medications observed in rigorous research studies (in which nearly all the patients take the medications as directed) are often not seen in medical practice (where fewer than half of patients take the medication appropriately). Poor adherence to medical therapy is associated with suboptimal disease management and increased morbidity and mortality. Poor adherence also leads to more frequent hospital admissions and readmissions, particularly for chronic conditions like congestive heart failure.

KEY POINTS: SAFE AND APPROPRIATE MEDICATION USE

1. ADEs are very common among hospitalized patients. They are costly both economically and in terms of patients' quality of life.

2. ADEs may be caused by errors at any stage of the prescription-fulfillment process, from the prescription writing to the actual administration of the medication to the patient. However, most ADEs are caused by prescription errors.

3. Use of nonstandardized abbreviations and illegible handwriting are common and easily preventable causes of medication errors.

4. Patients with altered metabolism such as patients with renal or hepatic dysfunction and older patients are at particularly high risk for ADEs.

5. Patient nonadherence to prescribed medication regimens is very common and is a frequent cause of suboptimal treatment results.

16. **How can physicians assess patient adherence?**
Asking patients a leading, yes/no question like, "Are you taking all your medicines?" is *not* an effective way to assess patient adherence. More effective techniques include:
- Asking patients about medication use in a non-threatening manner. Example: "A lot of my patients tell me they occasionally forget to take their medications. When is the last time you missed one of your pills?"
- Confirming refill dates with the patient or pharmacy (e.g., a patient who last filled a 30-day supply of medication 6 weeks ago probably is not taking it every day).
- Counting the number of pills remaining in a container and comparing this to the number that *should* be left, based on the last refill date.

17. **What are some effective techniques to improve patient adherence?**
Involving patients in the decision-making process is an important first step to improving adherence. For example, instead of telling patients that you want them to start a new medication, explain to them why it is necessary and get their "buy in." When possible, prescribe medications that are dosed once a day instead of several times a day. When starting a new medication, describing common side effects can help patients know what to expect, and this knowledge reduces the chance they will simply stop the medicine upon experiencing any new symptoms. Confirming patient comprehension of side effects and dosing instructions is important, particularly when changes are made. An effective way to do this is to ask the patient to repeat back key instructions. Finally, encouraging use of pill boxes and other reminder systems can significantly improve adherence.

BIBLIOGRAPHY

1. Bates DW, Cullen DJ, Laird N, et al: Incidence of adverse drug events and potential adverse drug events: Implications for prevention. JAMA 274:29–34, 1995.
2. Beers MH: Explicit criteria for determining potentially inappropriate medication use by the elderly: An update. Arch Intern Med 157:1531–1536, 1997.

3. Brennan TA, Leape LL, Laird NM, et al: Incidence of adverse events and negligence in hospitalized patients: Results of the Harvard Medical Practice Study. N Engl J Med 324:370–376, 1991.

4. Gurwitz JH, Field TS, Avorn J, et al: Incidence and preventability of adverse drug events in nursing homes. Am J Med 109:87–94, 2000.

5. Haynes RB, Yao X, Degani A, et al: Interventions to enhance medication adherence. Cochrane Database of Systematic Reviews 2005(4).

6. Lesar TS, Briceland L, Stein DS: Factors related to errors in medication prescribing. JAMA 277:312–317, 1997.

CHAPTER 4

MEDICOLEGAL ISSUES IN HOSPITAL MEDICINE

Natalie G. Correia, DO, MA

Note: This chapter is not intended to substitute for legal counsel with respect to individual cases. Many laws and regulations vary in different jurisdictions. All decisions should be made with the appropriate legal and/or ethics consultations as needed.

1. **What is medical malpractice?**

   Legally speaking, medical negligence, also known as *medical malpractice,* is a *tort.* A tort is a civil wrong—an action that causes injury to person or property for which the plaintiff may seek redress through the courts. Unlike a criminal action, for which the prosecution must prove guilt "beyond a reasonable doubt," the burden of proof in a tort action is "by a preponderance of the evidence" or "more likely than not."

2. **What is standard of care?**

   The term *standard of care* is defined by each state and, therefore, specific language may vary somewhat. However, the generally accepted definition is "that which a reasonably well qualified physician would do under the same or similar circumstances." It is important to note that this allows for different standards in different settings and different practice types. Thus, the standard of care in a university medical center is different than in a rural hospital.

3. **Who decides what the standard of care is?**

   With regard to medical management issues, all too often, the standard of care becomes a battle of expert witnesses at a trial. In these cases, it is left to the jury to determine which expert they believe has articulated the accepted standard. As we begin to develop evidence-based protocols and best practice standards, it is possible these will become the benchmarks for standard of care.

4. **What specific criteria must be met to prove medical negligence?**

   The plaintiff must prove four elements in order to prevail in a malpractice claim:
   - **Duty was owed to the patient:** This is generally held to mean that a physician-patient relationship existed. Physicians who do not have a defined physician-patient relationship such as pathologists and radiologists also owe a duty.
   - **Deviation from the standard of care:** See question 3.
   - **Sustained injury:** A mistake does not rise to the level of negligence unless it results in damage. For example, a patient reports a penicillin allergy but inadvertently receives the drug without ill effects.
   - **Proximate cause:** It must be shown that the alleged action caused the injury. Proximate cause is defined as a cause that, in a natural and continuous sequence, unbroken by any intervening events, would produce the injury. In other words, *but for the action*, the injury would not have occurred.

5. **What are "chart wars"?**

   In the game of chart wars, individuals and hospital services point fingers at one another around patient care issues and responsibility for that care. This is done in the mistaken belief that it absolves the writer of liability for adverse events. In its most common form, a physician records that he has paged another individual or service without response. Far from protecting the writer from responsibility, these recordings demonstrate that the writer did not take the next step by trying other means to locate the required consultant. Chart wars are inappropriate and unprofessional.

6. **How significant are adverse drug events?**
    According to the Institute of Medicine, 1 of every 50 hospital admissions results in a significant adverse drug event. A substantial percentage of these events result from unclear handwriting leading to misinterpretation of a drug name, dose, timing, or route of administration. Computerized physician order entry (CPOE) has been shown to decrease the frequency of these events.

7. **If my hospital doesn't have CPOE, How can I decrease the frequency of drug errors?**
    There are several simple procedures that have been shown to decrease errors.
    - If your handwriting is illegible, print drug names.
    - Avoid trailing zeros—5 mg, *not* 5.0 mg, which can be easily mistaken for 50 mg.
    - Use leading zeros before decimals—0.5 mg is less likely to be mistaken as 5 mg.
    - Use mcg rather than μg for micrograms.
    - Spell out the word "units" instead of "u."
    - Spell out "morphine sulfate" rather than MSO_4.
    - Avoid verbal orders whenever possible.
    - Sign all orders and prescriptions and print your name and pager or phone number.
    - Avoid "accidental drowning." Every intravenous fluid order should have a built-in stop—either a total volume to be infused or a time limit.

8. **Who should be notified if I have an adverse outcome or there is a question of negligence?**
    Your insurance carrier and hospital risk manager should be notified as soon as possible. Depending on the specifics of your insurance policy, you may invalidate your coverage if you do not notify the carrier.

9. **Should adverse events be discussed with patients and families?**
    Honesty is virtually always the best policy. Candid discussions about adverse outcomes and events have not increased the frequency of litigation and, in many cases, have probably averted litigation. If there is an adverse event in the hospital, patients almost always hear about them one way or another. It is better to provide the information than give the appearance of trying to hide or cover up the incident. In fact, some states have enacted legislation that allows physicians to apologize for an adverse event without admitting liability.

10. **How and where should an adverse event be documented?**
    It is important to write a candid chronology of events and any other pertinent information as soon as possible after an adverse event or unexpected outcome. Memory fades with time, and critical pieces of information are often lost. After you have recorded your recollections, the names of witnesses, and any other significant information, the document should be sealed and a copy sent to your attorney and hospital risk manager. You should *not* retain a copy or put a copy in the hospital chart. Documents and notes in your possession are discoverable in the event of litigation. The same documents, if held by your attorney, risk manager, or insurance carrier are considered *work product* and are not discoverable.

11. **Can I discuss an adverse event or litigation with other physicians?**
    Unless the discussion is in the context of a morbidity and mortality conference or a quality assurance/improvement initiative, the answer is "no." Every state protects the process of quality review and improvement from discovery during litigation. However, discussions between

physicians outside that process are discoverable. As tempting as it is to decompress and validate your position, it is best to avoid discussions with colleagues.

12. How long after an event can a lawsuit be filed?

The *statute of limitations* defines a finite period of time during which litigation for medical malpractice can be filed. The period is determined by each state and, therefore, can vary. In most states, the statute of limitations is either 2 or 3 years for adults. It begins to run at the time of the event or at the time the patient knew, or reasonably should have known, that an adverse event has occurred.

13. Is the statute of limitations different for children?

Yes. State laws recognize the nature and extent of injuries to children may not be immediately apparent. In most states, the statute of limitations for children ranges from 6 to 8 years after the injury occurred. This applies to those who have not reached the age of majority as defined by the state—usually persons younger than 18 years.

14. What happens if documents or evidence are destroyed or concealed from the patient?

Intentional withholding of information or destruction of evidence is considered fraud, and the legal system does not look kindly on such behavior. In the case of fraudulent concealment, the statute of limitations begins to run from the time the fraud is discovered. There are substantial penalties for fraud. There are also specific instructions given to the jury in a case involving fraud that penalize the defendant.

15. Can I change a record or document after it is completed?

No. The medical record is a legal document that is intended to represent a contemporaneous recitation of the treatment provided to a patient. The only way additional information can be added is by specifically identifying the entry as an addition (e.g., "Late Entry" or "Addendum") and referring back to the original entry. Late entries should be timed and dated when they were written.

16. How much patient care documentation is enough?

In general, if you didn't write it, it didn't happen. All significant events should be memorialized in the patient's chart. If there are difficult interactions with patients or challenging clinical decisions, the details should be documented. This is particularly true when a patient refuses treatment that the physician deems necessary. Documentation may not prevent the filing of a lawsuit, but it may prevent a guilty verdict.

17. Is there any way to protect myself from litigation?

The best protection against litigation is a good relationship with your patient. This can be challenging when the hospitalist steps in to assume a role that many patients expect will be filled by their primary care physician. Time spent talking with a patient and his or her family is a good investment both from a risk management and from a patient care perspective.

18. Is sign-out between providers discoverable?

Yes. Whether sign-out is handwritten or communicated by e-mail, it is potentially discoverable in the event of litigation. It is important that all sign-outs be factual and avoid disparaging or unflattering remarks about patients, their conditions, or their families. Try to imagine sitting in a courtroom reading your sign-out to a jury. If it doesn't sound professional, you need to do some censoring.

19. How should I document informed consent?

Different hospitals have different protocols for the documentation of informed consent. Some favor detailed forms that enumerate specific risks and benefits. Other hospitals favor a simple statement such as "risks, benefits, and alternatives discussed with patient." Even if a specific form is the preferred method in your hospital, it may be beneficial to document the discussion in the progress notes.

20. **What is the difference between "claims-made" and "occurrence" liability insurance?**

    Claims-made insurance covers you for litigation that is filed during the years in which the insurance was in force regardless of the year in which the alleged incident occurred. Occurrence coverage insures you for any event that occurred while the insurance was in effect regardless of the year in which the litigation is filed. Because occurrence insurance continues to protect you for events during the covered period even after the coverage has terminated, it does not require "tail coverage" and is, therefore, much more expensive.

KEY POINTS: MEDICOLEGAL ISSUES IN HOSPITAL MEDICINE

1. The job isn't finished until the paperwork is done.

2. Anyone can bring a lawsuit for anything, but it does not mean they will prevail in court.

3. Never destroy or alter a document.

4. Communication and a good relationship with your patient are the best risk management strategies.

5. Confidentiality is everyone's concern: "Loose lips sink ships."

21. **What is tail coverage?**

    This is a form of insurance that is generally purchased at the time a claims-made policy terminates. It provides coverage for incidents that occurred while the claims-made policy was still active but that are not reported until after the policy has terminated.

22. **What are the limits of insurance coverage?**

    Policies may be purchased in varying amounts. The higher the policy limits, the more expensive the coverage. The most common packages are $1 million/$3 million and $2 million/$4 million. The first number refers to the maximum amount that will be paid for any one incident. The second number refers to the maximum amount that will be paid out during the policy year in the event of multiple suits.

23. **Do I have the right to refuse to settle a case out of court?**

    That depends on how your insurance policy is written and is something to consider when purchasing insurance coverage. Although an out-of-court settlement may be more cost-effective for the insurance carrier, settlements are reported to the National Practitioner Databank and can affect your future licensure and hospital privileges. On the other hand, it is difficult to be objective when your professional care is questioned, and the insurance carrier may provide a more objective and experienced view.

24. **What is HIPAA?**

    The Health Insurance Portability and Accountability Act (HIPAA) mandates that anyone belonging to a group health insurance plan must be allowed to purchase health insurance within an interval of time beginning when the previous coverage is lost. It also protects the confidentiality of personal medical information from disclosure—written or verbal—without the explicit consent of the patient.

25. Does HIPAA prevent me from obtaining medical information without written consent?
No. In emergency situations, hospitals and physicians can provide information necessary for the care of a patient who is unable to give consent. In nonemergent situations, written consent is always required.

26. Can I provide condition updates to family members of hospitalized patients?
You are free to discuss a patient's condition and care with any individual designated by the patient. However, specific consent by competent patients is required. Obviously, care can be discussed with a designated guardian or power of attorney for health care. This should be documented in the hospital chart.

WEBSITES

1. McCullough, Campbell & Lane, Summary of Malpractice Law
   http://www.mcandl.com/states.html

2. Institute of Medicine of the National Academies
   http://iom.edu

3. Centers for Medicare & Medicaid Services, U.S. Department of Health and Human Services
   http://www.cms.hhs.gov/hipaa/hipaa1

BIBLIOGRAPHY

1. Levinson W, Roter DL, Mullooly JP, Dull VT, Frankel RM: Physician-patient communication: The relationship with malpractice claims among primary care physicians and surgeons. JAMA 277:553–559, 1997.
2. In Prosser W, Keaton WP, Dobbs DB, et al (eds): Prosser and Keeton on the Law of Torts, 5th ed. St. Paul, MN, West Publishing, Co, 1984.

CHAPTER 5

COMMUNICATING WITH PATIENTS AND FAMILIES

Kathleen Finn, MD, MPhil

1. How does communication with patients and families in the hospital differ from the clinic?

Hospital communication occurs during an acute illness, which can be a very stressful time for patients and their families. Information about the illness and prognosis needs to be imparted quickly with enough details so that the patient and family can make decisions about care. The communication is often done by physicians who have no prior relationship with the patient and occurs in the setting of strong emotions like fear and anxiety.

2. What role does communication play in the care of a hospitalized patient?

Communication is the basis of any patient-doctor relationship and is *vital* during a hospitalization. Honest, intelligible, and timely information is very important to patients and families. It provides comfort and support and helps the patient and family feel more in control. It also is vital to creating a therapeutic bond and building trust. Poor communication is the number one cause of patient complaints and has been shown to adversely affect care and decision making.

3. Who should do the communicating?

Although any caregiver may communicate, it is important that everyone give the same message. Hospital care is provided by a team of people, which can be overwhelming to patients and their families. It is often worth communicating first with the care team so that everyone is on the same page. Although they do not all need to agree, it is important to explain this openly and clearly to patients. Patients and families report dissatisfaction if they perceive caregivers are not communicating with each other.

4. How should communication begin?

Begin with introductions of all the care providers, including their role and level of involvement. Identify the attending physician so the family knows who is leading the team. Remind the patient and family who you are each time you meet with them if there are many caregivers. Patients and families report dissatisfaction when they do not know who is caring for them.

5. What information should you communicate?

Patients and families want information about the clinical situation: possible diagnoses, plans for testing, treatment options, and prognosis. Unfortunately, studies have shown only 50% of patients and families understand the information given, and caregivers could not predict which families had a poor understanding. Do not spend a great deal of time on details or pathophysiology. This leads to confusion and causes the family to focus on minutiae rather than the big picture. It is best to explain things several times and in multiple ways.

6. Should you communicate expectations about the hospitalization?

Yes. Setting expectations not only helps the patient and family feel they have some control, but it can also minimize conflicts. Explain how long the work-up may take, including timing of tests, and what they should anticipate in terms of improvement and course of illness. It is important to identify how long the patient may be hospitalized and discuss post-discharge plans. Patients and families cling to the information given by the team. Conflict may arise if the patient is told discharge will be in a few days and then later informed he or she can now leave. Given the shortened length of stay in hospitals, it is also important to caution patients they may not be feeling back to baseline at the time of discharge.

7. When should communication occur, and how frequently?

There are two ways to communicate with patients and their families. The first is the traditional family meeting that is planned ahead of time and tries to include as many family members as possible along with the entire care team. The second is the less formal meeting where you provide daily updates and plans. Although not every patient needs a family meeting, there should be daily informal communication either to the patient or a family member. Multiple short meetings over time are better than one long meeting. If the patient has many family members, ask one person to be the spokesperson for the family to minimize having to repeat the care plan to numerous relatives.

8. Who should have a family meeting?

- Patients with complex medical conditions or a length of stay greater than 2 days
- Patients needing to make complicated decisions or to have an end-of-life discussion
- Patients with a change in his or her medical status
- Families in which a conflict is present, or situations in which the patient/family request a meeting

9. What if the patient does not have decision-making capacity?

When patients cannot speak for themselves, a surrogate or designated health care proxy will need to speak for them. The appointed surrogate has the legal or moral authority to make decisions for the patient. This changes the doctor-patient relationship and clearly raises other challenges of communication. Besides providing the surrogate with the same medical information you would provide the patient, it is also important to help him or her make decisions that the patient would want. It is often difficult for surrogates to separate what they would choose from the patient's wishes. Phrases such as, "If your dad was sitting here now, what would he say?" can help tease apart conflicting feelings.

10. Are there techniques that allow for better communication?

The best communicators are actually the best listeners. Start by asking the patient and family their understanding of the situation. Ask them to repeat things back and modify your explanations based on their understanding. Use of written material, video, or brochures can help. Do not use medical jargon. Translate medical language into plain English and explain things at a ninth-grade level. Given the stress of hospitalization, the patient and family will be limited as to what they can take in. State no more than three new pieces of information at a time, and allocate sufficient time for questions and answers.

11. How can I be a better communicator?

Create a sense of trust, openness, curiosity, and respect by actively listening and being self-aware. Active listening means truly hearing, accepting, and validating what the patient and family are saying, including their emotions and concerns. Physicians are taught to minimize emotions. However, it is the avoidance of emotions, both the patient's and your own, that limit your ability to communicate. Self-awareness of emotions can help you avoid projecting personal feelings onto patients and families and getting upset or angry when they project their feelings on you. It also helps you engage in conversation with patients and families about their fears, concerns, and emotions.

KEY POINTS: COMMUNICATION WITH PATIENTS AND FAMILIES

1. Communication with patients and their families is fundamental to good patient care and a vital part of a patient-physician relationship.

2. You should communicate information about the clinical situation, treatment options, and prognosis in plain English at a ninth-grade level, focusing on the big picture.

3. Setting clear and reasonable expectations helps guide a patient and family through a hospitalization.

4. The best communicators are actually the best listeners.

5. Essential to communicating is learning to understand your own emotions and accepting the emotions of patients and their families.

12. What about emotions? How do I deal with the patients' or families' emotions?

Hospitalization brings out strong emotions in patients and families. They react in many different ways. Some are angry and upset and want to blame, others have a flight or fight response or become withdrawn and sad. Each family has its own "functional" way of handling stress. Your role is to provide support by listening and acknowledging their emotions. If possible, name the emotion, show understanding and respect, and help the family members explore their feelings. Do not hesitate to refer them to members of the care team who can provide more support. Acknowledge that their feelings are normal. Above all, do not take their emotions personally.

13. How do I communicate with non–english-speaking patients and families?

Communication becomes even more difficult when the physician and patient do not speak the same language. Use translators who are trained in medical communication. Having family members translate should be avoided because they will often answer for the patient, and privacy issues are a concern. When translators are unavailable, there are telephone translators available through phone companies.

14. How do I discuss prognosis and maintain hope?

Patients and families want to know the prognosis but also feel there is hope. Balancing this can be difficult, for although you want to provide hope, you also want to be truthful. Focusing solely on a positive prognosis misses opportunities for patients and families to explore emotions of loss and end-of-life issues. Focusing solely on a negative prognosis can make the family perceive the care team is giving up too early. It is recommended to give both the best and worst situations by saying "we are hoping for the best, but preparing for the worst." Although the patient and family may not be ready to deal with loss, the seed is planted. Yet it also indicates that you, too, are hoping for the best for them.

15. Are there phrases that can help in patient/family communication?

See Table 5-1.

TABLE 5-1. HELPFUL PHRASES IN SPECIFIC SITUATIONS

Emotional family	"It sounds like you are feeling (name emotion). Can you tell me about it?"
Angry patient	"I am sorry that you are so angry. Could you tell me what is bothering you?"
Talkative patient	"I am eager to hear about your sister's health, but I'm not sure we are getting to the facts that I need most now. Could you tell me about your cough?"
Crying patient	"You look like you are feeling sad. Can you tell me what is bothering you?"
Hypochondriac patient	"I see that you are very worried, but I feel confident we are not dealing with a serious physical problem. We will need to work together to help you through these symptoms."
Health care proxy	"Sometimes what you want is different from what your family member would want. I realize it's very difficult to separate the two and focus on her wishes."
End-of-life issues	"I am hoping that your illness will improve, and we are doing everything we can to support you. I also want to be prepared if it does not respond to treatment."

BIBLIOGRAPHY

1. Back AL, Arnold RM, Quill TE: Hope for the best, and prepare for the worst. Annals 138:439–443, 2003.
2. Billings JA, Stoeckle JD: The Clinical Encounter. Chicago, Year Book, 1989.
3. Chaitin E, Arnold RM: Communication in the ICU: Holding a family meeting. UpToDate Online 12.3. Available at: http://www.utdol.com/utd/content/topic.do?topicKey=genr_med/32430&type=A&selectedTitle=1~2.
4. McLeod ME: Doctor-patient relationship: Perspectives, needs and communication. Am J Gastroenterol 93:676–680, 1997.
5. Quill TE: Recognizing and adjusting to barriers in doctor-patient communication. Ann Intern Med 111:1–57, 1989.

CHAPTER 6

PROFESSIONAL COMMUNICATION

John Nelson, MD

1. **Why does communication between health care professionals in hospitalist systems matter?**
   Hospitalist systems have a built-in discontinuity between the patient and his or her usual outpatient provider. This increases the risk that important clinical information can "fall through the cracks" as the patient moves back and forth from inpatient to outpatient settings.

2. **What are the important communication issues at the time of admission and discharge?**
   - Ensure the patient's usual outpatient provider is made aware of the admission or discharge in a timely way (e.g., by phone/voicemail/e-mail or via stat transcription of the admit note that is faxed to the outpatient provider on the day of admission).
   - Develop a protocol to request patient information from the outpatient provider and/or other hospitals where the patient has received care. Always dictate/write the admission and discharge reports on the day the patient is seen. Never put these off for another day.

3. **How much detail should be included in the discharge report?**
   The three most important principles of good discharge summaries are that they are timely (e.g., available within 24 hours of discharge), thorough, and succinct. Avoid repeating lengthy descriptions of the history of present illness and initial physical examination, etc., that were detailed in the admission note. To decrease the chance that important details are forgotten, consider including specific sections under their own heading such as "test results that are pending at discharge" (and will need to be reviewed by the outpatient provider in the future) and "recommended follow-up studies" (e.g., a reminder that the patient had a heme positive stool for which future colonoscopy is indicated but was not done during the hospital stay, or the need to repeat a chest x-ray in 3 months to reassess a lung nodule).

4. **What information do primary care providers say they need in a discharge summary?**
   Primary care doctors indicate the following information is extremely important to them:
   - Discharge medications (a complete list with doses and frequency)
   - Discharge diagnoses
   - Procedure results
   - Scheduled follow-up visits
   - Key lab results

   Pantilat SZ, Lindenauer PK, Katz PP, Wachter RM: Primary care physician attitudes regarding communication with hospitalists. Am J Med 111:15S–20S, 2001.

5. **What communication should occur between hospitalists and other providers during the patient's hospital stay (i.e., other than at admission and discharge)?**

   Be sure the patient's usual outpatient provider, with whom he or she might have a close relationship, is made aware (usually via a phone call) if there are significant unexpected changes in the patient's condition or if complex decisions need to be made. Examples include unanticipated transfer to the intensive care unit, a decision by the patient to pursue only palliative care in anticipation of a natural death, or a patient/family struggling to decide whether to pursue high-risk surgery. Outpatient providers should always be notified in a timely manner when a patient dies.

6. **What is the best way to request a consult?**

   Speak with the person you are consulting and clearly communicate the issue or question you want the consultant to address, and the urgency of the consult.

7. **What are some useful principles to follow when serving as a consultant?**
   - Gather important patient data yourself rather than relying on what you have been told by the person requesting the consult.
   - Provide a brief written report that offers very specific recommendations, and make yourself available to discuss these if necessary.
   - Avoid vague recommendations such as "consider adding an anti-hypertensive agent."

8. **How can patients help in facilitating inpatient-outpatient provider communication?**

   Consider providing patients with a copy of their discharge summary. It can provide them with another reminder of follow-up visits that were planned, as well as the need to check on test results that were pending at discharge, and ensure that important follow-up tests are completed as planned. The patient can show the report to any caregivers that the hospitalist was not aware of (and did not send a report to) such as home nursing services and other doctors that the patient may see.

KEY POINTS: PROFESSIONAL COMMUNICATION

1. Develop a standard approach to communication with other health care providers and patients, and follow this approach for every patient.

2. Admission and discharge notes should be prepared on the day the patient is seen and transmitted immediately to the outpatient provider.

3. Consider providing patients with a copy of the discharge summary and phoning them within a couple weeks of discharge to see how they are doing.

---

9. **What contact should the hospitalist have with patients after discharge?**

   Consider phoning all patients within a couple weeks of their discharge. The call can provide a time to:
   - Review test results that were not final when the patient left the hospital.
   - Clarify any misunderstandings the patient may have had about the findings during the hospital stay, and the treatment and follow-up plans.
   - Detect treatment failures or side effects.
   - Increase patient satisfaction (patients *love* these calls, and they usually take the doctor only 2–4 minutes).

Doctors who make such calls find the experience very gratifying. It is common that the main outcome of the call is a chance for the patient to express gratitude for the call and the care delivered during the hospital stay.

Nelson J: The importance of postdischarge telephone follow-up for hospitalists: A view from the trenches. Am J Med 111:435–436, 2001.

WEBSITE

Society of Hospital Medicine: http://www.hospitalmedicine.org

BIBLIOGRAPHY

1. Geehr E, Nelson J: Hospitalist Program Essentials, 2nd ed., 2003. Available at http://www.hospitalmedicine.org/presentation/, 2003.

2. Nelson J: The importance of postdischarge telephone follow-up for hospitalists: A view from the trenches. Am J Med 111:435–436, 2001.

3. Nelson J, Whitcomb W: Organizing a hospitalist program: An overview of fundamental concepts. Med Clin North Am 96:887–909, 2002.

4. Pantilat SZ, Lindenauer PK, Katz PP, Wachter RM: Primary care physician attitudes regarding communication with hospitalists. Am J Med 111:15S–20S, 2001.

CHAPTER 7

HANDOFFS

Joseph Ming Wah Li, MD, and Sunil Kripalani, MD, MSc

1. **What is a handoff? When do handoffs occur?**

   The *handoff* refers to the reciprocal communication that occurs when clinical responsibilities are transferred from one provider to another. Given the rapid growth of hospital medicine and residency work hour reforms, handoffs are increasingly common. Most commonly, handoffs occur between a primary care provider (outpatient) and an inpatient provider (e.g., hospitalist). Additional handoffs may occur between providers in the hospital (e.g., ward patient transferred to an ICU provider). Finally, handoffs occur when a patient's care is transferred to a provider covering nights or weekends. This type of handoff is referred to as *cross-coverage.*

2. **Why are handoffs important?**

   Effective handoffs are essential to delivering high-quality, efficient care by health care teams. Fumbled handoffs, typically involving missing or incorrect information, can lead to medical error. One study found 6 times the odds of a preventable adverse event during cross-coverage, as opposed to regular provider coverage. Overall, 26% of adverse events occurred during cross-coverage.

   Petersen LA, Brennan TA, O'Neil AC, et al: Does housestaff discontinuity of care increase the risk of preventable adverse events? Ann Intern Med 121:866–872, 1994.

3. **How should handoffs occur?**

   Ideally, the exchange of information should occur at the time responsibility for patient care is transferred, with both the transferring and accepting providers present. Information must be easily understood, accounting for the recipient's baseline knowledge. In addition to the face-to-face interaction, the same information should be transferred between providers on a durable and easily accessible medium (e.g., on paper or computer). Using a standardized template helps to ensure that all the relevant information is communicated. Use of a computerized sign-out can decrease the likelihood of an adverse event.

   Petersen LA, Orav EJ, Teich JM, O'Neil AC, Brennan TA: Using a computerized sign-out program to improve continuity of inpatient care and prevent adverse events. Jt Comm J Qual Improv 24:77–87, 1998.

4. **Why is it necessary to list more than just the patient name as an identifier?**

   Listing more than one unique patient identifier is essential to prevention of identity error. This is one of the Joint Commission on Accreditation of Healthcare Organization's National Patient Safety Goals.

5. **List other common problems involved with handoffs.**

   - Incorrect or missing information
   - Illegible writing
   - Use of shorthand or colloquialisms
   - Not written down/not easily accessible
   - Participants don't show up
   - Not timely—information is outdated
   - Ineffectively communicated—meeting is rushed or environment is not conducive to effective communication

KEY POINTS: COMPONENTS OF AN EFFECTIVE HANDOFF

1. Patient identifiers: name, age, gender, date of birth, and medical record number

2. Names of patient's other inpatient and outpatient providers

3. Names of patient's family and health care proxy, with contact information

4. Problem list

5. Reason for hospitalization and hospital course

6. Allergies

7. List of current medications, doses, and schedules

8. Current active issues (e.g., mental status, fall risk, nutritional status)

9. Code status/advanced directives

10. Pending questions/active issues/things to be done

6. **Who should have access to the information in handoffs?**
   All providers involved in the patient's care should have timely access to this information.

7. **Comment on the use of abbreviations, acronyms, and symbols.**
   Abbreviations, acronyms, and symbols can result in medical error with dire consequences if they are misunderstood by different providers. Each organization should have a standard list of abbreviations, acronyms, and symbols that should *not* be utilized. (See Chapter 3 for more details.)

8. **What is pre- and post-hospitalization medicine reconciliation?**
   A patient's medication list changes frequently during his or her hospital stay. To minimize error, it is important to review the medication list with each handoff. At the time of hospital discharge, it is vital to compare the list of discharge medicines to the list of medicines at the time of hospital admission to make sure no medicines were inadvertently omitted and that correct dosages are being prescribed.

CHAPTER 8

DISCHARGE PLANNING AND TRANSITIONS OF CARE

Jennifer S. Myers, MD, and Sunil Kripalani, MD, MSc

1. **When should one start planning for discharge?**

   Physicians should begin thinking about discharge planning during a patient's admission evaluation. Obtaining information about a patient's social support systems, physical limitations, insurance status, and primary care provider (PCP) will assist the inpatient multidisciplinary care team in preparing for transitions of care upon discharge.

2. **Why is managing the patient's transition to discharge a crucial skill for hospital-based physicians?**

   Because many outpatient PCPs no longer provide inpatient care for their hospitalized patients, medical information must be communicated in a timely manner, preferably before or around the time of hospital discharge. If information is inaccurate or not communicated at all during the discharge process, an information "voltage drop" may occur, and this could lead to medical errors.

3. **List the potential forms of communication between the hospital physician and the PCP during the discharge process.**

   Communicating in more than one fashion and considering the communication modalities preferred by the PCP will help to ensure that information is transferred completely and accurately. Methods of communication include:

   - **Discharge summary:** Mailed, faxed, or posted on an electronic medical record
   - **Telephone call at the time of discharge**
   - **E-mail communications:** Used if using a HIPAA-protected site*
   - **Hand-delivered information:** Patient or caregiver serves as courier of information

4. **What is the purpose of the discharge summary?**

   The discharge summary has historically served as the standard document for recording and retrieving the vital details of a patient's hospital course. When created in a succinct and organized fashion, the summary should contain enough information for a PCP to assume longitudinal care of his or her patient. In addition, the Joint Commission on Accreditation of Hospital Organizations (JCAHO) requires discharge summaries for all hospitalizations.

5. **List the essential components of a discharge summary.**

   - **General information*:** Includes the patient's name and a second personal identifier (i.e., medical record number, date of birth), the attending physician name, and the name of practitioner dictating the summary
   - **Admission and discharge dates***
   - **Principal diagnosis*:** Reason for hospitalization†
   - **Secondary diagnoses***
   - **Brief history***
   - **Hospital course*:** Significant findings†

---

* Items required by JCAHO.

† HIPAA = Health Insurance Portability and Accountability Act of 1996. A HIPAA-protected site is one in which the security and privacy of health information is guaranteed.

- **Procedures*:** Procedures or treatment rendered
- **Discharge instructions*:** Instructions to patient and family, including discharge medications (highlighting changes to admission regimen) and follow-up care plan (highlighting appointments that have been scheduled or need to be scheduled and test results that require follow-up)
- **Functional status*:** Patient's condition at discharge

Items required by JCAHO are indicated by an asterisk.

6. **What are some common problems associated with discharge summaries?**
   Discharge summaries are often incomplete, lacking the important medical information detailed above. They may also arrive to the PCP too late to be useful. The average time to follow up with the PCP is 6 days after discharge, whereas discharge summaries are often not available for a few weeks due to delayed dictation, transcription, or delivery. Incomplete, delayed, or inaccurate communication of relevant information from the hospitalization limits the outpatient provider's ability to provide good follow-up care.

7. **What is a hospital care team?**
   A hospital care team is a collaborative group that assists the hospital physician in planning for a patient's post-discharge needs. The group may include physicians, nurses, therapists (e.g., physical, occupational, and/or speech pathology), clinical pharmacists, social workers or case managers, and palliative care providers.

8. **How does health insurance coverage affect discharge planning?**
   Patients who lack health insurance have limited resources available to them after discharge, and as such, they are prone to increased use of hospital services and readmissions. Health insurance coverage dictates the accessibility of all medical care, including office visits, home health care, prescription drugs, laboratory and radiologic studies, and durable medical equipment. Therefore, knowledge of a patient's health insurance coverage at the time of hospital *admission* is crucial to managing a patient's hospital *discharge*.

9. **How do Americans get health insurance?**
   The vast majority of insured Americans receive health insurance through their employers. A smaller percentage of people obtain coverage from the military, purchase insurance individually (also known as "nongroup" coverage), or receive federal coverage. Medicare and Medicaid are the two largest federally sponsored health insurance programs.

10. **What is the difference between Medicare and Medicaid?**
    Unlike most government health care programs, eligibility for Medicare does not depend on a person's assets. Medicare covers persons older than 65 years if they or their spouses are eligible for Social Security payments, people younger than 65 years who receive Social Security payments due to a disability, and all patients with end-stage renal disease regardless of age. In contrast, Medicaid is a major source of health care coverage for the underprivileged population. Because Medicaid is funded by both the state and federal governments, eligibility rules are complex and vary based on state requirements. Medicaid's coverage is very limited for adults. Only low-income adults who are parents, pregnant, or severely disabled are eligible. Medicaid also pays for nearly half of all long-term care services in the United States, including custodial nursing home care.

11. **Who are the uninsured in America?**
    Nearly 44 million people in the United States lack health coverage. According to the U.S. Census Bureau, about 1 in 5 adults aged 18–64 years old were uninsured in 2004. Compared with the general population, the uninsured tend to be younger, have lower incomes, and have fewer years of schooling. As a consequence of the Medicaid eligibility rules outlined above, childless adults

and men with low incomes have a higher uninsured risk compared with children, parents, or pregnant women in similar low-income tax brackets. A common misconception is that those who lack health insurance also lack jobs. The truth is that the majority of the uninsured are actively in the labor force but either cannot afford employer-sponsored coverage or have jobs that do not offer coverage. Another myth is that most uninsured persons in the United States are minorities. Blacks and whites make up almost half of the uninsured in the United States (Fig. 8-1 and Table 8-1).

U.S. Census Bureau. Health Insurance Coverage in the United States: 2002. U.S. Census Bureau, 2003. Available at http://www.census.gov/hhes/www/hlthins/hlthins.html

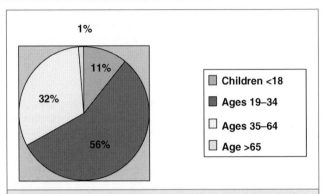

Figure 8-1. Uninsured by age groups, 2003, U.S. Census Bureau. Adults aged 19–34 years represent 56% of the uninsured. Their chances of being uninsured are high because they are more likely to be single or to have low incomes.

TABLE 8-1. PERCENTAGES OF PEOPLE WITHOUT HEALTH INSURANCE COVERAGE BY RACE, 2002–2004, U.S. CENSUS BUREAU

Race	Percent Uninsured*
Hispanic	33%
American Indian and Alaskan Native	29%
White	26%
Native Hawaiian and other Pacific Islander	22%
Black	20%
Asian	18%

*Numbers do not sum to 100. Federal surveys now give respondents the option of reporting more than one race.

12. **What is transitional care? How is the need for such care assessed in the hospital?**
Transitional care is care that occurs after a patient's hospitalization. It may be a permanent transition (e.g., nursing home placement, assisted-living facility) or a temporary health care

transition (e.g., rehabilitation center, short-term nursing facility) between hospital and home. Assessment of transitional care needs should begin at the time of admission and continue to be discussed by the multidisciplinary care team throughout the hospitalization. Knowledge of a patient's baseline level of functioning; level of physical, medical, or cognitive decline (if any) in the hospital; social support systems; and individual wishes will all play a role in determining whether another level of care is needed after discharge.

13. **What are activities of daily living (ADLs)?**
ADLs are activities that are usually performed for oneself during the course of a day. The ability to perform ADLs is necessary for someone who is living alone or without assistance from others. Examples of ADLs include bathing, dressing, eating, walking, using the telephone, and taking medications.

14. **List the types of transitional care facilities available after hospital discharge.**
See Table 8-2.

TABLE 8-2. EXAMPLES OF TRANSITIONAL CARE	
Nursing home	Facility where custodial care and skilled nursing care can be provided. Residents may be in the nursing home for extended/permanent periods or for short rehabilitation stays (*see* SNF).
Skilled nursing facility (SNF)	Facility where skilled nursing and/or rehabilitative care is given from licensed health professionals. SNF care is often provided in nursing homes.
Physical rehabilitation center	Facility focused on acute physical and occupational rehabilitation. Some of these centers are specialized to include specific diagnoses (e.g., stroke, spinal cord injuries).
Assisted-living facility/personal care homes	Facility providing housing and personal health care for persons who require assistance with ADLs and cannot live independently, but do *not* require 24-hour care.
Hospice	Program available to help terminally ill patients live their remaining days with dignity. Hospice can be provided either in a home or in an SNF/nursing home setting.

15. **What services can home health care provide?**
Some post-hospitalization medical needs can be performed in a patient's home environment. Home health services may include part-time skilled nursing care, health aides, physical, occupational, or speech therapy, social services, and the placement of medical equipment (e.g., wheelchairs, hospital beds, oxygen) in the home.

16. **What is hospice?**
Hospice is a concept of care (rather than a physical site of care) for patients with a terminal illness. Although hospice care is usually provided in a patient or caregiver's home, it is sometimes administered in a nursing home or hospital setting. Hospice care emphasizes pain control and symptom management rather than focusing on life-sustaining treatments. Hospice services are designed to address the physical needs of terminally ill patients as well as the psychosocial needs of patients and their loved ones. (See Chapter 92 for more details.)

KEY POINTS: FORMS OF TRANSITIONAL CARE AFTER HOSPITAL DISCHARGE

1. Nursing home

2. Skilled nursing facility

3. Physical rehabilitation center

4. Assisted-living facility/personal care homes

5. Hospice

6. Home care

WEBSITES

1. 2004 Comprehensive Accreditation Manual for Hospital: The Official Handbook (CAMH)
   http://www.jcaho.org/accredited+organizations/hospitals/standards/hospital+faqs/
   faq+index.htm

2. Health care coverage in America: Understanding the issues and proposed solutions
   http://www.CoverTheUninsured.org/Materials

3. Kaiser Family Foundation. An informative website with frequently asked questions about the
   federal health insurance programs.
   http://www.kff.org

4. Eldercare. Information about transitions of care and other community services and
   resources for the elderly.
   http://www.eldercare.gov

5. National Hospice and Palliative Care Organization
   http://www.nhpco.org

BIBLIOGRAPHY

1. Manning RT: Dictation of the discharge resume: A forgotten link between the spoken and written word. J Gen Intern Med 4:453–456, 1989.

2. Whitcomb WF, Nelson JR: Hospital Interfaces. In Wachter RM, Goldman L, Hollander H (eds): Hospital Medicine. Philadelphia, Lippincott, 2000, pp 9–14.

CHAPTER 9

EVIDENCE-BASED MEDICINE

Lisa S. Kettering, MD

1. What is evidence-based medicine (EBM)?

EBM is an approach to patient care: best research evidence, clinical expertise, and patient values (the "EBM Trilogy") are integrated in the practice of EBM to make decisions about the care of individual patients.

2. Why is it important to practice EBM?

An exploding volume of medical literature, the rapid introduction of new technologies, and increasing attention to the quality and outcomes of medical care are current, significant forces influencing the practice of medicine; new evidence is constantly emerging that may change the way patients are treated. Concomitantly, evidence-based databases and information systems have been created that allow clinicians rapid access to current and valid information about diagnosis, prognosis, therapy, and prevention. The result of this progress is that traditional approaches to medical education no longer provide physicians with the skills necessary to efficiently access and incorporate current, best evidence into patient care.

3. What are the limitations to practicing EBM?

The practice of EBM has several recognized limitations:
- Limited time for busy clinicians to master EBM skills
- Limited availability of resources required for rapid access to evidence
- The need to develop new skills in literature searching and critical appraisal
- Lack of evidence that EBM improves patient outcomes

KEY POINTS: EVIDENCE-BASED MEDICINE: ESSENCE AND OPPORTUNITY

1. EBM emphasizes the examination of evidence from clinical research and the integration of that evidence with clinical expertise and patient values.

2. Instruction in EBM methodology is essential; physicians must incorporate an exploding volume of medical literature, focused on quality and outcomes, into their practices.

3. Skill development, time and resource availability management, and accumulation of evidence that EBM alters patient outcomes provide opportunities for advancement in the practice of evidence-based health care.

4. What are the six essential components of the practice of EBM?

1. Defining the patient problem/clinical question
2. Defining what information is required to efficiently answer the question
3. Finding the current, best evidence that answers the question
4. Critically appraising the evidence (with an understanding of essential statistics)

5. Integrating the clinical message(s) from the evidence with clinical expertise and the individual patient's biology and values

6. Evaluating the effectiveness of the EBM process

5. Why is it important to define the patient problem or clinical question?
Access to current information regarding patient care management is a consistent requirement for physicians; clinical questions arise up to five times per in-patient encounter. Since clinicians have more questions than they have time to answer them, decisions must be made as to which question(s) take priority for a search. Efficiency in the EBM process may be enhanced by carefully selecting which questions merit search time and effort.

6. What factors should be considered when deciding which question(s) merit a search?
- The relevance of the question to the patient's welfare
- Questions related to a clinical decision about whether to use a therapeutic, diagnostic, or preventive intervention may warrant the most search time
- The relevance of the question to the learner's needs
- The frequency with which the clinical question will recur in practice and its relevance to the practice

7. Must all six components of the EBM process be considered each time a clinical question is determined to deserve a search?
For conditions commonly encountered in hospital medicine, all six steps of the process deserve attention. For conditions encountered less frequently, consideration should be given to seeking answers to questions through resources that have undergone rigorous critical appraisal before publication such as the Cochrane Database of Systematic Reviews, the Cochrane Central Register of Controlled Trials, ACP Journal Club, and Clinical Evidence. This approach abbreviates the time-consuming step 4 (see question 4). For conditions encountered infrequently or those for which best evidence is lacking, seeking expert opinion from clinical authorities may replace a literature search.

KEY POINTS: THE PRACTICE COMPONENTS OF EVIDENCE-BASED MEDICINE

1. There are six essential practice components to the practice of evidence-based medicine.

2. Whether all six steps of the evidence-based medicine process are deserving of the clinician's time and effort depends on the relevance of the question to the patient's welfare and to the clinician's practice and learning needs, as well as on the availability of best evidence in response to the question.

8. Why is it important to define the information required to efficiently answer the question?
Carefully defining the necessary information is key to the practice of EBM and entails structuring the question so as to optimize the efficiency of the search and enhance the search retrieval.

9. What elements of a clinical question should be defined to most effectively answer it?
- The question should be placed into a multiple-component format: a "PICO" format.
- The question should be identified as "background" or "foreground."
- The question should be "mapped" to guide the search for evidence.

10. **What does the acronym *PICO* stand for, and why is it important?**
P stands for the patient or problem being addressed, *I* for the intervention or exposure being considered, *C* for the comparison intervention or exposure, when relevant, and *O* for the clinical outcome(s) of interest.
   Identifying the PICO components of the question identifies the search terms most relevant to the question, thereby providing the structure for a focused, efficient search. For example, when the clinical question "Does using a nasogastric or percutaneous endoscopically placed gastrostomy (PEG) tube for feedings in a patient with dysphagic stroke prevent aspiration pneumonia?" is structured as a PICO question as follows: "In [P] patients with dysphagic stroke, do [I] PEG tube feedings, compared with [C] nasogastric tube feedings, prevent [O] aspiration pneumonia?" Major search terms, as underlined, are identified.

11. **Define and differentiate *background* versus *foreground* clinical questions.**
   - **Background** questions ask for general knowledge about a disorder and have two essential components: (1) A question root (who, what, where, when, why) with a verb and (2) a disorder, or an aspect of a disorder. Example: "When do complications of acute pancreatitis usually occur?"
   - **Foreground** questions ask for specific knowledge about managing patients with a disorder and use the "PICO" components. Example: "In older patients with heart failure from isolated diastolic dysfunction, does adding digoxin to standard diuretic and angiotensin-converting enzyme inhibitor treatment yield enough reduction in morbidity and/or mortality to be worth its adverse effects?" (See Fig. 9-1.)

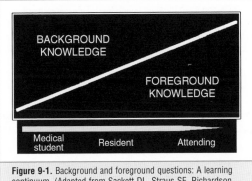

Figure 9-1. Background and foreground questions: A learning continuum. (Adapted from Sackett DL, Straus SE, Richardson WS, et al: Evidence-Based Medicine: How to Practice and Teach EBM, 2nd ed. New York, Churchill Livingstone, 2000.)

12. **Why is it important to classify a question as "background" or "foreground"?**
This classification provides guidance as to where to look for the answer, increasing the efficiency of the search. Answers to background questions are most likely to be found in text-based or reference databases or from expert opinion. Answers to foreground questions are usually found in medical literature or EBM databases.

13. **How is a question "mapped" to guide the search for evidence?**
A clinical question is "mapped" to guide the search for an answer in two ways. The first is by matching the question to a question type, placing it on the "Clinical Map." (Table 9-1). The "clinical map" is a list of central issues involved in the care of patients from which most clinical questions arise. Placing the question in one of the areas of the clinical map increases the efficiency of the search process by prompting the searcher to use map-identified MEDLINE search engine "limits" and methodology filters ("preselected" search strategies that can be

TABLE 9-1. THE CLINICAL MAP

Manifestations of disease	Therapy
Clinical findings	Harm/risk
Differential diagnosis	Prevention
Etiology/cause	Quality of life
Diagnosis	Cost-effectiveness
Prognosis	Education

Adapted from Sackett DL, Straus SE, Richardson WS, et al: Evidence-Based Medicine: How to Practice and Teach EBM, 2nd ed. New York, Churchill Livingstone, 2000.

applied to a search to retrieve articles with high-quality evidence relating to map-defined areas). In addition, mapping a clinical question prompts the searcher to match the type of information/ evidence desired to the study design best suited to answer it.

14. **How is the desired information/evidence matched to the study design best suited to answer it?**
To be able to map the information that is the target of the search to the study design that provides it, the types of information used as evidence, from the strongest to the weakest, and appropriate for a question type, must be understood. This hierarchy of evidence is illustrated in the *Evidence Pyramid,* a model of study design and grading of evidence. For comprehensive information on study design and the Evidence Pyramid, reference the following Websites:
- State University of New York Downstate Medical Center EBM Tutorial, Medical Research Library of Brooklyn: http://library.downstate.edu/ebm/2toc.htm
- Centre for Evidence-Based Medicine, University of Oxford: http://www.cebm.net/ study_designs.asp

KEY POINTS: OPTIMIZING THE SEARCH

1. Defining three elements of each clinical question will optimize the efficiency of the search and enhance search retrieval.

2. First, the clinical question should be placed into the PICO format to identify the search terms most relevant to the question.

3. Second, the question should be identified as background or foreground to provide guidance as to database selection for most favorable retrieval.

4. Third, the question should be placed on the clinical map to prompt the searcher to use map-identified search limits, to apply methodology filters to the search process, and to consider the type of study design that might be used as evidence to answer it.

15. **What is essential to "finding the best evidence" when answering a clinical question?**
Answering a clinical question requires awareness of the clinical resources available at the point of care, selection of the best background or foreground clinical resource(s) from which to answer the question, development of competence in the skills necessary to execute an efficient search, and selection of the best, most relevant material from the search result.

16. **What search strategies should be used to optimize the search for an answer to background and foreground questions?**
There is no particular search strategy for finding an answer to a background question. Rather, it is recommended that the clinician become well acquainted with two-to-three background question-appropriate databases of personal preference. To most efficiently search for an answer to a foreground question, follow a four-step approach (Fig. 9-2).

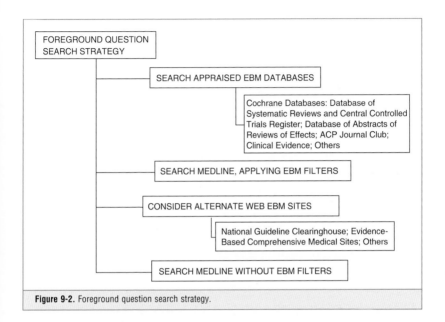

Figure 9-2. Foreground question search strategy.

17. **Why is it important to use a search strategy when looking for an answer to a foreground question?**
The foreground strategy prompts the clinician to search in critically appraised databases first; the information in these databases is analyzed, synthesized, and critically evaluated for the reader. Such value-added resources require much time and effort to create—time and effort the searching clinician often need not duplicate with a successful retrieval in these databases.

18. **What are quality or methodology filters?**
Quality filters are generic search strategies incorporating research methodology terms. These filters have been designed and tested to retrieve study types appropriate to diagnosis, prognosis, therapy, etiology, or harm/risk. Therefore, filters conform to the specific types of clinical questions identified on the clinical map and help restrict the citations found to the types of studies that are likely to provide valid answers to those questions. The "Clinical Queries" mode in PubMed uses stored search strategies that serve as quality filters.

19. **Describe search methods that will result in an efficient retrieval for a foreground question in a MEDLINE-associated database.**
Once a resource has been selected, the next step is to develop an efficient search. This involves converting the question to a format that is understandable by the database(s)' search engine(s). The goal is to develop high-sensitivity and high-specificity search strategies from the question. For high sensitivity, use a very broad search strategy to maximize retrieval and not miss any pertinent references. For high specificity, use a more precisely defined strategy to yield fewer but more

relevant results. The challenge is to find the point of balance between these two requirements. Devise an initial strategy based on PICO search terms for foreground questions, with attention to placement of the question on the clinical map. Then evaluate, refine, and adapt the strategy until the question is answered or there is reasonable certainty that the information does not exist.

Strategies for successful searching within EBM databases can be found on the following website:

- Finding the Best Evidence: EBM Tutorial, Exempla-Saint Joseph Hospital, Denver. http://www. exempla.org/courses/FindBestEBM/strategies/stratebm

Tutorials for successful search strategies within MEDLINE are located at the following sites:

- http://www.exempla.org/courses/FindBestEBM/strategies/medline
- National Library of Medicine PubMed Tutorial: http://www.nlm.nih.gov/bsd/pubmed_tutorial/ m1001.html

20. **Once the search is complete, what should be considered to select the best, most relevant studies for further review?**
An initial selection of studies should be based on consideration of the EBM trilogy, with consideration given to further review of articles that will allow the integration of evidence, clinical expertise, and patient values at the bedside.

KEY POINTS: FINDING CURRENT BEST EVIDENCE

1. Maximize the potential for best evidence retrieval by becoming aware of available clinical resources and selecting the optimal resource for each clinical question.

2. For foreground questions, search initially in EBM, critically appraised databases. Apply methodology filters to MEDLINE searches to enhance search quality.

3. Initiate a search based on PICO search terms, optimal background or foreground resource selection, clinical map prompts, and the foreground search strategy when appropriate; evaluate and refine the search as necessary.

4. Select, review, and critically appraise resources for integration into patient care; employ the EBM trilogy by integrating best research evidence with clinical expertise and patient values.

21. **The understanding of what statistical concepts is essential to critically appraise the literature?**
Tables 9-2 through 9-6 review the essential statistical concepts required to critically appraise the literature.

TABLE 9-2.	MEASURES OF PRECISION	
Statistical Term	**Definition**	**Comments**
P Value	P represents the probability that the result of a study could have been obtained by chance alone (could have been a "false positive").	$P \leq .05$ is "statistically significant"; the scientific community is willing to take a 5% risk that a false positive error has occurred.
Confidence Interval (CI)	The range of values within which the true value of the result of the study probably lies.	Usually reported as a 95% CI; one can be sure that the true value lies somewhere within the stated interval.

TABLE 9-3. MEASURES OF TEST ACCURACY: USED IN REFERENCE TO DIAGNOSIS

Statistical Term	Definition	Calculation*
Sensitivity	The proportion of people with a target disorder who will test positive	$\dfrac{A}{A+C}$
Specificity	The proportion of people without a disorder who will test negative	$\dfrac{D}{D+B}$
Positive predictive value	The proportion of people with a positive test result who will have the target disorder	$\dfrac{A}{A+B}$
Negative predictive value	The proportion of people with a negative test result who are free of the target disorder	$\dfrac{D}{C+D}$
Likelihood ratio (LR)	The likelihood that a given test would be expected in a patient with the target disorder compared with the likelihood that the same result would be expected in a patient without the target disorder	LR Positive: The odds of a disease if the result of the test is positive. $\dfrac{Sensitivity}{1-Specificity}$ LR Negative: The odds of a disease if the result of the test is negative. $\dfrac{Sensitivity}{1-Specificity}$ $\dfrac{A+C}{A+B+C+D}$
Pretest probability	The probability of disease in a person, estimated before the results of a test are known	
Posttest probability	The probability of disease in a person after the results of a test are known	$\dfrac{(pretest\ prob/1-pretest\ prob)\ \times\ LR}{1+(pretest\ prob/1-pretest\ prob)\ \times\ LR}$

*See Table 9-4.

TABLE 9-4. REFERENCE TABLE FOR MEASURES OF TEST ACCURACY

	Disease Present	Disease Absent
Test Positive	A	B
Test Negative	C	D

TABLE 9-5. MEASURES OF ASSOCIATION USED IN REFERENCE TO TREATMENT AND HARM

Statistical Term	Definition	Calculation*	Comment(s)
Relative Risk (RR)	The ratio of the risk of an outcome in an exposed group to the risk of an outcome in an unexposed group	$\dfrac{\frac{A}{A+B}}{\frac{C}{C+D}}$	Also referred to as: $\dfrac{\textit{Experimental Event Rate (EER)}}{\textit{Control Event Rate (CER)}}$
Relative Risk Reduction (RRR) (Expressed as a %)	The proportional reduction in rates of outcomes between experimental and control groups	$1 - RR$	Also calculated as: $\dfrac{CER - EER}{CER} \times 100$
Absolute Risk Reduction (ARR) (Expressed as a %)	The absolute difference in the event rate between control and experimental groups	$\dfrac{C}{C+D} - \dfrac{A}{A+B}$	Also calculated as: $CER - EER$
Number Needed to Ttreat (NNT)	The number of patients that need to be treated (in a defined period) to prevent one adverse outcome	$\dfrac{1}{ARR}$	
Odds Ratio (OR)	The ratio of the odds of having the target disorder in the experimental group relative to the odds in favor of having the target disorder in the control group	$\dfrac{\frac{A}{B}}{\frac{C}{D}}$	

*See Table 9-6.

TABLE 9-6. REFERENCE TABLE FOR MEASURES OF ASSOCIATION

	Outcome Occurs	Outcome Does Not Occur
Exposed to treatment (experimental)	A	B
Not exposed to treatment (control)	C	D

22. **What resources provide instuction on critical appraisal of the literature?**
   - Centre for Evidence Based Medicine, University of Toronto: www.cebm.utoronto.ca
   - Centre for Evidence Based Medicine, University of Oxford: www.cebm.net
   - Users' Guide to Evidence Based Practice
   - Centre for Health Evidence, University of Alberta: www.cche.net

23. **Once the most relevant study has been selected, reviewed, and critically appraised, what is the next step?**
   The next step in the EBM process is to integrate the best research evidence with your clinical expertise and the patient's values to make decisions about the care of the individual patient.

24. **What are some guiding questions that can help to incorporate the patient's biology and values into the EBM process?**
   - Is the patient so different from those in the study that the results cannot apply?
   - What are the patient's potential harms and benefits from the therapy?
   - What are the patient's values and expectations for both the outcome we are trying to prevent and the treatment we are offering?

25. **What are approaches to self-evaluation of the practice of EBM?**
   The final practice component of EBM is evaluating the effectiveness of the process. A critical aspects of this evaluation is self-evaluation. All six components of the practice of EBM are recommended domines for self-evaluation. For specific approaches to self-evaluation in these domains, visit www.cebm.utoronto.ca and follow the "Practising EBM" link to "Evaluation."

WEBSITES

1. ACP Journal Club, American College of Physicians: http://www.acpjc.org

2. Centre for Evidence-Based Medicine, University of Oxford: http://www.cebm.net

3. Centre for Evidence Based Medicine, University of Toronto: http://www.cebm.utoronto.ca

4. Centre for Health Evidence: Users' Guides to Evidence-Based Practice, University of Alberta: http://www.cche.net/usersguides/main.asp

5. Clinical Evidence, BMJ Publishing Group: http://www.clinicalevidence.com

6. Cochrane Library: http://www.cochrane.org

7. Condon J: Finding the Best Evidence. Exempla-Saint Joseph Hospital: http://www.exempla.org/courses/FindBestEBM

8. McMaster University: Health Sciences Library Evidence Based Medicine Practice Resources: http://hsl.lib.mcmaster.ebpractice.htm

9. National Library of Medicine: PubMed Tutorial: http://www.nlm.nih.gov/bsd/pubmed_tutorial/m1001.html

10. State University of New York Downstate Medical Center: Evidence-Based Medicine Course. Medical Research Library of Brooklyn: http://library.downstate.edu/ebm/2toc.htm

BIBLIOGRAPHY

1. Covell DG, Uman GC, Manning PR: Information needs in office practice: Are they being met? Ann Intern Med 103:596–599, 1985.

2. Osheroff JA, Forsythe DE, Buchanan BG, et al: Physicians' information needs: Analysis of questions posed during clinical teaching. Ann Intern Med 114:576–581, 1991.

3. Sackett DL, Straus SE, Richardson WS, et al: Evidence-Based Medicine: How to Practice and Teach EBM, 2nd ed. New York, Churchill Livingstone, 2000.

4. Smith R: What clinical information do doctors need? BMJ 313:1062–1068, 1996.

5. Straus SE, McAlister FA: Evidence-based medicine: A commentary on common criticisms. CMAJ-JAMC 163:837–841, 2000.

CONVENTIONAL AND NONINVASIVE VENTILATION

Sheri Chernetsky Tejedor, MD

CHAPTER 10

1. **What is mechanical ventilation?**
Modern mechanical ventilation involves the delivery of a preset volume or pressure to the lungs. The main goals are to correct refractory hypoxemia or hypercapnia, reduce the work of breathing, and protect the patient's airway. Table 10-1 reviews the common terms used in mechanical ventilation.

TABLE 10-1. MECHANICAL VENTILATION TERMS	
Tidal volume (V_T)	Volume of air delivered to the lungs with each breath. Increasing tidal volume will decrease PCO_2, increase pressures in the lungs, and possibly lead to breath stacking and auto-PEEP. Range: 5–10 mL/kg.
Respiratory rate (RR)	Rate of breaths delivered by the machine. Increasing the respiratory rate will decrease PCO_2 and can lead to auto-PEEP. Range: 10–20 breaths/min.
Fractional concentration of oxygen in inspired gas (FIO_2)	Fraction of inspired oxygen. This is the oxygen content in the delivered air. Range: 0.21 (room air) to 1.0. The goal is the lowest FIO_2 (<0.6 is ideal) to keep the oxygen saturation > 90% and PaO_2 > 60 mmHg.
Pressure support (PS)	A preset pressure delivered with each spontaneous, patient-initiated breath. It can be used alone as a ventilatory mode or with IMV. Increasing PS will increase tidal volume and decrease PCO_2. Range: 5–20 cmH_2O.
Extrinsic-PEEP	A back pressure applied by the ventilator at the end of exhalation that increases alveolar pressure and stents open the smaller airways. PEEP improves oxygenation allowing for the use of a lower FIO_2. PEEP increases intrathoracic pressure and can cause hypotension by decreasing preload. PEEP increases peak and plateau pressures. Range: 5–20 cmH_2O.
Auto-PEEP	Abnormally elevated pressures in the lungs at the end of exhalation due to incomplete emptying of the lungs (i.e., hyperinflation) from rapid breathing and obstruction (i.e., breath stacking).
Peak airway pressure	Pressure proportional to airway resistance and inversely related to lung compliance. Measured at the end of inspiration. Goal: < 45–50 cmH_2O.

Continued

TABLE 10-1. MECHANICAL VENTILATION TERMS—CONT'D	
Plateau pressure	Surrogate measure for peak alveolar pressure. Inversely related to lung compliance. Measured by cutting off airflow and measuring the pressure at the end of inspiration. Goal: < 30 cmH$_2$O.
Airway resistance	Proportional to peak airway pressure minus plateau pressure. Increased in the setting of obstruction, bronchospasm, excess secretions, or biting of ETT.
Lung compliance	Inversely proportional to plateau pressure. Is increased in the setting of ARDS, atelectasis, pulmonary edema, auto-PEEP, ARDS, CHF, atelectasis, pneumothorax, ETT in mainstem bronchus.

PEEP = Positive end-expiratory pressure, IMV = intermittent mandatory ventilation, ETT = endotracheal tube, ARDS = acute respiratory distress syndrome, CHF = congestive heart failure.

2. **What are the indications for mechanical ventilation?**
   The two general indications for mechanical ventilation are hypoxemic and hypercapnic respiratory failure. Hypoxemic respiratory failure is most commonly due to pulmonary airspace disease (e.g., pneumonia, pulmonary edema). Hypercapnic ventilatory failure is due to hypoventilation and is often seen in patients with respiratory muscle fatigue (e.g., obstructive lung disease, neuromuscular disease, severe sepsis) or altered mental status (e.g., drug overdose).

3. **Describe the main modes of mechanical ventilation.**
   The two main modes of ventilatory assistance are pressure support and volume cycled. During *pressure-support ventilation* (PSV), a preset pressure is delivered with each respiratory effort. The volume of air delivered to the lungs will depend on lung mechanics and patient effort. In volume-cycled ventilation, which includes *assist control* (AC) and *intermittent mandatory ventilation* (IMV) modes, a preset volume is delivered to the lungs with each machine breath; the pressures in the airways and alveoli will depend on patient factors (Table 10-2).

4. **Describe the differences between PSV, AC, and IMV modes.**
   In both AC and IMV modes of ventilation, a backup respiratory rate is set and a breath (machine breath) will be delivered if the patient has not initiated a breath within a specified period of time. In PSV, there is usually no set backup rate and the patient must trigger each breath. Pressure support is also often added to the IMV mode to assist with spontaneous breaths between scheduled machine breaths and to overcome the resistance of the ventilatory circuit. During AC mode, when the machine senses the patient is initiating a breath, it delivers the entire preset tidal volume (see Tables 10-1 and 10-2). Rapid breathing can therefore result in breath stacking, increased pulmonary pressures, and respiratory alkalosis. In the IMV mode, the preset tidal volume is delivered only with machine breaths at the set rate. With all other patient-initiated breaths, the volume delivered will depend on the respiratory effort of the patient and the amount of pressure support provided.

TABLE 10-2. MAIN MODES OF MECHANICAL VENTILATION

	AC	IMV	PSV
Tidal volume (V_T)	Set by the operator. The same V_T is given for spontaneous (patient-initiated) and machine breaths.	Set by the operator. The full V_T is given for machine breaths. V_T with spontaneous breaths will be determined by the pressure support, patient effort, and lung mechanics.	Not set by operator. Patient will determine V_T by effort and lung mechanics based on the amount of pressure support provided.
Respiratory rate (RR)	Set by the operator.	Set by the operator.	In general, no backup rate is provided.
Fraction of inspired oxygen (FIO_2)	Set by the operator.	Set by the operator.	Set by the operator.
Pressure support (PS)	Not used; all patient breaths get the full set tidal volume.	Often added to IMV to augment patient-initiated, spontaneous breaths in between machine breaths.	The amount of pressure support is the main fixed parameter in PSV mode.
Extrinsic-PEEP	Set by the operator, added to improve oxygenation.	Set by the operator, added to improve oxygenation.	Set by the operator, added to improve oxygenation.
Advantages	Full ventilatory support. Patient does not need to work to receive a full V_T breath. Support given is fixed (same V_T each breath).	Graded levels of assistance determined by patient effort and the machine's pressure support.	Increased patient control of breathing. Often used as weaning mode before extubation.
Disadvantages	Unsedated, rapid breathers may develop breath stacking, respiratory alkalosis, and hyperinflation (auto-PEEP).	Patient's effort generally greater than in AC mode, which may delay weaning.	Not used for patients who cannot breath spontaneously.

AC = Assist control, IMV = intermittent mandatory ventilation, PSV = pressure-support ventilation, PEEP = positive end-expiratory pressure.

KEY POINTS: MAIN MODES OF MECHANICAL VENTILATION

1. AC mode is volume cycled. The patient receives a preset volume at a specified rate. With any additional breaths over this set rate, the patient receives the entire preset tidal volume.

2. IMV mode is volume cycled. The patient receives a preset volume at a specified rate. Additional breaths may be taken, for which the tidal volume will be determined by the patient's effort, pressure support provided, and lung mechanics.

3. In pressure support ventilation, air is delivered at a preset pressure when the patient initiates a breath. The patient determines the duration of the breath, and the tidal volume is determined by effort and lung mechanics.

5. **What ventilator adjustments can be made to improve oxygenation?**
Increasing the fraction of inspired oxygen (FIO_2) will improve oxygenation in most patients (except in those with true shunt). Positive end-expiratory pressure (PEEP) is a preset pressure delivered by the ventilator that acts to stent open the smaller airways and alveoli. Increasing PEEP can improve oxygenation by recruiting alveoli.

6. **What adjustments can be made to improve ventilation and correct a respiratory acidosis?**
Ventilation and PCO_2 are improved by increasing alveolar ventilation, and this is accomplished via an increased respiratory rate or tidal volume. Because alveolar ventilation itself cannot be measured easily, the *minute ventilation* ($V_T \times RR$) is sometimes used as a surrogate (Fig. 10-1).

7. **What parameters are important to monitor in a ventilated patient?**
In addition to standard vital signs and arterial blood gas levels (ABGs), it is important to monitor lung pressures to avoid barotrauma. *Peak airway pressure* reflects the maximum pressure in the proximal airways during a delivered breath. *Plateau pressure* gives an estimate of transalveolar pressure. It is measured when airflow has ceased, an instant in which proximal airway pressure equals alveolar pressure. The relation between peak pressure and plateau pressure provides information about airway resistance and lung compliance. When peak pressures are elevated (>50 cmH$_2$O) and plateau pressures are normal (<30 cmH$_2$O) it suggests increased airway resistance. When both peak and plateau pressures are elevated it suggests decreased lung compliance. (See Table 10-1.)

8. **What are the hemodynamic effects of mechanical ventilation?**
Normal breathing is accomplished through negative inspiratory pressures created by contraction of the diaphragm. Mechanical ventilation utilizes *positive* inspiratory pressures, which raise intrathoracic pressure. This tends to reduce preload (ventricular filling in diastole) as well as afterload. These effects can be beneficial for the failing heart with systolic dysfunction and volume overload, because cardiac output improves with reduction in afterload. However, patients who are relatively preload dependent (e.g., those with a normal heart, hypovolemia and shock) may develop hypotension with positive pressure ventilation. This often responds to volume infusion.

9. **What is permissive hypercapnia?**
For patients with acute lung injury (ALI) or acute respiratory distress syndrome (ARDS), and those with underlying lung disease, lower tidal volume ventilation is the preferred strategy to

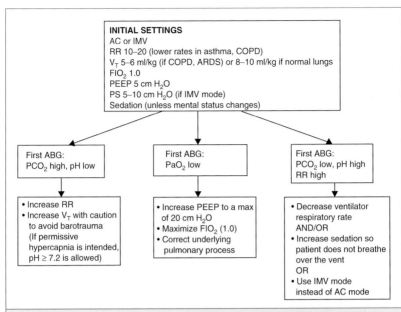

INITIAL SETTINGS
AC or IMV
RR 10–20 (lower rates in asthma, COPD)
V_T 5–6 ml/kg (if COPD, ARDS) or 8–10 ml/kg if normal lungs
FIO_2 1.0
PEEP 5 cm H_2O
PS 5–10 cm H_2O (if IMV mode)
Sedation (unless mental status changes)

First ABG:
PCO_2 high, pH low

First ABG:
PaO_2 low

First ABG:
PCO_2 low, pH high
RR high

- Increase RR
- Increase V_T with caution to avoid barotrauma (If permissive hypercapnia is intended, pH ≥ 7.2 is allowed)

- Increase PEEP to a max of 20 cm H_2O
- Maximize FIO_2 (1.0)
- Correct underlying pulmonary process

- Decrease ventilator respiratory rate AND/OR
- Increase sedation so patient does not breathe over the vent OR
- Use IMV mode instead of AC mode

Figure 10-1. Adjusting the ventilator based on clinical parameters. RR = Respiratory rate, COPD = chronic obstructive pulmonary disease, ARDS = acute respiratory distress syndrome, PS = pressure support, ABG = arterial blood gas.

avoid barotrauma. Tidal volumes of 5–6 mL/kg and a lower FIO_2 (< 0.6) are used in these patients, with higher levels of PEEP to improve oxygenation. Plateau pressures are maintained less than 30 cmH2O. The consequence is often a respiratory acidosis from CO_2 accumulation (i.e., permissive hypercapnia), which is tolerated as long as the pH is greater than 7.2. Hypercapnia is also permitted in ventilated patients with underlying chronic obstructive pulmonary disease (COPD) with baseline chronic, compensated hypercapnia.

10. **List the complications of mechanical ventilation.**
Invasive mechanical ventilation can lead to lung injury from high pressures and volumes delivered to the lungs (e.g., barotrauma, volutrauma). There is also evidence that the high oxygen concentrations delivered by the ventilator ($FIO_2 > 0.6$) can be toxic to the lungs. The endotracheal tube can cause tracheal injury, leading to stenosis or vocal cord dysfunction. Most importantly, up to 25% of patients acquire ventilator-associated pneumonia.

11. **How can ventilator-associated pneumonia (VAP) be prevented?**
The most important interventions necessary to avoid VAP are hand hygiene, prompt removal of the nasogastric and endotracheal tubes, elevation of the head of the bed, subglottic suctioning (in specific groups of patients), and avoidance of gastric overdistention and nasal intubation. Pharmacologic suppression of gastric acid for stress ulcer prophylaxis appears to increase the risk of VAP and should be avoided in patients at low risk for gastrointestinal tract bleeding.

12. **Describe the diagnosis and management of VAP.**
The diagnosis of VAP requires new signs of infection (e.g., leukocytosis, fever, increased oxygen requirement), increased purulent secretions, and a new or persistent infiltrate exhibited on chest

radiograph. Management of VAP involves obtaining a sputum specimen or bronchial washing of the lower airways via bronchoscopy and antibiotics to cover nosocomial pathogens (with consideration of resistant *Staphylococcus* and *Pseudomonas* organisms). Antibiotic coverage is narrowed based on culture results. (See Chapter 55 for more details.)

KEY POINTS: COMPLICATIONS OF MECHANICAL VENTILATION

1. Ventilator-associated pneumonia

2. Hypotension

3. Tracheal injury

4. Lung injury from barotrauma, volutrauma, and oxygen toxicity

---

13. **When is it appropriate to attempt to wean a patient?**
    Weaning from the ventilator is appropriate when the patient has met the following conditions: resolution of the inciting event, hemodynamic stability, minimal oxygen requirements ($PaO_2 > 60$ mmHg on $FIO_2 < 0.5$ and PEEP < 7.5 cm H_2O), and the patient is alert and following commands. The rapid shallow breathing index is a useful predictor of weaning success. A respiratory rate (bpm)/tidal volume (liters) < 105 bpm/L during spontaneous breathing (T-piece) predicts successful weaning.

14. **Describe the methods of weaning a patient from mechanical ventilation.**
    There are multiple modes of weaning. During IMV mode, reducing the backup rate of delivered breaths allows the patient to take more breaths on his own, with some pressure support. Alternatively, pressure support can be used alone with no backup rate. During a spontaneous breathing trial (e.g., T-piece trial) the patient breathes spontaneously without any backup rate or pressure support. Pressure support and spontaneous breathing trials are typically only performed for one half hour at a time, once daily. At the end of this period, a blood gas measurement may be drawn and the patient's vital signs reviewed, as suitability for extubation is determined. The use of once-daily T-piece trials appears to lead to more rapid extubation.

    Esteban A, Frutos F, Tobin M, et al: A comparison of four methods of weaning patients from mechanical ventilation. N Engl J Med 332:345–350, 1995.

15. **What are the indications for a tracheostomy?**
    Tracheostomy is considered after 11–14 days of tracheal intubation and earlier if it is clear that the patient is unlikely to be extubated promptly. There is limited data available to establish clear guidelines on this.

16. **What is noninvasive mechanical ventilation (NIMV)?**
    NIMV is a mode of ventilatory assistance used for acute and chronic respiratory failure. It is, simply put, mechanical ventilation without intubation, typically using a tightly affixed facial mask. NIMV can be bilevel (cycling in both inspiration and expiration) or simply involve a constant pressure throughout the breathing cycle.

17. **How does NIMV compare with invasive mechanical ventilation?**
    NIMV is similar to pressure support mode in invasive mechanical ventilation, but the terminology is slightly different. In bilevel NIMV, the inspiratory positive airway pressure is

equivalent to the sum of pressure support and PEEP, and the expiratory positive airway pressure is the equivalent of PEEP. When NIMV is used to apply a constant pressure through inspiration and expiration, it is called *continuous positive airway pressure* (CPAP). This is similar to using PEEP alone. CPAP can be used for patients with hypoxemia in the absence of hypoventilation because it does not provide additional inspiratory support. By comparison, bilevel NIMV is useful for hypoventilation and hypoxemia.

18. What are the advantages and disadvantages of face and nasal masks for NIMV?
Nasal masks make it easier to remove oral secretions and may reduce the likelihood of aspiration. Patients are able to speak and eat with nasal masks. Facial masks permit the use of higher ventilatory pressures, avoid leakage from the mouth, require less patient cooperation, and permit mouth breathing; however, they may be more uncomfortable. A reasonable strategy is to use a full-face mask for initial treatment and later switch to a nasal mask as the patient's condition improves.

19. Which machines are available for NIMV?
NIMV can be administered through portable/home devices, mechanical ventilators, or bilevel pressure generators. Portable machines are typically used for chronic respiratory failure and are not ideal for acute applications. Standard intensive care unit ventilators, when used for NIMV, can provide exact FIO_2 blends but may alarm with small air leaks around the face mask, requiring adjustments to their settings. Bilevel pressure generators allow high flow rates, good patient monitoring, and some have oxygen blenders to permit exact FIO_2 titration up to 1.0.

20. What are the specific indications for NIMV for acute respiratory failure?
NIMV has been extensively studied in patients with acute hypercapnic respiratory failure from COPD exacerbation. When compared with standard medical therapy and oxygen alone, NIMV reduced the intubation rate by 28% and also reduced the incidence of nosocomial pneumonia, length of stay, and mortality (10% reduction). NIMV has also been studied in other groups with hypoxemic and hypercapnic respiratory failure from pulmonary edema and pneumonia with good results. Clinical improvement in the first hour, an initial $pH > 7.1$ and $PCO_2 < 92$ mmHg, few secretions, intact dentition, a quickly reversible process, and young patient age all predict eventual success with NIMV (Table 10-3).

Keenan SP, Sinuff T, Cook DJ, Hill NS: Which patients with acute exacerbation of chronic obstructive pulmonary disease benefit from noninvasive positive-pressure ventilation? A systematic review of the literature. Ann Intern Med 138:861, 2003.

Liesching T, Kwok H, Hill NS, et al: Acute applications of noninvasive positive pressure ventilation. Chest 124:699–713, 2003.

KEY POINTS: MAIN INDICATIONS FOR NIMV

1. COPD exacerbation with $pH < 7.35$ or $PCO_2 > 45$ mmHg

2. CHF (CPAP alone may be used for hypoxemia and tachypnea, but if hypercapnia is present, bilevel NIMV may be preferred)

3. Community-acquired pneumonia with minimal secretions (especially in patients with COPD)

21. Which patients are not appropriate candidates to receive NIMV?
Patients must be carefully selected for NIMV. Contraindications include:
- Need for immediate intubation because of cardiopulmonary arrest
- High risk of aspiration because of mental status changes or vomiting

- Failed extubation from conventional ventilation
- Inability to tolerate face mask or nasal mask
- Anatomic facial abnormalities
- Pneumothorax without a chest tube
- Severe upper airway obstruction
- Refractory hypoxemia (PaO_2 < 60 mmHg on FIO_2 1.0)
- Recent gastrointestinal surgery (relative contraindication)

Esteban A, Frutos-Vivar F, Ferguson ND, et al: Noninvasive positive-pressure ventilation for respiratory failure after extubation. N Engl J Med 350:2452–2560, 2004.

TABLE 10–3. RECOMMENDATIONS FOR THE USE OF NIMV IN SPECIFIC CLINICAL SCENARIOS	
Recommendation	Setting of Respiratory Failure
NIMV recommended	Pulmonary edema from CHF with (bilevel settings) or without hypercapnia (CPAP alone)
	Community-acquired pneumonia (especially with COPD)
	Weaning COPD patients from ventilator
	Immunosuppressed and organ transplant patients
NIMV not clearly beneficial	Acutely decompensated obstructive sleep apnea, chest wall deformity, or neuromuscular disease
	ARDS/ALI
	Pneumocystis carinii pneumonia (PCP)
	Do not intubate order
	After lung resection
	Asthma, cystic fibrosis, bronchiectasis

CHF = congestive heart failure, ARDS = acute respiratory distress syndrome, ALI = acute lung injury.
Modified from Liesching T, Kwok H, Hill NS, et al: Acute applications of noninvasive positive pressure ventilation. Chest 124:699–713, 2003.

22. **What are the complications of NIMV?**
Major complications are rare with NIMV and occur less frequently than with invasive ventilation. However, it is critical to carefully select and monitor patients so that intubation is not delayed in patients who fail to respond to NIMV. Complications include pneumothorax, pneumonia, hemodynamic changes, rebreathing in the mask, hypoxemia, and aspiration. Minor complications can occur from the pressure of the mask on the face resulting in skin ulceration, which can be avoided with an artificial skin dressing. Dry mucous membranes can be treated with humidified air, nasal steroids, or saline. Gastric distention may be reduced by a reduction in inflation pressures. Claustrophobia and anxiety may be unavoidable in some patients.

BIBLIOGRAPHY

1. Dodek P, Keenan S, Cook D, et al: Evidence-based clinical practice guideline for the prevention of ventilator-associated pneumonia. Ann Intern Med 141:305–313, 2004.

2. International Consensus Conferences in Intensive Care Medicine: Noninvasive positive pressure ventilation in acute respiratory failure. Am J Respir Crit Care Med 163:283, 2001.

3. Marino PL: The ICU Book, 2nd ed. Baltimore, MD, Williams & Wilkins, 1998.

4. Tobin MJ: Advances in mechanical ventilation. N Engl J Med 344:1986–1996, 2001.

CHAPTER 11

VASOPRESSORS, INOTROPES, AND VASODILATORS

Christin H. Ko, MD

1. **Describe the principles of resuscitation in a hypotensive patient.**
   The first priority is to aggressively restore volume. The use of a vasoconstricting agent without adequate volume repletion may be ineffective or even worsen end-organ perfusion. Next, search for and treat underlying causes of the hypotension and select a vasoactive agent based on the suspected etiology of the hypotension. Add a second medication if the patient is unresponsive to the first drug. Place an arterial line for blood pressure monitoring, and titrate the drug to an endpoint.

2. **Describe the mechanism of action of common vasopressors.**
   Vasopressors, such as dopamine, norepinephrine, and epinephrine, exert their effects by vasoconstriction, which increases the *mean arterial blood pressure* (MAP).

   $$MAP = [\text{systolic arterial pressure} + 2(\text{diastolic arterial pressure})] \div 3$$

   The characteristics of common vasopressors are summarized in Table 11-1.

3. **What is the mechanism of action of common inotropes? In what clinical situations are they used?**
   Inotropes, such as dobutamine and milrinone, exert their effects by increasing contractility of the heart. They are used in severe congestive heart failure and as bridge therapy to cardiac transplantation. Dobutamine can provide symptomatic relief, but there is no improvement in mortality rates. Some data even suggest an *increased* risk of death. Ventricular arrhythmias are a potential complication with some inotropes. The characteristics of common inotropes are summarized in Table 11-2.

4. **Many drugs have *both* vasopressor and inotropic features. Provide examples.**
   Dopamine is an inotrope at intermediate doses (β-adrenergic effect) and essentially a vasopressor at high doses (α-adrenergic effect). At low doses, norepinephrine has a positive inotropic effect. With increasing doses, the vasoconstrictive effects overshadow the inotropic effects. So, in general, the vasopressor effects predominate at the higher doses.

5. **What are the adrenergic receptors relevant to vasopressor use?**
   The types of adrenergic receptors important to vasopressor use are α_1, β_1, and β_2. Adrenergic receptors bind norepinephrine. α_1 receptors are present in the smooth muscle cells of many vascular beds as well as the heart. Stimulation of these receptors in the blood vessels causes vasoconstriction. In the heart it produces positive inotropy, an increase in the force of muscular contraction. β_1 receptors are predominant in the heart, and stimulation causes a positive inotropic and chronotropic response (i.e., increase in heart rate). β_2 stimulation causes relaxation of smooth muscle cells in bronchial, gastrointestinal, and uterine muscles, as well as vasodilation in skeletal muscle blood vessels.

TABLE 11-1.   CHARACTERISTICS OF COMMONLY USED VASOPRESSORS*

Drug	Dose	Receptor	Indications	Contraindications/ Precautions	Adverse Effects
Dopamine	*Start:* 1 μg/kg/min IV *Maintenance:* Increase by 1–4 μg/kg/min every 10 min PRN *Maximum:* 20–50 μg/kg/min	Dopamine β–1 α–1	Hypotension, sepsis, congestive heart failure (in conjunction with dobutamine)	Hypovolemia, pheochromocytoma, monoamine oxidase inhibitors, concurrent administration with IV phenytoin	Tachyarrhythmias; renal failure; skin necrosis; myocardial, limb, and intestinal ischemia
Norepinephrine	*Start:* 0.5–1 μg/min IV *Maximum:* 30 μg/min IV	α–1 β–1	Hypotension, hyperdynamic sepsis, neurogenic shock	Hypovolemia, concurrent administration with some anesthetics	Tachyarrhythmias; renal failure; skin necrosis; myocardial, limb, and intestinal ischemia
Epinephrine	*Start:* 1 μg/min IV *Maintenance:* 1–4 μg/min IV *Maximum:* 10 μg/min IV	α–1 β–1 β–2	Anaphylaxis, third-line sepsis agent, cardiac arrest	Caution with beta blockers because unopposed alpha constriction may occur	Tachyarrhythmias; renal failure; skin necrosis; myocardial, limb, and intestinal ischemia; hypertension; cerebral hemorrhage

Continued

TABLE 11-1. CHARACTERISTICS OF COMMONLY USED VASOPRESSORS*—CONT'D

Drug	Dose	Receptor	Indications	Contraindications/ Precautions	Adverse Effects
Phenylephrine	*IV bolus:* Start: 0.1–0.5 mg IV bolus, then every 15 min PRN Maximum: 0.5 mg for initial dose *IV infusion:* Start: 100–180 μg/min Maintenance: 40–60 μg/min	α–1 β	Anesthesia-induced hypotension, neurogenic shock, supraventricular tachycardia	Severe hypertension, ventricular tachycardia	Arrhythmias, reflex bradycardia
Ephedrine	Start: 5–25 mg IV every 10 min PRN Maximum: 150 mg/24 h	α–1 β	Anesthesia-induced hypotension	Arrhythmias	Arrhythmias, hypertension, seizures

IV = Intravenous, PRN = as needed.
* Please note the use of units in all drug dosing. They can differ considerably in the starting, maintenance, and maximum doses of a drug.

TABLE 11-2. CHARACTERISTICS OF COMMONLY USED INOTROPES*

Drug	Dose	Receptor	Indications	Contraindications/Precautions	Adverse Effects
Dobutamine	*Start:* 0.5–1 µg/kg/min IV *Maintenance:* 2.5–20 µg/kg/min IV *Maximum:* 40 µg/kg/min	β–1 β–2	Refractory heart failure, cardiogenic shock	Diastolic dysfunction, idiopathic hypertrophic subaortic stenosis, severe aortic stenosis	Hypertension, tachycardia, ventricular tachycardia
Milrinone	*Start:* 50 µg/kg IV over 10 min *Maintenance:* 0.375 µg/kg/min IV *Maximum:* 0.75 µg/kg/min	N/A	Refractory heart failure	Severe obstructive aortic or pulmonic valve disease, acute myocardial infarction	Ventricular arrhythmias, thrombocytopenia, hepatotoxicity
Inamrinone	*Start:* 0.75 mg/kg IV over 2–3 min *Maintenance:* 5–10 µg/kg/min IV *Maximum:* 10 mg/kg/day	N/A	Refractory heart failure	Hypotension, severe aortic or pulmonic valve disease, acute myocardial infarction	Arrhythmias, hypotension, thrombocytopenia, hepatotoxicity, increased mortality with long-term use
Digoxin	*Start:* loading dose 0.5 mg IV (divided as 0.25 mg initially, then 0.125 mg every 6–12 h × 2)	N/A	Congestive heart failure, atrial fibrillation	Renal failure, heart block, bradycardia, hypokalemia	Heart block, bradycardia
Isoproterenol	*Start:* 2–10 µg/min IV infusion	β–1 β–2	Hypotension due to bradycardia	Arrhythmias, tachycardia	Arrhythmias

IV = Intravenous.
* Please note the use of units in all drug dosing. They can differ considerably in the starting, maintenance, and maximum doses of a drug.

6. **What are dopaminergic receptors, and what are the effects when they are stimulated?**
   Dopaminergic receptors bind dopamine. They are located in the renal, mesenteric, cardiac, and cerebrovascular beds. Stimulation of these receptors causes vasodilation and natriuresis (i.e., excretion of urinary sodium).

7. **What is the relationship between drug dose and receptor selectivity?**
   Different doses of a drug may activate different receptors. For example, dopamine stimulates dopaminergic receptors at low doses (<5 µg/kg/min), β_1 receptors at intermediate doses (5–10 µg/kg/min), and α receptors at high doses.

8. **Name some nonadrenergic vasopressors and inotropes.**
   Some agents produce vasoconstriction or inotropy through nonadrenergic mechanisms. Examples include phosphodiesterase inhibitors (e.g., amrinone), which mediate their effects by increasing calcium concentration in cells, thus enhancing inotropy. Vasopressin causes vasoconstriction of vascular smooth muscle via stimulation of V_1 receptors. It may play a future role in refractory septic shock by acting as a third-line vasopressor.

9. **How do vasodilators exert their effects? What are the indications for their use?**
   Vasodilators, such as nitroglycerin, nesiritide, diltiazem, and enalaprilat, dilate arteries or veins. They are typically used in treating exacerbations of congestive heart failure. Some may be used in hypertensive crises and tachyarrhythmias. The characteristics of common vasodilators are summarized in Table 11-3.

10. **What agent is emerging as the preferred choice in septic shock?**
    Although dopamine traditionally has been used as the first-line agent, there is mounting evidence that it is associated with a decrease in splanchnic mucosal blood flow and increased risk of gastrointestinal bleeding. Norepinephrine is now the preferred first-line agent. Vasopressin is also an emerging option for refractory septic shock. However, it is too early to recommend broad use of the drug as a vasopressor.

11. **What is the ultimate goal in using vasopressors and inotropic agents?**
    Adequate tissue and organ perfusion is the goal, not an absolute blood pressure. Clinical parameters to assess and monitor include:
    - **Mental status:** Patient should be awake and alert
    - **Urine output:** Greater than 0.5 cc/kg/h
    - **Heart rate:** Less than 100 beats/min
    - **Skin:** Warm, with brisk capillary refill
      Practically, this translates into a mean arterial blood pressure of about 60 mmHg or a systolic blood pressure of about 100 mmHg.

KEY POINTS: PRINCIPLES OF USING VASOPRESSORS

1. Adequate volume resuscitation should come first.

2. Either dopamine or norepinephrine is a good first choice.

3. Norepinephrine is the preferred vasopressor in sepsis.

4. A mean arterial pressure of 60 mmHg is a reasonable target.

5. The ultimate goal is tissue perfusion.

TABLE 11–3. CHARACTERISTICS OF COMMONLY USED VASODILATORS*

Drug	Dose	Indication	Contraindication/Precautions	Adverse Effects
Nitroglycerin	*Start:* 5 μg/min IV, *Maintenance:* Increase by 5 μg/min every 5 min *Maximum:* 20–200 μg/min	Congestive heart failure	Hypotension, right ventricular myocardial infarction, concurrent use with phosphodiesterase 5 inhibitors (e.g., sildenafil)	Hypotension, headache, tachyphylaxis, methemoglobinemia
Nitroprusside	*Start:* 0.25–0.3 μg/kg/min *Maintenance:* Increase by 0.5 μg/kg/min to goal, usually 3 μg/kg/min *Maximum:* 10 μg/kg/min	Hypertensive crisis, congestive heart failure	Compensatory hypertension (e.g., coarctation of aorta), increased intracranial pressure, hepatic or renal dysfunction	Hypotension, cyanide toxicity
Nesiritide	*Start:* 2 μg/kg IV *Maintenance:* 0.01 μg/kg/min, may increase by 0.005 μg/kg/min every 3 h PRN *Maximum:* 0.03 μg/kg/min	Congestive heart failure	Hypotension, cardiogenic shock, significant valvular stenosis, severe renal failure, sepsis	Hypotension, ventricular tachycardia, renal failure

Continued

TABLE 11-3. CHARACTERISTICS OF COMMONLY USED VASODILATORS*—CONT'D

Drug	Dose	Indication	Contraindication/Precautions	Adverse Effects
Enalaprilat	*Start:* 0.625–1.25 mg IV every 6 h PRN	Hypertension, congestive heart failure	Renal failure, hyperkalemia, bilateral renal artery stenosis	Hypotension, renal failure, hyperkalemia, angioedema
Hydralazine	*Start:* 10–40 mg IV every 4–6 h PRN	Hypertension, preeclampsia, congestive heart failure	Hypotension	Hypotension, tachycardia, lupus-like syndrome with prolonged use
Diltiazem	*Start:* 0.25 mg/kg IV over 2 min *Maintenance:* 0.35 mg/kg over 2 min if needed, then 5–15 mg/h × 24 h	Atrial fibrillation, supraventricular tachycardia	Hypotension, heart block, concomitant use with beta blocker or digoxin	Hypotension, bradycardia, edema, atrioventricular block
Nicardipine	*Start:* 5 mg/h *Maintenance:* Increase by 2.5 mg/h every 15 min *Maximum:* 15 mg/h	Hypertensive emergency except with congestive heart failure	Advanced aortic stenosis, hypotension, cardiogenic shock, ventricular tachycardia	Tachyarrhythmias, headache, flushing

IV = Intravenous.
* Please note the use of units in all drug dosing. They can differ considerably in the starting, maintenance, and maximum doses of a drug.

12. **Which vasodilator is associated with cyanide toxicity?**
    Nitroprusside may cause cyanide toxicity through the formation of thiocyanate. Doses above 2 μg/kg/min and treatment over several days may lead to this adverse effect. Signs of cyanide toxicity include cyanosis, psychosis, seizures, an almond odor, bright red venous blood, and death. Sodium nitrite, amyl nitrite, and sodium thiosulfate (in addition to discontinuation of the drug) are the treatment options for this condition.

13. **Which vasodilator is associated with methemoglobinemia?**
    Nitroglycerin oxidizes hemoglobin to methemoglobin so that it is unable to bind oxygen. Cyanosis occurs, although patients may not appear acutely ill. Altered mental status usually occurs with high levels of methemoglobin. The arterial oxygen level on the arterial blood gas measurement should be *normal* even though the blood appears chocolate brown. The pulse oximetry reading may be *unreliable*. If you are suspicious that methemoglobinemia is present, look for a "saturation gap" where the arterial blood gas oxygen saturation is *greater* than the pulse oximetry saturation. Methemoglobinemia is treated with intravenous methylene blue.

14. **How is drug extravasation with subsequent skin necrosis treated?**
    When a vasoconstricting agent extravasates into the surrounding skin, local skin necrosis and sloughing may occur. Phentolamine can be injected subcutaneously at the site to limit the damage. This should be done immediately because it becomes ineffective after 12 hours.

15. **Does low-dose dopamine provide renal protection?**
    No. Although some animal studies suggest dopamine may improve renal blood flow, the evidence is less clear in human subjects. Currently, there are no data to support the routine use of dopamine for prophylaxis against or treatment of renal failure in severely ill patients.

16. **What is the preferred agent for a pregnant patient with hypotension?**
    Pregnant patients who receive spinal anesthesia before delivery may experience vasodilation and subsequent hypotension. While supine, the patient should be tilted 15 degrees to the left to shift the fetus off the inferior vena cava. If the blood pressure remains low, start the administration of intravenous fluids and consider administering ephedrine because it does not appear to compromise uterine blood flow (Table 11-4).

TABLE 11-4. PREFERRED VASOACTIVE AGENTS FOR CERTAIN CLINICAL SITUATIONS	
Clinical Situation	**Preferred Agent**
Sepsis	Norepinephrine
Congestive heart failure	Nitroglycerin
Cardiogenic shock	Dobutamine with dopamine
Anaphylaxis	Epinephrine
Hypertensive emergency	Nitroprusside *or* labetalol
Aortic dissection	Nitroprusside *and* labetalol
Anesthesia-induced hypotension	Phenylephrine, ephedrine
Pregnant patient with hypotension	Ephedrine

WEBSITES

1. Lexi-Comp: http://www.lexi.com

2. Epocrates Rx Drug Reference: http://www.epocrates.com

BIBLIOGRAPHY

1. Beale RJ, Hollenberg SM, Vincent JL: Vasopressor and inotropic support in septic shock: An evidence-based review. Crit Care Med 32:S455–S465, 2004.

2. Dennis P: Methemoglobinemia. In Goldfrank (ed): Goldfrank's Toxicologic Emergencies, 7th ed. New York, McGraw-Hill, 2002, pp 1–15.

3. Felker GM, Benza RL, Chandler AB: Heart failure etiology and response to milrinone in decompensated heart failure: Results from the OPTIME-CHF study. J Am Coll Cardiol 41:997–1003, 2003.

4. Freeman BD, Natanson C: Hypotension, shock and multiple organ failure. In Wachter, Goldman, Hollander (eds): Hospital Medicine. Philadelphia, Lippincott, Williams & Wilkins, 2000, pp 123–131.

5. Gooneratne N, Manaker S: Physiology and principles of the use of vasopressors and inotropes. In Rose BD (ed): Up to Date, 2004.

6. Hollenberg SM, Ahrens TS, Djillali A: Practice parameters for hemodynamic support of sepsis in adult patients: 2004 update. Crit Care Med 32:1928–1948, 2004.

7. Tabaee A, Givertz MM: Pharmacologic management of the hypotensive patient. In Irwin, Rippe (eds): Intensive Care Medicine, 5th ed. Philadelphia, Lippincott, Wilkins, & Williams, 2003, pp 296–302.

CHAPTER 12

PULMONARY ARTERY CATHETERS AND INTRA-AORTIC BALLOON PUMPS

Julia Feliz Alvarado, MD

1. **What is a pulmonary artery (PA) catheter?**

   A PA catheter, also known as a *Swan-Ganz* or a *right heart catheter* is a balloon-tipped catheter used to directly measure pressures within the right side of the heart and PA. A standard catheter has a proximal lumen for the measurement of right atrial pressures and infusion of fluids, a lumen to introduce air into a balloon at the distal tip, a thermistor for measurement of cardiac output, and a distal lumen to record PA wedge pressure and mixed venous oxygen saturation.

2. **What are the indications for PA catheter use?**

   The decision to use a PA catheter in a critically ill patient balances the risk of proceeding with therapy without invasive hemodynamic information versus the risk associated with the use of the PA catheter. Frequently, the clinical question (e.g., "Is this patient hypotensive due to cardiogenic shock?") can be answered noninvasively. However, a PA catheter is frequently used in patients with complex physiology (e.g., cardiogenic shock with sepsis) or patients who do not respond to the initial therapeutic approach (e.g., diuresis or volume resuscitation).

3. **Which clinical conditions can be diagnosed with the assistance of a PA catheter?**

   PA catheters can be helpful in the diagnosis of pulmonary edema, shock, oliguric renal failure, lactic acidosis, pulmonary hypertension, ventricular septal defect, right ventricular infarction, pericardial tamponade, tricuspid regurgitation, constrictive pericarditis, and tachyarrhythmia.

4. **What are the complications of PA catheter use?**

   Complications of PA catheter use can be related to both achieving vascular access and insertion and use of the catheter. The most frequent complications of PA catheter use and the associated rates of occurrence are:

   - Ventricular tachycardia or premature ventricular contractions during insertion (11–68%)
   - Thrombosis of the insertion site or catheter (common but rarely clinically significant)
   - Transient right bundle branch block (0.5–5%)
   - Ectopy requiring antiarrhythmic therapy, chest thump, or cardioversion (1.5%)
   - Pulmonary infarction (0–1.4%)
   - PA rupture (0.06–0.2%)

5. **How can these complications be minimized?**

   Since the bulk of these events occur during catheter insertion, the incidence of complications can be reduced by correcting arrhythmogenic conditions before catheter insertion, using the full 1.5 mL of air to inflate the balloon during placement, and keeping catheterization time as short as possible. Prophylactic administration of lidocaine, heparin, or external pacemakers is not recommended. Avoid overinflation of the balloon, and secure the catheter firmly so that it does not migrate. Once the wedge position is found, the balloon should *always* be deflated between pulmonary capillary wedge pressure (PCWP) measurements. Another potential complication of PA catheter use is misinterpretation of the measurements or misuse of the clinical information obtained. Minimize both types of complications by interpreting the information with the assistance of a person with significant experience.

6. **What direct measurements can be made with a PA catheter?**
Pressure waveforms can be transduced at every point between catheter insertion and placement of the inflated balloon in a branch of the PA (Table 12-1).

TABLE 12-1. DIRECT MEASUREMENTS OF THE PA CATHETER: NORMAL VALUES	
Measurement	Normal Value
Right atrial pressure	0–8 mmHg
Right ventricular pressure (systolic/diastolic)	15–30 mmHg/0–8 mmHg
Pulmonary artery pressure (systolic/diastolic)	15–30 mmHg/3–12 mmHg
Pulmonary capillary wedge pressure	5–15 mmHg
Mixed venous oxygen saturation	65–75%

7. **What additional values can be *derived* from measurements made with a PA catheter?**
See Table 12-2.

TABLE 12-2. PA CATHETER-DERIVED MEASUREMENTS: FORMULA OF DERIVATION AND NORMAL VALUES		
Measurement	Formula	Normal Value
CO	Stroke volume $\times$ heart rate	5–8 L/min
CI	CO/body surface area	2.5–4.0 L/min/m^2
SVR	[(Mean arterial pressure $-$ RAP) $\times$ 80]/CO	1200–1600 dyn $\times$ sec/cm^5
PVR	({MPAP $-$ PCWP} $\times$ 80)/CO	200–400 dyn $\times$ sec/cm^5
Arterial oxygen content	(Hgb $\times$ 1.36 $\times$ SaO$_2$) + (0.0031 $\times$ PaO$_2$)	16–22 mL O$_2$/100 mL
Oxygen consumption	(Arterial oxygen content $-$ CVO$_2$) $\times$ CI $\times$ 10	100–175 mL/min/m^2
Oxygen delivery	CI $\times$ 10 $\times$ arterial oxygen content	500–750 mL/min/m^2

CO = Cardiac output, CI = cardiac index, SVR = systemic vascular resistance, RAP = right atrial pressure, dyn = dyne, PVR = pulmonary vascular resistance, MPAP = mean pulmonary arterial pressure, PCWP = pulmonary capillary wedge pressure, Hgb = hemoglobin, SaO$_2$ = percentage of hemoglobin saturation with oxygen, CVO$_2$ = mixed venous oxygen content.

8. **How is PCWP measured? What does it mean?**
PCWP is measured via placement of the inflated balloon in a branch of the PA, creating a static column of blood between the catheter tip and the left atrium. During normal cardiac diastole the pressures within the left atrium and ventricle equalize, allowing the PCWP to be used as a

surrogate for left ventricle end-diastolic pressure (LVEDP). Finally, the LVEDP approximates the left ventricular end diastolic volume. Therefore, the PCWP is considered to be a reflection of the volume in, and function of, the left ventricle.

9. **How can the cause of shock be differentiated using a PA catheter?**
See Table 12-3.

TABLE 12-3. PA CATHETER MEASUREMENT CHANGES SEEN IN SHOCK				
Disease State	CI	PCWP	CVP	SVR
Septic shock/anaphylactic shock	Increased	Decreased	Decreased	Decreased
Cardiogenic shock (left ventricular failure)	Decreased	Increased	Increased	Increased
Hypovolemic shock	Decreased	Decreased	Decreased	Increased
Pericardial tamponade	Decreased	Increased	Increased	Increased

CI = Cardiac index, PCWP = pulmonary capillary wedge pressure, CVP = central venous pressure, SVR = systemic vascular resistance.

10. **What is an intra-aortic balloon pump (IABP)?**
An IABP is a cylindrical balloon that can be temporarily inserted into the aorta via the femoral artery to provide mechanical assistance to the heart. The balloon pump deflates during ventricular systole, thereby reducing afterload and in turn reducing myocardial oxygen demands. Balloon pump inflation, during ventricular diastole, augments diastolic pressure, improving myocardial oxygen supply. This may result in increased stroke volume, cardiac output, and coronary perfusion (Figs. 12-1 and 12-2).

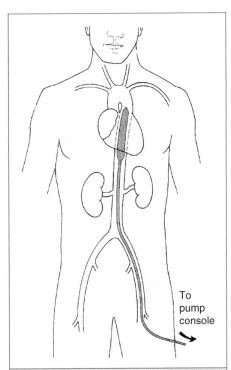

To pump console

Figure 12-1. IABP placement: balloon tip is distal to the left subclavian artery and the balloon end is proximal to the renal arteries. (From Flynn J, Bruce N: Introduction to Critical Care Skills. St. Louis, Mosby, 1993, p 262.)

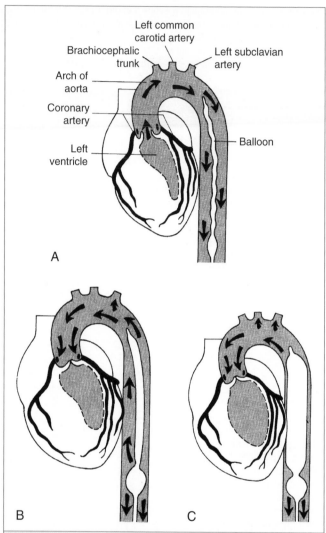

Figure 12-2. *A,* Balloon deflation decreases left ventricular afterload. ***B*** and ***C,*** Balloon inflation increases coronary perfusion pressure. (From Flynn J, Bruce N: Introduction to Critical Care Skills. St. Louis, Mosby, 1993, p 262.)

11. **What are the clinical indications for balloon pump placement?**
   Use of an IABP is considered in the settings of refractory unstable angina, cardiogenic shock, postoperative hemodynamic compromise, acute myocardial infarction with severe mitral regurgitation or ventricular septal defect, intractable ventricular tachycardia due to myocardial ischemia, cardiac surgery for left main or three-vessel disease, and high-risk percutaneous transluminal coronary angioplasty for a total occlusion.

KEY POINTS: PULMONARY ARTERY CATHETER INTERPRETATION

1. The hallmark of hypovolemic shock is a decreased PCWP.

2. The hallmark of cardiogenic shock is a decreased cardiac output/cardiac index.

3. The hallmark of distributive shock is a decreased SVR.

4. The hallmark of cardiac tamponade is an equalization of right atrial pressure, right ventricular diastolic pressure, and PCWP.

12. **What are the contraindications for IABP placement?**
Situations in which an IABP is ill advised include anatomic abnormality of the femoral-iliac artery, iliac or aortic atherosclerotic disease impairing blood flow runoff, moderate to severe aortic regurgitation, aortic dissection, aortic aneurysm, patent ductus arteriosus, history of bypass grafts to femoral arteries or aorta, bleeding diathesis, and sepsis.

13. **What are the complications of IABP Use?**
The most common major complication of IABP use is lower extremity ischemia due to placement of the IABP in a branch of the femoral artery, causing occlusion. An IABP should always be placed in the common femoral artery. Hemolysis, thrombosis, balloon rupture, acute renal failure, arterial dissection, and hematoma can all occur. Sepsis is a contraindication to placement but rarely a complication.

14. **How can you tell whether the IABP deflation is timed properly?**
The balloon of the IABP should be timed to deflate just after the closure of the aortic valve. This is indicated on the aortic waveform by the dicrotic notch. With a 2:1 timed inflation of the IABP, the waveform should demonstrate a decrease in the systolic blood pressure and an increase in the diastolic blood pressure (Fig. 12-3).

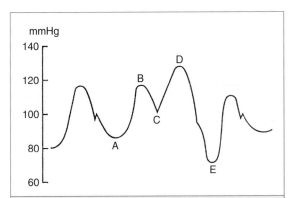

Figure 12-3. IABP waveform. A = End-diastolic pressure, B = systolic pressure, C = dicrotic notch (balloon inflates), D = augmented diastolic pressure, E = assisted end-diastolic pressure. (From Flynn J, Bruce N: Introduction to Critical Care Skills. St. Louis, Mosby, 1993, p 269.).

KEY POINTS: INTRA-AORTIC BALLOON PUMPS

1. IABPs should only be placed or removed by a specialist experienced in these procedures.

2. Patients with an IABP in place should have serial lower extremity pulse measurements for early detection of limb ischemia and a daily chest radiograph to ensure proper placement of the IABP above the renal arteries and below the takeoff of the subclavian artery.

3. Approximately 10% of patients will experience complications due to IABP use. However, less than 5% of patients will experience permanent morbidity, and the incidence of IABP-related mortality is less than 1%.

BIBLIOGRAPHY

1. Albert RK, Spiro SG, Jett JR: Clinical Respiratory Medicine. Philadelphia, Mosby, 2004.

2. Cooper AB, Doig GS, Sibbald WJ: Pulmonary artery catheters in the critically ill: An overview using the methodology of evidence-based medicine. Crit Care Clin 12:777–794, 1996.

3. Swan HJC, Ganz W, Forrestr J, et al: Catheterization of the heart in man with the use of a flow-directed balloon-tipped catheter. N Engl J Med 283:447, 1970.

CHAPTER 13

BRAIN DEATH AND ORGAN DONATION

Barbara Cleary, MD

1. **What is brain death?**
   Brain death is the *irreversible* loss of function of the entire cerebrum and brain stem.

2. **What are the differences between cardiac arrest, cardiac death, and brain death?**
   Cardiac arrest is the acute cessation of heart function, with the possibility of resuscitation. *Cardiac death* is the irreversible cessation of heart function; *brain death* inevitably follows. Brain death without cardiac death, which may occur with head trauma and in other situations, allows the body to be sustained on life support for possible organ donation.

3. **What is consciousness?**
   Consciousness consists of both awareness and alertness in an individual. Table 13-1 summarizes the different states of consciousness and brain death.

4. **Who can pronounce brain death?**
   An attending physician familiar with the brain death examination is required for pronouncement. Hospital policy may require that a neurologist or neurosurgeon be involved.

5. **What conditions must be met before brain death can be determined?**
   - Exam findings demonstrate brain death (see question 6)
   - There is a plausible cause of brain death (see question 8)
   - Irreversibility is established
   - There is an absence of confounding variables (see question 9)
   - Optional studies are performed when indicated (see question 10)

6. **What exam findings demonstrate loss of function of the cerebrum and brain stem?**
   - **Loss of cerebral function:** No motor function in response to painful stimulus.
   - **Loss of all brain stem function:** No pupillary light reflex, corneal reflex, occulocephalic, or occulovestibular reflex.
   - **Apnea test:** Patient remains apneic off ventilator, with adequate oxygenation, despite an appropriate time to induce hypercarbic respiratory drive.

7. **Does the presence of spinal reflexes argue against a diagnosis of brain death?**
   No. Spinal reflexes, such as deep tendon reflexes, do not depend on brain function and may persist for a time after brain death.

8. **What are some common causes of brain death?**
   Trauma, anoxic insult from cardiac or pulmonary arrest, subarachnoid bleed, brain stem or cerebral herniation, and hydrocephalus.

| | | Wake | Brain Stem | |
Condition	Awareness	Cycles	Reflexes	General
Sedation or paralytic agent	Variable	Variable	Variable	Should recover
Locked-in syndrome	Present	Present	Present	Recovery depends on etiology
Minimally conscious state	Low level, reproducible, consistent	Present	Present	Better chance of recovery than vegetative state
Vegetative state	Absent	Present	Present	Termed *persistent vegetative state* after 1 month; *permanent* after 1 year after trauma or 3 months after anoxic injury
Coma	Absent	Absent	Variable	Must persist at least 1 hour to differentiate between syncope or other loss of consciousness
Brain death	Absent	Absent	Absent	No recovery

TABLE 13-1. DIFFERENT STATES OF CONSCIOUSNESS AND BRAIN DEATH

Modified from Laureys S, Owen AM, Schiff ND: Brain function in coma, vegetative state, and related disorders. Lancet Neurol 3:537–546, 2004.

9. **What confounding variables must be ruled out before brain death is declared?**
   - Hypothermia (temperature must be >32°C)
   - Extreme electrolyte, acid-base, and endocrine disturbances
   - Sedatives, narcotics, overdoses, and paralytic agents

10. **Under which circumstances should brain death be confirmed by additional studies?**
    If the cause of coma is unknown or insufficient to explain the exam findings, a confirmatory test is indicated. Confirmatory tests include:
    - Electroencephalogram isoelectric at maximum gain for 30 minutes
    - Absent brain stem–evoked potentials
    - Cerebral angiography without cerebral blood flow
    - Radionuclide study showing a total lack of cerebral circulation

11. **Can brain death be pronounced if a study verifies lack of cerebral blood flow?**
    Yes. A patient is brain dead if no circulation reaches the brain. In this case, exam findings, assessment of confounding variables, and determination of cause of brain death are not necessary to make the diagnosis.

KEY POINTS: STEPS TO DECLARE BRAIN DEATH ✓

1. The physician must be familiar with the brain death exam.

2. The exam findings must be consistent with the mechanism of injury.

3. Medications, drugs, hypothermia, and metabolic derangement alter exam findings.

4. Confirmatory tests are needed if exam findings are not consistent with the mechanism of injury.

12. **How are organ donors classified?**
    Living donors may donate one of a paired set of organs or part of an organ that is not necessary for the donor's health. Donors *after cardiac death* may donate certain organs such as kidneys or corneas. Most organs do not remain viable for transplant after cardiac death. Donors *after brain death* whose organs are preserved artificially may donate many organs for transplant including heart, liver, lungs, kidneys, pancreas, and eyes.

13. **How are organ donors identified?**
    All states provide a system to identify organ donors such as the back of the driver's license or an organ donor card available from the Federal Division of Transplantation or the Coalition on Donation. Family or interested persons must also give consent for organ donation.

14. **Who should approach families about the idea of organ donation?**
    All families should be offered the opportunity of organ donation if a family member dies. Hospital policy may determine who approaches the family—a physician versus an organ donation team.

15. **Who decides whether organs are usable?**
    Organ donation teams are specially trained to make this determination.

WEBSITES

1. Coalition on Donation: http://www.shareyourlife.org

2. Federal Division of Transplantation: http://www.organdonor.gov

BIBLIOGRAPHY

1. Booth CM, Boone RH, Tomlinson G, et al: Is this patient dead, vegetative, or severely neurologically impaired? Assessing outcome for comatose survivors of cardiac arrest. JAMA 291:870–879, 2004.

2. Corr CA: Organ donation: Ethical issues and issues of loss and grief. In Doka KJ, Jennings B, Corr CA (eds): Living with Grief: Ethical Dilemmas at the End of Life. Hospice Foundation of America, 2005, pp 251–266.

3. Eelco FM, Wijdicks: The diagnosis of brain death. N Engl J Med 344:1215–1221, 2001.

4. Laureys S, Owen AM, Schiff ND: Brain function in coma, vegetative state, and related disorders. Lancet Neurol 3:537–546, 2004.

STROKE AND TRANSIENT ISCHEMIC ATTACKS

Sylvia C.W. McKean, MD

CHAPTER 14

1. What are the definitions of *stroke* and *transient ischemic attack* (TIA)?
A stroke is a cerebral infarction resulting from reduced blood flow to a portion of brain or retina. A TIA is a brief episode of neurologic dysfunction caused by focal ischemia without imaging evidence of acute infarction. Historically, TIAs were distinguished from stroke by the duration of the deficit (<24 and ≥24 hours, respectively). This time limit for the diagnosis of TIAs has been abandoned with the advent of radiographic imaging. Duration of symptoms of TIA are typically <30 minutes, and the majority of TIAs fully resolve within 60 minutes. For those patients with symptoms exceeding 60 minutes, more than 85% will turn out to be cerebral infarctions. *Reversible ischemic neurologic deficit* represents a TIA that improves after 24 hours. It has little use now that the current definition of TIA depends on neuroimaging.

2. How common are cerebrovascular events in the United States?
The annual incidence of stroke is approximately 750,000 events, costing approximately $45 billion for stroke-related care. Death from stroke remains the third leading cause of mortality. Ten-year follow-up of >400,000 patients without a history of prior acute myocardial infarction link relative risk of stroke with diastolic blood pressure. The incidence, prevalence, and type of stroke also vary according to geographic region. The National Stroke Association reports that ischemic strokes, which include thrombosis (51.5%) and embolism (31.5%), account for 83% of all strokes; the remainder are hemorrhagic strokes (17%). The prognosis and cost of ischemic strokes may be altered by early, critical treatment according to criteria published by the National Institutes of Neurologic Disorders and Stroke (NINDS). A meta-analysis of tissue plasminogen activator (tPA) trials reported 140 fewer dead or dependent per 1000 patients treated with tPA within 3 hours of symptom onset.

Albers GW, Amarenco P, Easton JD, et al: Antithrombotic and thrombolytic therapy for ischemic stroke. The 7th ACCP Conference on Antithrombotic and Thrombolytic Therapy. Chest 126:483S–512S, 2004.

3. What are the risk factors for stroke/TIA?
Risk factors that cannot be altered include age, sex, race/ethnicity, family history, and prior stroke/TIA. Risk factors that may be altered include hypertension, atrial fibrillation, smoking, elevated lipid levels, diabetes, carotid stenosis, and heavy alcohol use.

4. What is the initial evaluation of a patient with stroke/TIA?
Time is of the essence, so begin with a rapid triage history and examination focusing on the key neurologic symptoms and signs. If apparent stroke or TIA is present, commence neuroimaging and prepare for possible thrombolytic therapy. A comprehensive history and physical examination can be completed at any point before thrombolytic therapy is given. Identify a health care proxy and code status. Talk with witnesses if any are available. Rule out conditions that may be confused with stroke/TIA. Try to localize the ischemic event and confirm the presence of an occlusion. Estimate whether an embolic cause of stroke is more likely based on the presence of multiple infarctions in different vascular territories, prior history of systemic emboli, altered consciousness, or speedy recovery from major loss of neurologic function. Onset, progression, or involved vascular territory do not discriminate an embolic mechanism of stroke from other stroke subtypes.

5. **What other conditions may mimic acute stroke/TIA?**

Seizure may be confused with TIA, and electroencephalography is infrequently diagnostic of seizure. Cardiogenic causes of *syncope* may lead to symptoms consistent with TIA, and the patient may experience a seizure due to inadequate cerebral perfusion. In patients with preexisting vascular disease, decreased cerebral perfusion of abnormal cerebrovascular territories and metabolic abnormalities may unmask deficits from prior strokes. The symptoms of *migraine* may be confused with TIA, and often patients with stroke experience headaches. Risk factors for stroke/TIA, time course, and the type of symptoms (loss of function) are helpful in determining whether the symptoms are consistent with ischemic disease. *Metabolic disturbances* are generally easy to identify and the clinician should routinely check electrolytes, blood sugar, and other metabolic parameters as part of the admission work-up. A prior history of *multiple sclerosis* and *myasthenia gravis* raise the possibility of these diagnoses as the cause of the neurologic deficit. A patient with a prior history of falls may have a *subdural hematoma*, which would be identified as part of the diagnostic work-up of stroke/TIA.

KEY POINTS: DISEASE STATES THAT CAN MIMIC AN ACUTE STROKE

1. Dissection of a major cerebral vascular supply

2. Brain tumor

3. Infection, including septic emboli from bacterial endocarditis

4. Migraine headache

5. Subdural hematoma, subarachnoid hemorrhage, intraparenchymal hemorrhage

6. Toxic metabolic encephalopathy

7. Seizure with Todd's paralysis (weakness of affected limb or limbs after motor seizure)

8. Metabolic derangements

9. Multiple sclerosis and myasthenia gravis

6. **What imaging studies should be performed in the evaluation of stroke/TIA?**

Noncontrast computed tomography (CT) and multimodal magnetic resonance imaging (MRI) are used to evaluate cerebral tissue. The density of subarachnoid or intraparenchymal hemorrhage differs with normal brain mass and hence is easily identified on head CT. The parenchymal changes associated with nonhemorrhagic stroke are less apparent than hemorrhage and may not be seen initially. The location of the neurologic event also influences the sensitivity of noncontrast CT, which is significantly lower for lacunar and posterior fossa strokes. The signal of diffusion-weighted imaging in multimodal MRI is inversely proportional to the diffusion of water molecules. Because the diffusion is restricted with edema caused by ischemia, the signal intensity is increased in areas of ischemia compared with normal brain tissue. T2-weighted MRI can also be used to diagnose cerebral hemorrhage (parenchymal and subarachnoid) even within the initial 6 hours after the onset of stroke symptoms. Noncontrast head CT is the preferred imaging modality to rule out acute hemorrhage in the setting of stroke for thrombolysis protocols. Although minor or subtle radiographic changes do not increase the risk of intracerebral hemorrhage from thrombolysis, the presence of greater than one-third middle cerebral artery territory and reported hypodensity on CT is an exclusion criterion for thrombolysis (Table 14-1).

TABLE 14-1. COMPARISON OF IMAGING MODALITIES IN ACUTE CEREBROVASCULAR DISEASE

Imaging Study	Noncontrast Head CT	Multimodal MRI, Including DWI
Advantages	Universal availability Rapid performance High sensitivity for acute hemorrrhagic events	Superior in identifying acute stroke, posterior fossa stroke, small vessel lacunar infarcts, clarifying time course of stroke (acute, subacute)
Disadvantages	May be normal immediately after onset of neurologic deficit	Not always available Takes longer to perform Contraindicated or not tolerated by some patients Greater interobserver variability

CT = computerized tomography, MRI = magnetic resonance imaging, DWI = diffusion-weighted imaging.

7. **What imaging modalities are used to evaluate the vascular supply to the brain?**

Helical scanners rapidly evaluate the aortic arch, carotid system, and intracranial vasculature with one injection of intravenous contrast. Compared with catheter angiography, CT angiography has an 80–100% accuracy. MR angiography is an acceptable alternative to CT angiography and catheter angiography for those patients who cannot receive intravenous contrast. Compared with catheter angiography, MR angiography has a sensitivity of 70–100% but is less reliable in identifying distal or branch occlusions and may overestimate stenoses. Ultrasound techniques that include Doppler insonation of the extracranial carotid vasculature and transcranial Doppler are limited by the difficulty in imaging through bony structures and the relative lack of availability.

8. **What additional studies can be performed as soon as TIA/stroke is suspected?**

Routine laboratory studies include complete blood count, coagulation studies (e.g., prothrombin time, activated partial thromboplastin time), complete metabolic profile (electrolytes, blood urea nitrogen, creatinine, blood sugar), electrocardiography (ECG), and chest radiography. If a patient has a hematocrit count <25%, an acute subdural hematoma will not appear hyperacute on head CT. In the emergency department, cervical spine imaging is routinely obtained to rule out cervical trauma in all patients who may have fallen because of an acute neurologic deficit. An erythrocyte sedimentation rate is often obtained because vasculitis and septic emboli to the central nervous system would require different management.

9. **What ECG abnormalities can be seen in acute stroke?**

Abnormalities suggesting myocardial ischemia (e.g., ST-segment depression or elevation, abnormal T and U waves) and/or prolongation of the QT interval can be detected in up to 75% of patients with subarachnoid hemorrhage and more than 90% of unselected patients with either ischemic stroke or intracerebral hemorrhage. The specificity of these ECG abnormalities to identify acute myocardial ischemia are low during acute stroke. However, the 6-month mortality rate is higher in patients with ECG changes. All kinds of ECG changes, including heart block (right side) and supraventricular tachycardia (left side), can be seen with insular cortex infarcts.

10. **What is the time frame for use of thrombolytics, and what needs to happen in the interim?**

The role of thrombolytics in the treatment of acute stroke is still evolving. When given within 3 hours of onset of symptoms, the benefit of intravenous tPA outweighs the risk of hemorrhage. To achieve this benefit, patients must be appropriately screened and diagnosed within a very narrow time frame. Neuroimaging plays a pivotal role in the decision to use thrombolysis. Start by ruling out any conditions that may be confused with stroke/TIA so that you can rapidly tailor your diagnostic work-up and treatment. Immediately order imaging studies to distinguish cerebral hemorrhage from ischemia/infarction, and factor in the size of the infarct. Determine the cause of the stroke, which varies according to age, risk factors, and underlying comorbid conditions. Confirm your suspicion of a vascular cause of stroke/TIA through review of neuroimaging and correlation with your targeted history and physical examination. You should then be able to provide an early prognosis and initiate appropriate treatment, which may include the use of thrombolytics, transfer to a stroke center, or admission to an intensive care unit. Intra-arterial administration of thrombolytic agents has a longer window of efficacy (6 hours and perhaps longer versus 3 hours with systemic thrombolysis) but there are no head-to-head comparisons, no evidence that it is safer or more effective, and intra-arterial administration of thrombolytics requires a stroke center and time to mobilize resources.

KEY POINTS: USE OF THROMBOLYTIC AGENTS IN ACUTE STROKE

1. The patient has to have an arterial occlusion to benefit from thrombolytics.

2. Appropriate imaging tests must be performed quickly to rule out hemorrhage.

3. The size of the infarct influences the likelihood of hemorrhagic complications.

4. Failure to improve is more likely with the presence of cortical infarction, hyperglycemia, and longer length of time to treatment.

5. Higher mortality is associated with older age, decreased levels of consciousness, and occasions when treatment does not occur in a stroke center.

11. **When is heparin indicated in the treatment of acute stroke/TIA?**

No randomized controlled trial has been published regarding the use of anticoagulation within 12 hours of the onset of neurologic symptoms from stroke. To date, there is no evidence that heparin improves neurologic outcomes and no evidence—even among patients with suspected cardioembolism—that heparin lowers the risk of early recurrent stroke. Although the use of long-term anticoagulation with warfarin reduces the risk of stroke in patients with atrial fibrillation, there does not appear to be any benefit to initiating this therapy early in the course of an acute, atrial fibrillation–related stroke. In fact, emergent anticoagulation therapy for stroke/TIA has been associated with increased intracranial and systemic bleeding. Most patients with acute stroke/TIA do not benefit from treatment with heparin.

12. **What is the role of antiplatelet therapy in acute and chronic stroke management?**

After a patient experiences a TIA or stroke, the most likely cause of death becomes a subsequent stroke rather than myocardial infarction (the overall number one cause of death). Many stroke survivors, however, often die of subsequent vascular events including myocardial infarction. Antiplatelet agents have a role in the secondary prevention of stroke and myocardial infarction, but ongoing research is needed to determine which antiplatelet agent is preferred and whether switching to another antiplatelet drug improves outcomes in patients already taking aspirin. Limited data suggest that the risk of hemorrhagic transformation is less with antiplatelet agents than with warfarin or heparin. For noncardioembolic stroke/TIA, start with aspirin as initial therapy: 160–325 mg/day within 48 hours of stroke onset. Use 50–100 mg/day for patients at higher risk of bleeding.

Alternatively, more expensive regimens include aspirin 25 mg with extended-release dipyridamole 200 mg twice a day, or clopidogrel 75 mg daily. For patients with noncardioembolic events and defined prothrombotic disorders such as the anti-phospholipid syndrome, oral anticoagulation may be preferred over antiplatelet agents. For patients with atrial fibrillation, long-term anticoagulation with warfarin is indicated with a target international normalized ratio of 2.5 (range, 2–3).

13. **What are stroke vital signs? What measures can be taken to improve prognosis?**
    In addition to the ABCs of cardiac resuscitation (i.e., airway, breathing, circulation) and stabilization of the cervical spine pending imaging, an elevated glucose level and fever are modifiable poor prognostic factors. Stroke patients with hyperglycemia should have tight glucose control, preferably in an intensive care unit setting with intravenous insulin. Fever should be aggressively treated.

14. **When should hypertension be treated?**
    Current stroke guidelines do not recommend treating elevated blood pressure during the initial hospitalization for acute stroke unless the blood pressure is very elevated or the patient has suffered a hemorrhagic stroke. Hypertension in ischemic stroke may be a mechanism to maintain cerebral blood flow. Abruptly lowering blood pressure to "normal levels" may increase the ischemic territory and worsen outcomes. Preferred agents include labetalol or esmolol with enalapril being used in patients with significant bradycardia. The guideline recommendations depend on the setting (i.e., presence of hemorrhage versus ischemia) and whether thrombolytics are used. The NINDS trial excluded patients whose blood pressure required aggressive management to meet target endpoints. This trial reported strict algorithms for blood pressure treatment and monitoring to reduce the incidence of intracerebral hemorrhage as a complication of thrombolysis.
    1. First 24 hours after thrombolytic therapy: treatment as per NINDS guidelines
       - Treat when mean arterial blood pressure >120 mmHg
       - Target blood pressure: systolic blood pressure <180 mmHg, diastolic blood pressure <105 mmHg
    2. Evidence of end-organ damage: treatment as per NINDS guidelines
       - Treat in patients with hemorrhagic transformation of stroke, myocardial ischemia, hypertensive encephalopathy, arterial dissection, and acute renal failure, and in pregnant patients with eclampsia, or other end-organ damage.
    3. Ischemic stroke patients not receiving thrombolysis (Mayo Clinic protocol)
       - No treatment unless mean arterial pressure >130 mmHg
       - Target blood pressure: systolic blood pressure <220 mmHg, diastolic blood pressure <120 mmHg

    For stroke complicated by cerebral hemorrhage, use nicardipine 5–15 mg/h to maintain systolic blood pressure according to published guidelines (i.e., <160 mmHg). Labetalol may be more difficult to titrate to optimum blood pressure, and nitroprusside (Nipride) carries the risk of cyanide toxicity effects on the ischemic brain. Long-term management of hypertension is required to prevent subsequent stroke. It is estimated that 360,000 strokes could be prevented annually by long-term blood pressure control based on an estimated 731,000 annual incidence of stroke.

Gorelick PB: Stroke prevention. Arch Neurol 52:347–355, 1995.

Marler JR, Tilley BC, Lu M, et al: Early stroke treatment associated with better outcome: The NINDS rt-PA stroke study. Neurology 55:1649–1655, 2002.

15. **Do all stroke patients require imaging of their carotids and heart?**

Imaging of the carotids and heart is not required for all stroke patients; however, there is not universal agreement as to how to select patients for additional testing. The key question to ask is whether the results of the testing will influence management. For example, anterior circulation TIA/stroke requires the evaluation to identify those patients who might benefit from carotid endarterectomy. Echocardiography is not required in patients who are already anticoagulated for atrial fibrillation. It would be considered for patients who are not already anticoagulated to look for cardiac conditions for which warfarin has been shown to be more efficacious than antiplatelet agents for recurrent stroke prevention.

KEY POINTS: STEPS IN THE MANAGEMENT OF ACUTE STROKE

1. Reestablish blood flow to ischemic but viable brain tissue as quickly as possible but *within 3 hours* of stroke onset, following strict protocols.

2. Consider intra-arterial thrombolytic therapy as an option *within 6–12 hours* of stroke onset for patients with occlusion of major anterior circulation or basilar artery.

3. Triage to a stroke center may improve outcomes including mortality and functional recovery and is required for intra-arterial thrombolysis.

4. Avoid emergent anticoagulant therapy with heparin for most patients with ischemic stroke/ TIA, including patients with suspected cardioembolism.

5. Follow the American College of Chest Physicians guidelines recommending antiplatelet therapy to reduce the risk of stroke and other vascular events. Options include aspirin 50–325 mg daily, aspirin and extended-release dipyridamole 25/200 mg twice daily or clopidogrel 75 mg daily.

6. Use chronic warfarin therapy in cases of cardiogenic embolism documented by the presence of atrial fibrillation or structural heart disease.

7. Consider carotid endarterectomy for extracranial carotid stenosis of 70–99%.

16. **What steps can be taken to prevent adverse hospital events?**

Initial management includes protection of the airway and assessment of swallowing, sometimes with a video swallowing study. For patients with impaired swallowing, a gastrostomy tube may be indicated with the anticipation that these patients may recover over a period of several months. Stroke patients require intravenous hydration with normal saline. Dextrose should be avoided because persistent post-stroke hyperglycemia is independently associated with infarct expansion and worse clinical outcomes. Free water administration should be avoided because it may worsen the presentation of the syndrome of inappropriate anti-diuretic hormone that is often associated with stroke. Institute prophylactic measures to prevent aspiration (e.g., positioning, special diets), venous thromboembolism, malnutrition, and decubitus ulcers.

17. **What important follow-up issues need to be addressed before the patient is discharged?**

Appropriate secondary preventive therapy should be started, and the specifics of new medications should be addressed. If anticoagulation therapy is prescribed, appropriate education and follow-up need to be prescribed. Parameters for management of hypertension, lipids, and diet need to be discussed. Follow-up with a primary care physician and neurologist should be established and measures to optimize post-discharge function, including home safety evaluation, physical therapy, and elder services, should be prearranged as appropriate.

WEBSITE

National Institute of Neurological Disorders and Stroke: http://www.ninds.nih.gov

BIBLIOGRAPHY

1. Albers GW, Amarenco P, Easton JD, et al: Antithrombotic and thrombolytic therapy for ischemic stroke. The 7th ACCP Conference on Antithrombotic and Thrombolytic Therapy. Chest 126:483S–512S, 2004.

2. Baird TA, Parsons MW, Phanh T, et al: Persistent post stroke hyperglycemia is independently associated with infarct expansion and worse clinical outcome. Stroke 349:2208–2214, 2004.

3. Bogousslavsky J, Cachin C, Regali F: Cardiac sources of embolism and cerebral infarction: Clinical consequences and vascular concomitants: The Louisanne Stroke Registry. Neurology 41:855–859, 1991.

4. Bruno A, Saha C, Williams LS, Shankar R: IV insulin during acute cerebral infarction in diabetic patients. Neurology 54:1441–1442, 2004.

5. Castillo J, et al: Blood pressure decrease during the acute phase of ischemic stroke is associated with brain injury and poor stroke outcome. Stroke 352:520, 2004.

6. Flemming KD, Brown RD, Petty GW, et al: Evaluation and management of transient ischemic attack and minor cerebral infarction. Mayo Clin Proc 79:1071–1086, 2004.

7. Fulgham JR, Ingall TJ, Stead LG, et al: Management of acute ischemic stroke. Mayo Clin Proc 79:1459–1469, 2004.

8. Kidwell C, Chalela JA, Saver JL, et al: Comparison of MRI and CT for detection of acute intracerebral Hemorrhage. JAMA 292:1823–1830, 2004.

9. Marler JR, Tilley BC, Lu M, et al: Early stroke treatment associated with better outcome: The NINDS rt-PA stroke study. Neurology 55:1649–1655, 2002.

10. National Institute of Neurologic Disorders and Stroke rt-PA. Stroke Study Group: Tissue plasminogen activator for acute ischemic stroke. N Engl J Med 333:1581–1587, 1995.

11. Oiveria-Filho J, et al: Detrimental effect of blood pressure reduction in the first 24 hours of acute stroke onset. Neurology 618:1047, 2003.

12. Reith J, Jorgensen HS, Pedersen PM, et al: Body temperature in acute stroke: Relation to stroke severity, infarct size, mortality, and outcome. Lancet 17:422–425, 1996.

CHAPTER 15

SEIZURES

Yvette M. Cua, MD, and Suzette LaRoche, MD

1. **What is the difference between a seizure and epilepsy?**

   A seizure is a paroxysmal alteration in behavior or perception; it is a *symptom* that warrants further investigation for a cause. Epilepsy is a *disease* characterized by spontaneous recurrent unprovoked seizures.

2. **How is epilepsy classified?**

   By *seizure type* (based on clinical presentation and electroencephalogram [EEG]) or by *epilepsy syndrome* (based on seizure type, age of onset, genetics, possible etiologies, neurologic examination, magnetic resonance imaging [MRI], and EEG). Table 15-1 lists seizure types. Both classification systems assist in determining the most effective anti-epileptic drug (AED), but classification by epilepsy syndrome also provides prognostic information.

TABLE 15-1. CLASSIFICATION BY SEIZURE TYPE
Partial onset* ("focal seizures")
Simple partial: "aura" (no alteration of awareness)
Complex partial (with alteration of awareness)
Secondarily generalized
Generalized onset
Absence: typical and atypical
Tonic-clonic
Tonic
Clonic
Myoclonic
Atonic
Infantile spasm
Unclassified

   * Each type of partial onset can be furthered subclassified as: **m**otor, **a**utonomic, **p**sychic, **s**ensory.

3. **How can absence and complex partial seizures be differentiated clinically?**

   See Table 15-2.

4. **What is status epilepticus?**

   Although there is no universally accepted definition, it is a medical emergency traditionally defined as ≥30 minutes of continuous clinical or electrical seizure activity *or* repetitive seizures with incomplete neurologic recovery interictally. Many propose shortening the time criteria for diagnosis from ≥30 minutes to 5 minutes.

TABLE 15–2. DIFFERENTIATING ABSENCE AND COMPLEX PARTIAL SEIZURES

Attribute	Absence	Complex Partial
Age	Childhood, rarely adulthood	All ages
Automatisms*	Absent	Common
Before seizure, "aura"	Absent	Occasional
Confusion, "postictal"	Absent	Present
Duration of seizure	10–20 seconds	1–2 minutes
EEG findings	3-Hz generalized spike/wave	Normal or focal spikes
Frequency of seizures	Several per day	Can be daily, weekly, or monthly

*Examples of automatisms: lip smacking, nose rubbing, repeated swallowing, repetition of a word, coughing, grunting, picking at one's clothing, purposeless hand movements, or even singing.

KEY POINTS: DEFINITION AND CLASSIFICATION OF SEIZURES

1. A seizure is *a sign* of epilepsy or of another condition and should never be the diagnostic endpoint of an evaluation.

2. Seizure classification by both type and syndrome is ideal for optimal AED selection.

3. Status epilepticus is a medical emergency requiring prompt recognition and intervention.

5. **Describe the etiology of new-onset seizures.**
Only one-third of new-onset seizures have an identifiable cause, which may include structural, metabolic, and toxic factors (Fig. 15-1 and Table 15-3). Other drugs that can provoke seizures include antipsychotic medicines, bupropion, lithium, penicillin, selective serotonin reuptake inhibitors, theophylline, and tricyclic antidepressants.

6. **What are some common causes of status epilepticus?**
Acute central nervous system (CNS) injury (50%), medication changes in patients with epilepsy (20%), and idiopathic causes (30%).

7. **What are some common seizure triggers?**
The mnemonic *SEIZE* summarizes common seizure triggers:
- **S:** Stress
- **E:** EtOH (i.e., alcohol)
- **I:** Illness
- **Z:** ZZ (i.e., sleep deprivation)
- **E:** Estrogen level fluctuation/menses

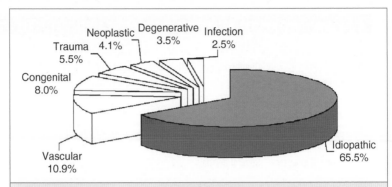

Figure 15-1. Etiology of new-onset seizures. (From Hauser WA, Annegers JF, Kurland LT: Incidence of epilepsy and unprovoked seizures in Rochester, Minnesota; 1935–1984. Epilepsia 34:453–468, 1993, with permission.)

TABLE 15-3. CAUSES OF NEW-ONSET SEIZURES

Acquired structural lesions: Use the mnemonic *VITAMIN*

Vascular (hemorrhage, arteriovenous malformation, venous thrombosis, cavernous angiomas)

Infectious (meningitis, encephalitis, abscess, neurocystercercosis, HIV/AIDS)

Trauma

Autoimmune (systemic lupus erythematosus, polyarteritis nodosum)

Mesial temporal sclerosis

Ischemic stroke

Neoplasm (primary CNS, metastatic)

Metabolic: Use the mnemonic *UH's*

Uremia

Hypoglycemia* and hyperglycemia

Hyponatremia

Hypocalcemia

Hypomagnesemia

Hypothyroid myxedema

Hepatic failure

Hypoxia

Hyperosmolar states

High fever

Drugs/toxins: The mnemonic *ABCD* includes the four most common:

Alcohol withdrawal*

Benzodiazepine withdrawal

Cocaine

Demerol

*Most common in its category.

KEY POINTS: SEIZURE ETIOLOGY

1. Most cases of new-onset epilepsy have no underlying identifiable cause.

2. By comparison, single, provoked seizures by definition have an identifiable metabolic or toxic cause.

8. **What other diseases may mimic a seizure?**
   The mnemonic *STAMP* summarizes diseases that may mimic a seizure:
   - **S: S**yncope (i.e., vasovagal, arrhythmia), **s**leep disorder (e.g., narcolepsy, REM behavior disorder)
   - **T: T**ransient ischemic attack, **t**etany
   - **A: A**mnesia (i.e., transient global)
   - **M: M**igraine, **m**ovement disorders (e.g., myoclonus, familial paroxysmal dystonia, choreoathetosis, hemiballismus, tremor)
   - **P: P**aroxysmal vertigo, **p**sychogenic (e.g., panic attack, attention deficit hyperactivity disorder, posttraumatic stress disorder, hyperventilation syndrome, fugue state, conversion disorder)

9. **What clues help differentiate an epileptic seizure from syncope?**
   Seizures but not syncope typically have a postictal state (i.e., transient period of decreased neurologic function as the brain recovers after a seizure); can cause retrograde amnesia, incontinence, and tongue biting; and have more forceful prolonged tonic-clonic movements than the "twitches" that can accompany (convulsive) syncope.

10. **What differentiates psychogenic seizures from epileptic seizures?**
    Psychogenic seizures usually last longer than epileptic seizures (>5 minutes, often waxing and waning), are not usually associated with incontinence or physical injury, are often associated with pelvic thrusting and turning the head side to side, and are refractory to AEDs.

11. **What historical elements aid in classifying seizures?**
    The mnemonic *AURA* summarizes helpful historical elements:
    - **A: A**utomatisms (i.e., repetitive purposeless activity), **a**ura (i.e., unusual smells, epigastric sensation), **a**ltered consciousness/**a**cute confusional postictal state (typically occurs with all seizures except simple partial, myoclonic, and absence seizures; atypical postictal phenomena include neurogenic pulmonary edema [usually after status epilepticus] and Todd's paralysis [transient focal neurologic deficits lasting <48 hours]), **a**ccidents (e.g., incontinence, tongue biting)
    - **U: U**nprovoked (usually not triggered by emotional stimuli)
    - **R: R**etrograde amnesia
    - **A: A**brupt onset, brief duration (<90–120 seconds). Observers often overestimate duration.

12. **Which other items should be included in the patient history?**
    Personal or family history of psychiatric illness or seizures; frequency and pattern of occurrence; childhood febrile seizures; congenital abnormalities; previous stroke, CNS infection, or head trauma; diabetes, renal or hepatic disease, sickle cell, human immunodeficiency virus (HIV)/acquired immunodeficiency syndrome (AIDS), malignancy; medications (including over-the-counter and herbal remedies), recent changes in dosing, new medicines, adherence; drug or alcohol use; and sleep deprivation.

13. **What are the key physical exam findings to look for?**
    - **Postictal findings:** Hyperreflexia, Babinski's reflex, dilated pupils, Todd's paralysis
    - **Consequences of a convulsive seizure:** Incontinence, hyperthermia, hypertension (initially) followed by hypotension, arrhythmias, pulmonary edema, tongue biting, ecchymoses, fractures, dislocations

14. **Which studies should be obtained in patients with new-onset seizures?**
    Oxygen saturation, glucose, sodium, calcium, magnesium, blood urea nitrogen, creatinine, liver enzymes, hemoglobin, platelets, white blood cell count with differential, urinalysis, syphilis testing, and toxicology screen. Consider HIV testing in high prevalence areas or if risk factors exist. All patients with new-onset seizures should have a head computed tomography [CT] or MRI performed at the time of presentation to exclude structural lesions. If the initial study is a CT scan, a follow-up outpatient MRI should be scheduled.

15. **What abnormalities in laboratory study results may be seen after a generalized tonic-clonic seizure?**
    Metabolic acidosis, hypoglycemia/hyperglycemia, hypoxia, leukocytosis, hyperprolactinemia (first 10 minutes), disseminated intravascular coagulation, rhabdomyolysis.

16. **How does an EEG help in diagnosis?**
    An EEG can aid in seizure/syndrome classification, can help localize the region of seizure onset, and may confirm a diagnosis of epileptic seizure versus nonepileptic event. However, a normal EEG does not exclude the possibility of epilepsy. Repeat EEGs can increase the sensitivity for detecting epileptiform activity.

17. **When should an EEG be done emergently?**
    In cases of (1) persistent altered mental status or unresponsiveness after a witnessed seizure to exclude ongoing nonconvulsive status epilepticus, (2) refractory status epilepticus being treated with anesthetic coma or pharmacologic paralysis, or (3) altered mental status of unknown cause.

18. **When is a lumbar puncture indicated?**
    In all patients with a seizure who have HIV, fever, or otherwise high suspicion for infectious etiology (e.g., bacterial meningitis, neurosyphilis, herpes, tuberculosis, fungus).

19. **What other tests can be done if the presentation is unclear?**
    Electrocardiography, Holter monitor, tilt-table test, sleep study, and EEG-video monitoring.

20. **Describe the initial management of a witnessed seizure.**
    Protect the patient from self-injury. Help him or her to the ground if standing, cushion the area if possible, stabilize the patient's neck, immobilize the neck if there is a question of spinal injury. Do not place anything in the patient's mouth. Roll the patient on his or her side, and clear the airway at the end of the seizure. Treat the underlying cause, if known. The majority of seizures are self-limited. If it continues for >5 minutes, consider initiating abortive therapy (e.g., benzodiazepines).

21. **Describe the general management of status epilepticus**
    The primary goal is to abort the seizure as quickly as possible to minimize complications because seizure duration is the major determinant of morbidity and mortality. Management includes protecting the patient's airway (intubate if necessary); establishing intravenous access and drawing appropriate studies; giving thiamine plus dextrose, and administering intravenous

benzodiazepines followed by phenytoin or fosphenytoin. If seizures persist, EEG monitoring and treatment with phenobarbital, pentobarbital, midazolam, or propofol is appropriate. Patients should be monitored continuously and admitted to the intensive care unit with neurologic consultation.

KEY POINTS: DIAGNOSTIC EVALUATION OF SEIZURES

1. All patients with new-onset seizures should have a head CT or MRI performed at the time of presentation to exclude acute structural lesions.

2. A normal interictal EEG does not exclude the possibility of underlying epilepsy.

3. Persistent altered mental status after a witnessed seizure is an indication for emergent EEG.

4. All HIV-positive patients with a new-onset seizure require a lumbar puncture.

22. **What is the difference between phenytoin and fosphenytoin?**
Fosphenytoin is the highly water-soluble pro-drug of phenytoin and can be administered more rapidly with fewer risks of hypotension, cardiac arrhythmias, and thrombophlebitis.

23. **When should patients be started on an AED?**
AEDs are indicated with recurrent, unprovoked seizures (epilepsy). Consider initiating therapy with an AED after a single seizure in the following situations: underlying CNS structural lesion or infection, EEG shows epileptiform activity, family history of epilepsy, acutely ill or unstable patients in which having additional seizures may induce serious metabolic and cardiovascular consequences, after status epilepticus if no obvious reversible cause found, and in HIV-positive patients without an obvious reversible cause.

24. **What factors influence the choice of AED?**
The choice of AED is affected by comorbid medical conditions that could affect the patient's metabolism, current medications (potential drug interactions), side effects, dosing frequency, cost of medication, and insurance formulary. Two-thirds of seizures are controlled with AEDs; maintain a high index of suspicion for medication nonadherence if treatment fails (Table 15-4).

    Kwan P, Brodie MJ: Early identification of refractory epilepsy. N Engl J Med 342: 314–319, 2000.

25. **What special instructions are required for patients with seizure disorders?**
    - ***Do not drive.*** Check state laws. Most require patients to be seizure free for 6–24 months before driving again.
    - Avoid heavy lifting, operating large machinery, climbing ladders or ropes, and swimming or bathing alone. More seizure patients die in bathtubs than in motor vehicle accidents annually.
    - Avoid drugs that lower the seizure threshold (e.g., cocaine, alcohol).
    - Get adequate sleep.
    - Check for drug interactions with any newly prescribed medicines.
    - Epileptic caregivers of babies should change and feed them on the floor and have another adult present when bathing the infant.
    - Invest in a medical bracelet stating "seizure disorder."

TABLE 15-4. INDICATIONS FOR ANTIEPILEPTIC DRUGS BY SEIZURE TYPE

Generalized or Partial-Onset (Broad Spectrum)	Partial-Onset Only
Old drugs	**Old drugs**
Ethosuximide (Zarontin): absence only	Carbamazepine (Tegretol)
Valproate (Depakote)	Phenobarbital
	Phenytoin (Dilantin)
	Primidone (Mysoline)
New drugs	**New drugs**
Felbamate (Felbatol)*	Gabapentin (Neurontin)
Lamotrigine (Lamictal)	Levetiracetam (Keppra)
Topiramate (Topamax)	Oxcarbazepine (Trileptal)
	Pregabalin (Lyrica)
	Tiagabine (Gabitril)
	Zonisamide (Zonegran)

*Not considered first-line treatment due to risk of aplastic anemia and hepatotoxicity.

KEY POINTS: TREATMENT OF SEIZURES

1. Most seizures are self-limited. Consider abortive therapy if seizure persists for >5 minutes.

2. Fosphenytoin is preferred over phenytoin due to its safer side effect profile and more rapid administration.

WEBSITES

1. Epilepsy Information Center: http://www.neuroland.com/sz

2. Evidence-Based Epilepsy, an Epilepsy Reference Source: http://www.neuro.wustl.edu/epilepsy/pediatric/EvidenceBasedEpilepsy-TC.html

3. North Pacific Epilepsy Research: http://www.seizures.net

BIBLIOGRAPHY

1. Engel J Jr, Pedley TA (eds): Epilepsy: A Comprehensive Textbook. Philadelphia, Lippincott-Raven, 1998.
2. Foldvary-Schaefer N, Wyllie E: Epilepsy. In Goetz CG (ed): Textbook of Clinical Neurology, 2nd ed. 2003, pp 1155–1186.
3. LaRoche SM, Helmers SL: The new antiepileptic drugs. JAMA 291:615–620, 2004.

CHAPTER 16

SYNCOPE
Michael J. Pistoria, DO

1. **What is syncope? How does it differ from presyncope?**
   - *Syncope* is defined as a transient loss of consciousness and postural tone due to an acute reduction in cerebral blood flow. This is also known as "going to ground." It is important to remember that syncope is a symptom and not a disease. One must always work to diagnose the underlying cause of a syncopal episode.
   - *Presyncope* encompasses the symptoms that may precede a syncopal episode such as the classic "tunnel vision" (i.e., progressively blurred vision that leads to transient blindness), dizziness, feeling warm, diaphoresis, nausea, and lightheadedness. However, in presyncope alone, these symptoms are not accompanied by loss of consciousness or postural tone.

2. **How often does syncope occur?**
   The incidence of syncope is 6.2 per 1000 person-years. Over a 10-year period, the cumulative incidence is roughly 3–6%. Between one and two million patients are evaluated each year for syncope in the United States alone. Syncope accounts for 3–5% of all emergency department visits and 1–6% of hospital admissions.

3. **Name key cardiac and noncardiac causes of syncope.**
   There are four basic categories of causes of syncope: reflex-mediated, cardiac, neurologic, and every student's favorite, "other" (Table 16-1).

4. **Who should be hospitalized for syncope?**
   A patient should be hospitalized for evaluation of syncope if there is risk of adverse outcome with any delay in diagnostic testing and treatment of the underlying cause. Cardiac causes fall into this category and are also the most lethal, so both the history and physical examination must probe for findings consistent with structural heart disease, arrhythmia, or ischemia. It may be helpful to think in terms of risk groups for cardiac causes of syncope when determining the need for admission. Any patients at high risk for cardiac syncope should be admitted for further evaluation, and clinical judgment should be used for patients at moderate and low risk. A patient with severe orthostasis is another in whom hospitalization is prudent because of the risk of further syncopal episodes and potential injury. Patients in whom there is a concern for transient ischemic attack or seizure should also be admitted for observation and consideration of therapy (Table 16-2).

KEY POINTS: COMMON MECHANISMS OF SYNCOPE

1. Reflex-mediated

2. Cardiac

3. Neurologic

4. Psychiatric

TABLE 16-1. CAUSES OF SYNCOPE			
Basic Category	Cause	High-Yield History Findings	High-Yield Physical Exam Findings
Reflex-mediated	Vasovagal	Presyncopal symptoms after sudden unpleasant experience	Unexplained bruising or injury
	Situational (e.g., cough, defecation)	Specific activity before episode	Unexplained bruising or injury
	Orthostatic	Rising from recumbent position, anti-hypertensive or diuretic use	Pulse and blood pressure changes consistent with orthostasis
Cardiac	Valvular or outflow tract obstruction	History of CHF, exertional dyspnea	Cardiac murmur
	Arrhythmia	History of CAD, no prodromal symptoms	Unexplained bruising or injury. Lack of prodrome often results in significant injury
	MI, coronary spasm	History of CAD, chest pain, or exertional dyspnea	Diaphoresis, pallor
Neurologic	Seizure	Witnessed episode, postictal confusion	Tongue injury or loss of bowel/ bladder function
	TIA	Motor or speech deficits	Neurologic deficits
	Migraine	Headache (may have vertigo or dysarthria with basilar migraine)	Photo- or sonophobia, neurologic deficits
Other	Psychiatric	Frequent episodes without clear cause	Lack of referable physical findings

CHF = congestive heart failure, CAD = coronary artery disease, MI = myocardial infarction, TIA = transient ischemic attack.

5. **What is the best means of diagnosing the underlying cause of syncope?**
   Thankfully for fans of Osler who still value the basics, an accurate history and physical examination remains the best method of diagnosing the cause of syncope. Multiple studies have

TABLE 16-2.   RISK GROUPS FOR CARDIAC SYNCOPE

High-Risk Group	Moderate-Risk Group	Low-Risk Group
Suspicion of MI	History of heart disease, but no findings consistent with an acute cardiac event	No history of cardiac disease
Acute CHF	Family history of unexplained sudden death	History or examination findings consistent with reflex-mediated syncope
Moderate/severe valvular disease by examination or echocardiogram		Normal cardiovascular and neurologic examination
History of ventricular arrhythmias		Normal ECG findings
Abnormal ECG (e.g., ischemic changes, old infarcts, arrhythmias, prolonged QT, or conduction blocks)		

MI = myocardial infarction, CHF = congestive heart failure, ECG = electrocardiogram.

reported a diagnostic yield with history and physical examination alone of between 50% and 70%. Further diagnostic testing should be targeted to findings on history or physical examination.

6. **What questions are important to ask as part of the history-taking?**
See Table 16-3.

7. **What should be checked on physical examination?**
A thorough physical examination should always be performed. However, there are certain elements to which one should pay particular attention in evaluating a patient with syncope. When taking the vital signs, one should check for changes in pulse and blood pressure consistent with orthostasis. Measure the blood pressure in each arm because subclavian steal syndrome and aortic dissection can cause differences in pulse and blood pressure between arms. Examining the skin for unexplained bruising or injury (i.e., tongue lacerations from bites) is important. Carefully auscultate the chest for murmurs (either consistent with valvular disease or an outflow tract obstruction like hypertrophic cardiomyopathy or atrial myxoma) or changes in heart sounds (e.g., an S4 or accentuated P2, which can be signs associated with pulmonary embolism). Carotid sinus massage should be done in patients in whom there is no contraindication. Performing this maneuver as part of the initial evaluation has been shown to improve the overall diagnostic yield. Lastly, a thorough neurologic examination is important. Pay attention to subtle findings like neuropathy (particularly diabetic) or loss of muscle tone (from deconditioning) that may be associated with orthostatic hypotension.

TABLE 16-3. QUESTIONS TO ASK A PATIENT WITH SYNCOPE

Question	Comment
How many episodes have you experienced?	Patients with syncope from arrhythmias often report multiple episodes. Repeated, unexplained episodes are also seen in patients with an underlying psychiatric disorder.
Have you experienced associated symptoms?	Chest pain or exertional dyspnea suggests MI or structural heart disease. Neurologic findings are associated with TIA and migraine.
Was there a prodrome?	Patients with vasovagal syncope often have classic presyncopal symptoms. Those with syncope due to arrhythmia usually have no prodromal symptoms.
Was the episode witnessed?	This is often helpful in eliciting evidence of seizure activity.
Was there any positional effect?	Patients who relate having had a syncopal episode after a change in position should prompt investigation into orthostatic hypotension.
What were the preceding events?	Patients with situational syncope (cough, micturition, defecation) provide a history of those activities immediately prior to their syncopal episode.
What was the duration of the LOC?	This can often be helpful in evaluation of arrhythmia (brief LOC) and seizure (LOC lasting for minutes).
How quick was the recovery?	Patients with syncope due to seizure often have prolonged postictal confusional states.

MI = myocardial infarction, TIA = transient ischemia attack, LOC = loss of consciousness.

8. **What diagnostic tests should be ordered?**
   There are two basic studies that should be done in all patients presenting with syncope—an electrocardiogram (ECG) and blood glucose. These are readily available and low-cost initial tests. Although the yield of each test may be low (<5% for ECG, for example), the combination of these with a thorough history and physical examination can increase diagnostic yield and point toward additional diagnostic tests that can lead to the final diagnosis. In general, basic laboratory testing such as a complete blood count and basic metabolic profile are not indicated. Specific cardiovascular testing is warranted in the event that something in the history, physical examination, or ECG results suggests an underlying cardiac cause. For example, an echocardiogram should be obtained in patients with a history of valvular or structural heart disease, or in whom the physical examination reveals a previously unevaluated murmur. Ambulatory monitoring (such as Holter or event monitoring) can be done in patients with known or suspected arrhythmias. Neurologic testing such as computed tomography (CT), electroencephalography (EEG), and transcranial or carotid Doppler imaging are often performed as part of the initial evaluation. However, the diagnostic yield of each of these tests is very low. For example, EEG and CT provide new information regarding the cause of syncope in <5% of cases (at substantially greater cost than the aforementioned ECG). Additionally, there are often findings in the history or physical examination that would have prompted the physician to subsequently

order the CT or EEG. So, in the absence of history or physical examination details pointing toward a specific neurologic cause, routine neurologic evaluation for syncope is not warranted.

Linzer M, Yang EH, Estes NA III, et al: Diagnosing syncope. Part 1. Value of history, physical examination, and electrocardiography: Clinical Efficacy Assessment Project of the American College of Physicians. Ann Intern Med 126:989–996, 1997.

KEY POINTS: DIAGNOSTIC EVALUATION OF SYNCOPE

1. History

2. Physical examination (including orthostatics, carotid sinus massage, and full neurologic examination)

3. Serum blood glucose

4. Electrocardiogram

9. **How often is the underlying cause of syncope diagnosed?**
   The underlying cause of syncope often goes undiagnosed. Several published reports place the incidence of undiagnosed syncope as high as nearly 40%. Algorithms can help lower this rate while minimizing unnecessary diagnostic evaluation. The important thing as a clinician is to try and identify those patients at high risk for death from their underlying cause and to ensure they receive a prompt, evidence-directed diagnostic evaluation.

   Kapoor WN: Current evaluation and management of syncope. Circulation 106:1606–1609, 2002.

BIBLIOGRAPHY

1. Kapoor WN: Current evaluation and management of syncope. Circulation 106:1606–1609, 2002.

2. Kapoor WN: Syncope. N Engl J Med 343:1856–1862, 2001.

3. Linzer M, Yang EH, Estes NA III, et al: Diagnosing syncope. Part 1: Value of history, physical examination, and electrocardiography: Clinical Efficacy Assessment Project of the American College of Physicians. Ann Intern Med 126:989–996, 1997.

4. Linzer M, Yang EH, Estes NA III, et al: Diagnosing syncope. Part 2: Unexplained syncope: Clinical Efficacy Assessment Project of the American College of Physicians. Ann Intern Med 127:76–86, 1997.

5. Sarasin FP, Louis-Simonet M, Carballo D, et al: Prospective evaluation of patients with syncope: A population-based study. Am J Med 111:177–184, 2001.

6. Shen WK, Decker WW, Smars PA, et al: Syncope evaluation in the emergency department study (SEEDS). Circulation 110:3636–3645, 2004.

7. Soteriades ES, Evans JC, Larson MG,, et al: Incidence and prognosis of syncope. N Engl J Med 347:878–885, 2002.

CHAPTER 17

MENINGITIS AND ENCEPHALITIS

Gentian Scheer, MD

1. **Define meningitis and encephalitis.**
   - *Meningitis* is an inflammation of the meninges.
   - *Encephalitis* is inflammation of the brain parenchyma and is characterized by cognitive deficits.

2. **What is the incidence of bacterial meningitis? Of aseptic meningitis?**
   In U.S. adults, the incidence of bacterial meningitis is 2.5–10 cases/100,000 population with an increase in winter and early spring. *Aseptic meningitis* refers to a patient with clinical and laboratory evidence of meningeal inflammation with negative bacterial cultures. The incidence of aseptic meningitis is the same as bacterial with a spike in summer and fall due to enteroviral and arboviral trends.

3. **What is the mortality rate associated with bacterial meningitis?**
   The mortality rate varies based on the host's age and immune status as well as the organism involved. Overall, the mortality rate is 25%, with mortality from meningitis caused by *Streptococcus pneumoniae* 21–32%, *Listeria monocytogenes* 15–28%, and *Neisseria meningitidis* 3–10%.

   Durand ML, Calderwood SB, Weber DJ, et al: Acute bacterial meningitis in adults: A review of 493 episodes. N Engl J Med 328:21–28, 1993.

4. **How has the epidemiology of acute bacterial meningitis changed in the last 15 years?**
   There has been a marked decline in incidence of meningitis caused by *Haemophilus influenzae* type B due to the introduction of programs for the immunization of infants.

5. **What are the most common causes of acute bacterial meningitis in adults?**
   See Table 17-1.

6. **What are the most common causes of nonbacterial meningitis?**
   See Table 17-2.

7. **What are the noninfectious causes of meningitis?**
   Posterior fossa syndrome after neurosurgery, carcinomatous meningitis, sarcoidosis, systemic lupus erythematosus, Behçet's disease, drugs (e.g., trimethoprim-sulfamethoxazole, nonsteroidal anti-inflammatory drugs, muromonab-CD3 [OKT3]), and Mollaret's meningitis, which is a chronic meningitis often associated with herpes simplex virus (HSV) infection.

8. **What historical information should be obtained when evaluating a patient for meningitis?**
   Inquire about exposure to someone with meningitis, recent infection, travel to areas with endemic disease, intravenous drug use, progressive petechial or ecchymotic rash, recent head trauma, neurosurgery or cerebrospinal fluid (CSF) shunt, and any known immunodeficiency (e.g., AIDS).

TABLE 17-1. MOST COMMON CAUSES OF BACTERIAL MENINGITIS	
Up to the Age of 18–60 years old	*Streptococcus pneumoniae* (60%)
	Neisseria meningitidis (20%)
	Haemophilus influenzae (10%)
	Listeria monocytogenes (6%)
	Group B *Streptococcus* (4%)
Age >60 years	*S. pneumoniae* (70%)
	L. monocytogenes (20%)
	N. meningitidis, Group B *Streptococcus* and
	H. influenzae (3–4% each)
Patients with underlying neoplastic disease, organ transplant recipients, or those receiving corticosteroids	*L. monocytogenes*
Patients with HIV/AIDS	*Cryptococcus neoformans*
	S. pneumoniae
	L. monocytogenes
Nosocomial bacterial meningitis	Gram-negative rods (*Escherichia coli, Klebsiella* species, *Pseudomonas aeruginosa, Acinetobacter* species, *Enterobacter* species)
	Staphylococcus
	Streptococci other than *S. pneumoniae*

9. **What is the classic symptomatic triad of bacterial meningitis? What percent of patients with bacterial meningitis have all three in the triad? What percent of patients have at least one in the triad?**

Fever, neck stiffness, and altered mental status. Approximately 45% of patients will present with all three. Between 99% and 100% of patients will have at least one sign or symptom from the triad such that a lack of all three effectively rules out meningitis.

10. **What findings should be sought on physical examination?**
    - **Nuchal rigidity:** Involves an inability to touch chin to chest.
    - **Kernig's sign:** Patient is in supine position with hips and knees flexed 90 degrees; pain is elicited with passive extension of knees.
    - **Brudzinski's sign:** Passive flexion of the neck will cause involuntary flexion of the hips while patient is in supine position.
    - **Jolt accentuation of headache:** Worsening of headache occurs with horizontal rotation of the head at a rate of 2–3 rotations/sec.
    - **Evaluate mental status and for focal neurologic deficit**.

    See also Table 17-3.

11. **Can meningitis be effectively ruled out based on the information revealed in the clinical presentation and physical examination?**

    A patient without one of the signs or symptoms of the classic triad can be effectively ruled out for meningitis with 99–100% sensitivity. All others need further clinical evaluation.

TABLE 17-2. CAUSES OF NONBACTERIAL MENINGITIS

Cause	Comments
Viral	
Enteroviruses (e.g., Coxsackie, echovirus, other nonpolio enteroviruses)	Most common cause of viral meningitis overall. Increased incidence in summer and fall. Viral culture of CSF positive in 40–80%.
HSV–1 and HSV–2	HSV–2 usually causes meningitis and is almost always associated with acute primary genital herpes infection. HSV–1 usually causes encephalitis.
EBV	
HIV	May be presenting symptom in HIV. Suspect this in anyone with risk factors for HIV.
HHV–6, –7, and –8	More common in transplant recipients.
Lymphocytic choriomeningitis virus	Most common in young adults in autumn with exposure to aerosols or rodents.
VZV	Occurs during winter and spring. More common in immunocompromised hosts.
CMV	More common in immunocompromised hosts.
Paramyxoviruses (e.g., measles, mumps)	Consider in patient with fever, nausea, and vomiting with parotitis.
Arboviruses (e.g., St. Louis encephalitis virus, California encephalitis virus, Colorado tick fever)	More common in summer and early fall.
Nonviral	
Tuberculosis	More common in immunocompromised patients. Onset is typically subacute over weeks. Hypoglycorrhagia found on CSF analysis.
Treponema pallidum	Meningitis typically occurs during primary or secondary stage.
Borrelia burgdorferi	Agent of Lyme disease. Typical onset is 2–10 weeks after rash of erythema nodosum.
Cryptococcus neoformans	More common in patients with AIDS and in transplant recipients.
Aspergillus species	
Coccidioid immitis	Fatal if untreated. Eosinophil levels may be elevated in CSF.
Candida species	

HSV = Herpes simplex virus, EBV = Epstein-Barr virus, HIV = human immunodeficiency virus, HHV = human herpes virus, VZV = varicella zoster virus, CMV = cytomegalovirus, CSF = cerebrospinal fluid.

TABLE 17-3. PHYSICAL EXAMINATION FINDINGS IN BACTERIAL MENINGITIS

Presenting Manifestation or Physical Examination Finding	Frequency of Finding in Patients with Bacterial Meningitis
Fever	77–95%
Nuchal rigidity	83–94%
Altered mental status	69–95%
	51% confused or lethargic
	22% responsive only to pain
	6% unresponsive to all stimuli
Headache	43–94%
Kernig's sign	Needs further evaluation with prospective study
Brudzinski's sign	Needs further evaluation with prospective study
Jolt accentuation of headache	97%
	Needs confirmation with prospective study
	Based on one study of 34 patients

Data from De Gans J, Van De Beek D: Dexamethasone in adults with bacterial meningitis. N Engl J Med 347:1549–1556, 2002; Durand ML, Calderwood SB, Weber DJ, et al: Acute bacterial meningitis in adults: A review of 493 episodes. N Engl J Med 328:21–28, 1993; Van de Beek D, de Gans J, Spanjaard L, et al: Clinical features and prognostic factors in adults with bacterial meningitis. N Engl J Med 351:1849–1859, 2004; and Attia J, Hatala R, Cook D, Wong JG: Does this adult patient have acute meningitis? JAMA 281:175–181, 1999.

12. **What other clinical manifestations of bacterial meningitis can occur?**
Photophobia, nausea, rash, seizures, hearing loss, and focal neurologic deficits including cranial nerve palsy, hemiparesis, and aphasia.

13. **How does the presentation of viral meningitis differ from that of bacterial meningitis?**
The clinical presentation is difficult to differentiate. However, viral infections tend to be more nonspecific with fever, headache, nausea, vomiting, photophobia, and stiff neck.

14. **Describe the rash that is typically found with meningococcal infection. Is this rash specific for meningococcus?**
The rash is typically petechial (minute hemorrhagic spots that do not blanch with pressure) and may develop into purpura (i.e., papular hemorrhages within the skin, mucous membrane, or serosal surface). This rash is not specific for meningococcal disease and can also be seen with *S. pneumoniae* and *Staphylococcal* meningitis. A maculopapular rash can also be seen with meningococcus.

15. **If meningitis is suspected, based on clinical picture and physical examination, what is the next step in evaluating a patient for meningitis?**
A sample of CSF should be obtained via a lumbar puncture. Consider whether a head computed tomography (CT) scan needs to be done before a lumbar puncture is performed. Remember, this needs to be done quickly because delays in therapy can cause an increase in adverse outcomes.

16. **What are the indications for performing a head CT before doing a lumbar puncture? Why is doing a CT scan necessary in these instances?**
A CT scan should be done before a lumbar puncture in certain clinical situations to rule out a mass effect and to prevent post–lumbar puncture cerebral herniation. A head CT scan is indicated in patients with coma, abnormal altered level of consciousness, papilledema, focal neurologic findings, papilledema, a history of impaired cellular immunity, previous central nervous system disease, or a seizure within the previous week.

17. **How often will head CT reveal an abnormality that will contraindicate performance of a lumbar puncture?**
Three to five percent will have focal or nonfocal abnormalities with mass effect. If a lumbar puncture is contraindicated, the patient should be treated empirically for meningitis.

18. **If a head CT scan is indicated, what steps should be taken *before* performing the CT scan?**
Blood culture specimens should be obtained, adjuvant dexamethasone should be considered and given before antibiotics if indicated, and empiric antibiotic therapy should be initiated immediately before the patient is sent to receive a head CT scan. Data has shown that a short elapsed time before antibiotics are administered is important to prevent negative outcomes.
See Table 17-5 for more information on choosing empiric antibiotics.

19. **Who should receive adjuvant dexamethasone? What dose is recommended, and when? What are the benefits of using adjuvant dexamethasone?**
If used appropriately, dexamethasone has been associated with improved morbidity (15% dexamethasone versus 25% placebo) and mortality (7% dexamethasone versus 15% placebo) at 8 weeks. Dexamethasone has proved beneficial for patients with *S. pneumoniae*, but not for patients with *N. meningitides*. Adults with suspected bacterial meningitis who have a Glasgow coma score of 8–11 should be given dexamethasone intravenously (0.15 mg/kg every 6 hours) prior to the administration of antibiotics and continued for 4 days. It can be discontinued if the culture is negative or shows an organism other than *S. pneumoniae*.

De Gans J, Van De Beek D: Dexamethasone in adults with bacterial meningitis. N Engl J Med 347:1549–1556, 2002.

20. **A lumbar puncture is the next step in evaluating a patient with suspected bacterial meningitis. What CSF findings do you see in bacterial meningitis and aseptic meningitis?**
See Table 17-4.

21. **What should be done when it is not clear whether the patient has bacterial or viral meningitis?**
Treat empirically with antibiotics for bacterial meningitis and wait until culture results are available (24–48 hours). If the patient is symptomatically improved and culture results are negative, the antibiotics can be stopped in most cases. If the patient has not improved, a repeat lumbar puncture should be considered. Although no controlled trials have proved the efficacy of antiviral agents in the treatment of HSV meningitis, there is anecdotal evidence of clinical improvement. Therefore, if HSV meningitis is a consideration, then empiric acyclovir (10 mg/kg intravenous every 8 hours) can be given until results of CSF analysis for HSV by polymerase chain reaction (PCR) results are available.

22. **If the Gram stain and culture results remain negative, but your suspicion of bacterial meningitis is high, what further tests can be undertaken?**
A latex agglutination test to detect antigens of *S. pneumoniae, N. meningitidis, H. influenzae* type B, group B *Streptococcus,* and *Escherichia coli* can be performed with specificity of

TABLE 17-4.	CSF FINDINGS IN MENINGITIS		
Finding	Reference Range	Bacterial Meningitis	Viral Meningitis
Opening pressure	<200 mmH$_2$O	Usually elevated; 80% have pressure >180 mm 20% have pressure >400 mm	Normal or slightly elevated
White cell count (total)	<5/mm^3	Typically 1000–5000/mm^3; range <100 to >10,000/mm^3	Typically <250/mm^3; range, 50–1000/mm^3
Differential of white cell count	Lymphocytes, 60–70%; monocytes, 30–50%; neutrophils, 0%	Neutrophils, >50–80%	Early in infection, neutrophils may dominate; changes to lymphocytic predominance in 6–48 hours into infection
Glucose	>40 mg/dL	<40 mg/dL	Normal
CSF:serum glucose ratio	>60%	<40%	>40%
Protein	<45 mg/dL	100–500 mg/dL; >45 mg/dL in 90% of patients	20–80 mg/dL
Gram stain	Negative	Positive in 60–90% of patients	Negative
Culture	Negative	Positive in 70–85% of patients	Negative

CSF = Cerebrospinal fluid.

95–100% for *S. pneumoniae* and *N. meningitidis*. It is therefore virtually diagnostic if the result is positive. The sensitivity for latex agglutination is lower, so a negative test result does not exclude the diagnosis.

23. **Which type of *bacterial* meningitis can be associated with a CSF lymphocytosis and negative Gram stain result?**
The CSF from patients with *L. monocytogenes* commonly has >25% lymphocytes. Gram stain has a low sensitivity of 0–40% for this organism. Therefore, consider *Listeria* in a patient with a negative Gram stain result but acute lymphocytic meningitis, especially if the patient is immunosuppressed.

24. **What other tests can be sent to confirm the etiology in viral meningitis?**
PCR for the enteroviruses, HSV, cytomegalovirus, Epstein-Barr virus, and varicella zoster virus.

25. **What should be done for patients with lymphocytic predominant CSF and negative bacterial cultures who fail to improve with conservative therapy?**
Repeat CSF analysis for fungal and mycobacterial cultures. Consider HIV testing, Lyme serology, Venereal Disease Research Laboratory (for syphilis), and central nervous system imaging with magnetic resonance imaging or CT to rule out an abscess or other structural anomaly. Consider noninfectious causes of meningitis. Continue treatment with antibiotics and antiviral agents until a diagnosis is made.

KEY POINTS: MENINGITIS

1. Nearly 100% of patients with bacterial meningitis will have at least one sign or symptom from the "classic triad" of fever, neck stiffness, or altered mental status.

2. Although *S. pneumoniae* and *N. meningitidis* are the most common causes of bacterial meningitis in adults, *L. monocytogenes* should be considered in patients older than 50 years, organ transplant recipients, patients taking corticosteroids, and those with underlying neoplastic process.

3. Dexamethasone decreases morbidity and mortality associated with bacterial meningitis caused by *S. pneumoniae.*

4. Chemoprophylaxis is required for people exposed to patients with meningitis caused by *N. meningitidis* and *H. influenzae.*

26. **What is the recommended empiric antibiotic regimen for an adult with suspected bacterial meningitis?**
Third-generation cephalosporin. Vancomycin should be added if there has been β-lactam resistance noted locally. If the patient is older than 50 years, then add ampicillin to cover *Listeria* infection.

27. **What is the recommended treatment regimen based on Gram stain and culture of CSF?**
See Table 17-5.

28. **What is the recommended empiric antibiotic regimen for an adult with a nondiagnostic Gram stain of CSF who has impaired cellular immunity? What if the patient has a history of head trauma, neurosurgery, or CSF shunt?**
In the case of impaired cellular immunity, consider *L. monocytogenes* or gram-negative bacilli as the infecting agent and treat empirically with ampicillin, ceftazidime, and vancomycin.
A history of head trauma, neurosurgery, or CSF shunt increases the likelihood of staphylococci, gram-negative bacilli, pseudomonas, or *S. pneumoniae,* so empiric treatment should include vancomycin and ceftazidime.

29. **What is the recommended treatment for suspected aseptic meningitis?**
Consider empiric antibiotics if the patient is elderly or immunocompromised or if he or she has recently received antibiotics because these patients may actually have bacterial meningitis. Empiric acyclovir 10 mg/kg administered intravenously every 8 hours can be given for empiric treatment of suspected HSV meningitis until results of a PCR are available. The patient may be admitted for observation until symptoms improve.

TABLE 17-5. TREATMENT OF BACTERIAL MENINGITIS

Type of Bacteria	Choice of Antibiotic
On Gram staining	
Cocci	
Gram-positive	Vancomycin plus third-generation cephalosporin. If adjunctive dexamethasone is given in adults, the preferred regimen is ceftriaxone plus rifampin.
Gram-negative	Penicillin G
Bacilli	
Gram-positive	Ampicillin or penicillin G plus aminoglycoside
Gram-negative	Third-generation cephalosporin plus aminoglycoside. If the patient has recent head trauma or neurosurgery, or for those with CSF shunts, ceftazidime is recommended.
On Culture	
S. pneumoniae	Vancomycin plus third-generation cephalosporin. If MIC for cefotaxime or ceftriaxone is >0.5 μg/mL, then continue vancomycin with third-generation cephalosporin.
H. influenzae	Ceftriaxone
N. meningitidis	Penicillin G
L. monocytogenes	Ampicillin plus gentamicin
Streptococcus agalactiae	Penicillin G
Enterobacteriaceae	Broad-spectrum cephalosporin plus aminoglycoside
Pseudomonas aeruginosa or *Acinetobacter*	Ceftazidime plus aminoglycoside

CSF = Cerebrospinal fluid, MIC = minimal inhibitory concentration.

30. **What are the risk factors for an adverse outcome from bacterial meningitis?**
    Patients who are older than 50 years or who present with hypotension, seizures, or focal neurologic findings are at high risk for adverse outcomes. Additionally, a Glasgow Coma Scale score of <10 or an Acute Physiology and Chronic Health Evaluation (APACHE) II score of >13 portends a bad prognosis.

31. **What neurologic complications can result from bacterial meningitis?**
    Up to 23% of patients can experience seizures. An additional 28% will develop focal neurologic deficits such as hemiparesis, aphasia, or gaze preference. Sensorineural hearing loss complicates 12% of cases. All complications are more common with *S. pneumoniae* meningitis than with *N. meningitidis*. Specifically, 27% of patients with pneumococcal meningitis will develop neuropsychologic impairment compared with only 4% with *Neisseria* infection.

32. **What infections require chemoprophylaxis for contacts, and to whom do you provide chemoprophylaxis?**
    - ***N. meningitidis***: Close contacts of an isolated case of invasive meningococcal infection including household members and other intimate contacts, children in school environments,

coworkers in the same office, young adults in dormitories, and recruits in military training centers. Health care workers do not require prophylaxis unless there is direct exposure to respiratory secretions, such as with suctioning or intubation. The Centers for Disease Control and Prevention recommends rifampin 600 mg PO q12 h × 4 doses, ciprofloxacin 500 mg PO once, or ceftriaxone 250 mg IM once.

- **H. influenzae**: Chemoprophylaxis for household or day-care classroom contacts of patients with *H. influenzae* disease should be directed at both vaccinated and unvaccinated contacts because immune persons may asymptomatically carry and transmit the organism. If every child in a household or day-care classroom has been fully vaccinated, chemoprophylaxis is unnecessary. The suggested regimen is rifampin 20 mg/kg with maximum of 600 mg/day for 4 days.

33. **What is the incidence of encephalitis in the United States?**
Approximately 20,000 reported cases per year, with the actual number likely being much higher.

34. **How does the clinical picture of encephalitis differ from that of meningitis?**
A patient with encephalitis commonly has confusion, behavioral abnormalities, altered level of consciousness, and evidence of focal or diffuse neurologic signs. Altered consciousness may range from lethargy to deep coma.

35. **What are the most common causes of encephalitis?**
See Table 17-6.

TABLE 17-6.	CAUSES OF ENCEPHALITIS	
Common	**Less Common**	**Rare**
HSV–1	CMV	Adenovirus
Arboviruses	EBV	CTFV
Enteroviruses	HIV	Hepatitis C
	Mumps	Influenza A
		LCMV
		Rotavirus
		Rubella

HSV = Herpes simplex virus, CMV = cytomegalovirus, EBV = Epstein-Barr virus, HIV = human immunodeficiency virus, CTFV = Colorado tick fever virus, LCMV = lymphocytic choriomeningitis virus.

36. **What are the CSF findings in persons with encephalitis?**
A lumbar puncture should be performed in all patients with suspected encephalitis, unless contraindicated. CSF findings in persons with encephalitis are indistinguishable from viral meningitis and are characterized by lymphocytic pleocytosis with white blood cell count of 5–100 cm^3, a mildly elevated protein level, and a normal glucose level.

37. **What confirmatory tests are done to diagnose the cause of encephalitis?**
CSF PCR has become the primary diagnostic test for HSV, Epstein-Barr virus, varicella zoster virus, and enteroviruses. Culture is usually not helpful in viral encephalitis. Detection of West Nile virus by immunoglobulin M is diagnostic.

38. What is the empiric treatment for a patient with encephalitis?
Acyclovir (10 mg/kg) should be given intravenously every 8 hours for 14 days. Ganciclovir or foscarnet may be used for cytomegalovirus-related encephalitis.

39. Is there any specific antiviral therapy for West Nile virus?
No, only supportive care.

BIBLIOGRAPHY

1. Attia J, Hatala R, Cook D, Wong JG: Does this adult patient have acute meningitis? JAMA 281:175–181, 1999.

2. De Gans J, Van De Beek D: Dexamethasone in adults with bacterial meningitis. N Engl J Med 347:1549–1556, 2002.

3. Durand ML, Calderwood SB, Weber DJ, et al: Acute bacterial meningitis in adults: A review of 493 episodes. N Engl J Med 328:21–28, 1993.

4. Flores-Cordero JM, Amaya-Villar R, Rincon-Ferrari MD, et al: Acute community-acquired bacterial meningitis in adults admitted to the intensive care unit: clinical manifestations, management and prognostic factors. Intens Care Med 29:1967–1973, 2003.

5. Gopal AK, Whitehouse JD, Simel DL, Corey GR: Cranial computed tomography before lumbar puncture: A prospective clinical evaluation. Arch Intern Med 159:2681, 1999.

6. Hasbun R, Abrahams J, Jekel J, Quagliarello VJ: Computed tomography of the head before lumbar puncture in adults with suspected meningitis. N Engl J Med 345:1727–1733, 2001.

7. Quagliarello VJ, Scheld WM: Treatment of bacterial meningitis. N Engl J Med 336:708–716, 1997.

8. Van de Beek D, de Gans J, McIntyre P, Prasad K: Corticosteroids in acute bacterial meningitis. Cochrane Database Syst Rev, 2003. CD004305

9. Van de Beek D, de Gans J, Spanjaard L, et al: Clinical features and prognostic factors in adults with bacterial meningitis. N Engl J Med 351:1849–1859, 2004.

CHAPTER 18

DELIRIUM AND DEMENTIA IN THE HOSPITALIZED PATIENT

Melissa L.P. Mattison, MD

1. What is dementia, and how common is it in hospitalized patients?

Dementia is a syndrome of acquired, progressive, permanent, cognitive, functional, psychiatric, and behavioral decline most commonly seen in the elderly population. A person with dementia develops the condition gradually over time and is not otherwise suffering from a delirious state. Approximately 6% of patients aged 65–69 years old admitted to the hospital are said to suffer from moderate-severe dementia, increasing to nearly 21% in patients aged 80 years or more.

> Erkinjuntti T, Autio L, Wikstrom J: Dementia in the medical wards. J Clin Epidemiol 41:123–126, 1988.

2. Is a patient with dementia prone to a longer length of stay (LOS)?

Yes. One study found the mean LOS was 10.4 days for demented patients compared with 6.5 days for those without dementia. Patients with dementia are also more prone to develop delirium, which is also associated with a longer LOS. In fact, another study showed that up to 41% of patients with dementia were delirious at the time of admission.

> Erkinjuntti T, Wikstrom J, Palo J, Autio L: Dementia among medical inpatients: Evaluation of 2000 consecutive admissions. Arch Intern Med 146:1923–1926, 1986.
> Lyketsos CG, Sheppard JM, Rabbins PV: Dementia in elderly persons in a general hospital. Am J Psychiatry 157:704–747, 2000.

3. What are the potentially reversible causes of cognitive impairment?

Cognitively impaired patients should undergo testing for potentially reversible causes. Many disorders can cause cognitive impairment such as delirium, hypothyroidism, depression, vitamin B_{12} (cobalamin) deficiency, and drug toxicity. Depending on the patient's clinical history, other causes that might be considered include tertiary syphilis, subdural hematoma, normal pressure hydrocephalus, infection, malignancy, and hypercalcemia. Only when the clinical criteria are met and there is no potentially reversible cognitive impairment should a patient be diagnosed with dementia.

4. Is dementia treatable? If so, should the administration of medication be started in the hospital?

If a patient has suspected multi-infarct dementia, risk modification with aspirin and/or hydroxymethylglutaryl (HMG)–CoA reductase inhibitor (i.e., a "statin") should be considered. Pharmacologic treatments to slow or palliate cognitive decline such as cholinesterase inhibitors are a treatment option in most patients with a diagnosis of dementia. As always, it is best to start a new medication when a patient is otherwise stable and not suffering from a new medical problem or exacerbation of a chronic illness. Appropriate follow-up to monitor for adverse effects and the need for upward titration in 2–4 weeks should be arranged.

5. Is there a cure for dementia? What is the life expectancy of a patient diagnosed with dementia?

There is no cure for dementia. Most patients are not diagnosed until 1–3 years after their symptoms begin. The rate of cognitive decline varies from person to person, but the average length of time a person suffers from dementia is approximately 10–12 years (Table 18-1).

	Mini-Mental Status Examination Score	Years from Onset of Symptoms	Findings
Stage			
Preclinical	26–30	–	Mild language or executive dysfunction
Mild	22–28	1–3	Disoriented to time; trouble recalling recent events; poor insight; personality changes
Moderate	10–21	2–8	Disoriented to time and place; getting lost; trouble with self care; behavioral disturbances
Severe	0–9	6–12	No memory; unable to care for self; generally unable to communicate verbally; behavioral disturbances

TABLE 18-1. STAGES OF DEMENTIA

Adapted from Reuben DB, Herr KA, Pacala JT, et al. Geriatrics at Your Fingertips, 7th ed. The American Geriatrics Society, 2005. Available at: http://www.geriatricsatyourFingertips.org/ebook/gayf_9. asp#c9s3_PROGRESSION_OF_AD.

6. **Does artificial feeding (e.g., via a gastrostomy or jejunostomy tube) prolong the life expectancy of a person with dementia or stop recurrent aspiration?**
No. Studies have shown that patients with dementia who are carefully hand fed live as long as demented patients fed artificially. Moreover, gastrostomy and jejunostomy tubes do not decrease the risk of aspiration pneumonia. Studies evaluating patients with metastatic cancer have shown that with proper mouth care and nursing, there is little to no report of discomfort associated with poor oral intake.

KEY POINTS: DEMENTIA

1. All patients suspected of suffering from dementia should undergo testing for potentially reversible forms of cognitive impairment.

2. Patients with dementia commonly develop super-imposed delirium during hospitalization.

7. **Define *delirium*.**
Delirium is an acute confusional state. The *Confusion Assessment Method* is used to diagnose delirium. The patient must have features 1 and 2 and either 3 or 4:
1. Acute onset and fluctuating course
and
2. Inattention
and either
3. Disorganized thinking
or
4. Altered level of consciousness

Inouye, SK, van Dyck CH, Alessi CA, et al: Clarifying confusion: The Confusion Assessment Method: a new method for detection of delirium. Ann Intern Med 113:941–948, 1990.

8. **How common is delirium in a hospitalized patient? How frequently does it go undetected by clinicians?**

Delirium is very common in hospitalized patients, especially in the geriatric population. For example, it occurs in up to two-thirds of all patients admitted to the hospital with a hip fracture. It is a costly and morbid diagnosis and increases a patient's LOS significantly. There are three types of delirium: hyperactive (25%), hypoactive (50%), and mixed (25%). Up to 70% of cases of delirium may be unrecognized, in part because many cases of delirium are of the hypoactive subtype. These patients may be quiet and not actively drawing attention to their deficits or confused state. The clinician must have a heightened level of suspicion to diagnose delirium in these patients. Patients who suffer hyperactive symptoms are more readily identified by staff because they frequently call out, are agitated (e.g., pulling at their bed sheets, intravenous lines, or catheters), and may wander, if able.

9. **What are the common causes of delirium in a hospitalized patient?**

See Table 18-2.

TABLE 18-2.	COMMON CAUSES OF DELIRIUM
D	Drugs (e.g., sedatives, opiates, anticholinergics)
E	Electrolyte abnormalities (e.g., sodium imbalance, hypercalcemia, dehydration)
L	Lack of drugs (e.g., pain relief, withdrawal)
I	Infection (e.g., UTI, pneumonia)
R	Reduced sensory input (e.g., hearing or visual impairment)
I	Intracranial event (e.g., stroke, SDH)
U	Urinary retention/fecal impaction
M	Myocardial (e.g., ischemia, arrhythmia, CHF)

UTI = urinary tract infection, SDH = subdural hematoma, CHF = congestive heart failure.

10. **Which drugs are most commonly associated with delirium?**

Prescribing drugs in an elderly and/or delirious patient should be undertaken with caution. Many drugs can exacerbate or even cause confusion in the elderly, including analgesics, anticholinergics, antiepileptics, benzodiazepines and other sedatives, digoxin, dopamine-activating drugs, and H_2-receptor blockers. In addition, the use of three or more new medications increases a patient's risk of developing delirium.

Fick DM, Cooper JW, Wade WE, et al: Updating the Beers Criteria for Potentially Inappropriate Medication Use in Older Adults. Arch Intern Med 163:2716–2725, 2003.

Inouye SK, Charpentier PA: Precipitating factors for delirium in hospitalized elderly persons: Predictive model and interrelationship with baseline vulnerability. JAMA 275:852–857, 1996.

11. **Name some risk factors for developing delirium.**

Polypharmacy, dehydration, severe illness, the presence of physical restraints, bladder catheterization, malnourishment, and cognitive, visual, or hearing impairment all increase a patient's risk of developing delirium.

12. **Describe how to evaluate and manage a patient with suspected delirium.**

Determine and treat underlying causes. A thorough medical assessment for potentially reversible causes should be undertaken. This should include a physical examination and may include blood chemistries, a complete blood cell count, electrocardiography, and chest x-ray.

Stop the administration of unnecessary or potentially inappropriate medications. Remember that a delirious state may take days to weeks to resolve fully. Reorient, redirect, and restore a calm, quiet environment. Restore day-night orientation. Have family or a familiar person stay with the patient. Avoid restraints, and do not prescribe a therapy until the patient has been fully evaluated and a cause found.

13. **How can delirium be prevented?**
See Table 18-3.

TABLE 18-3. DELIRIUM PREVENTION	
Risk Factor	**Intervention to Prevent Delirium**
Cognitive impairment, as defined by MMSE score of <20	Orientation: Present a board with names of care-team members and the day's schedule; provide communication to reorient patient to surroundings. Activities: Introduce cognitively stimulating activities several times daily.
Sleep deprivation	Establish a nonpharmacologic sleep protocol at bedtime (e.g., warm milk, relaxation tapes or music, back massage). Institute unit-wide noise reduction (e.g., silent pill crushers, vibrating beepers, and quiet hallways) and schedule adjustments to allow sleep (e.g., rescheduling of medications and procedures).
Immobility	Early mobilization: Ambulation or active range of motion exercises should be performed three times daily, with minimal use of immobilizing equipment (e.g., bladder catheters or physical restraints).
Visual impairment: for patients with <20/70 visual acuity on binocular near vision testing	Provide visual aids (e.g., glasses or magnifying glasses) and adaptive equipment (e.g., large illuminated telephone keypads, large-print books, and fluorescent tape on call bell) with daily reinforcement on their use.
Hearing impairment: patients hearing ≤6 of 12 whispers on Whisper Test	Provide portable amplifying devices, earwax disimpaction, and special communication techniques, with daily reinforcement of these adaptations.
Dehydration: patients with ratio of blood urea nitrogen to creatinine of ≥18	Encourage oral intake of fluids.

MMSE = mini-mental status examination.
Adapted from Inouye SK, Bogardus ST, Charpentier PA, et al: A multicomponent intervention to prevent delirium in hospitalized older patients. N Engl J Med 340:669–676, 1999.

14. **How can delirium be prevented in the perioperative period specifically?**
Early identification of at-risk patients is imperative. Postoperative pain control can be particularly challenging. Scheduling around-the-clock acetaminophen as well as offering small doses of

morphine (e.g., 1–2 mg given intravenously or subcutaneously) periodically can be helpful. Starting a good bowel regimen to avoid constipation and early removal of indwelling urinary catheters may help. Additionally, have physical therapy and nursing personnel work to mobilize the patient as soon as possible postoperatively.

15. **Should physical restraints be used?**
When a patient is confused and agitated, caregivers often feel the need to physically restrain a patient for safety. Restraints include side-rails and vest and wrist restraints. Physically restraining a patient is dangerous and can contribute to patient injury, strangulation, and falls and should be avoided. Providing 1:1 supervision with a "sitter" is often a better solution. If a patient wishes to walk or "wander" through the unit and it is medically safe for him or her to do so, allow the patient to wander in the company of the sitter.

KEY POINTS: DELIRIUM

1. Delirium is common, costly, and morbid.

2. The risk of developing delirium can be lowered by identifying high-risk patients early in the course of their hospitalization and implementing nonpharmacologic delirium prevention treatments.

3. Medication to treat delirium should be used as a last resort, after the patient has been fully examined and a cause found.

16. **How can aspiration be prevented?**
A patient should be sitting upright at at least a 30-degree angle in bed. This will help prevent aspiration of gastric contents. A patient should only be offered food or liquid when he or she is fully awake and with an intact gag reflex. If there is any doubt, a test performed by a swallowing expert may be indicated. Alternatively, cautiously offer a trial of thickened liquids and soft solids with supervision. Of note, thin liquids (e.g., water) are the most difficult to swallow without aspiration and should not be offered if there is concern for aspiration.

17. **What drugs are used to treat delirium and agitation associated with dementia?**
Neuropsychiatric symptoms of dementia (e.g., agitation, wandering, hallucinations, repetitive behaviors or vocalizations) and delirium can be troubling to caregivers. Nonpharmacologic treatments should be considered first. Medications, particularly antipsychotic agents, have been used to help control these types of behavior, although their effects seem to be minimal. Medication use should be limited and its necessity and effectiveness readdressed at short intervals (Table 18-4).

Sink KM, Holden KF, Yaffe K: Pharmacologic treatment of neuropsychiatric symptoms of dementia. JAMA 293:596–608, 2005.

WEBSITE

Geriatrics At Your Fingertips:
http://www.geriatricsatyourfingertips.org/

TABLE 18-4. DRUGS USED TO TREAT DELIRIUM

Drug	Mechanism of Action	Starting Dose	Frequency	Titration	Clearance	Some Potential Adverse Effects
Typical Antipsychotic						
Haloperidol	Exact mechanism of action unknown; selectively antagonizes dopamine D2 receptors	0.5 mg po	Up to 4× daily	0.5 mg/dose; maximum dose, 100 mg/day*	Liver; CYP450:2D6 substrate/inhibitor 3A4 substrate; half-life, 21–24 hours	Extrapyramidal side effects (EPS), neuroleptic malignant syndrome (NMS), tardive dyskinesia, arrhythmias, hypotension, seizures, jaundice
Atypical Antipsychotics						
Olanzapine	Exact mechanism of action unknown; thought to antagonize dopamine D2 receptors, serotonin 5-HT2 receptors	2.5 mg po	Once or twice daily	Increase by 2.5 mg/dose every 1–2 days; maximum dose, 20 mg/day*	Liver; CYP450:2D6 substrate with active metabolite	EPS, NMS, somnolence, weight gain, insomnia, and agitation
Quetiapine	Exact mechanism of action unknown; thought to antagonize dopamine D2 receptors, serotonin 5-HT2 receptors	12.5 mg po	Twice daily	Increase by 12.5 mg/dose every 1–2 days; maximum dose, 800 mg/day*	Liver extensively; CYP450:3A4 substrate	EPS, NMS, somnolence, weight gain, insomnia, and agitation

Continued

TABLE 18-4.   DRUGS USED TO TREAT DELIRIUM—CONT'D

Drug	Mechanism of Action	Starting Dose	Frequency	Titration	Clearance	Some Potential Adverse Effects
Risperidone	Exact mechanism of action unknown; thought to antagonize dopamine D2 receptors, serotonin 5-HT2 receptors	0.25 mg po	Daily	0.25–0.5 mg per day every 2–7 days; maximum dose, 16 mg/day*; risk of EPS > 6 mg/day	Liver, CYP450:2D6 substrate with active metabolite; half-life, 20 hours	EPS, NMS, somnolence, weight gain, insomnia, and agitation
Short- to Medium-Acting Benzodiazepines						
Alprazolam	Bind to benzodiazepine receptors and enhance GABA effects	0.25 mg po	Up to tid	0.25 mg/dose; maximum dose, 4 mg/day	Liver	Sedation, weakness, syncope, respiratory depression, confusion, hypotension
Lorazepam	Bind to benzodiazepine receptors and enhance GABA effects	0.5 mg po or IV	Up to tid	0.5 mg/dose; maximum dose, 10 mg/day	Liver	Sedation, weakness, syncope, respiratory depression, confusion, hypotension
Oxazepam	Bind to benzodiazepine receptors and enhance GABA effects	10 mg po	Up to 4× daily	10 mg/dose	Liver	Sedation, weakness, syncope, respiratory depression, confusion, hypotension

*Maximum dose listed as generally published in the pharmaceutical literature for use in acute psychosis. One should aim for a significantly smaller dose in the elderly as a maximal dose for use in the setting of neuropsychiatric features of delirium and dementia is not known. Higher doses of these medications are not likely to be more effective and may be associated with significant adverse effects.

BIBLIOGRAPHY

1. Hazzard WR, Blass JP, Hlater JB, et al: Principles of Geriatric Medicine and Gerontology.
2. Landefeld CS, Palmer R, Johnson MA, et al: Current Geriatric Diagnosis and Treatment.

EVALUATION OF THE PATIENT WITH DYSPNEA OR HYPOXIA

James H. Williams, Jr, MD

CHAPTER 19

1. **What is dyspnea? What stimulates it?**
   Dyspnea, or the sensation of being "short of breath," is primarily driven by three stimuli:
   - **Hypoxia:** Sensed by multiple baroreceptors, hypoxia is generally the result of perfusion of poorly ventilated regions of the lung (low ventilation-perfusion mismatch [V/Q]). This problem is magnified by low venous oxygen saturation (SvO_2) returning to the lung to shunt through these poorly ventilated regions, which can result from low oxygen delivery (DO_2) and/or increased oxygen consumption (VO_2).
   - **Acidosis:** Primarily sensed by a receptor in the brain stem sensitive to pH (cerebrospinal fluid [CSF] > blood), acidosis occurs when a rise in blood pCO_2 crosses the blood-brain barrier to acutely drop CSF pH, which gradually is corrected by production of bicarbonate. Hypercapnia alone is a weak stimulus, after CSF pH has been corrected over time with increased bicarbonate.
   - **Insufficient chest inflation:** This occurs via stretch receptors in lung and chest wall.

2. **What are some common, rapidly treatable causes of acute hypoxia?**
   These may be organized into several categories, outlined in Table 19-1, based on similar etiology and approach to acute management. The use of positive pressure ventilation (PPV) via noninvasive ventilation (NIV) with a mask or invasive ventilation with an endotracheal tube (ETT) is covered in more detail in Chapter 10. Poor matching of ventilation (V) and perfusion (Q) is the usual cause of dyspnea, with low V/Q causing hypoxia from shunting of venous blood, high V/Q causing hypercapnia from wasted ventilation, and low V causing both hypercapnia and hypoxia because of inadequate ventilation.

3. **What are five physiologic causes of hypoxia?**
   - V/Q mismatch
   - Frank shunt (V/Q = 0) (Fig. 19-1)
   - Diffusion abnormalities (usually less impact than V/Q mismatch)
   - Hypoventilation
   - Low FiO_2 (e.g., at high altitude)

4. **Can the A-a gradient be used to differentiate causes of hypoxia?**
   Not reliably, although a larger (A-a) gradient generally reflects increased lung areas of low V/Q, particularly shunt (V/Q = 0). The A-a gradient represents the difference between the partial pressure of oxygen in the alveolar (A) and arterial (a) spaces, calculated as follows: $A - a (O_2) = (FiO_2 \times (P_{atm} - 47 \text{ mmHg}) - (PaCO_2/0.8) - PaO_2$. In this equation, FiO_2 is the fraction of oxygen in the inspired gas (%/100), P_{atm} is barometric pressure in that location, 47 mmHg represents water vapor pressure at 37°C at sea level, 0.8 represents the estimated respiratory quotient for production of CO_2 from O_2 during metabolism, and partial pressure in mmHg of carbon dioxide and oxygen in blood are designated $PaCO_2$ and PaO_2, respectively.

   Unfortunately, these variables are not reliably known in a given patient. More importantly, arterial PaO_2 is affected by factors other than shunt fraction. In particular, the partial pressure of oxygen in mixed venous blood (PvO_2) on passing through the shunt bed has a proportionally greater impact on mixed arterial saturation (low PvO_2 reduces PaO_2) after admixing in the left

TABLE 19-1. COMMON CAUSES AND TREATMENT OF HYPOXIA

General Problem	Specific Problem	Management (General Rx and Then Specific Rx)
Airway obstruction		Clear airway (suction), apply oxygen, consider PPV
	Bronchospasm	Neb, bronchodilators (albuterol + ipratropium = DuoNeb)
	Laryngospasm	Neb (racemic epinephrine), head positioning, consider ETT/trach
	Posterior tongue	Oral airway, body position up, head to side, consider ETT
	Foreign body	Remove foreign body (forceps, laryngoscope, bronchoscope), consider ETT
	ETT malposition	Check position (18–24 cm at teeth, avg 21–22 cm), listen to BS: *High:* balloon above cords → air leak at throat *Low:* near carina left lung weak BS, lower → RUL (right upper lobe) poor BS
	Mucus plugging	Hydrate airway, neb [DuoNeb, mucolytic (20% NAC× 2–3 mL)], and heparin 5000 or 10,000 units in 1 mL, max 30–40,000 U/day)
Low ventilation ($\uparrow PCO_2$)		Support ventilation (PPV) as needed, Rx specific problem
	Weak effort	Reverse sedation, consider PPV (NIV if mild, reversible)
	Pleural fluid or air	Thoracentesis (14G or larger catheter) or indwelling tube
	Tension pneumothorax	Thoracentesis (14G or larger catheter) or indwelling tube, preferably after CXR to confirm safe location
High and low V/Q ($\uparrow PCO_2$ and $\downarrow PO_2$)	COPD/asthma	Nebs (DuoNeb) and steroids, if PPV, use shorter I-time, less PEEP, note nasal rather than full face mask usually tolerated better here
Low V/Q ($\downarrow PO_2$)		Supplemental oxygen (O_2), ± PPV, as NIV with mask, or intubation (ETT)
	Atelectasis	Stimulate cough and deep breath, reverse sedation, evacuate fluid or air if accumulating in pleural space, PPV as IPPB (intermittent positive pressure breathing), CPAP/BIPAP mask, ETT ventilation
	Pulmonary edema	Diuresis, PPV
	ARDS	Diuresis, PPV (longer I-time, PEEP), see O_2 delivery issues on following page
	Thromboemboli	Thrombolysis improves gas exchange faster than heparin alone, but 3× the risk of hemorrhage limits overall impact
	Pneumonia	May respond to PPV, mucus Rx, pending antibiotic response

TABLE 19-1. COMMON CAUSES AND TREATMENT OF HYPOXIA—CONT'D

General Problem	Specific Problem	Management (General Rx and Then Specific Rx)
Low DO_2	Cardiac ischemia	Nitrates, ASA, beta blockers as tolerated
	Low preload	IV fluids, and if PPV, reduce rapidly as possible to promote venous return (e.g., no PEEP, pressure support ventilation, or shortest I-time possible, at lowest pressure adequate)
	Cardiomyopathy	Inotropes if not ischemic, vasodilators if not hypotensive
	Anemia	Correct to Hb $\geq$ 10, consider higher if severe hypoxia
High VO_2		Decrease metabolic needs
	Fever	Antipyretics, anti-infectives
	Agitation	Sedation, paralysis only if sedation alone inadequate

Rx = treatment, PPV = positive pressure ventilation, neb = nebulize, DuoNeb = albuterol + ipratropium nebulization, ETT = endotracheal tube, trach = tracheostomy, BS = breath sounds, NAC = N-acetylcysteine (e.g., Mycomyst), NIV = noninvasive ventilation, CXR = chest x-ray, COPD = chronic obstructive pulmonary disease, V = ventilation, Q = perfusion, V/Q = matching of ventilation and perfusion where high V/Q = wasted ventilation or dead space and low V/Q = poor oxygen uptake or shunt, CPAP = continuous positive airway pressure (implies one set pressure), BIPAP = bilevel positive airway pressure, ARDS = adult respiratory distress syndrome, I-time = inspiratory time (inspiratory time in pressure control = [inversely] peak flow in volume control [slower flow = longer time]), PEEP = positive end-expiratory pressure, O_2 = oxygenation, DO_2 = delivery of oxygen (to body), ASA = aspirin, IV = intravenous, Hb = hemoglobin, VO_2 = consumption of oxygen (by body).

atrium with blood from well-ventilated regions, also with progressively more impact as V/Q declines in various units. Raising the FiO_2 has more impact on dissolved blood oxygen tension than total oxygen content of arterial blood (CaO_2) because hemoglobin saturation (SaO_2) is the primary carrier of oxygen in blood, unless the hemoglobin concentration [Hb gm/dL] is very low. Regardless, the response to supplemental oxygen provides some insight into the degree of low V/Q areas, which at its most severe reflects a shunt. As such, noting the PaO_2/FiO_2 can be more helpful. Largely shunted blood (perfusion of unventilated regions, or intracardiac shunt) leads to marked hypoxia, refractory to increasing FiO_2, so oxygen saturation remains low even if the FiO_2 is increased. Examples include dense alveolar filling such as occurs in acute respiratory distress syndrome (ARDS) or a cardiac septal defect in the face of rising right-sided pressures. The PaO_2/FiO_2 is often <200. Mixed patterns of milder V/Q mismatch, with little frank shunt, tend to be more easily corrected with oxygen supplementation. Examples include mild asthma and chronic obstructive pulmonary disease (COPD) and "walking pneumonia," wherein hypoxic vasoconstriction has adequately redistributed blood to an adequate remaining supply of near normal V/Q units. The PaO_2/FiO_2 is commonly 300–500.

5. **What are important symptoms of hypoxia?**
General symptoms of hypoxia include dyspnea, fatigue, and confusion. Chest pain of various types may emerge, including pain from increased work of breathing (often an ache under ribs), cardiac ischemia, and pleuritis (e.g., pneumonia, pericardial inflammation, pulmonary embolism). Ischemic pain may also occur in other marginally perfused organs such as the gut and lower extremities.

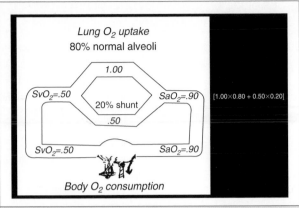

Figure 19-1. Impact of small (20%) shunt with low venous oxygen saturation (SvO_2). Clinical examples include dehydrated patients and febrile patients with pneumonia. Note the following: (1) Shunted blood not oxygenated ($= SvO_2$) mixes with oxygenated blood and lowers hemoglobin saturation (SaO_2). (2) Febrile illness increases oxygen consumption and lowers SvO_2 entering the shunt. (3) Dehydration reduces oxygen delivery, further lowering SvO_2 entering shunt.

6. **What are important signs of hypoxia?**

   Cyanosis is most often recognized at the lips and nail beds. Cardiovascular signs normally include tachycardia and hypertension as a normal sympathetic response, or bradycardia and hypotension as an abnormal response if the patient has an ischemic heart. Inadequate oxygenation of various organs may lead to altered mental status with absent focal neurologic signs and occasional seizures. Metabolic acidosis may emerge, with accumulation of lactate.

7. **When might pulse oximetry be misleading in the evaluation of patients with dyspnea or hypoxia?**

   Pulse oximetry provides a very limited view of gas exchange, estimating oxyhemoglobin and deoxyhemoglobin directly by light absorption, but not discriminating methemoglobin (met-Hb) and carboxyhemoglobin (CO-Hb) and not providing any direct information regarding PCO_2 and pH. Therefore, an arterial blood gas is usually needed to adequately evaluate patients with dyspnea or unexplained changes in mental status that might mask ineffective ventilation. If an arterial sample is not obtainable, a venous blood gas measurement can be used to estimate arterial pH and PCO_2 in most patients. Two examples in which pulse oximetry would be misleading include the following:

   - Respiratory alkalosis augments hemoglobin saturation at a lower PO_2, masking hypoxia driving hyperventilation (e.g., $pH/pCO_2/pO_2 = 7.56/20/58 = SaO_2 = 92–93\%$, but inspired oxygen should be increased).
   - Conversely, respiratory acidosis lowers SaO_2 ($pH/PCO_2/PO_2 = 7.25/60/74$, then $SaO_2 = 92–93\%$). Symptoms might include altered mental status, with or without dyspnea, and treatment should focus on increasing ventilation rather than supplemental oxygen.

8. **When applying oxygen therapy, what oxygen saturation (SpO_2) should be targeted?**

   Sufficient oxygen should be provided for adequate tissue oxygenation. Approximately 93–95% is usually desirable, but this varies with the patient's condition. For example, a higher SpO_2 is desirable with severe anemia, particularly with evidence of insufficient tissue oxygenation.

A lower SpO_2 may be adequate if the patient is comfortable and with low oxygen demands, but inadequate delivery can increase acidosis and respiratory muscle fatigue, leading to increased risk of intubation.

9. **Should one limit oxygen supplementation to avoid blunting hypoxic drive?**
Oxygen supplementation only occasionally promotes progressive acidosis from hypercapnia. Decreased ventilation normally is associated with a rise in $PaCO_2$ and a decline in PaO_2, both of which stimulate respiratory drive; supplemental oxygen blunts the hypoxic drive, and (theoretically) bronchodilation induced by increased airway oxygen concentration may increase ventilation to high-V/Q (dead space) areas, thereby both tolerating and promoting CO_2 retention. Limiting oxygen levels increases respiratory drive in patients with hypercapnia. However, this increases the work of breathing in a fatiguing patient and compromises oxygen delivery to fatiguing respiratory muscles and other organs risking cardiac ischemia, arrhythmias, and altered mental status, which can promote aspiration and seizures in susceptible patients. Therefore, adequate oxygenation needs to be maintained regardless, commonly targeting a PaO_2 of 60–70 or an SpO_2 of 90–93, or higher if tissue hypoxia is still evident.

10. **What are the causes of tissue hypoxia (DO_2 < metabolic needs [VO_2])?**
These include both global and local factors. Global factors include decreased PaO_2 and decreased SaO_2. When hemoglobin saturation exceeds 90% ($SaO_2 > 90$), dissolved oxygen adds little to arterial oxygen content, unless there is severe anemia or abnormal Hb binding (CO-Hb, met-Hb, sickle cell, severe acidosis). Dissolved oxygen adds more importantly to blood oxygen content in these settings. DO_2 to tissues is then dependent on cardiac output and local tissue perfusion. In healthy, young persons, cardiac output increases by several fold (from 5 to 15–20 L/min) with increasing oxygen consumption and anemia, and a limited cardiac response may lead to global tissue ischemia. Abnormal (injured) blood vessels can more selectively diminish local oxygen delivery to the tissues, exceeding metabolic demands.

11. **How does poor cardiac function cause PaO_2 and SaO_2 to change?**
There are two major ways in which cardiac performance affects arterial oxygenation. The adverse impact of pulmonary edema on oxygenation is widely appreciated, if not always recognized. Alveolar edema increases shunt (low V/Q units) in the lung. Less often recognized is the impact of decreased cardiac output on arterial oxygen levels. Both limited DO_2 and elevated metabolic needs lead to decreased SvO_2. A low SvO_2 amplifies the impact of existing alveolar shunt, decreasing mixed arterial PaO_2 and SaO_2. Extra oxygen dissolved in blood exposed to a high FiO_2 in well-ventilated regions has little impact because the oxygen content of arterial blood (CaO_2) is largely bound to hemoglobin, as the following formula shows: $CaO_2 = (Hb \times SaO_2 \times 1.34) + (PaO_2 \times 0.003)$.

12. **When are the hemodynamic effects of mechanical ventilation likely to be clinically important?**
Most commonly, PPV critically reduces preload in patients with dehydration, a condition common among patients who present with dyspnea. The further decrease in preload is proportional to the duration and magnitude of the positive pressure, which impedes venous return, commonly causing hypotension and worsening oxygenation as cardiac output falls (Fig. 19-2). On the other hand, PPV is beneficial for patients with fluid overload, maintaining alveolar inflation, diminishing pulmonary capillary hypertension, and providing time for adequate diuresis.

13. **Can NIV be used to avoid ETT intubation in patients with dyspnea?**
In general, good candidates for NIV are those with respiratory insufficiency without frank failure, as best demonstrated with congestive heart failure (CHF; responds to continuous positive airway pressure using full face mask effectively), and COPD (responds to bilevel positive airway pressure [BIPAP] with nasal mask better tolerated). Most also agree that patients with

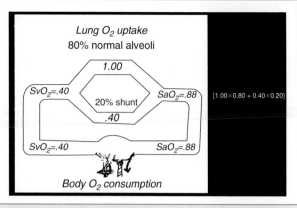

Figure 19-2. Positive pressure ventilation can worsen hemoglobin saturation (SaO_2), and declining venous oxygen saturation (SvO_2) worsens impact of shunt. Note the following: (1) PPV decrease oxygen delivery by decreasing preload (auto–positive end expiratory pressure with dehydration. (2) Oxygen consumption is increased (e.g., agitation, stimulants).

pneumonia are likely to benefit if the system can reliably provide blended oxygen at necessary concentrations, usually as BIPAP with full face mask. The role of NIV for patients after extubation is more controversial. Benefits have been reported when applied early among patients with marginal weaning parameters, but when applied late in patients already failing with hypercapnic acidosis, outcomes may be worsened by delaying intubation. In general, if patients are not improving in 1–2 hours, most clinicians would proceed to intubation. Others often excluded from NIV include patients with heavy secretions, upper gastrointestinal tract hemorrhage, facial deformities, and altered mental status.

KEY POINTS: ACUTE DYSPNEA AND HYPOXIA

1. Oxygen deprivation is an emergency that, in most circumstances, requires rapid intervention—in a matter of minutes, not hours.

2. Pulse oximetry provides a useful but sometimes misleading assessment of gas exchange that is best used to track trends in oxygenation, not to replace arterial blood gases for assessment of abnormal gas exchange in the lungs.

3. Cardiopulmonary interactions require consideration of both organ systems, as well as blood oxygen carrying capacity (Hb), for effective management of hypoxia and dyspnea.

4. Focus first on quickly treatable problems in a hypoxic patient, pursing less quickly treatable problems later.

14. **What are important initial considerations for managing a *nonintubated* patient with acute hypoxia?**
The following provides a quick list of things to do in this setting, from first to last:
1. **Increase the FIO_2:** to maintain the $SaO_2 > 93\%$, or higher.

2. **Check the arterial blood gas immediately (*do not wait* 15–30 minutes):** This confirms an adequate SpO_2 and supplemental O_2. It also potentially identifies continued distress (respiratory alkalosis) or ventilatory insufficiency (respiratory acidosis).

3. **Stimulate deep breathing and cough, and consider suctioning as needed:** Mucous plugs are a common cause of hypoxia in patients with pneumonia, COPD, sedation, and hypoventilation; atelectasis is common with pain medications and sedation.

4. **Listen and percuss the chest:** Wheezes suggest a role for a nebulized bronchodilator, or diuresis if CHF is present. Crackles suggest a role for diuresis if CHF is present. Diminished breath sounds suggest obstructed airway, atelectasis, effusion, or pneumothorax (although decreased blood pressure and tachycardia are more common with tension pneumothorax). Hollow percussion suggests pneumothorax or acute obstruction

5. **Order a chest x-ray.**

6. **Obtain an electrocardiogram:** Look for consequences of hypoxia, particularly if no other obvious cause of hypoxia evident because ischemia can lead to CHF, and decreased cardiac output can worsen the impact of an existing shunt by decreasing venous oxygenation.

7. **Check a hematocrit:** Consider acute gastrointestinal tract bleeding, which by decreasing cardiac output and Hb progressively can also lower venous O_2 and worsen the impact of existing pulmonary shunt

8. **Consider contrast pulmonary embolism study:** This can be a computed tomography (CT) angiogram or a conventional angiogram, particularly if abnormal breath sounds or plain chest film suggest ventilation-perfusion nuclear scanning would be hard to interpret.

15. **What (in addition to the above) should be considered when evaluating an *intubated and mechanically ventilated* patient with rapidly progressive hypoxia by pulse oximetry?**

   - **Suction the airway:** This will potentially clear the airway and demonstrate a clear path to the lower airways.
   - **Check ETT position:** First inspect the mouth, where the markings at the teeth should be at about 20–22 cm (varies with height). Order a stat chest x-ray to confirm the position, and listen to chest. Diminished breath sounds can reflect a ETT that is low on the opposite side (commonly, the left side is diminished). The percussion is initially hallow if acute and progressively becomes dull with atelectasis.
   - **Consider ventilator changes; this often requires trial and error:** For example, consider increased positive end-expiratory pressure (PEEP) and/or inspiratory time for CHF, ARDS, and atelectasis *but* decrease PEEP and/or inspiratory time for COPD, or if the patient appears intravascularly volume deplete. A decline in peak pressure when increasing peak flow during volume control ventilation often indicates breath stacking from inadequate exhalation time. Similarly, a rise in volume when decreasing inspiratory time in pressure control ventilation indicates stacking from inadequate exhalation time.

BIBLIOGRAPHY

1. Desai MH, Mlcak R, Richardson J, et al: Reduction in mortality in pediatric patients with inhalation injury with aerosolized heparin/N-acetylcystine therapy. J Burn Care Rehabil 19:210–212, 1998.

2. Fraser RS, Colman N, Mulle NL, Pare PD: Diagnoses of the Chest, 4th ed. Philadelphia, W.B. Saunders, 1999.

3. Smith RM: Evaluation of arterial blood gases and acid-base hemeostasis. In Bordow RA, Ries AL, Morris TA (eds): Manual of Clinical Problems in Pulmonary Medicine, 5th ed. Philadelphia, Lippincott Williams & Wilkins, 2001, pp 27–35.

CHAPTER 20

COMMUNITY-ACQUIRED PNEUMONIA

Loreno Di Francesco, MD, and Alpesh N. Amin, MD, MBA

1. **How common is community-acquired pneumonia (CAP)?**

   In the United States, there are close to 5 million cases of CAP managed each year in outpatient clinics, emergency departments, and hospitals. Four million are managed as outpatients, with the remaining 1 million patients requiring hospitalization for treatment.

2. **What is the mortality rate for CAP?**

   The estimated mortality rate for CAP is <1–5% in the outpatient setting, approximately 12% in patients requiring hospitalization, and nearly 40% in patients in the intensive care unit (ICU).

3. **What are the common symptoms of CAP?**

   The classic presentation—sudden onset of rigors followed by fever, pleurisy, and productive sputum—is found in approximately 80% of patients. Cough is present in 90% of patients and is often productive of purulent sputum. Other common symptoms include chest discomfort or pleurisy (present in 30% of patients), chills, and rigors. Atypical symptoms may include fatigue, myalgias, arthralgias, abdominal pain, nausea and vomiting, acute diarrhea, anorexia, and headache.

4. **What are the common signs of CAP?**

   Common signs of CAP include tachycardia (heart rate > 90 beats/min), tachypnea (respiratory rate > 20 breaths/min), fever (present in 80% of patients), hypoxia (pulse oximetry < 90%), and focal rales (present in 30% of patients) with signs of consolidation including increased fremitus, egophony, and whispered pectriloquy.

5. **How does one diagnose CAP?**

   There is technically no gold standard for the diagnosis of CAP. There are a number of other pulmonary and nonpulmonary processes that can mimic the presentation of CAP. Thus, the clinical diagnosis of CAP should fulfill the following four criteria:
   - Symptoms of an acute pulmonary parenchymal infection
   - Not a hospital-acquired pneumonia (HAP) or a healthcare-associated pneumonia (HCAP) or a ventilator-associated pneumonia (VAP) as defined below.

     HAP: pneumonia that occurs 48 hrs or more after hospital admission, which was not incubating at the time of admission.

     HCAP: any patient who was hospitalized in an acute care hospital for 2 or more days within 90 days of the current "pneumonia"; resided in a nursing home or long-term care facility; received recent intravenous antibiotic therapy, chemotherapy, or wound care within the past 30 days of the current infection; or attended a hospital or hemodialysis clinic.

     VAP: pneumonia that arises more than 48–72 hrs after endotracheal intubation.
   - Presence of an acute infiltrate on the chest radiography consistent with a pneumonia
   - Any CAP mimickers clinically ruled out

6. **Which common conditions can mimic CAP?**

   See Table 20-1.

TABLE 20-1. COMMUNITY-ACQUIRED PNEUMONIA MIMICKERS

Atelectasis
Cardiogenic pulmonary edema
Noncardiogenic pulmonary edema
Pulmonary embolus
Malignancy
Tuberculosis
Fungal pneumonia
Sarcoidosis
Interstitial lung disease
Vasculitis
Bronchiolitis obliterans with organizing pneumonia
Endocarditis with septic pulmonary emboli
Hypersensitivity pneumonitis
Lipoid pneumonia
Eosinophilic pneumonia

TABLE 20-2. COMMON IDENTIFIABLE CAUSES OF CAP IN NORTH AMERICA

	Percentage (%)
Bacteria	
Streptococcus pneumoniae	20-60
Haemophilus influenzae	3–10
Staphylococcus aureus	3–5
Gram-negative bacilli	3–10
Miscellaneous	10–20
Atypical bacteria	
Legionella species	2–8
Mycoplasma pneumoniae	1–6
Chlamydia pneumoniae	4–6
Viruses	2–15
Aspiration (anaerobic bacteria)	6–10

7. **What are the most common causes of CAP in the United States?**
In the most sophisticated studies, researchers are only able to definitively identify infectious causes of CAP in 50% of patients. The most common identifiable causes of CAP in North America are shown in Table 20-2.

8. **What is atypical CAP? Can it be clinically differentiated from typical CAP?**
Atypical CAP refers to CAP traditionally caused by the nonpyogenic bacteria such as *Chlamydia pneumoniae*, *Mycoplasma pneumoniae*, and *Legionella* species, as well as other rarer CAPs. The clinical presentation of a patient with typical pyogenic CAP and a patient with "atypical" CAP overlaps, and distinction cannot be made accurately on clinical grounds (e.g., history, physical examination, chest radiography, or standard laboratory data).

9. **What are risk factors for CAP caused by drug-resistant *Streptococcus pneumoniae* (DRSP), gram-negative bacteria, or *Pseudomonas* species?**
   - Risk factors for **DRSP** include age older than 65 years, β-lactam antibiotic use within the last 3 months, alcoholism, immunosuppression, multiple medical comorbidities, and exposure to child care facilities.
   - **Gram-negative pneumonia** risk factors include pulmonary comorbidities (e.g., asthma, chronic bronchitis), previous hospital admission for 48 hours within the last 30 days, previous antibiotics within the last 30 days, aspiration, and witnessed high-risk behavior (e.g., delirium, abnormal gag or swallow response).
   - **Pseudomonal** pneumonia risk factors include structural lung disease, corticosteroids >10 mg prednisone/day or its equivalent, antibiotic use for >7 days in past month, and malnutrition.

10. **What key epidemiologic clues might suggest the underlying CAP pathogen?**
    See Table 20-3.

TABLE 20-3. EPIDEMIOLOGIC CLUES IN CAP

Clue	Infectious Agent
Recent travel to the Southwestern United States	*Coccidioides immitis*
Exposure to bats or soil enriched with bird droppings	*Histoplasma capsulatum*
Exposure to domestic birds	*Chlamydia psittaci*
Exposure to farm animals or parturient cats	*Coxiella burnetii* (Q fever)
Exposure to rabbits	*Francisella tularensis* (tularemia)
Exposure to infected mouse urine, saliva, or stool	Hantavirus

11. **What medical risk factors predispose patients to particular respiratory pathogens?**
    See Table 20-4.

TABLE 20-4. PREDISPOSING PATIENT RISKS FOR PARTICULAR RESPIRATORY PATHOGENS

Patient Condition	Respiratory Pathogen(s)
Alcoholism	*S. pneumoniae*, anaerobes, gram-negative bacteria
COPD/smoker	*S. pneumoniae, H. influenzae, Moraxella catarrhalis, Legionella* sp.
Post-influenza	Influenza A/B, *S. aureus, S. pneumoniae*
Splenectomy (functional or surgical)	*S. pneumoniae, Neisseria menigitidis, Escherichia coli, H. influenzae*
Poor oral hygiene	Anaerobes
Aspiration risk	Anaerobes or chemical pneumonitis
Bronchiectasis, cystic fibrosis	*Pseudomonas* species, *S. aureus*
Endobronchial obstruction	Postobstructive pneumonia (anaerobes)
Nursing home resident	*S. pneumoniae, H. influenzae,* gram-negative bacteria, *S. aureus,* anaerobes
Recent broad-spectrum antibiotics	*Pseudomonas* species, gram-negative bacteria

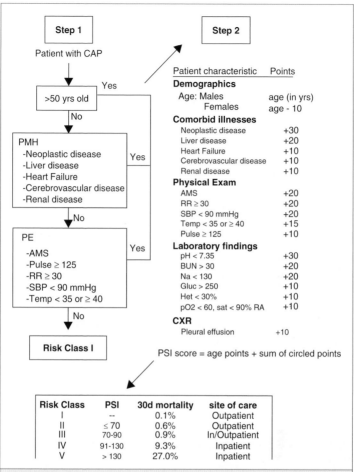

Figure 20-1. Algorithm for risk stratification using the pneumonia severity index (PSI) score in patients with community-acquired pneumonia (CAP). PMH = past medical history, PE = physical exam, AMS = altered mental status, RR = respiratory rate, SBP = systolic blood pressure, Temp = temperature, BUN = blood urea nitrogen, Na = sodium, Gluc = glucose, Hct = hematocrit, pO_2 = arterial blood oxygenation, RA = room air, CXR = chest x-ray.

12. **What is the pneumonia severity index (PSI)?**
   The PSI is a validated score performed at the time a patient presents with CAP that uses clinical, laboratory, and chest radiographic data to place patients into one of five risk classes (classes I–V). It is calculated in a two-step process outlined in Fig. 20-1. Each risk class has been validated to accurately predict a patient's 30-day risk of death and, more recently, has been found to be a reasonable triage tool to determine potential site of care (i.e., outpatient or inpatient).

13. **What are "auto admission criteria"?**
   Although many patients may seem to be at low risk according to their PSI score and risk class, there are a number of situations that increase the risk for a poor outcome that are not appropriately accounted for in the PSI. Patients with the following characteristics warrant initial

hospitalization despite a low PSI score and risk class: altered mental status, hypoxia, hypotension, intractable vomiting, suspected metastatic infectious complications (e.g., meningitis, septic arthritis, endocarditis), immunocompromised state (HIV infection, lung cancer), suspected tuberculosis or fungal pneumonia, homelessness, or elderly age with poor social support.

14. **Which patients should be admitted to the ICU?**
Patients who require mechanical ventilation or noninvasive positive pressure ventilation (i.e., bilevel positive airway pressure), those with septic shock, and those with two of the following three features (systolic blood pressure < 90 mmHg, multilobar infiltrates, or oxygenation failure with PaO_2/FiO_2 < 250) should be admitted directly to the ICU.

15. **What constitutes the basic evaluation of a patient with CAP?**
All patients being admitted to the hospital should have the following: a complete chemistry panel, complete blood count with differential and platelets, two sets of blood cultures, sputum Gram stain and culture (ideally before antibiotics), *Legionella* urinary antigen testing (all ICU patients and those at high risk), HIV testing for patients with risk factors, oxygenation determination by pulse oximetry or arterial blood gas, posteroanterior and lateral chest radiographs and lateral decubitus chest films (in patients with suspected parapneumonic effusions on posteroanterior chest radiograph).

16. **How useful is sputum Gram staining?**
Clinically, sputum Gram staining is often not very useful in guiding diagnosis or therapy. Adequate sputum samples are only attainable in approximately one third of patients. An adequate sample has <10 squamous epithelial cells and >25 polymorphonuclear cells per low-power field. One study found that sputum Gram staining had a sensitivity of 35% and specificity of 97% for identifying culture-proven *S. pneumoniae* and a sensitivity of 43%, and specificity of 99% for *Haemophilus influenzae*. The sensitivity and specificity for other organisms is currently not known.

Roson B, Carratala J, Verdaguer R, et al: Prospective study of the usefulness of sputum Gram stain in the initial approach to community-acquired pneumonia requiring hospitalization. Clin Infect Dis 31:869–874, 2000.

17. **What is the appropriate management of CAP in a patient with parapneumonic effusion?**
All CAP patients with a possible pleural effusion in association with their pneumonia (i.e., parapneumonic effusion) need to undergo evaluation to rule out a complicated pleural space infection. If a patient's lateral decubitus radiograph shows at least a 1-cm layering of pleural fluid, a diagnostic thoracentesis should be done. If the effusion does not layer, then a computed tomography scan of the chest can be used to evaluate for loculated fluid collections that require drainage. Drainage criteria for a parapneumonic effusion include pleural pus (empyema), pleural pH < 7.21, gram-positive pleural fluid, and culture-positive pleural fluid (except if *S. pneumoniae*). See Chapter 84 for more details.

18. **Initial administration of which antibiotics is recommended for hospitalized patients with CAP?**
Low-risk CAP patients (PSI score < 91) without significant cardiopulmonary disease who are admitted to the hospital can be treated with either azithromycin or a respiratory fluoroquinolone (e.g., levofloxacin, moxifloxacin, gatifloxacin) as long as they have not received that class of antibiotic in the last 90 days (to avoid potential antibiotic-resistance issues). High-risk CAP patients (PSI score > 90) with cardiopulmonary disease and patients admitted to the ICU should receive treatment with one of the following intravenous antibiotic options (as long as they have not received that class of antibiotic in the last 90 days): nonpseudomonal β-lactam (e.g.,

ceftriaxone) plus a macrolide or nonpseudomonal β-lactam plus a respiratory fluoroquinolone. Patients with risk factors for pseudomonas pneumonia (see question 9) should receive two intravenous antibiotics with adequate pseudomonas coverage (see Chapter 52 for more details.)

19. **What are the Joint Commission on Accreditation of Healthcare Organization (JCAHO) core measures for all hospitalized patients with CAP?**
    JCAHO is a quality-oversight body for health care organizations and managed care. It periodically assesses and accredits hospitals in the United States. JCAHO requires that hospitals track particular performance measures for certain common diseases in what are called "core measures," most of which have been shown to be associated with improved patient outcomes. (See Chapter 2 for more details.) The core measures for all hospitalized patients with CAP include the following:
    - Oxygenation assessment within 24 hours of admission
    - Blood cultures performed before the initiation of treatment with antibiotics
    - Antibiotic timing (triage to intravenous dose <4 hours)
    - Antibiotics consistent with Infectious Disease Society of America guidelines
    - Influenza and pneumococcal vaccine screening and administration in eligible patients before discharge
    - Smoking cessation and counseling, if patient is a tobacco user, during his or her hospital stay

20. **When is it safe to convert a patient from intravenous to oral antibiotics?**
    Hospitalized patients with CAP who reach clinical stability rarely (<1%) decompensate in the hospital and can be switched to oral antibiotics. *Clinical stability* is defined by improvement in symptoms, mental status at baseline, ability to tolerate oral medications, systolic blood pressure > 90 mmHg, heart rate < 100 beats/min, respiratory rate < 20 respirations/min, temperature < 100°F, and oxygen saturation > 90%.

KEY POINTS: COMMUNITY-ACQUIRED PNEUMONIA

1. CAP is the sixth-leading cause of death and the number one cause of infectious death in the United States.

2. Risk stratification techniques such as the PSI should be used to stratify appropriate treatment plans and location for treating CAP.

3. All patients should have a determination of their oxygenation within 24 hours of admission, blood cultures before antibiotic treatment, appropriate antibiotics within 4 hours of admission, appropriate smoking counseling, and influenza and pneumococcal vaccinations (or documentation of prior immunization) before discharge.

4. Conversion of intravenous to oral antibiotics can be used safely to optimize efficiency of inpatient management while maintaining quality of care for patients with CAP.

21. **What factors influence the choice of antibiotics when discharging a patient from the hospital?**
    - Adjust antibiotics for any definitive organism that has been isolated.
    - If an atypical pneumonia is still a possible cause, be sure to cover with a macrolide or fluoroquinolone for an appropriate length of therapy.
    - If no definitive organism was isolated, choose an oral formulation of the parenteral antibiotic used or an oral agent with a similar spectrum of activity.

22. **When is it safe to discharge a patient with CAP from the hospital?**
Most patients are candidates for early discharge from the hospital if they are clinically stable, did not have a high-risk pneumonia (e.g., *Staphylococcus* species, *Pseudomonas* species), sustained no life-threatening complications (e.g., heart failure, myocardial infarction), and have no additional reason for continued hospitalization.

23. **What patient education instructions should a CAP patient receive at the time of discharge?**
Stress the importance of compliance with the follow-up appointment, of using the full course of medications, and of smoking cessation.

24. **What is the natural history of symptom resolution in CAP patients?**
Most patients with CAP recover slowly. Despite their often quick clinical response, up to 64% of patients continue to experience >1 CAP-related symptom such as cough, shortness of breath, sputum production, chest pain, fever, or fatigue up to 6 weeks after therapy. Repeat chest radiographs are not recommended unless there is high suspicion of lung cancer or underlying structural lung disease. Depending on age and comorbidities, chest radiographic improvement may occur as fast as 2 weeks in young healthy patients, but may take up to 12 weeks for older, chronically ill patients with multilobar CAP.

Marrie TJ, Lau CY, Wheeler SL, et al: Predictors of symptom resolution in patients with community-acquired pneumonia. Clin Infect Dis. 31:1362–1367, 2000.

BIBLIOGRAPHY

1. Fine MJ, Auble TE, Yealy DM, et al: A prediction rule to identify low-risk patients with community-acquired pneumonia. N Engl J Med 336:243–250, 1997.
2. Mandell LA, Bartlett JG, Dowell SF, et al: Update of practice guidelines for the management of community-acquired pneumonia in immunocompetent adults. Clin Infect Dis 37:1405–1433, 2003.
3. Niederman MS, Mandell LA, Anzueto A, et al: For the American Thoracic Society. Guidelines for the management of adults with community-acquired pneumonia. Diagnosis, assessment of severity, antimicrobial therapy, and prevention. Am J Respir Crit Care Med 163:1730–1754, 2001.

CHAPTER 21

CHRONIC OBSTRUCTIVE PULMONARY DISEASE

Daniel D. Dressler, MD, MSc

1. **What is the definition of chronic obstructive pulmonary disease (COPD)?**
   COPD is a progressive airflow limitation that is not completely reversible and is associated with an abnormal airway inflammatory response of the lungs. It consists of small airway disease (obstructive bronchiolitis) and parenchymal destruction (emphysema).

2. **What is the impact of COPD on our society and health care system?**
   COPD is the fourth leading cause of death in the United States, resulting in more than 100,000 deaths per year. There are more than 500,000 hospitalizations and more than 16 million office visits per year due to COPD.

KEY POINTS: IMPACT OF COPD

1. Fourth leading cause of death in the United States

2. Results in more than 100,000 deaths per year

3. Leads to over 500,000 hospitalizations per year

3. **What are the common causes of COPD?**
   Although smoking is responsible for 85–90% of all cases of COPD, only a fraction of smokers acquire the disease. Other less common causes include passive smoke exposure, occupational exposures (e.g., dusts, chemicals), air pollution, and α_1 antitrypsin deficiency.

4. **What are chronic bronchitis and emphysema?**
   - **Chronic bronchitis:** Represents small airway inflammation in association with enlargement of the submucosal glands. It presents clinically with cough and sputum production for most days of at least 3 months per year over the course of 2 consecutive years.
   - **Emphysema:** Indicates destruction of alveoli and surrounding parenchyma leading to air trapping and hyperexpansion.
   The contributions of each of these processes to individual cases of COPD are variable and determine the disease presentation.

5. **What pathophysiologic changes are characteristic of COPD?**
   Peripheral small airways are the major site of obstruction, due to structural changes as well as inflammation (including airway edema and mucus hypersecretion). However, lung parenchyma, pulmonary vasculature, and larger airways are affected as well. The usual order of disease progression is as follows:
   Mucus hypersecretion $\rightarrow$ ciliary dysfunction $\rightarrow$ airflow limitation $\rightarrow$ pulmonary hyperinflation $\rightarrow$ abnormal gas exchange (ventilation-perfusion [V/Q] mismatch and hypoxia) $\rightarrow$ pulmonary hypertension $\rightarrow$ cor pulmonale

Worsening of the V/Q mismatch occurs during exacerbations due to increased airway inflammation, edema, and hypersecretion, as well as hypoxic bronchoconstriction of arterioles.

6. **What are the clinical features of a COPD exacerbation?**
   - **Cardinal symptoms:** Increased shortness of breath (dyspnea), increased sputum volume, and increased sputum purulence (or change in color)
   - **Other features**: Increased cough frequency or severity, wheezing, increased heart rate and/or respiratory rate, fever, malaise, fatigue, hypoxia, and confusion

7. **What are the common precipitants of a COPD exacerbation?**
   See Table 21-1.

TABLE 21-1. COMMON INFECTIOUS AND NONINFECTIOUS PRECIPITANTS OF COPD EXACERBATION

Infectious	Noninfectious
Tracheobronchitis	Medication nonadherence
Viral	Environmental irritants (e.g., smoke, smog,
Bacterial (*Haemophilus influenza* >	workplace exposures)
Streptococcus pneumoniae >	Overuse or inappropriate use of sedating
Moraxella catarrhalis)	medications or beta-blocking agents
Atypical bacteria (*Mycoplasma*	CHF or arrhythmias
species and *Chlamydia pneumoniae*;	Pulmonary embolism
<10% of cases causing exacerbation)	Rib fracture, chest trauma, pneumothorax
Pneumonia	Thick bronchial secretions (e.g., dehydration)

CHF = congestive heart failure.

8. **What testing is recommended for patients being evaluated for a presumptive COPD exacerbation?**
   See Table 21-2.

9. **Is spirometry (pulmonary function tests or peak flow measurements) indicated in the setting of a COPD exacerbation?**
   No. Unlike asthma exacerbations (in which peak flow information can be valuable), there is no demonstrated value of spirometry in the acute COPD exacerbation. It should be reserved for outpatient evaluation of stable COPD.

10. **What factors influence the decision for hospital admission in exacerbations of COPD?**
    The decision to admit a patient to the hospital is often subjective. Most often, patients should be given a trial of therapy in the emergency department or clinic and admitted if they don't respond. Strong consideration for admission should be given to patients with severe COPD at baseline, significant comorbid conditions, older age, and a marked increase in symptom severity or new physical examination findings (e.g., increased work of breathing or use of accessory respiratory

TABLE 21-2. RECOMMENDED WORK-UP OF A PATIENT WITH COPD EXACERBATION

Test	Potential Findings
Chest x-ray	16–21% have abnormalities (e.g., infiltrate or pulmonary edema, blebs, flat diaphragms)
Arterial blood gas	May identify hypercapnia, acidemia, and hypoxemia
Complete blood count	May identify secondary polycythemia
Sputum culture	Can identify bacterial pathogens and their sensitivities to antibiotics
Electrocardiogram	Common abnormalities include right-sided strain (RVH, tall P waves in lead II), MAT, or low voltage

RVH = right ventricular hypertrophy, MAT = multifocal atria tachycardia.

musculature). Additionally, the presence of new arrhythmias (e.g., atrial fibrillation, supraventricular tachycardia, or multifocal atrial tachycardia) or severe hypoxia or hypercapnia warrants hospital admission.

11. **What factors influence the decision for intensive care unit (ICU) admission in cases of exacerbation of COPD?**
Patients with severe symptoms that do not respond to initial emergent therapies or the presence of confusion or lethargy should be monitored in an ICU setting. The presence of severe hypercapnia, acidosis, or hypoxemia despite supplemental oxygen therapy also indicates ICU admission. Finally, patients initiating the use of noninvasive mechanical ventilation (NIMV) or those with impending respiratory failure are best cared for in an ICU environment.

12. **What therapies for COPD exacerbations are supported by robust randomized controlled trial evidence?**
Bronchodilators, oxygen, systemic corticosteroids, antibiotics (for some patients; see question 16), and NIMV are all supported by strong evidence.

13. **What respiratory therapies do *not* bear adequate randomized controlled trial evidence to support their use in COPD exacerbations?**
Mucolytic agents (e.g., guaifenesin), chest physical therapy, and methylxanthine agents (e.g., theophylline or aminophylline) have not shown definitive benefit.

14. **Which bronchodilator has the greatest efficacy in COPD exacerbations?**
Short-acting $beta_2$ agonists (e.g., albuterol) have equal efficacy to short-acting anticholinergic bronchodilators (e.g., ipratropium). Anticholinergic agents, however, have fewer adverse effects.

15. **What is the optimal dosing and duration for systemic corticosteroids for COPD exacerbations?**
Studies have shown that systemic steroid use is beneficial and that 8 weeks of therapy is no better or worse than 2 weeks. Beyond that, the optimal dosing or duration has not been well studied. Although high doses of steroids (e.g., methylprednisolone 125 mg given intravenously every 8 hours) are often initiated, it appears that lower doses (30–60 mg of prednisone or methylprednisolone daily) provide a reasonable efficacy without the unnecessary increase in adverse effects that may result from higher dosing regimens. Steroids should be tapered over a

10–14-day total course. There is no role for inhaled corticosteroids in the setting of acute COPD exacerbation.

16. **Which patients with a COPD exacerbation benefit from antibiotics? What first-line antibiotics should be considered?**
    ■ Patients with three of three (or possibly two of three) cardinal symptoms (see question 6)
    or
    ■ Patients admitted to the hospital for exacerbation of COPD
    First-line antibiotics include trimethoprim/sulfamethoxazole or doxycycline. Other acceptable options include higher-generation macrolides (e.g., azithromycin, clarithromycin), cephalosporins, or higher-generation quinolones (e.g., levofloxacin, moxifloxacin, or gatifloxacin). A 7-day course is typically adequate.

17. **Do hypoxic patients with COPD exacerbation benefit from oxygen therapy?**
    Oxygen therapy is beneficial because it relieves pulmonary vasoconstriction and right heart strain, resulting in a survival benefit in controlled trials. Only enough oxygen should be administered to relieve hypoxemia, using nasal canula or precisely titratable face mask (e.g., Venturi mask) to achieve low normal oxygen saturation (e.g., 89–94%). Patients should be monitored closely for altered mental status and respiratory depression because patients with chronic hypercapnia may depend on hypoxia to stimulate their respiratory drive.

KEY POINTS: EVIDENCE-BASED THERAPIES FOR COPD EXACERBATION

1. Bronchodilators (e.g., albuterol and ipratropium)

2. Oxygen, if patient is hypoxic

3. Systemic corticosteroids

4. Antibiotics (if two of the following three are present: increased shortness of breath, sputum volume, or sputum purulence)

5. NIMV (for certain patients)

18. **How does NIMV help reduce intubation rate, mortality, and hospital length of stay?**
    NIMV reduces patient work to breathe by assisting with and improving ventilation through pressure support applied externally through a nasal mask or face mask. It reduces CO_2 levels, improves pH, and reduces the likelihood of intubation and its complications. It can also improve oxygenation by providing positive end-expiratory pressure. (See Chapter 10 for more details.)

KEY POINTS: BENEFITS OF NONINVASIVE MECHANICAL VENTILATION FOR COPD EXACERBATION

1. Reduces intubation rate

2. Reduces mortality

3. Reduces hospital length of stay

19. **Is there an ideal pH range within which patients with COPD exacerbation more frequently benefit from NIMV?**
Yes, pH 7.2–7.35. Many patients with pH < 7.2 may be too ill for a trial of NIMV (although it is not absolutely contraindicated), and these persons may require intubation. Patients with pH > 7.35 typically will not gain additional benefit from NIMV therapy, despite an elevated pCO_2.

20. **What interventions may be used to assist with management of COPD patients requesting end-of-life care?**
Discussions with patients and family should be undertaken at the time of admission to the hospital to assess wishes regarding medical care, use of invasive interventions (e.g., intubation), and end-of-life wishes. Opiate analgesic medications (e.g., morphine or hydromorphone) may be used to relieve symptoms of dyspnea or work of breathing during end-of-life care. Support services including social service and spiritual or pastoral care should be provided to support the end-of-life decision.

21. **What factors influence mortality for patients admitted to the hospital with a COPD exacerbation?**
Patients requiring intubation (>25% inpatient mortality) and ICU admission (10–25% inpatient mortality and nearly 50% 1-year mortality) are at increased risk of death.

22. **What percentage of patients admitted to the hospital for COPD exacerbation is readmitted within 6 months?**
Fifty percent.

23. **What criteria should be met before a patient with a COPD exacerbation is discharged from the hospital?**
   - Patient is clinically stable (including stable oxygen saturation) for 12–24 hours.
   - Patient requires bronchodilator treatment *no more often than* every 4 hours.
   - Patient is able to eat and ambulate.
   - Patient is able to sleep without frequent awakening by dyspnea.
   - Patient or caregiver has received metered-dose inhaler and medication teaching.
   - Follow-up and home care have been established.

24. **What prevention measures should be administered before the patient is discharged?**
Smoking cessation counseling, pneumonia vaccine, and influenza vaccine should be documented in the record prior to discharge.

KEY POINTS: PREVENTIVE MEASURES AT DISCHARGE AFTER COPD EXACERBATION

1. Smoking cessation counseling

2. Pneumococcal vaccine (administer prior to discharge or document that patient has previously received)

3. Influenza vaccine (as seasonally appropriate)

25. **What are the indications for home oxygen therapy?**
   - $PO_2 \leq 55$ or pulse oximetry < 88%
   or

- $PO_2 < 60$ with stigmata of chronic hypoxia (e.g., cor pulmonale, persistent lower extremity edema, or polycythemia)

WEBSITE

Global Initiative for Chronic Obstructive Lung Disease (GOLD) Guidelines: Global Strategy for the Diagnosis, Management, and Prevention of Chronic Obstructive Pulmonary Disease: NHLBI/WHO Workshop Report. National Heart, Lung, and Blood Institute, National Institutes of Health; April 2001: http://www.goldcopd.com

BIBLIOGRAPHY

1. Anthonisen NR, Manfreda J, Warren CP, et al: Antibiotic therapy in exacerbations of chronic obstructive pulmonary disease. Ann Intern Med 106:196–204, 1987.
2. Bach PB, Brown C, Gelfand SE, et al: Management of acute exacerbations of chronic obstructive pulmonary disease: A summary and appraisal of published evidence. Ann Intern Med 134:600–620, 2001.
3. Keenan SP, Sinuff T, Cook DJ, Hill NS: Which patients with acute exacerbation of chronic obstructive pulmonary disease benefit from noninvasive positive pressure ventilation? A systematic review of the literature. Ann Intern Med 138:861–870, 2003.
4. Niewoehner DE, Erbland ML, Deupree RH, et al: Effect of systemic glucocorticoids on exacerbations of chronic obstructive pulmonary disease. Department of Veteran Affairs Cooperative Study Group. N Engl J Med 340:1941–1947, 1999.
5. Saint S, Bent S, Vittinghoff E, Grady D: Antibiotics in chronic obstructive pulmonary disease exacerbations: A meta-analysis. JAMA 273:957–960, 1995.
6. Snow V, Lascher S, Mottur-Pilson C, et al: Evidence base for management of acute exacerbations of chronic obstructive pulmonary disease. Ann Intern Med 134:595–599, 2001.

CHAPTER 22

ASTHMA

Preetha Basaviah, MD

1. What is *asthma*, and how is it categorized?

Asthma is a chronic inflammatory airway disorder. It is classified as "mild intermittent," "mild persistent," "moderate," or "severe," based on the frequency and severity of symptoms, the impact on pulmonary function, and the necessity for treatment (Table 22-1). Generally, the frequency and severity of exacerbations are variable. However, patients at any level of severity may experience severe, life-threatening attacks.

2. Which precipitating factors play a role in asthma exacerbations?

Approximately 20–30% of asthmatics presenting for emergency care require hospitalization. The most common triggers are viral upper respiratory infections, especially rhinovirus. However, infections with other respiratory pathogens, such as influenza, parainfluenza, respiratory syncytial viruses, adenoviruses, and *Mycoplasma pneumoniae* and *Chlamydia pneumoniae* can also precipitate flares. Other common precipitants include allergens (e.g., animal dander, dust mites, cockroaches, pollen, molds), noncompliance with medications, exercise, cold air, stressful situations, nonsteroidal anti-inflammatory medicines, occupational irritants, and gastroesophageal reflux.

3. Describe common clinical features of asthma.

The signs and symptoms of asthma correlate poorly with the severity of airflow obstruction. Consider asthma as a diagnosis in patients with a history of recurrent wheezing, shortness of breath, chest tightness, cough (particularly if worse at night), exercise intolerance, or symptoms worsening with exposure to an allergen such as weather changes, airborne chemicals, or animal dander.

4. Which diagnostic studies should be performed to assess the extent of an asthma flare?

Assessment of air flow, commonly done by checking the peak expiratory flow (PEF) with a peak flow meter, is the quickest and easiest method of assessing the severity of an asthma attack. Reversible airway obstruction can also be documented by measuring forced expiratory volume in 1 second (FEV_1). Serial measurements help clinicians assess response to therapy and help avoid both unnecessary hospital admissions and premature discharge. Airway obstruction is indicated by a decreased FEV_1 and decreased ratio of FEV_1 to forced vital capacity relative to predicted values. An increase in FEV_1 after bronchodilator treatment indicates reversible obstruction. Performing this maximal inspiratory-expiratory maneuver can itself provoke bronchoconstriction. Therefore, in patients suffering an apparent severe acute attack, it is wise to wait 1–2 hours after treatment before the first measurement of FEV_1 or peak flow.

5. Are chest radiographs necessary when an asthma exacerbation is being considered?

A chest radiograph is not required in the routine assessment of a patient with an asthma attack. It may be warranted if a clinician suspects infection on examination (possibly indicated by rales and egophony) or entertains other possible diagnoses, such as pulmonary embolism, pneumothorax, or heart failure.

TABLE 22-1. CLASSIFICATION OF ASTHMA SEVERITY: CLINICAL FEATURES BEFORE TREATMENT

	Mild Intermittent	Mild Persistent	Moderate Persistent	Severe Persistent
Symptom frequency	≤2×/week	>2×/week, <1×/day	Daily	Continuous
Exacerbations	Brief	Limit activity	≥2×/week	Frequent
Nighttime symptoms	≤2×/month	>2×/month	>1×/week	Frequent
Usual symptoms	Asymptomatic with normal lung fxn	Asymptomatic with normal lung fxn	>1×/week	Limit activity
FEV_1 and PEFR	≥80% predicted	≥80% predicted	61–79% predicted	≤60% predicted
PEFR variability	<20%	20–30%	>30%	>30%
Long-term control	No daily medication needed	**Low-dose inhaled steroid, e.g., 200–500 μg/day or cromolyn (Intal) or nedocromil** Alternatives: 1. Leukotriene modifier, e.g., zafirlukast (Accolate) or zileuton (Zyflo) may be considered in patients ≥12 years old 2. Theophylline (serum level 5–15 μg/mL) is an alternative but not preferred	**Medium-dose inhaled steroid, e.g., 800–2000 μg/day** Alternatives: 1. Low- to medium-dose inhaled corticosteroid 2. Long-acting bronchodilator, e.g., salmeterol (Serevent) 3. Long-acting beta₂ agonist tablets 4. Theophylline	**Inhaled steroid 800–2000 μg and long-acting bronchodilator, e.g. salmeterol (Serevent)**, long-acting beta₂ agonist tablets, or theophylline *And* oral steroid (2 mg/kg/day, generally NTE 60 mg)
Quick relief	Short-acting inhaled beta₂ agonists as needed*	Short-acting inhaled beta₂ agonists as needed*	Short-acting inhaled beta₂ agonists as needed*	Short-acting inhaled beta₂ agonists as needed*

FEV_1 = forced expiratory volume in 1 second, PEFR = peak expiratory flow rate, fxn = function, NTE = not to exceed.
Patients should be assigned to the most severe group in which any feature occurs.
*Daily or more frequent use indicates need for additional long-term control therapy.
Preferred treatments in **boldface**.
Modified from: National Asthma Education and Prevention Program, Expert Panel Report 2. Guidelines for the Diagnosis and Management of Asthma. NIH publication No. 97-4051, April 1997.

6. **Should clinicians measure arterial blood gases (ABG) when evaluating asthmatic patients with acute symptoms?**

   ABG assessment is rarely needed in the initial assessment. Patients with mild attacks usually present with mild hypoxemia with normal oxygen saturation (PaO_2, 66–69 mmHg), hypocapnia ($PaCO_2$, 33–36 mmHg), and respiratory alkalosis. The main reason to measure an ABG is to detect CO_2 retention (hypercapnia). The peak flow rate is a poor predictor of hypoxemia but is a useful tool to assess for hypercapnia, which typically occurs only when the peak flow rate drops below 25% of normal. Respiratory drive is usually increased in asthma attacks, so a normal value for PCO_2 may indicate severe airflow obstruction ($FEV_1 < 15$–20% of predicted value) and respiratory muscle fatigue.

7. **Discuss critical "can't miss" conditions in the differential diagnosis and initial evaluation of patients presenting with cough, shortness of breath, or wheezing.**
   - **Asthma exacerbation**
   - **Pneumonia:** Wheezing is localized and usually associated with sputum production.
   - **Pulmonary edema:** Acute elevations in left atrial pressure can cause airway narrowing and wheezing (i.e., "cardiac asthma").
   - **Pulmonary embolism:** Wheezing is possible but the frequency is likely overestimated.
   - **Acute bronchitis:** Similar to acute bronchitis presentations, acute asthma exacerbations may present with productive cough and dyspnea associated with acute inflammation of the bronchial mucosa. However, the diagnosis is insufficient, and the typical treatment (i.e., antibiotics) is inappropriate and ineffective in patients with asthma.
   - **Mechanical obstruction of the upper airway:** Consider when patients present with dysphonia, inspiratory stridor, and monophasic wheezing over the lung fields that is loudest over the neck.

8. **What are the first priorities when treating a patient with an asthma exacerbation?**

   Initial management remains the same regardless of the precipitant (Fig. 22-1). The first steps include oxygen, inhaled beta$_2$ agonist, and systemic corticosteroids. The dose and frequency of administration and assessment of the patient's response may vary. An inhaled short-acting beta$_2$ agonist should be administered promptly and is usually given via a nebulizer (albuterol 2.5–5.0 mg in 1.5–2.0 mL isotonic saline) powered by a compressed oxygen-air mixture every 20 minutes for the first hour and hourly thereafter, or until improvement occurs. For severe exacerbations, an anticholinergic agent (0.5 mg of ipratropium bromide) should be added to the nebulized beta$_2$ agonist. For moderate to severe exacerbations not completely responsive to initial therapy, begin an oral corticosteroid "burst" regimen (e.g., 40–60 mg of prednisone per day) given in single or divided doses for 3–7 days. Despite the fact that steroids do not take effect for at least 6 hours, they have been proven to reduce the rates of hospitalization. Both prednisone and methylprednisone are well absorbed when taken orally, so intravenous administration is not necessary. Methylxanthines (e.g., theophylline) are no longer recommended in acute flare-ups because they appear to add no benefit to optimal inhaled beta$_2$ agonist therapy and may increase adverse events. For long-term control of mild persistent or greater-severity asthma, alternatives to inhaled steroids include leukotriene modifiers (e.g., zafirlukast [Accolate] or zileuton [Zyflo]) or, least preferred, sustained-release theophylline to serum concentration of 5–15 µg/mL (Table 22-2).

   Recent trials offer preliminary evidence that leukotriene receptor blockade could be an effective therapy for acute asthma in adults. In a randomized controlled trial of 201 adults with acute asthma and a $FEV_1 < 70\%$ predicted after an albuterol nebulized treatment, patients receiving montelukast therapy (7 or 14 mg given intravenously) experienced a 15% increase in FEV_1 at both dosages, compared with a 4% increase in patients treated with placebo. A larger randomized controlled trial evaluated the effect of zafirlukast (120 mg orally given in the emergency department) on 641 adults with acute asthma and found patients were less likely than those receiving placebo to require prolonged observation or hospital admission (10% and

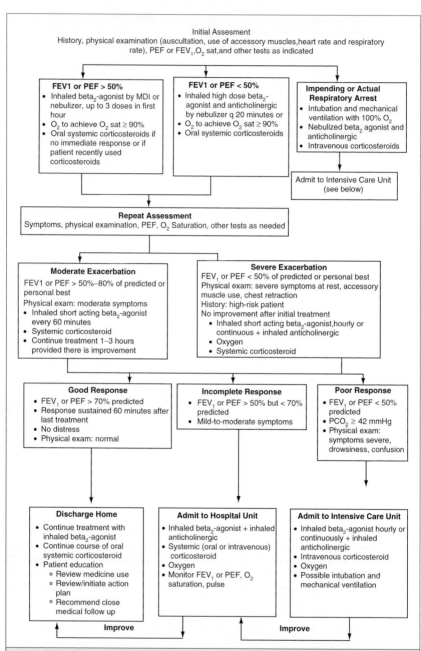

Figure 22-1. Management of asthma exacerbations in the emergency department and hospital. PEF = peak expiratory flow, FEV$_1$ = forced expiratory volume in 1 second, PEFR = peak expiratory flow rate, MDI = metered dose inhaler. (Modified from National Asthma Education and Prevention Program, Expert Panel Report 2: Guidelines for the Diagnosis and Management of Asthma. NIH publication No. 97–4051, April 1997.)

TABLE 22-2. SYMPTOM RELIEVERS USED FOR TREATING BRONCHOCONSTRICTION

Short-acting beta$_2$ agonists

Albuterol (Proventil, Ventolin)	2–4 puffs q4–6h prn sx or before exercise or 4 puffs (100 µg/puff) every 10–20 minutes for up to 3 hours for acute asthma exacerbations
Terbutaline (Brethine, Brethaire)	2–4 puffs q4–6h prn sx; 5 mg po tid (in adults)
Pirbuterol (Maxair)	1–2 puffs q4–6h prn—asthma sx
Metaproterenol (Alupent)	2–3 puffs q3–4h prn—asthma sx
Albuterol (nebulized)	0.1–0.15 mg/kg (e.g., 5–10 mg of albuterol for adults) given every 20 minutes for 1–3, along with nebulized ipratropium 500 µg given every 20 minutes for 1–3 hours

Long-acting beta$_2$ agonists

Salmeterol (Serevent)	2 puffs qd to bid (NEVER exceed 4 puffs/24 h)

Methylxanthines

Theophylline (Theodur and others)	100–400 mg po bid; follow serum levels

Anticholinergics

Ipratropium bromide—Atrovent, nebulized Ipratropium bromide—aerosolized	500 µg given every 20 minutes for 1–3 hours (to be given with nebulized albuterol) 4 puffs of ipratropium (20 µg per puff) every 10–20 minutes for up to 3 hours for acute asthma exacerbations; 2–4 puffs q6h prn maintenance

prn = as needed, sx = symptom, po = by mouth, tid = three times daily, qd = once daily, bid = twice daily.

15%, respectively). Furthermore, patients given zafirlukast 20 mg/day for 6 days after discharge from the emergency department were less likely than patients receiving placebo to require medical care for relapse during a 28-day follow-up period (24% and 29%, respectively).

9. **Which asthmatic patients should be hospitalized?**
   Generally, patients with an incomplete response to therapy in the emergency department (e.g., FEV$_1$ or PEF > 50% but < 70% of predicted value or "personal best") and persistence of mild to moderate symptoms need an individualized determination regarding hospitalization. Those with an FEV$_1$ < 50% after 2 or 3 hours of initial treatment most often require hospitalization. Other considerations in the decision to admit include duration and severity of symptoms, course and severity of prior exacerbations, medication use, access to medical care and medications, adequacy of support and home conditions, and presence of comorbidities.

10. **Which patients need admission to an intensive care unit (ICU)?**
    Patients experiencing an asthma attack that is unresponsive to treatment (i.e., status asthmaticus) or who demonstrate severe airway obstruction and impending respiratory arrest are best cared for in an ICU setting. Suggestive clinical features include altered level of consciousness, apparent clinical exhaustion, cyanosis or severe hypoxia (PaO$_2$ ≤ 60 mmHg), pulsus paradoxus > 15 mmHg, diminished breath sounds on examination ("silent chest"),

tachycardia (i.e., > 130 beats/min), low arterial pH with a high $PaCO_2$, FEV_1 < 0.6 L, or a PEF rate < 60 L/min that is unresponsive to bronchodilator therapy.

KEY POINTS: ASTHMA

1. Asthma is a disease of chronic airway inflammation triggered by a wide array of precipitants.

2. Initial assessment should include assessment of airflow by measuring FEV_1 or PEF.

3. The primary therapies (i.e., oxygen, inhaled beta$_2$ agonist, and systemic corticosteroids) remain the cornerstones, but the dose and frequency of administration and the frequency of assessing the patient's response may vary.

4. Because viral respiratory infections are the most common trigger of asthma attacks, antibiotics should not be prescribed routinely.

5. Hospitalization for an asthma exacerbation is a predictor of increased risk for readmission for subsequent attacks and for death from asthma. Hospitalization presents an opportunity to educate patients about the disease, treatment, and self-monitoring.

11. **Identify risk factors for death from asthma.**
    Patients at high risk for asthma-associated death need intensive monitoring, education, and medical care. Factors suggestive of high risk for asthma-related mortality include past history of sudden severe exacerbations, prior intubation for asthma, prior ICU admission for asthma, ≥2 hospitalizations for asthma in the past year, three or more emergency care visits for asthma in the past year, use of >2 canisters per month of inhaled short-acting beta$_2$ agonist, current use of or recent withdrawal from treatment with systemic corticosteroids, difficulty perceiving airflow obstruction or its severity, comorbidity (e.g., cardiovascular diseases, chronic obstructive pulmonary disease), serious psychiatric disease, low socioeconomic status and urban residence, illicit drug use, and sensitivity to *Alternaria* (a species of mold).

12. **What issues should be considered at discharge?**
    - **Discharge criteria:** Symptoms and physical findings significantly improved. PEF or FEV_1 remains above 70% of the predicted or "personal best" value for 3 or 4 hours after beta$_2$ agonist administration.
    - **Patient education:** Before discharge, patients should receive training on proper inhaler and peak flow techniques. Smoking cessation and indicated vaccinations are key elements of the discharge plan. Furthermore, clinicians should reinforce the need for maintenance therapy, avoidance of triggers, and development of self-assessment skills (e.g., routine assessment of peak flow).
    - **Discharge medications:** Patients and clinicians should review the types and purposes of prescribed medications, especially focusing on proper inhaler technique and use of peak flow meters. Treatment with inhaled corticosteroids and possibly a long-acting beta$_2$ agonist should be initiated. Residual airflow obstruction may persist for several days even when symptoms and peak expiratory flow rate have improved. A short course of oral corticosteroids (e.g., 8-day taper beginning with methylprednisolone 64 mg/day) significantly reduces the likelihood of relapse, emergency department reevaluation, and persistence of severe symptoms within the subsequent 2 weeks.
    - **Discharge follow-up:** This includes a follow-up visit and an action plan for steps to determine whether symptoms, signs, and peak expiratory flow rates indicate airflow obstruction.

WEBSITES

1. Comprehensive summary of links to resources for the diagnosis and management of asthma provided by the National Library of Medicine.
http://www.nlm.nih.gov/medlineplus/asthma.html

2. Teach Your Patients about Asthma: A Clinician's Guide. A helpful clinician's guide to teaching patients about asthma from the National Asthma Education Program Office of Prevention, Education, and Control, National Heart, Lung and Blood Institute, National Institute of Health. Publication No. 92–2737, October 1992.
http://www.meddean.luc.edu/lumen/MedEd/medicine/Allergy/Asthma/asthtoc.html

3. The National Center for Chronic Disease Prevention and Health Promotion of the CDC provides a helpful database focusing on chronic disease prevention.
http://www.cdc.gov/nceh/asthma/default.htm

4. New Guidelines for the Diagnosis and Management of Asthma from the National Asthma Education and Prevention Program updating the 1991 Expert Panel Report of the National Heart, Lung, and Blood Institute. July 1997. NIH Pub. No. 97–4051.
http://www.nhlbi.nih.gov/guidelines/asthma/asthgdln.pdf

BIBLIOGRAPHY

1. Boushey HA: Exacerbations of asthma. In Wachter RM, Goldman L, Hollander H (eds): Hospital Medicine, 2nd ed. Philadelphia, Lippincott Williams & Wilkins, 2005, pp 539–548.

2. Camargo CA Jr, Smithline HA, Malice MP, et al: A randomized controlled trial of intravenous montelukast in acute asthma. Am J Respir Crit Care Med 167:528, 2003.

3. Fanta C: Treatment of acute exacerbations of asthma. In Up-to-Date, 2005. Available at: http://www.utdol.com/utd/content/topic.do?topicKey=asthma/12318&type=A&selectedTitle=7~230.

4. Kalltrom TJ: Evidence-based asthma management. Respir Care 49:783–792, 2004.

5. McFadden ER Jr: Acute severe asthma. Am J Respir Crit Care Med 168:740–759, 2003.

6. National Institutes of Health/National Heart, Lung, and Blood Institute/National Asthma Education and Prevention Program: Practical Guide for the Diagnosis and Management of Asthma. Bethesda, MD, National Institutes of Health/National Heart, Lung, and Blood Institute/National Asthma Education and Prevention Program, 1997.

7. Plotnick LH, Ducharme FM: Combined inhaled anticholinergics and beta$_2$-agonists for initial treatment of acute asthma in children. Cochrane Database Syst Rev 2000; CD000060.

8. Silverman RA, Nowak RM, Korenblat PE, et al: Zafirlukast treatment for acute asthma: Evaluation in a randomized, double-blind, multicenter trial. Chest 126:1480, 2004.

CHAPTER 23

PNEUMOTHORAX

Adam L. Friedlander, MD

1. What is a pneumothorax? How are pneumothoraces classified?

The presence of free air between the visceral and parietal pleura is a pneumothorax. Those occurring without a precipitating event are considered spontaneous. Spontaneous pneumothoraces are further classified based on the presence or absence of underlying lung disease. A *primary spontaneous pneumothorax* occurs in a patient without clinical lung disease; these are usually the result of a previously unrecognized subpleural bleb (commonly due to smoking). A *secondary spontaneous pneumothorax* occurs as a complication of preexisting lung disease. *Iatrogenic pneumothorax* results from a complication of a diagnostic or therapeutic intervention, such as thoracentesis. *Traumatic pneumothorax* is caused by penetrating or blunt trauma to the chest, such as alveolar rupture from chest compressions.

2. How are simple, tension, and open pneumothoraces differentiated?

Pneumothoraces are also described in terms of pathophysiologic presentation and repercussions:

- In a *simple pneumothorax,* the pleural pressure becomes slightly more positive than the pleural pressure in the contralateral hemithorax but still remains subatmospheric (Fig. 23-1).
- With a *tension pneumothorax,* the intrapleural pressure exceeds atmospheric pressure, particularly in expiration. The resulting "check valve" mechanism promotes the inspiratory accumulation of air and pressure in the pleural space, with eventual respiratory failure from compression of the normal lung (Fig. 23-2).
- A chest wall defect can cause an *open pneumothorax,* in which ambient air enters the injured hemithorax during inspiration. This forms a "sucking wound," with mediastinal shift toward the normal side. During expiration, the mediastinum swings to the injured side, and expiratory air from the normal lung enters the collapsed lung, often resulting in respiratory failure.

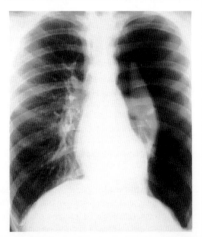

Figure 23-1. Left-sided simple pneumothorax. Note the complete collapse of the left lung (evidenced by the loss of lung markings between the chest wall and the visceral pleural line), which is retracted to the left hilum. The intrapleural pressure on the left has remained subatmospheric. (From Hansell DM, Padley SPG: Imaging. In Albert RK, Spiro SG, Jett JR [eds]: Clinical Respiratory Medicine, 2nd ed. St. Louis, Mosby, 2004, p 42, Fig. 1.86a.)

3. What are the common causes of a pneumothorax?

Almost every lung disease can be associated with a secondary spontaneous pneumothorax. However, most pneumothoraces are due to chronic obstructive lung disease or *Pneumocystis jiroveci* infection in patients with AIDS (Table 23-1).

4. **How do patients with a pneumothorax typically present?**
The clinical hallmark of a pneumothorax is unilateral pleuritic chest pain and dyspnea. Primary spontaneous pneumothorax typically occurs in tall, thin males between the ages of 10 and 30 years and rarely occurs in persons over the age of 40 years. Onset is acute and usually begins at rest, with symptom resolution within 24 hours even if the pneumothorax remains untreated. Secondary spontaneous pneumothorax occurs later in life, with a peak incidence of 60–65 years. Since patients with underlying lung disease have less pulmonary reserve, symptoms are generally more severe and dyspnea is nearly always present. Symptoms do not resolve spontaneously and may be associated with life-threatening hypoxia, hypercapnia, and/or hypotension.

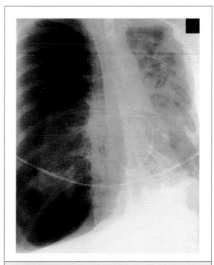

Figure 23-2. Tension pneumothorax after insertion of a Swanz-Ganz catheter. Note the shift of the mediastinum toward the left and reversal of the normal contour of the right hemidiaphragm. The intrapleural pressure on the right is greater than atmospheric pressure. (From Hansell DM, Padley SPG: Imaging. In Albert RK, Spiro SG, Jett JR [eds]: Clinical Respiratory Medicine, 2nd ed. St. Louis, Mosby, 2004, p 42, Fig. 1.87.)

5. **Describe the characteristic physical findings in a patient with a pneumothorax.**
The classic physical findings when a large pneumothorax is present are decreased chest excursion, diminished breath sounds, and hyperresonant percussion on the affected side. These findings may be absent when the pneumothorax is small (i.e., involves <15% of the hemithorax). Tachycardia is the most common physical finding. A tension pneumothorax should be suspected when tachycardia >135 bpm, hypotension, or cyanosis is present. In patients with a secondary spontaneous pneumothorax, expected physical findings may be subtle and masked by the underlying lung disease.

6. **Discuss the major radiologic features of a pneumothorax.**
A white visceral pleural line separated from the parietal pleura by an avascular collection of air is the classic radiologic feature of a pneumothorax. Lung and vascular markings are absent between the chest wall and the visceral pleural line (Figs. 23-3 and 23-4).

7. **What are the mechanisms of impaired gas exchange in a patient with a large pneumothorax?**
Collapsed and poorly ventilated portions of lung continue to receive significant perfusion, commonly resulting in hypoxia from a low ventilation-perfusion ratio and shunting. In primary spontaneous pneumothorax, hypercapnia is unusual because underlying lung function is normal and adequate alveolar ventilation is maintained in the contralateral lung.

TABLE 23-1. CLASSIFICATION OF PNEUMOTHORAX ACCORDING TO CAUSE

Spontaneous
Primary
Secondary
  Chronic obstructive pulmonary disease
  Cystic fibrosis
  Asthma
  Pneumocystis jiroveci pneumonia
  Necrotizing pneumonia
  Tuberculosis
  Sarcoidosis
  Idiopathic pulmonary fibrosis
  Langerhans' cell histiocytosis
  Lymphangiomyomatosis
  Tuberous sclerosis
  Ankylosing spondylitis
  Polymyositis and dermatomyositis
  Marfan's syndrome
  Sarcoma
  Pleural malignancy
  Thoracic endometriosis (catamenial)

Iatrogenic
Chest aspiration (thoracentesis)
Intercostal nerve block
Subclavian cannulation
Transbronchial biopsy
Needle aspiration lung biopsy
Positive pressure ventilation

Traumatic
Penetrating chest wounds
Chest compression injury

Adapted from Vanderschueren R: Pneumothorax. In Albert RK, Spiro SG, Jett JR (eds): Clinical Respiratory Medicine, 2nd ed. St. Louis, Mosby, 2004, p 721; and Sahn SA, Heffner JE: Spontaneous pneumothorax. N Engl J Med 342:868–874, 2000.

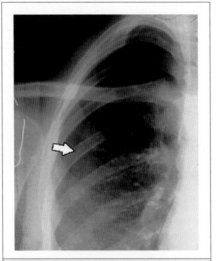

Figure 23-3. Shallow right pneumothorax.
A discrete pleural white line is seen (arrow).
Peripheral to this, there are no lung markings.
(From Hansell DM, Padley SPG: Imaging. In Albert RK,
Spiro SG, Jett JR [eds]: Clinical Respiratory Medicine,
2nd ed. St. Louis, Mosby, 2004, p 42, Fig. 1.85a.)

8. **What are the management options for pneumothoraces?**
With any pneumothorax, the goals are to remove air from the pleural space and to decrease the likelihood of recurrence. The best treatment method is controversial and depends on the presentation, the size of the pneumothorax, and the presence of bullae. Choices include observation (with supplemental oxygen therapy); simple aspiration with a catheter; insertion of a chest tube; pleurodesis (procedure by which chemical or mechanical sclerosing agents are introduced into the pleural space to adhere the surfaces of the visceral and parietal pleurae); thoracoscopy (including video-assisted thorascopic surgery); and thoracotomy. In cases of life-threatening pneumothorax, immediate insertion of a large-bore needle anteriorly through the second intercostal space in the mid-clavicular line should be done. The definitive treatment procedure can be performed later.

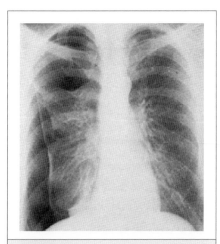

Figure 23-4. Partial pneumothorax with adhesions. When there are adhesions between the pleurae, the lung cannot collapse completely. (From Vanderschueren R: Pneumothorax. In Albert RK, Spiro SG, Jett JR [eds]: Clinical Respiratory Medicine, 2nd ed. St. Louis, Mosby, 2004, p 720, Fig. 62.3.)

KEY POINTS: MANAGEMENT OPTIONS FOR A PNEUMOTHORAX

1. Observation (with supplemental oxygen therapy)

2. Simple aspiration with a catheter (with immediate removal of the catheter)

3. Insertion of a chest tube

4. Pleurodesis

5. Thoracoscopy (including video-assisted thorascopic surgery)

6. Thoracotomy

9. **When is observation alone appropriate in the management of a pneumothorax?**
Observation alone with supplemental oxygen therapy is appropriate only for small (<15% of the hemithorax) primary pneumothoraces. Supplemental oxygen accelerates by a factor of four the reabsorption of air by the pleura, which occurs at a rate of 2% per day when breathing room air.

Northfield TC: Oxygen therapy for spontaneous pneumothorax. BMJ 4:86–88, 1977.

WEBSITE

American Thoracic Society: http://www.thoracic.org

BIBLIOGRAPHY

1. Baumann MH, Strange C, Heffner JE, et al: Management of spontaneous pneumothorax: An American College of Chest Physicians Delphi consensus statement. Chest 119:590–602, 2001.

2. Devanand A, Koh MS, Ong TH, et al: Simple aspiration versus chest-tube insertion in the management of primary spontaneous pneumothorax: A systematic review. Respir Med 98:579–590, 2004.

3. Hansell DM, Padley SPG: Imaging. In Albert RK, Spiro SG, Jett JR (eds): Clinical Respiratory Medicine, 2nd ed. St. Louis, Mosby, 2004, pp 1–60.

4. Primrose WR: Spontaneous pneumothorax: a retrospective review of aetiology, pathogenesis management. Scott Med J 29:15–20, 1984.

5. Sahn SA, Heffner JE: Spontaneous pneumothorax. N Engl J Med 342:868–874, 2000.

6. Vanderschueren R: Pneumothorax. In Albert RK, Spiro SG, Jett JR (eds): Clinical Respiratory Medicine, 2nd ed. St. Louis, Mosby, 2004, pp 719–722.

CHAPTER 24

PLEURAL EFFUSION

Joseph Ming Wah Li, MD, and David Feinbloom, MD

1. **Describe the normal production and reabsorption of pleural fluid.**
   The visceral and parietal pleura form a potential space between the lung and chest wall called the *pleural space*. This space normally contains 0.1–0.2 mL/kg of pleural fluid. The pleural membrane produces pleural fluid at approximately 0.6 mL/h, and the pleural lymphatic system absorbs the fluid at the same rate. When production exceeds resorption, pleural fluid accumulates, resulting in a pleural effusion.

2. **What is the normal pleural fluid cell count, differential, and protein concentration?**
   Normal pleural fluid has a white blood cell count of 1700/mm^3 with a differential of 75% macrophages and 23% lymphocytes. The protein concentration is typically 1 gm/dL or approximately 15% of plasma protein concentration.

   Noppen M, De Waele M, Li R, et al: Volume and cellular content of normal pleural fluid in humans examined by pleural lavage. Am J Respir Crit Care Med 162:1023, 2000.

3. **Describe the physical signs associated with a pleural effusion.**
   Pleural fluid attenuates the transmission of sound during auscultation such that percussion results in a dull sound. Although bronchial breath sounds may be heard near the top of a large effusion, the remainder of the lung fields will have decreased or no breath sounds. Transmitted voice sounds, such as egophony, are usually decreased or absent but may be increased at the top of a large effusion.

4. **Differentiate between an exudative and transudative pleural effusion.**
   Pleural inflammation, due to infection or injury, causes exudative effusions, whereas changes in hydrostatic and oncotic pressures cause transudative effusions. The presence of any of the following is diagnostic of an exudative pleural effusion:
   - Pleural fluid protein/serum protein ratio > 0.5
   - Pleural fluid lactic dehydrogenase (LDH)/serum LDH ratio > 0.6
   - Pleural fluid LDH > two thirds normal serum LDH
   - Pleural fluid protein > 2.9 gm/dL

   The inflammatory fluid found in exudative effusions may become loculated, leading to chronic pleural changes. Because of this, exudative effusions generally require removal by thoracentesis or insertion of a chest tube. Common causes of exudative and transudative pleural effusions are summarized in Table 24-1.

   Light RW, Macgregor MT, Luchsinger PC, et al: Pleural effusions: The diagnostic separation of transudates and exudates. Ann Intern Med 77:507, 1972.

5. **What is normal pleural fluid pH and why should it be measured?**
   The pH of normal pleural fluid is approximately 7.60. Transudates typically have a pH of 7.40–7.55, whereas exudates range from 7.30 to 7.45. An exudative effusion with a pH < 7.3 suggests an empyema, cancer, tuberculosis, esophageal rupture, systemic lupus erythematosus or rheumatoid-associated pleural disease.

TABLE 24-1.   COMMON CAUSES OF EXUDATIVE AND TRANSUDATIVE PLEURAL EFFUSIONS

Exudates	Transudates
Pneumonia	Heart failure
Pulmonary embolism	Pulmonary embolism
Empyema	Cirrhosis
Cancer	Nephrotic syndrome
Tuberculosis	
Asbestosis	
Sarcoidosis	

Sahn SA: Pleural fluid pH in the normal state in diseases affecting the pleural space. In Chretien J, Bignon J, Hirsch A (eds): The Pleura in Health and Disease. New York, Marcel Dekker, 1985, pp 253–266.

6. **Estimate the size of pleural effusion necessary to be seen on the chest radiograph.**
   - 75 mL will obliterate the posterior costophrenic sulcus on an upright x-ray
   - 175 mL will obscure the lateral costophrenic sulcus on an upright x-ray
   - 500 mL will obscure the diaphragmatic contour
   - 1000 mL is present if the effusion reaches the fourth rib

   Decubitus radiographs are often helpful in determining whether sufficient fluid is present for a thoracentesis (tap). With these radiographs, the patient lays flat on the side of the pleural effusion. Effusions that layer >1.0 cm against the lateral chest wall are large enough to tap.

   Moskowitz H, Platt RT, Schachar R, et al: Roentgen visualization of minute pleural effusion: An experimental study to determine the minimum amount of pleural fluid visible on a radiograph. Radiology 109:33, 1973.
   Stark P: The pleura. In Taveras JM, Ferruci JT (eds): Radiology. Diagnosis Imaging, Intervention. Philadelphia, Lippincott, 2000, pp 1–29.

7. **What is the difference between a complicated and an uncomplicated parapneumonic effusion?**
   Forty percent of all pneumonias are complicated by the development of a parapneumonic effusion. An uncomplicated parapneumonic effusion is an exudative effusion that results from pleural inflammation associated with a pneumonia. These effusions are generally benign and resolve with treatment of the pneumonia. In contrast, a complicated parapneumonic effusion occurs when there is persistent bacterial invasion into the pleural space with neutrophil recruitment, acidosis, and fibrin deposition. If untreated, this will become an empyema, an infected pus collection. All parapneumonic effusions should be sampled to exclude a complicated parapneumonic effusion or empyema. The exceptions to this rule are parapneumonic effusions that are free-flowing and are <1 cm on a lateral decubitus radiograph. Parapneumonic effusions that require chest tube drainage include:
   - Loculated effusions
   - Effusions that layer >1 cm on a lateral decubitus radiograph
   - Effusions with a thickened parietal pleural or laboratory studies suggestive of empyema

   Colice GL, Curtis A, Deslauriers J, et al: Medical and surgical treatment of parapneumonic effusions: An evidence based guideline. Chest 118:1158, 2000.

8. **How do glucose and amylase levels in pleural fluid help in the differential diagnosis?**
   - **Low glucose level (<60 mg/dL):** A low level in the pleural fluid or a pleural fluid/serum glucose ratio of <0.5 suggests tuberculosis, cancer, rheumatoid pleuritis, esophageal rupture, parapneumonic effusion, or empyema.
   - **Elevated amylase levels:** Elevated levels in the pleural fluid suggest a pancreatic disorder (e.g., cancer, pancreatitis, or pseudocyst) or esophageal rupture.

9. **How does the white blood cell differential help in the differential diagnosis?**
   Pleural fluid lymphocytosis suggests cancer, tuberculosis, sarcoidosis, yellow nail syndrome, chylothorax, or rheumatoid pleuritis. The majority of carcinomatous pleural effusions have lymphocytosis.

10. **What is a hemorrhagic pleural effusion?**
    The presence of approximately 10,000 red blood cells/μL of pleural fluid is defined as a *hemorrhagic effusion*. A *hemothorax* is present if the pleural fluid hematocrit is >50% of the serum hematocrit. In the absence of trauma, a bloody pleural fluid is worrisome for a pulmonary embolism or malignancy.

11. **Describe the characteristics of pleural effusion caused by tuberculosis.**
    The fluid may be serous to serosanguineous with a white blood cell count of 5000–10,000 cells/μL with lymphocytic predominance and a red blood cell count typically <10,000 cells/μL. The pH is usually >7.3 and the glucose is <50 mg/dL in one-third of cases, whereas the protein concentration is usually >4.0 gm/dL. Because acid fast bacilli testing and tuberculous cultures often have negative results, pleural biopsies are required to make the diagnosis.

    Frye MD, Pozsik CJ, Sahn SA: Tuberculous pleurisies and HIV disease. Chest 108:102S, 1995.

KEY POINTS: SIZING OF PLEURAL EFFUSIONS WITH DECUBITUS CHEST RADIOGRAPHS

1. Small effusions: <1.5 cm

2. Moderate effusions: 1.5–4.5 cm

3. Large effusions: >4.5 cm

BIBLIOGRAPHY

1. Heffner JE, Brown LK, Barbieri CA: Diagnostic value of tests that discriminate between exudative and transudative pleural effusions. Chest 111:970–980, 1997.

2. Light RW, Macgregor MI, Luchsinger PC, Ball WC Jr: Pleural effusions: The diagnostic separation of transudates and exudates. Ann Intern Med 77:507–513, 1972.

3. Noppen M, De Waele M, Li R, et al: Volume and cellular content of normal pleural fluid in humans examined by pleural lavage. Am J Respir Crit Care Med 162:1023–1026, 2000.

CHAPTER 25

PULMONARY HYPERTENSION

James H. Roum, MD,ᶜPhD

1. **What is pulmonary hypertension (PH)?**
   PH is defined by a mean pulmonary artery pressure >25 mmHg at rest or >30 mmHg with exertion.

2. **How is PH classified?**
   An *old classification* scheme divided PH into "primary PH" (no identifiable cause/risk) and "secondary PH" (identifiable cause/risk present).

   A *new classification* scheme (Venice Clinical Classification; Table 25-1) has general categories that include pulmonary arterial hypertension (PAH), PH associated with left heart disease, PH associated with pulmonary disease or hypoxemia, PH due to chronic thrombotic/embolic disease, and PH due to miscellaneous other causes. Of special interest is the PAH category, in which each disease is characterized by a progressive increase in pulmonary vascular resistance, leading to right ventricular failure (and death), and has similarities in pathophysiology, clinical presentation, and therapeutic options. Thus, differentiating PAH from other PH types has important clinical implications.

TABLE 25-1.   CLINICAL CLASSIFICATION OF PULMONARY HYPERTENSION (PH) (VENICE 2003)

Pulmonary arterial hypertension (PAH)
- Idiopathic PAH (IPAH)
- Familial PAH (FPAH)
- Associated with PAH (APAH)
    - Connective tissue disorder (CTD)
    - Congenital systemic to pulmonary shunts
    - Portal hypertension
    - Drugs/toxins
    - HIV
- Venous or capillary involvement
    - Pulmonary veno-occlusive disease (PVOD)
    - Pulmonary capillary hemangiomatosis (PCH)

Associated with left heart disease
- Left atrial or ventricular failure
- Left-sided valvular dysfunction
- Congenital heart disease—Eisenmenger's syndrome

Associated with pulmonary disease or hypoxemia
- Emphysema/chronic obstructive pulmonary disease
- Interstitial lung disease
- Hypoxemia, sleep-disordered breathing, obstructive sleep apnea

---

> **TABLE 25-1. CLINICAL CLASSIFICATION OF PULMONARY HYPERTENSION (PH) (VENICE 2003)—CONT'D**
>
> - Alveolar hypoventilation disorders
> - Chronic high-altitude exposure
> - Developmental disorders
>
> **Due to chronic thrombotic and/or embolic disease**
>
> - Thromboembolic obstruction of proximal or distal pulmonary arteries
> - Nonthrombotic pulmonary emboli (e.g., tumor, parasites, foreign material)
>
> **Miscellaneous**
>
> - Sarcoidosis
> - Histiocytosis X
> - Lymphangioleiomyomatosis
> - Compression of vessels (adenopathy, tumor, fibrosing mediastinitis)

3. **List some risk factors for PAH.**
   Various drugs, toxins, demographics, medical conditions, and diseases have definite, probable, or possible associations with PAH (Table 25-2).

> **TABLE 25-2. RISK FACTORS FOR PULMONARY ARTERIAL HYPERTENSION**
>
> **Drugs/toxins**
>
> - Definite: aminorex, fenfluramine, dexfenfluramine, toxic rapeseed oil
> - Probable: amphetamines, L-tryptophan
> - Possible: meta-amphetamines, cocaine, chemotherapeutic agents
>
> **Demographics/medical conditions**
>
> - Definite: sex (female)
> - Possible: pregnancy, systemic hypertension
> - Unlikely: obesity alone
>
> **Diseases**
>
> - Definite: HIV
> - Probable: portal hypertension/liver disease, connective tissue disorders, congenital systemic-pulmonary cardiac shunts
> - Possible: thyroid dysfunction, asplenia, sickle cell disease, β-thalassemia, chronic myeloproliferative disorders, von Gierke's disease, Gaucher's disease, Osler-Weber-Rendu disease

4. **When should PH be suspected?**
   - **Symptoms:** These may include breathlessness without overt signs of heart or lung disease or out of proportion to the underlying disease when heart or lung disease is present. Also, fatigue, weakness, angina, syncope, or abdominal distension may be seen.
   - **Physical signs:** These may include parasternal lift, accentuated cardiac S2 heart sound, pan-systolic tricuspid regurgitant murmur, diastolic pulmonary insufficiency murmur, right ventricular S3 heart sound, jugular venous distention, hepatomegaly,

hepatojugular reflux, peripheral edema, ascites, cool extremities, and central or peripheral cyanosis.
- **Associated conditions:** These may include connective tissue disorders (CTDs, especially scleroderma/systemic sclerosis), portal hypertension, HIV infection, congenital heart disease, and known or suspected ingestion of drugs or toxins.
- **Incidental abnormal study results:** Abnormal results may be the product of an electrocardiogram (e.g., right ventricular hypertrophy, right axis deviation), a chest radiograph (e.g., pulmonary arterial dilatation, "pruning" of peripheral blood vessels, enlargement of right atrium or ventricle), or an echocardiogram (e.g., estimated pulmonary artery systolic pressure from tricuspid regurgitant jet >35 mmHg, enlargement of right atrium or ventricle).

5. **How does one assess the severity of PAH?**
   - **New York Heart Association (NYHA) Class:** Determining the NYHA class (I–IV) is important in the initial evaluation, prognostic determinations, and decision when to treat PAH.
   - **Hemodynamic measurements:** Whether performed noninvasively by echocardiography or invasively by pulmonary arterial catheterization, these measurements can confirm the diagnosis of PAH, can help in assessing its severity, and are valuable in evaluating treatment success.
   - **The 6-minute walk test:** This test is inexpensive and simple to perform. It complements the NYHA functional classification, has prognostic value in PAH, and may also be used to evaluate treatment success.
   - **Cardiopulmonary exercise testing:** This test can also complement these other measures; maximal oxygen consumption is reduced in PAH, and a larger reduction correlates with a poorer prognosis.

6. **Which diagnostic procedures are helpful in evaluating PAH and in differentiating it from other causes of PH?**
   The most common tests are included in Table 25-3.

TABLE 25-3. USEFUL DIAGNOSTIC PROCEDURES IN EVALUATION OF PULMONARY ARTERIAL HYPERTENSION

Test	Features in PAH	Comments
Lung function testing	Normal lung volume and flow, a low DLCO, and ABG sometimes demonstrating hypoxemia	COPD and restrictive respiratory diseases can often be excluded using these tests
Exercise (6-minute walk)	Oxygen desaturation of >10% or distance walked <332 m predicts poorer survival in IPAH	While nonspecific, in PAH it is helpful for initial functional assessment and for treatment follow-up
Chest radiograph/ high-resolution chest CT	Large pulmonary arteries, normal lung parenchyma, large right heart	CT may rule out COPD or interstitial lung disease. CT pulmonary angiography may detect pulmonary emboli or saddle thrombus

TABLE 25-3.   USEFUL DIAGNOSTIC PROCEDURES IN EVALUATION OF PULMONARY ARTERIAL HYPERTENSION—CONT'D

Test	Features in PAH	Comments
Echocardiography	Large right heart, normal or "impinged" left heart (left heart restricted by large right heart), large pulmonary vessels, and tricuspid regurgitation. Estimated pulmonary artery systolic pressure from tricuspid regurgitant jet can be made (>35 mmHg is abnormal)	Left ventricular or valvular dysfunction can be assessed as causes of PH. Agitated saline "bubble" study can evaluate for right-to-left shunt as cause. The more sensitive transesophageal echocardiographic approach may enhance evaluation
Ventilation-perfusion scan	Normal or small peripheral nonsegmental defects on perfusion portion	Normal perfusion virtually rules out pulmonary embolus. Right-to-left shunt and other causes of lung disease can be detected
Polysomnography	Normal	Sleep-disordered breathing causing PH may be tested by this technique
Electrocardiogram	Right ventricular hypertrophy, right axis deviation	Although suggestive, it has low sensitivity and specificity for PAH
Right heart catheterization	Mean PAP > 25 mmHg with PCWP < 16, and PVR > 3 mmHg/L/min. Low CO and other values have prognostic implications	Left-sided dysfunction can often be excluded with a normal PCWP. Technique may be used to assess treatment options
Left heart catheterization	Normal or low CO	Used to confirm normal left ventricular end-diastolic pressures when right heart catheterization is inadequate for PCWP measurements. It may also be helpful for evaluation of pulmonary veno-occlusive diseases
Blood	Hyperuricemia and elevated BNP are seen in right ventricular pressure overload; these correlate with functional severity and poor prognosis	Serology is used to test for connective tissue disorders or HIV as cause of PAH

PAH = pulmonary arterial hypertension, DLCO = diffusion capacity of the lung for carbon monoxide; ABG = arterial blood gases, COPD = chronic obstructive pulmonary disease, IPAH = idiopathic PAH, CT = computed tomography, PAP = pulmonary artery pressure, PCWP = pulmonary capillary wedge pressure, PVR = pulmonary vascular resistance; CO = cardiac output, BNP = brain natriuretic peptide.

7. What are the treatment options for idiopathic PH?

Complexities of advanced testing and therapy dictate that a referral to an appropriate subspecialist (e.g., pulmonary, cardiology) should occur after background therapy and general measures are achieved. The various treatments have been evaluated mainly in sporadic idiopathic PAH (IPAH) and in PAH associated with scleroderma or anorexigen use. Acute vasoreactivity testing should be performed in all patients with PAH. Sustained response to calcium channel blockers (CCB) is defined as NYHA functional class I or II with near normal hemodynamics after several months of treatment. With NYHA functional class III patients, first-line therapy may include oral endothelin receptor antagonists, continuous intravenous epoprostenol, or prostanoid analogs. NYHA functional class IV patients in unstable condition may be better using the inhaled route for class IV with intravenous epoprostenol (Table 25-4).

TABLE 25-4. TREATMENT OPTIONS FOR IDIOPATHIC PULMONARY ARTERIAL HYPERTENSION

Category	Intervention	Comment
General measures	Avoid hypoxia	Take precaution with air travel and altitude
	Take precautions against infection	Avoid pneumonia; Pneumovax and influenza vaccinations are important
	Avoid pregnancy	Added hemodynamic stress is dangerous in PAH
	Avoid anemia or secondary polycythemia	PAH develops with chronic hypoxemia
		Phlebotomy for hct > 65% should be considered
	Avoid ACE inhibitors and beta blockade	There is concern for adverse hemodynamic effects with these agents
	Avoid elective surgery	
	Avoid positive-pressure mechanical ventilation	Monitor for suppressed cardiac output with increased intrathoracic pressures
"Traditional" interventions	Oxygen	Used to keep arterial saturation >90%
	Anticoagulants	Used to limit venous thromboembolism and pulmonary microcirculation thrombus. Adjust INR to 1.5–2.5. Weigh risk-benefit, especially with liver disease
	Diuretics	For symptomatic right heart failure treatment; avoid over-diuresis to prevent inadequate right-sided filling pressures with drop in cardiac output

TABLE 25-4. TREATMENT OPTIONS FOR IDIOPATHIC PULMONARY ARTERIAL HYPERTENSION—CONT'D

Category	Intervention	Comment
	Digitalis	Used to control rate in atrial arrhythmias; unclear benefit for right heart contractility
	Dobutamine	Used in end-stage patients to "bridge" to other treatments
Specific agents	Calcium channel blockers	Effective in <20% of cases of IPAH ("acute vasoreactivity" patients), thus most patients with IPAH should undergo this testing. Acute vasoreactivity predicts good prognosis. In contrast, these agents should not be used in "nonresponders"
	Prostaglandins	Synthetic prostacyclin and prostacyclin analogs are increasingly available in many forms (intravenous, subcutaneous, and now inhaled) and in general are effective for IPAH and other forms of PAH
	Inhaled nitric oxide	An effective vasodilator used for acute testing and treatment; not practical for long-term use
	Endothelin-1 receptor antagonists	Available for oral use. Effective in IPAH and some other forms of PAH
		Avoid in pregnancy (teratogen) and liver disease.
	Type 5 phosphodiesterase inhibitors	Sildenafil (oral preparation) was recently FDA approved for PAH
	Combination therapy	Two or more agents of different classes have been increasingly used in patients who have shown clinical deterioration on single-agent therapy

Continued

TABLE 25-4.   TREATMENT OPTIONS FOR IDIOPATHIC PULMONARY ARTERIAL HYPERTENSION—CONT'D

Category	Intervention	Comment
Surgical intervention	Balloon atrial septostomy	Creation of an atrial right-to-left shunt has been effectively used in selected end-stage patients as a "bridge" to lung transplantation
	Lung transplant, heart/lung transplant	Reserved for patients with advanced NYHA class III or IV symptoms that are refractory to other treatments. Limited long-term survival with transplant and variable organ donor availability makes timely referral to a transplant center essential

ACE = angiotensin-converting enzyme, hct = hematocrit, PAH = pulmonary arterial hypertension, INR = international normalized ratio, IPAH = idiopathic PAH, FDA = U.S. Food and Drug Administration, NYHA = New York Heart Association.

8. **What is the purpose of acute vasoreactivity testing for PAH?**
   Testing hemodynamics with inhaled nitric oxide, intravenous epoprostenol or adenosine can determine the responsiveness to CCB. CCB is a much less expensive treatment option, and responsiveness carries a much more favorable prognosis. Unfortunately, a low percentage of patients will show a positive result (i.e., decrease in mean pulmonary artery pressure to <40 mmHg and by at least 10 mmHg without a decrease in cardiac output).

9. **What is the prognosis for PH?**
   The presence of PH in related disorders (e.g., chronic obstructive pulmonary disease, interstitial lung disease) usually indicates the "end stage" of disease, and prognosis is generally poor. PAH, and particularly IPAH, were once almost uniformly fatal with a life expectancy of <2 years at diagnosis. Organ transplantation and an improved pharmacologic armamentarium have improved prognosis substantially.

10. **Describe characteristics of PAH in CTDs.**
    Systemic sclerosis (scleroderma) with calcinosis, Raynaud's phenomenon, esophageal involvement, sclerodactyly, and telangiectasia (CREST syndrome) is the CTD with the highest incidence (12% prevalence). It can also be seen in systemic lupus erythematosus, mixed connective tissue disease, rheumatoid arthritis, dermatopolymyositis, and primary Sjögren's syndrome.
    - **Pathogenesis:** Unknown; histopathology is virtually indistinguishable from IPAH.
    - **Clinical viewpoint:** The condition must be distinguished from CTD-associated interstitial lung disease (the two may coexist, however). PAH worsens the prognoses of systemic sclerosis. A yearly screening with echocardiography is suggested in patients with systemic sclerosis.
    - **Treatment:** Treatment with immunosuppression is not clearly beneficial for PAH; CCB sensitivity is lower than for IPAH. The benefit of chronic anticoagulation is unclear. Prostaglandins improve hemodynamics, symptoms, and exercise tolerance, but not survival. Treatment with an endothelin-1 receptor antagonist may be helpful.

KEY POINTS: PULMONARY HYPERTENSION

1. PAH is a subset of PH and includes disorders with similar histopathology and response to therapy.

2. PAH includes the following forms: idiopathic, familial, associated with (CTDs, shunt, portal hypertension, drugs/toxins, HIV), and venous capillary involvement.

3. Functional class is important in determining when to start many treatments in PAH; NYHA functional class is in common use. The 6-minute walk is a simple and inexpensive test.

4. Other forms of PH include those associated with left heart disease, pulmonary disease or hypoxemia, chronic embolic or thrombotic disease, and miscellaneous diseases.

5. Multiple new medical interventions are now available for PAH in addition to transplantation, including prostaglandin therapy, endothelin–1 receptor antagonism, and type 5 phosphodiesterase inhibitors.

BIBLIOGRAPHY

1. Galie N , Rubin R : Pulmonary arterial hypertension: Epidemiology, pathobiology assessment therapy. J Am Coll Cardiol 43(Suppl S), 2004.

2. Rubin L (Chair, ACCP Panel): Diagnosis and Management of Pulmonary Artery Hypertension: ACCP Evidence Based Clinical Practice Guidelines. Chest 126(Suppl), 2004.

3. Task Force on Diagnosis and Treatment of Pulmonary Arterial Hypertension of the European Society of Cardiology: Guidelines on diagnosis and treatment of pulmonary arterial hypertension. Eur Heart J 25:2243–2278, 2004.

EVALUATION OF THE PATIENT WITH CHEST PAIN

Daniel Robitshek, MD

1. **What is the most important first step in evaluating a patient with chest pain?**
   The most important first step is to *exclude a potentially life-threatening cause* by taking a brief problem-centered history and performing a focused physical examination.

2. **What are the five most important life-threatening causes of chest pain?**
   - Acute coronary syndrome (ACS)
   - Aortic dissection
   - Pulmonary embolism
   - Pneumothorax
   - Esophageal rupture

3. **What is the most common potentially life-threatening cause of chest pain?**
   The most common life-threatening cause of chest pain is unstable angina, comprising approximately 25–30% of patients presenting to emergency departments with acute chest pain. Acute myocardial infarction (AMI) is the second most common, comprising 10–15% of such patients.

4. **What is the mortality rate of patients with AMI mistakenly discharged from the emergency room?**
   The mortality rate of patients with AMI mistakenly discharged from an emergency department is approximately 25%, more than double the mortality expected of patients admitted to the hospital. The legal costs that can result from such cases constitute the largest category of losses from malpractice litigation in the emergency department.

5. **Describe the vital components of a good chest pain history.**
   A comprehensive chest pain history should include the characteristics of the pain (i.e., quality, location, radiation, associated symptoms, provoking or aggravating factors, and alleviating factors) and the timing of onset and duration of pain.

6. **Which historical components differentiate cardiac chest pain from other causes?**
   - **Quality:** Squeezing, tightness, pressure, burning, fullness, band-like, knot, lump in the throat, ache, heavy weight
   - **Location:** Substernal, diffuse, poorly localized chest discomfort
   - **Radiation:** Epigastrium, shoulders, arms, fingers, neck and throat, lower jaw and teeth (not upper jaw), rarely to the back
   - **Associated symptoms:** Shortness of breath, belching, nausea, indigestion, diaphoresis, dizziness, lightheadedness, clamminess, and fatigue
   - **Timing/duration:** Gradual in onset and usually lasting 5–20 minutes unless there is an AMI, then it can be persistent. If it lasts seconds or hours/days, it is unlikely to be cardiac ischemia.
   - **Provoking/aggravating factors:** Physical activity, cold, emotional stress, sexual intercourse

7. **List historical differences between AMI and unstable angina.**
   See Table 26-1.

TABLE 26-1. HISTORICAL DIFFERENCES BETWEEN UNSTABLE ANGINA AND ACUTE MYOCARDIAL INFARCTION

	Unstable Angina	Acute Myocardial Infarction
Chest pain onset	Waxes and wanes	Crescendo
Chest pain duration	Up to days	Minutes to hours
Past history of CAD	Common	Common or uncommon

CAD = coronary artery disease.

8. **What four physical examination signs increase the likelihood of the presence of an ACS?**
   - An S3 or S4 gallop (especially if new)
   - New murmur (especially mitral regurgitation)
   - Crackles on lung examination
   - Increased jugular venous distention

9. **Apart from the history and physical examination, what is the most important single source of data?**
   Apart from the history and physical exam, the most important single source of data is the 12-lead electrocardiograph (ECG). The ECG changes most commonly associated with an AMI include:
   - One millimeter or more of new ST-segment elevation in two or more contiguous leads; 80% prevalence of AMI
   - ST-segment depression and/or T-wave inversion not known to be old, 20% prevalence of AMI

10. **Describe the characteristics of the chest pain associated with aortic dissection.**
    The classic characteristics include sudden onset of severe tearing, ripping sensation radiating to the midscapular region. It is often associated with hypertension, a widened mediastinum on chest radiograph, and a radial pulse differential. (See Chapter 28, Acute Aortic Dissection, for more details.)

11. **What is the typical description of the chest pain associated with pulmonary embolism?**
    The typical description of the chest pain is pain with inspiration (pleuritic pain). Patients may also have dyspnea associated with tachycardia, tachypnea, and hypoxia. (See Chapter 57 for more details.)

12. **Which patients with chest pain should be admitted to the hospital?**
    Most patients with chest pain will not have a serious cause, yet the differential diagnosis includes many malignant causes. There are no adequately tested criteria to identify which patients should be considered for inpatient as opposed to ambulatory work-up. Based on history and examination, along with relevant diagnostic data, patients with an intermediate to high risk of clinically unstable causes of chest pain should be admitted for stabilization, diagnostic work-up, and/or observation. Alternatively, the risk of adverse outcomes and unwarranted procedures

in patients with low risk or with known stable etiologies should mitigate against hospitalizing these patients.

13. **How are patients who have been ruled out for an ACS risk stratified?**
Once you have excluded an ACS, the next step is to risk-stratify the patient into one of three categories: typical, atypical, and noncardiac chest pain. This distinction is based on the presence or absence of three characteristics: (1) substernal location of chest pain, (2) precipitation by exertion, and (3) alleviation by rest or nitroglycerin.
- *Typical* cardiac chest pain has all three characteristics.
- *Atypical* cardiac chest pain has either one or two of the characteristics.
- *Noncardiac* chest pain has none of the three characteristics.
    The presence of atypical chest pain does not rule out an AMI, it simply means it is less likely to result in an AMI than typical chest pain. Many patients (namely, women and patients with diabetes) often present with an AMI with atypical chest pain symptoms.

14. **What other factors should be taken into account when risk-stratifying patients who present with chest pain?**
The presence of any of the following cardiac risk factors increase the likelihood of true cardiac chest pain: advanced age, male sex, family history of early coronary artery disease (CAD) in a primary relative, or a personal history of diabetes, hypertension, hyperlipidemia or tobacco use.

15. **Which patients should have further noninvasive diagnostic testing to identify those for whom CAD is a cause of their chest pain?**
Patients with atypical cardiac chest pain are at intermediate risk of having CAD and yield the most information on noninvasive testing. This is the only group of the three that should have noninvasive testing for *diagnostic* purposes. You can perform noninvasive testing in the other two groups for *prognostic* purposes. Patients with typical chest pain have a very high pre-test probability of CAD (>90%) and therefore have such an appreciable false-negative rate that further noninvasive testing would not exclude CAD. Likewise, patients with noncardiac chest pain have a significantly low pre-test probability (<10%) and an unacceptably high false-positive rate and therefore should also not undergo noninvasive diagnostic testing.

KEY POINTS: CHEST PAIN

1. The most important first step in evaluating the patient with chest pain is to exclude a life-threatening cause.

2. Patients with cardiac chest pain often describe their discomfort as a poorly localized sensation of squeezing, tightness, pressure, burning, fullness, band, ache, or weight.

3. The single most important source of data in patients suspected of cardiac chest pain, apart from the history and examination, is the 12-lead ECG.

4. Noninvasive stress testing is not indicated for *diagnosing* CAD in patients with typical cardiac chest pain and those with noncardiac chest pain because the negative and positive predictive values, respectively, are poor in these groups.

5. Those patients with atypical cardiac chest pain should undergo diagnostic testing with a provocative stress test to exclude CAD.

6. The most common noncardiac causes of chest pain include gastrointestinal disorders, psychiatric disorders, and chest wall pain.

16. **List the types of noninvasive testing, and outline when they should be used.**
   All types of testing require a mechanism to *stress* the heart and a method to *detect myocardial ischemia.*

   The *stress* portion can be accomplished by exercising (most commonly on a treadmill) or with the use of chemical provocation (e.g., adenosine, dipyridamole [Persantine], or dobutamine). Adenosine and dipyridamole induce coronary vasodilatation. This causes a "steal phenomenon" of blood away from fixed stenotic lesions (which cannot vasodilate), inducing subsequent downstream ischemia. Exercise and dobutamine infusion cause an increased cardiac workload through adrenergic stimulation of the myocardium.

   The *imaging* portion can be accomplished by one of the following: (1) monitoring an ECG tracing for ST changes with or immediately after exertion; (2) an echocardiogram showing abnormal wall motion during stress as compared with rest; or (3) nuclear imaging such as thallium^{201} or technetium^{99m} or other markers of cardiac tissue perfusion showing a reduction in nuclear uptake during the stress portion compared with rest. Any combination of stress and imaging modalities can be used based on patient characteristics. Table 26-2 outlines key features of the various imaging modalities.

   - **Exercise treadmill testing (ETT):** This should be performed in patients who can exercise without significant limitation and do not have ECG findings that preclude the identification of cardiac ischemia (*see* below).
   - **Adenosine, dipyridamole, or dobutamine:** These medications are indicated instead of ETT in patients who are unable to adequately exercise. Caffeine antagonizes the effects of adenosine and dipyridamole and should be avoided before studies using these drugs. These agents can also induce bronchospasm and should be avoided in patients with severe chronic obstructive pulmonary disease or asthma. With left bundle branch block, dipyridamole is preferable to exercise or dobutamine, which may result in false-positive reversible septal defects. Dobutamine use is associated with more cardiac arrhythmias.
   - **Myocardial perfusion imaging or echocardiography:** These can be added to ETT or chemical stresses in patients who have had either prior coronary revascularization or the following baseline ECG abnormalities:
     - Preexcitation (Wolff-Parkinson-White) syndrome
     - Electronically paced ventricular rhythm

TABLE 26-2. CHARACTERISTICS OF CARDIAC IMAGING MODALITIES

	ECG Testing	Nuclear Imaging	Echocardiography
Sensitivity for detecting CAD	65%	85%	85%
Specificity for excluding CAD	85%	85%	85%
Accuracy in presence of baseline ST abnormalities, WPW, LBBB, or pacemaker	+	+++	+++
Localizing ischemia	+	+++	++
Estimating prognosis	++	+++	Limited studies
Cost	Inexpensive (relative)	Expensive	Modest

CAD = coronary artery disease, WPW = Wolff-Parkinson-White syndrome, LBBB = left bundle branch block, + = poor, ++ = good, +++ = very good.

- ST depression >1 mm at rest
- Complete left bundle branch block

17. **What are the most common causes of nonischemic chest pain?**
See Table 26-3.

TABLE 26-3. CAUSES OF NONISCHEMIC CHEST PAIN				
Nonischemic Cardiovascular	Pulmonary	Gastrointestinal	Chest Wall	Psychiatric
Pericarditis	Pneumonia	Biliary: Cholangitis Cholecystitis Choledocholithiasis	Cervical disc disease	Anxiety disorders: Panic disorder Generalized anxiety
Myocarditis	Pleuritis	Esophageal: Esophagitis Spasm Reflux Rupture	Costochondritis	Affective disorder: Depression
Mitral valve prolapse	Pulmonary embolism	Pancreatitis	Fibrositis	Somatoform disorder
Aortic dissection	Pneumothorax	Peptic ulcer	Herpes zoster Rib fracture Sternoclavicular joint pain Neuropathic	Psychosis/ delusions

18. **How does a patient with panic disorder present?**
A panic disorder is a discrete period of intense fear or discomfort, in which four (or more) of the following symptoms develop abruptly and reach a peak within 10 minutes:
- **Cardiopulmonary:** Chest pain, shortness of breath, palpitations
- **Neurologic:** Trembling, shaking, paresthesias, dizziness, lightheadedness or fainting
- **Psychiatric:** Derealization or depersonalization, fear of losing control or going crazy, fear of dying
- **Autonomic:** Sweating, chills, or hot flashes
- **Gastrointestinal:** Choking, nausea, or abdominal distress

BIBLIOGRAPHY

1. ACC/AHA/ACP Guidelines for the Management of Patients with Chronic Stable Angina. J Am Coll Cardiol 33:2092, 1999.
2. Braunwald E, Jones RH, Mark DB, et al: Diagnosing and managing unstable angina. Agency for Health Care Policy and Research. Circulation 90:613, 1994.

3. Diagnostic and Statistical Manual of Mental Disorders, 4th ed, Primary Care Version (DSM-IV-PC). Washington, DC, American Psychiatric Association, 1995.

4. Lee TH, Goldman L: Evaluation of the patient with acute chest pain. N Engl J Med 342:1187, 2000.

CHAPTER 27

ACUTE CORONARY SYNDROMES

Jennifer Kleinbart, MD

1. **Define *acute coronary syndromes* (ACS), and explain how these disorders are differentiated.**

   ACS includes the spectrum of disease resulting from acute coronary occlusion or stenosis, ranging from unstable angina to non–ST-segment elevation myocardial infarction (NSTEMI) to ST-segment elevation myocardial infarction (STEMI). Clinically, electrocardiogram (ECG) changes and cardiac markers are used to differentiate these disorders (Fig. 27-1; Table 27-1).

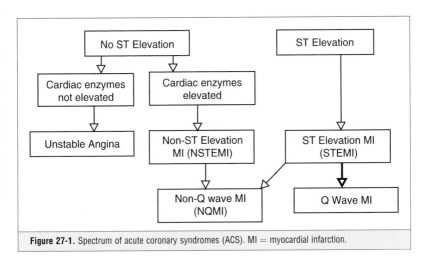

Figure 27-1. Spectrum of acute coronary syndromes (ACS). MI = myocardial infarction.

2. **What is the definition of *acute myocardial infarction* (MI)?**

   In 2000, the definition of *myocardial infarction* was revised to include troponins, which became available as an accurate marker of myocardial necrosis. MI is now defined by *either* number 1 *or* number 2 below:

   1. Typical rise and gradual fall (troponin) or more rapid rise and fall (creatine kinase, myocardial bound [CK-MB]) of biochemical markers of myocardial necrosis with at least one of the following:
      - Ischemic symptoms
      - Development of pathologic Q waves on the ECG
      - ECG changes indicative of ischemia (ST-segment elevation or depression) *or*
      - Coronary artery intervention (e.g., angioplasty)
   2. Pathologic findings of an acute MI

   Joint European Society of Cardiology/American College of Cardiology Committee: Myocardial infarction redefined: A consensus document of the Joint European Society of Cardiology/American College of Cardiology Committee for the Redefinition of Myocardial Infarction. J Am Coll Cardiol 35:959–969, 2000.

TABLE 27-1. FEATURES OF ACUTE CORONARY SYNDROMES			
	Unstable Angina	**NSTEMI**	**STEMI**
Arterial occlusion	Incomplete	Incomplete	Complete
Type of injury	Severe ischemia without infarction	Nontransmural infarction	Transmural infarction
Possible acute ECG changes	Normal Transient ST depression or T inversion	Normal ST depression Transient ST elevation T inversion	"Hyperacute" T waves (early) ST elevation New left bundle-branch block
Cardiac enzymes	Normal or mild troponin ↑ (<0.1 ng/mL)	Elevated	Elevated

3. **What is the pathophysiology of ACS?**
   ACS results when a coronary artery is acutely occluded or severely narrowed, resulting in inadequate blood flow to the myocardium it supplies. This may result from several mechanisms:
   - **Thrombus formation:** An existing nonobstructive atherosclerotic plaque ruptures, causing platelet activation and formation of an occluding thrombus; the most common cause of ACS
   - **Arterial constriction or spasm:** Focal spasm of a nonobstructed coronary artery (Prinzmetal's angina) or arterial vasoconstriction (as with cocaine)
   - **Progressive atherosclerosis or restenosis:** Occur after percutaneous intervention (without acute thrombus or spasm)
   - **Secondary unstable angina:** Increased oxygen demand due to underlying disease (e.g., sepsis, hyperthyroidism) or decreased supply (e.g., anemia) may cause acute ischemia in a patient with lesser degrees of coronary stenosis

4. **What are the major coronary arteries and the regions of myocardium they supply?**
   See Fig. 27-2 and Table 27-2.

KEY POINTS: DEFINITIONS AND CLASSIFICATION OF ACS

1. ACS includes the spectrum of disease that results from acute coronary stenosis or occlusion, ranging from unstable angina to NSTEMI to STEMI.

2. The pathophysiology of ACS usually involves rupture of a nonocclusive atherosclerotic plaque with thrombus formation.

3. NSTEMI is distinguished from unstable angina by the presence of elevated troponins.

4. The diagnosis of MI is made in the presence of a typical rise and gradual fall (troponin) or more rapid rise and fall (CK-MB) of cardiac enzymes along with one of the following: ischemic symptoms, development of pathologic Q waves on the ECG, ECG changes indicative of ischemia (ST-segment elevation or depression), or coronary artery intervention (e.g., angioplasty).

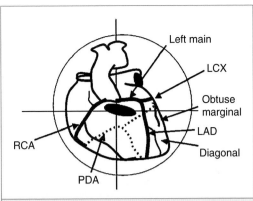

Figure 27-2. Major coronary arteries. RCA = right coronary artery, PDA = posterior descending artery, LCX = left circumflex artery, LAD = left anterior descending artery. Dashed lines indicate posterior aspect of the heart.

TABLE 27-2. MAJOR EPICARDIAL ARTERIES, THEIR BRANCHES, AND REGIONS OF HEART THEY SUPPLY

Major Epicardial Arteries	Major Branches	Regions Supplied
Right coronary artery	Posterior descending artery	Right ventricle
		Inferior and posterior LV
		Posterior septum
		Sinus node, AVN
Left circumflex	Obtuse marginal branches	Lateral wall
		Posterior wall
		AVN (10–15%)
Left anterior descending	Diagonal branches	Septum (anterior two-thirds)
		Anterior, anterolateral LV

LV = left ventricle, AVN = atrioventricular node.

5. **What are established risk factors for coronary artery disease?**
    Major independent risk factors include the following:
    - **Increasing age:** Men >45 years old, women >55 years old or postmenopausal without estrogen therapy
    - **Cigarette smoking**
    - **Hypertension:** Blood pressure >140/90 mmHg
    - **Family history of premature (coronary artery disease):** Definite MI or sudden cardiac death in first-degree relative before age 55 years (males) or 65 years (females)
    - **Coronary heart disease (CHD) risk equivalents:** Diabetes mellitus, chronic kidney disease (creatine >1.5 mg/dL or creatinine clearance < 60 mL/min), and cerebrovascular or

peripheral arterial disease; the risk of ACS among patients with these conditions is similar to that of patients with known CHD
- **Low high-density lipoprotein (HDL) cholesterol:** <40 mg/dL)
- **Elevated total and low-density lipoprotein (LDL) cholesterol:** Risk of cardiovascular disease increases with increasing total and LDL cholesterol, especially at levels over 200 mg/dL and 160 mg/dL, respectively; for patients with established coronary disease, diabetes, or renal disease, the goal should be to reduce LDL cholesterol below 70 mg/dL

Other risk factors include obesity, a sedentary lifestyle, and cocaine use. An elevated HDL (>60 mg/dL) and an active lifestyle protect against cardiovascular disease. An individual's 10-year risk of CHD can be estimated with the Framingham Risk Calculator, which is available at http://hin.nhlbi.nih.gov/atpiii/calculator.asp?usertype=prof.

6. **Which historical features are most useful for determining the likelihood that a patient's symptoms are due to acute MI?**
   History should address location and quality of chest pain, associated symptoms (e.g., nausea, shortness of breath), duration of symptoms, and precipitating/relieving factors. Ischemic pain is often described as a discomfort, tightness, heaviness, or pressure. *Typical* anginal pain is (1) substernal with radiation to the arm, neck or jaw; (2) precipitated by exertion or stress; and (3) relieved by rest or nitroglycerin within 10 minutes. Pain of *infarction* may occur at rest and last >20 minutes. *Atypical* symptoms are more common among women, persons with diabetes, and elderly persons, whose ischemia may manifest as dyspnea, nausea, or fatigue instead of pain. (See Chapter 19 for more details.)

7. **Which factors affect the likelihood that chest pain is due to CHD?**
   See Table 27-3.

8. **Which historical features lower the likelihood that chest pain is due to CHD?**
   Although atypical features lower the likelihood that symptoms are due to acute ischemia, keep in mind that patients with ACS may have atypical presentations. Chest pain that is pleuritic, is reproducible with palpation or movement of the upper body, is located primarily over the left chest (versus typical substernal pain) or mid-abdomen, radiates to the legs, or can be localized with one finger is atypical for ischemic pain. Likewise, pain that lasts for seconds or is constant for many hours (without objective evidence of myocardial injury) is unlikely to be due to CHD.

9. **Describe the Canadian Cardiovascular Society Classification (CCSC) for grading the severity of unstable angina.**
   See Table 27-4.

10. **Describe the three presentations of unstable angina.**
    - **Accelerating angina:** Increase in severity, frequency, or duration of symptoms, with an increase of at least one CCSC class to at least class III in the past 2 weeks
    - **New angina:** Within the past 2 weeks
    - **Rest angina**

11. **What are key elements of the physical examination in patients with suspected ACS?**
    Assess hemodynamic stability, evaluate for complications of AMI, and identify findings suggesting another etiology of chest pain.
    - **Hemodynamics:** Measure blood pressure in both arms and palpate all pulses. Cardiogenic shock is characterized by hypotension with signs of poor perfusion, such as cool extremities. Identify extracardiac vascular disease by palpating peripheral pulses and listening for carotid, renal, and femoral bruits.

TABLE 27–3. LIKELIHOOD THAT SIGNS AND SYMPTOMS REPRESENT AN ACS SECONDARY TO CHD

Feature	High Likelihood *Any of the following:*	Intermediate Likelihood *Absence of high-likelihood features and presence of any of the following:*	Low Likelihood *Absence of high- or intermediate-likelihood features but may have:*
History	Chest or left arm pain or discomfort as chief symptom reproducing prior documented angina Known history of CAD, including MI	Chest or left arm pain or discomfort as chief symptom Age >70 years Male sex Diabetes mellitus	Probable ischemic symptoms in absence of any of the intermediate likelihood characteristics Recent cocaine use
Examination	Transient mitral regurgitation, hypotension, diaphoresis, pulmonary edema, or rales	Extracardiac vascular disease	Chest discomfort reproduced by palpation
ECG	New, or presumably new, transient ST-segment deviation (≥0.05 mV) or T-wave inversion (≥0.2 mV) with symptoms	Fixed Q waves Abnormal ST segments or T waves not documented to be new	T-wave flattening or inversion in leads with dominant R waves Normal ECG
Cardiac markers	Elevated cardiac TnI, TnT, or CK-MB	Normal	Normal

Braunwald E, Mark DB, Jones RH, et al. Unstable angina: diagnosis and management. Rockville, MD: Agency for Health Care Policy and Research and the National Heart, Lung, and Blood Institute, US Public Health Service, US Department of Health and Human Services; 1994; AHCPR Publication No. 94-0602.

TABLE 27-4. CANADIAN CARDIOVASCULAR SOCIETY CLASSIFICATION OF ANGINA

Class	Description	Examples of Activity Level That Causes Symptoms
I	Ordinary activity does not cause angina	Rapid or prolonged exertion
II	Slight limitation of ordinary activity	Walking >2 blocks on level surface or climbing >1 flight of stairs at normal pace
III	Marked limitation of ordinary physical activity	Walking <2 blocks on level surface, climbing <1 flight of stairs
IV	Severe limitation	Any physical activity causes symptoms; may occur at rest

- **Complications:** Elevated jugular venous pressure with rales and an S3 is consistent with left ventricular (LV) failure and pulmonary edema. Elevated jugular venous pressure with hypotension occurs with cardiac tamponade and right ventricular (RV) infarction. A mitral regurgitation murmur may indicate acute papillary muscle or chordae rupture.
- **Signs of other diagnoses:** Unequal blood pressure between right and left arms and an aortic regurgitation murmur occur with aortic dissection. A friction rub indicates pericarditis. Chest wall or shoulder tenderness suggests musculoskeletal causes of pain. (See Chapter 19 for more details.)

KEY POINTS: HISTORY IN PATIENTS SUSPECTED OF ACS

1. Risk factors for atherosclerotic cardiovascular disease include increasing age, family history of premature coronary disease, hypertension, smoking, diabetes mellitus, renal disease, and dyslipidemia.

2. The initial evaluation of a patient with suspected ACS should focus on assessing the likelihood that a patient's symptoms represent ACS and the risk of short-term events.

3. Atypical symptoms are more common in women, elderly persons, and persons with diabetes.

4. Ischemic chest pain is typically worsened with exertion and relieved with rest, whereas pain of infarction may occur at rest and be prolonged.

12. **Describe the time course of the rise and fall of cardiac enzymes in ACS.**
    See Fig. 27-3.

13. **How accurate are myoglobin, troponins, and CK-MB for diagnosing acute MI?**
    At presentation, sensitivity of all markers is unacceptably *low* (60–78%). Serial enzymes in combination (both CK-MB *and* troponin T or I measured at presentation and 6–8 hours later) provides the highest sensitivity (98%) and specificity (93%). Myoglobin is a highly sensitive but nonspecific marker in the first 4–6 hours. Measuring the change in myoglobin during this time may allow earlier exclusion of acute MI.

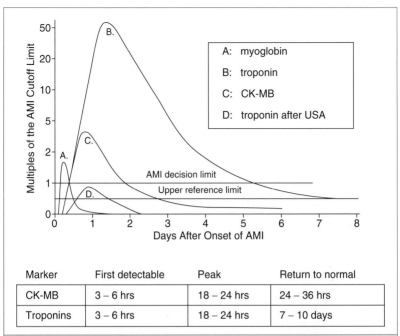

Figure 27-3. Time course of rise and fall of commonly used cardiac enzymes. AMI = acute myocardial infarction, CK-MB = creatine kinase, myocardial bound, USA = unstable angina. (With permission from the American College of Cardiology website: http://www.acc.org/clinical/guidelines/stemi/Guideline1/Images/figure11.jpg.)

14. **What other conditions may cause elevations in cardiac markers?**
    - **CK-MB:** Skeletal muscle injury or disease (e.g., surgery, trauma, myositis, rhabdomyolysis) and renal dysfunction. In these cases, the total creatine phosphokinase (CPK) is also elevated so that the ratio of CK-MB/CPK is not affected (normal ratios vary by laboratory, but typically range from 1% to 2.5%).
    - **Troponins:** Renal disease, pulmonary embolism, and decompensated heart failure
    - **Myoglobin:** Skeletal muscle injury or disease

15. **Which initial tests should be ordered in patients with suspected ACS?**
    Order cardiac enzymes (CK-MB, total CPK, and troponin T or I) and a 12-lead ECG on presentation, and repeat them 6–8 hours later. If a high suspicion of ACS is present, repeating the ECG in the first 3 hours may be useful for more prompt identification of infarction. Additional studies to order on presentation include complete blood cell count with platelets, complete metabolic profile (chemistry and hepatic panel), coagulation panel (partial thromboplastin time/international normalized ratio), lipid panel, β–human chorionic gonadotropin (for all premenopausal females), and chest x-ray. Consider a urinalysis to screen for hematuria, which would need to be monitored in patients receiving anticoagulation or in cases of infection. Consider a drug screen, especially if cocaine use is suspected.

16. **Describe the progression of ECG changes in STEMI.**
    See Table 27-5.

TABLE 27-5. SEQUENCE OF ECG CHANGES DURING AND AFTER ACUTE MI

Phase	Acute		Evolved	Chronic
Timing	Minutes	Minutes to hours	Hours to days	Weeks
Sample ECG				
ECG changes	Tall "hyperacute" T waves	ST-segment elevation and reciprocal ST-segment depression	ST segment gradually returns to baseline T-wave inversions	Q waves generally persist T-wave inversions may resolve

17. Know the ECG criteria to diagnose acute transmural MI by anatomic location. See Table 27-6.

TABLE 27-6. ECG FINDINGS IN ACUTE STEMI BY SITE OF INFARCT		
Area	Leads	Acute ECG Findings
Septal	V_1–V_2	ST-segment elevation >1 mm in two or more
Anterior	V_3–V_4	consecutive leads (using a cut-off of 2-mm
Lateral	I, aVL, V_5–V_6	elevation in anterior precordial improves
Inferior	II, III, aVF	diagnostic accuracy)
Posterior	V_1–V_2	Tall R waves, ST-segment depression
Right ventricle	V_1 or right-sided V_4	ST-segment elevation >1 mm

Adapted from Menown IB, Mackenzie G, Adgey AA: Optimizing the initial 12-lead electrocardiographic diagnosis of acute myocardial infarction. Eur Heart J 21:275–283, 2000.

18. Besides acute MI, what are other causes of ST-segment elevation?
 - **Pericarditis:** Diffuse ST-segment elevation and PR-segment depression except in lead aVR, which shows ST *depression* and PR *elevation*
 - **Early repolarization:** Seen with LV hypertrophy, in athletes, and in young men; ST segment is usually concave and upward
 - **Left bundle branch block, LV hypertrophy:** ST-segment elevation concave and upward in right precordial leads
 - **LV aneurysm:** Persistent ST-segment elevation in anterior leads after MI
 - **Hypothermia:** Prominent J-point elevation (marks beginning of ST segment) with resultant Osborne waves

19. Describe ECG changes that may be seen with non–ST-segment elevation ACS.
 ST-segment depression that is horizontal or downsloping and symmetric T-wave inversions represent subendocardial ischemia.

KEY POINTS: LABORATORY AND ECG EVALUATION OF ACS

1. Cardiac biomarkers may not be elevated at the time of initial presentation and must be repeated 6–8 hours later.

2. Acute MI is effectively ruled out by two negative sets of cardiac enzyme measurements (troponin and CK-MB) drawn 6–8 hours apart.

3. In STEMI, the area of infarct should be identified on ECG by the leads with ST-segment elevation.

20. **When should RV infarction be suspected?**
RV infarction should be suspected in patients with an inferior MI, especially if complicated by hypotension. RV infarction typically results from occlusion of the proximal right coronary artery, which supplies the right ventricle via the RV branch, as well as the inferior myocardium. ECG signs of acute RV infarction include ST-segment elevation in right-sided leads V_3 or V_4.

21. **Discuss important management issues in patients with RV infarction.**
RV infarction can lead to decreased RV compliance with impaired filling and decreased output to the left ventricle. This may result in hypotension, especially if nitrates are used, further decreasing preload. Patients with RV infarction who are hypotensive should be given intravenous fluids, and nitrates should be avoided.

22. **What are the overall mortality rates for patients with ACS?**
Overall in-hospital mortality for patients with unstable angina, NSTEMI, and STEMI is approximately 3%, 5%, and 8%, respectively. During the 6 months after discharge, another 3–6% of patients will die and approximately 20% of patients will be readmitted.

    Global Registry of Acute Coronary Events (GRACE) International ACS Registry 2005 Q-1 Data. Available at http://www.outcomes-umassmed.org/grace

23. **Which characteristics are associated with a higher risk of adverse outcomes in patients with ACS?**
Age >75 years and cardiogenic shock are the strongest predictors of mortality. Thirty-day mortality for patients with cardiogenic shock ranges from 45% to 80%. Other groups with higher mortality are women, persons with diabetes, those with stroke or heart failure during hospitalization, and patients with anterior or RV infarction. Mortality also increases with increasing baseline and peak levels of troponin.

24. **What are early complications of acute MI and their manifestations?**
   - **Mechanical complications:** Rupture of a papillary muscle, the ventricular septum, or LV free wall carries a very high mortality rate and requires emergent surgical repair. The incidence among patients with STEMI is <0.4% for septal rupture, 1–3% for papillary muscle rupture, and up to 6% for free wall rupture. Rupture generally occurs within the first 5 days after acute MI and should be suspected in the presence of a new systolic murmur, sudden hemodynamic collapse, acute pulmonary edema, electromechanical dissociation, or sudden death.
   - **Electrical complications:** Atrial and ventricular dysrhythmias may occur with STEMI. Spontaneous ventricular fibrillation or sustained ventricular tachycardia occurring after the first 48 hours is an indication for defibrillator placement. Inferior and RV infarctions are associated with sinus bradycardia, sinus node dysfunction, and atrioventricular block. Atrial fibrillation may complicate large or anterior infarctions and is also associated with higher mortality.

25. **Which therapies are indicated in the initial management of ACS?**
See Table 27-7.

26. **What are the benefits of reperfusion after acute MI?**
   - **STEMI:** Prompt reperfusion to restore flow to the occluded artery with either primary percutaneous coronary intervention (PCI) or thrombolytics decreases short- and long-term mortality in STEMI patients. When PCI can be performed within 90 minutes of hospital arrival, this is generally preferred over thrombolytic therapy. Otherwise, thrombolytic therapy should be administered if the onset of symptoms occurred within 12 hours and there are no contraindications (Table 27-8).

TABLE 27-7. INITIAL TREATMENT OF ACS

	NSTEMI	STEMI
Antiplatelet	Aspirin *Clopidogrel †Glycoprotein IIb/IIIa inhibitor	Aspirin
Anticoagulant	Enoxaparin SQ *or* Unfractionated heparin IV	Unfractionated heparin IV *or* enoxaparin SQ
Reperfusion	Primary PCI	Primary PCI *or* Thrombolytics
Anti-ischemic	Beta blocker (without intrinsic sympathomimetic effects)‡ Nitroglycerin Morphine for ongoing pain	
Other	HMG CoA–reductase inhibitor (statin) ACE inhibitor: especially if diabetes or LV systolic dysfunction is present	

* Clopidogrel should be used as initial treatment for patients with true aspirin allergy or in combination with aspirin for patients not planned to undergo angiography/revascularization.
† Glycoprotein IIb/IIIa inhibitors are indicated for patients with non–ST-segment elevation ACS who are planned for angiography/revascularization or who have elevated troponin levels or dynamic ST-segment depression on ECG.
‡ Metoprolol, atenolol, propranolol, esmolol.
SQ = subcutaneous, IV = intravenous, PCI = primary coronary intervention (balloon angioplasty or coronary stenting), HMG CoA = 3-hydroxy-3-methylglutaryl coenzyme A.

TABLE 27-8. CONTRAINDICATIONS TO THROMBOLYTIC THERAPY FOR STEMI

Contraindications	
Absolute	**Relative**
Prior intracranial hemorrhage	Blood pressure >180/110 mmHg
Cerebral vascular lesion (arteriovenous malformation)	Ischemic stroke >3 months prior
Intracranial neoplasm	Dementia
Ischemic stroke within 3 months (except acute ischemic stroke within 3 hours)	Traumatic or prolonged CPR (>10 minutes) within 3 weeks
Suspected aortic dissection	Major surgery or internal bleeding within 3 weeks
Active bleeding or bleeding diathesis (excluding menses)	Pregnancy
Significant closed-head or facial trauma within 3 months	Active peptic ulcer Current use of anticoagulants

CPR = cardiopulmonary resuscitation.

- **NSTEMI, unstable angina:** Early invasive management (i.e., routine angiography with revascularization when indicated, ideally within 24–48 hours) is recommended for patients at high risk for short-term adverse events as evidenced by ST-segment depression, troponin elevation, hemodynamic instability, angina at rest, recurrent ischemia, systolic dysfunction or signs of heart failure, PCI in the last 6 months, or sustained ventricular tachycardia. A noninvasive approach using medical management is appropriate for lower-risk patients.

27. **What type of risk factor modification and counseling should be addressed before the patient is discharged from the hospital?**
    Within 6 years of MI, 35% of women and 18% of men will experience a recurrent MI, and 46% of women and 22% of men will be disabled from heart failure. To reduce these risks, patients should be counseled about lifestyle modifications that include smoking cessation, diet (i.e., low fat/cholesterol, low sodium if hypertensive), exercise, and weight loss. Patients should be educated about medications, provided with follow-up appointments, and referred to a cardiac rehabilitation program.

    American Heart Association: Heart Disease and Stroke Statistics—2004 Update. Dallas, American Heart Association, 2003. Available at http://www.americanheart.org/presenter.jhtml?identifier=3000090.

KEY POINTS: TREATMENT OF ACS

1. All patients with suspected ACS should be given aspirin immediately on presentation.

2. Initial treatment of patients with ACS includes antiplatelet agents, anticoagulation, anti-ischemic therapy, and reperfusion (when indicated).

3. Prompt identification and treatment of patients with ACS reduces adverse events.

4. Patients with STEMI should undergo emergent reperfusion with PCI or thrombolytic therapy.

5. Primary PCI is recommended for high-risk patients with NSTEMI or unstable angina.

6. Provide education on risk factor modification (e.g., smoking cessation, diet, medication compliance) before hospital discharge.

28. **List standard discharge medications for patients with ACS.**
    Unless contraindicated, all patients with ACS should be discharged with aspirin, clopidogrel, a beta blocker, an angiotensin-converting enzyme (ACE) inhibitor (or angiotensin receptor blocker if ACE inhibitor not tolerated), and a statin. Lipid lowering should aim for an LDL < 70 mg/dL, and for most patients blood pressure should be <120/80 mmHg. In patients with STEMI, an ejection fraction <40% and symptomatic heart failure, aldosterone blockade (eplerenone or spironolactone) should be considered.

WEBSITES

1. TIMI Risk Calculator: http://www.timi.org

2. Grace Risk Calculator: http://www.outcomes-umassmed.org/GRACE/acs_risk.cfm

BIBLIOGRAPHY

1. Antman EM, Anbe DT, Armstrong PW, et al: ACC/AHA guidelines for the management of patients with ST-elevation myocardial infarction: executive summary: a report of the ACC/AHA Task Force on Practice Guidelines (Committee to Revise the 1999 Guidelines on the Management of Patients With Acute Myocardial Infarction). J Am Coll Cardiol 44:671–719, 2004. Available at http://www.acc.org/clinical/guidelines/stemi/, 2004.

2. Antman E, Antman EM, Beasley JW, et al: ACC/AHA 2002 guideline update for the management of patients with unstable angina and non–ST-segment elevation myocardial infarction: A report of the American College of Cardiology/American Heart Association Task Force on Practice Guidelines, Committee on the Management of Patients With Unstable Angina, 2002. Available at http://www.acc.org/clinical/guidelines/unstable/incorporated/index.htm., 2002.

CHAPTER 28

ACUTE AORTIC DISSECTION

Eric M. Siegal, MD

1. **Why is aortic dissection important?**
   Although an uncommon cause of acute chest pain, acute aortic dissection is highly lethal and frequently mistaken for less serious pathology. Up to 40% of aortic dissections are misdiagnosed at presentation. In the first 48 hours, the mortality rate for untreated aortic dissection is as high as 1% *per hour*, but survival exceeds 90% with prompt diagnosis and management. For these reasons, hospitalists must be able to rapidly identify aortic dissection, initiate care, and involve the appropriate consultants.

2. **What is an acute aortic dissection?**
   Aortic dissections result from tears in the aortic intima. Blood dissects across tissue planes into the aortic media, creating a false lumen, which may then propagate proximally or distally. Any dissection that is <14 days old is considered acute.

3. **Why are aortic dissections so lethal?**
   In their most dramatic presentation, aortic dissections rupture, causing rapid exsanguination and death. More frequently, aortic dissections impinge blood flow across aortic branch vessels or directly compromise the integrity of the pericardium or aortic valve.

4. **What are the major risk factors for aortic dissection?**
   Aortic dissection is primarily a disease of elderly men with hypertension. About 65% of aortic dissections occur in men over the age of 60 years. Hypertension, found in 72% of patients, is by far the most common risk factor. Other major risk factors include atherosclerosis (31%), history of prior cardiac surgery (18%), and known aortic aneurysm (16%).

5. **What are some other risk factors for dissection?**
   The following risk factors are generally more common in younger patients (<40 years old):
   - Marfan syndrome (present in 50% of young patients with dissection)
   - Bicuspid aortic valve (5–18-fold relative risk increase)
   - Aortic coarctation
   - Turner's syndrome
   - Strenuous exercise (e.g., weight lifting)
   - Large-vessel arteritis (e.g., giant cell and Takayasu's arteritis)
   - Sympathomimetic drug abuse (e.g., cocaine and methamphetamine)
   - Third-trimester pregnancy
   - Blunt chest trauma or high-speed deceleration injury
   - Cardiac catheterization (e.g., iatrogenic injury to the aortic endothelium)

6. **How are aortic dissections classified?**
   Aortic dissections are classified by anatomic location. The fundamental distinction is whether the dissection is proximal (involving the aortic root and/or ascending aorta) or distal (below the left subclavian artery). Proximal aortic dissections are surgical emergencies, whereas distal dissections can often be managed medically. The Stanford and DeBakey classification systems are most commonly used (Table 28-1; Fig. 28-1).

TABLE 28-1.   TRADITIONAL CLASSIFICATION OF AORTIC DISSECTION

Stanford:

Type A:	Ascending aorta
Type B:	Descending aorta, distal to left subclavian artery

DeBakey:

Type I:	Ascending and descending aorta
Type II:	Ascending aorta
Type III:	Descending aorta

a. Limited to the thoracic aorta

b. Extending to the abdominal aorta

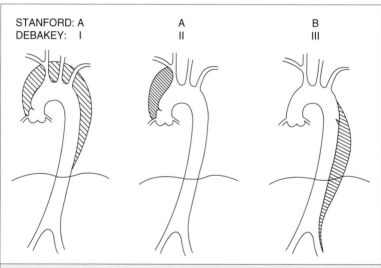

Figure 28-1. Stanford and DeBakey systems of classification of aortic dissection.

Some variants of aortic dissection are not described in either the Stanford or DeBakey systems. Aortic intramural hematomas are caused by intraluminal hemorrhage and thrombosis of the aortic wall without an identifiable intimal tear. Penetrating atherosclerotic ulcers are focal defects in the aortic wall with surrounding hematoma but no longitudinal tissue plane dissection. These variants may present similarly to aortic dissection but differ in their diagnostic and therapeutic implications. In recognition of these variants, a more comprehensive classification system has been proposed (Table 28-2; Fig. 28-2).

7. **What is the differential diagnosis of aortic dissection?**
    The differential diagnosis for aortic dissection is similar to any presentation of acute chest pain and includes acute coronary syndrome, pericarditis, pneumothorax, pneumonia, pulmonary embolus, acute pancreatitis, cholecystitis, esophageal spasm or rupture, and musculoskeletal pain.

TABLE 28-2.   PROPOSED CLASSIFICATION OF AORTIC DISSECTION

Class 1: Classical aortic dissection with intimal flap between true and false lumen
(Further subdivided according to Stanford or DeBakey classification)
Class 2: Aortic intramural hematoma without identifiable intimal flap
Class 3: Intimal tear without hematoma (limited dissection)
Class 4: Atherosclerotic plaque rupture with aortic penetrating ulcer
Class 5: Iatrogenic or traumatic aortic dissection (intra-aortic catheterization, high-speed
deceleration injury, blunt chest trauma)

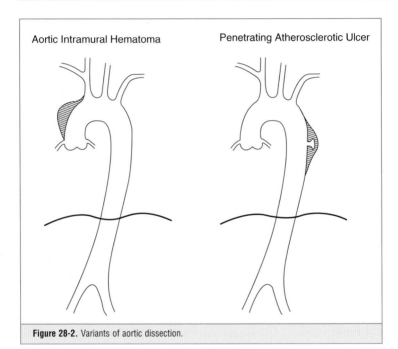

Aortic Intramural Hematoma   Penetrating Atherosclerotic Ulcer

Figure 28-2. Variants of aortic dissection.

8. **How does acute aortic dissection classically present?**
Aortic dissections are rarely asymptomatic. Upward of 90% of patients complain of the abrupt
onset of chest or back pain, usually very severe, that is classically described as "tearing" or
"ripping." Although hypertension is a common acute finding, about 15% of patients present with
hypotension or shock.

9. **What other findings may be seen in aortic dissection?**
Much of the pathology associated with aortic dissection results from dissection across blood
vessels that originate at the aorta, disrupting blood flow to end-organs. Clinical findings depend
on the anatomic location of the dissection and may include:
- Hypotension or shock due to:
  □ Hemopericardium and pericardial tamponade
  □ Acute aortic insufficiency due to dilatation of the aortic annulus
  □ Aortic rupture

- Acute myocardial ischemia/infarction due to coronary ostial occlusion
- Pericardial friction rub due to hemopericardium
- Syncope
- Pleural effusion or frank hemothorax
- Acute renal failure due to dissection across the renal arteries
- Mesenteric ischemia due to dissection across intra-abdominal arteries
- Neurologic deficits
  - Stroke due to occlusion of the arch vessels that supply the brain
  - Limb weakness
  - Spinal cord deficits due to cord ischemia
  - Horner syndrome due to compression of the superior sympathetic ganglion
  - Hoarseness due to compression of the left recurrent laryngeal nerve

The diagnosis of aortic dissection should be considered for any patient who presents with acute chest pain and acute neurologic deficits or end-organ injury.

10. Which three key clinical findings correlate strongly with aortic dissection?
1. Immediate onset of tearing or ripping chest pain
2. Mediastinal widening (>8 cm) or aortic enlargement/displacement on chest radiograph
3. Variable pulse pressure (>20 mmHg difference between arms)

If all three findings are absent, dissection is unlikely ($<7\%$). If either chest pain or radiographic findings are present, the likelihood is intermediate (31–39%). With any other combination of findings, dissection is likely ($>83\%$).

11. Does a normal chest radiograph exclude aortic dissection?
No. About 10% of patients with aortic dissection have a completely normal-appearing chest radiograph. Mediastinal widening and abnormal aortic contour, the "classic" findings in aortic dissection, are present in only 50–60% of cases. Nonspecific radiographic findings, most notably pleural effusion, may also be seen (Fig. 28-3).

12. Which imaging modalities definitively diagnose or rule out aortic dissection?
Four imaging modalities reliably identify or exclude aortic dissection. See Table 28-3 and Figs. 28-4 and 28-5.

13. How do I decide which study is right for my patient?
Computed tomography (CT), magnetic resonance angiography (MRA), and transesophageal echocardiography (TEE) are all excellent modalities for the evaluation of aortic dissection, with sensitivities and specificities approaching 100%. Therefore, the patient's condition, the information needed, and the resources and expertise available should drive the choice of study. MRA is the gold standard and the preferred modality for hemodynamically stable patients with suspected aortic dissection. Bedside TEE is an excellent choice for patients whose conditions are too unstable for MRA. Arch aortography is generally reserved to confirm questionable diagnoses or to specifically image branch arteries. In most hospitals, however, CT angiography is likely the most readily available imaging modality. Figure 28-6 is an algorithm summarizing the diagnostic approach to acute aortic dissection.

14. How is hypertension managed in acute aortic dissection?
About half of patients who present with acute aortic dissection are acutely hypertensive. This is a true hypertensive emergency that mandates immediate decrease in blood pressure to the lowest level that maintains organ perfusion as measured by such indicators as sensorium and urine output. As a rule, short-acting, parenteral, titratable antihypertensive agents should be used (Table 28-4).

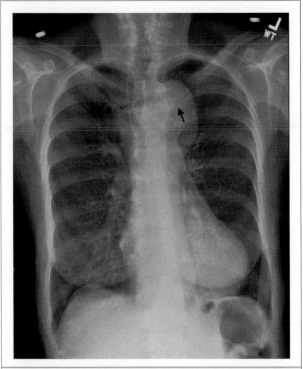

Figure 28-3. Chest radiograph of proximal aortic dissection, showing superior displacement of the aortic knob. (Courtesy Dr. E. Adib, UW Health and Meriter Hospital, Madison, WI.)

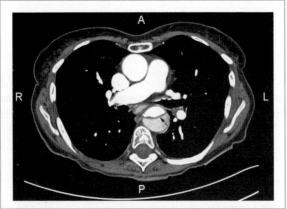

Figure 28-4. Axial view of a computed tomographic angiogram demonstrating proximal aortic dissection. (Courtesy Dr. E. Adib, UW Health and Meriter Hospital, Madison, WI.)

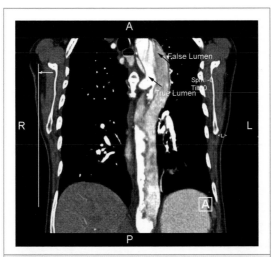

Figure 28-5. Transverse view of a computed tomographic angiogram demonstrating proximal aortic dissection. (Courtesy of Dr. E. Adib, UW Health and Meriter Hospital, Madison, WI.)

TABLE 28-3. IMAGING MODALITIES FOR AORTIC DISSECTION

Imaging Modality	Advantages	Disadvantages
Arch aortogram	Good views of the intimal flap, true and false lumen, coronary arteries and aortic valve	Invasive and time consuming Requires nephrotoxic contrast Cannot visualize aortic intramural hematoma. Sensitivity is lower than TEE, MRA, and CTA
Computed tomographic angiogram (CTA)	Readily available at most hospitals Very fast (<10 min)	Requires nephrotoxic contrast Limited ability to assess site of intimal flap or competency of aortic valve
Magnetic resonance angiography (MRA)	Extremely sensitive and specific No nephrotoxic contrast required Good visualization of branch vessels and variants of dissection	Slow (30–60 minutes) Inappropriate for unstable patients, who are largely inaccessible for duration of study May not be immediately available at many hospitals
Transesophageal echocardiogram (TEE)	Can be done at bedside Excellent view of intimal tear, aortic valves, pericardium	Invasive Requires rapid availability of a skilled operator

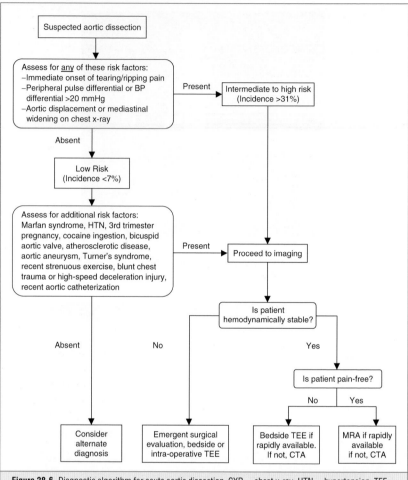

Figure 28-6. Diagnostic algorithm for acute aortic dissection. CXR = chest x-ray, HTN = hypertension, TEE = transesophageal echocardiography, MRA = magnetic resonance angiography, CTA = computed tomographic angiography.

- Intravenous beta blockers (e.g., labetalol, metoprolol, esmolol) are first-line therapy. Their negative inotropic/chronotropic effects decrease systolic shear stress and limit further propagation of the dissection.
- Vasodilators (e.g., nitroprusside, nitroglycerin) should be initiated if beta blockers prove insufficient to lower blood pressure. Vasodilators should never be used alone because they may cause reflex tachycardia, increasing intraluminal shear stress.
  Analgesia and anxiolysis further decrease blood pressure by controlling the severe pain and anxiety often associated with acute dissections.

15. **What is the significance of hypotension?**
    Hypotension, or shock, which develops in 15–30% of patients with acute aortic dissection, is an ominous finding that frequently portends hemodynamic collapse. The three most common

TABLE 28-4. ANTIHYPERTENSIVES IN ACUTE AORTIC DISSECTION

Name	Mechanism	Dose	Cautions/ Contraindications
Esmolol	Cardioselective beta$_1$ blocker	Load: 500 μg/kg IV Drip: 50 μg/kg/min IV Increase by increments of 50 μg/min	Asthma or bronchospasm Bradycardia Second- or third-degree AV block Cocaine or methamphetamine use
Labetalol	Nonselective beta$_{1,2}$ blocker Selective alpha$_1$ blocker	Load: 20 mg IV Drip: 2 mg/min IV	Asthma or bronchospasm Bradycardia Second- or third-degree AV block Cocaine or methamphetamine use
Enalaprilat	ACE inhibitor	0.625–1.25 mg IV q6h Max dose: 5 mg q6h	Angioedema Pregnancy Renal artery stenosis Severe renal insufficiency
Nitroprusside	Direct arterial vasodilator	Begin at 0.3 μg/kg/min IV Max dose: 10 μg/kg/min	May cause reflex tachycardia Cyanide/thiocyanate toxicity—especially in renal insufficiency
Nitroglycerin	Vascular smooth muscle relaxation	5–200 μg/min IV	Decreases preload— contraindicated in tamponade or other preload-dependent states Concomitant use of sildenafil or similar agents

IV = intravenous, AV = arteriovenous, ACE = angiotensin-converting enzyme.

causes of hypotension are acute aortic insufficiency, pericardial tamponade, and aortic rupture. Bedside transthoracic echocardiography is very useful for quickly evaluating the integrity of the pericardium and aortic valve. Tamponade and aortic rupture should be managed with fluid resuscitation. A small case series suggests that pericardiocentesis may actually worsen outcomes by accelerating exsanguination. Aortic insufficiency may be temporized with parenteral afterload reduction.

16. **What is the role of surgery in aortic dissection?**
    Proximal aortic dissections frequently compromise the pericardium, aortic valve, or great
    vessels of the aortic arch and therefore are surgical emergencies requiring immediate
    exploration and repair. Uncomplicated distal aortic dissections are usually managed medically.
    Hypotension, irrespective of the type of dissection, should prompt immediate surgical referral.

KEY POINTS: AORTIC DISSECTION

1. Hypertension is by far the most important risk factor for aortic dissection.

2. Look for three key findings when working up acute aortic dissection: immediate onset of
   tearing or ripping chest/back pain, mediastinal/aortic widening on chest radiograph, and
   variable pulse pressure.

3. Suspect aortic dissection in patients who present with acute chest pain and either acute
   neurologic deficits or acute end-organ damage.

4. A normal-appearing chest radiograph does *not* rule out aortic dissection. TEE, CT
   angiography, MRA, or arch aortogram must be performed to definitively rule out dissection.

5. Intravenous beta blockers are first-line therapy for patients who present with aortic
   dissection and hypertension.

17. **Are there alternatives to surgery?**
    Endovascular stent-grafting has been successfully used in patients with distal aortic dissections
    who would have otherwise required surgery. The stent-graft is deployed across the proximal
    intimal tear, obliterating the false lumen and allowing the aorta to heal. Preliminary studies
    suggest that endovascular stent-grafting may be safer and more efficacious than conventional
    surgery for type B dissections. However, long-term data are lacking and it remains unclear what,
    if any, complications may arise over the course of years.

18. **What is the prognosis in acute aortic dissection?**
    Despite significant medical and surgical advances, aortic dissection remains an extremely lethal
    disease (Table 28-5). In general, patients with proximal dissections are more likely to die than
    those with distal dissections. Medical treatment of proximal dissection is generally reserved for
    patients too ill, unstable, or frail to undergo surgery, hence the exceptionally high mortality rate.
    In contrast, the majority of patients with distal dissection are managed medically. Surgery is
    generally reserved for acute complications.

TABLE 28-5. MORTALITY IN ACUTE AORTIC DISSECTION BY TYPE OF MANAGEMENT				
	Proximal (DeBakey I, II; Stanford A)		Distal (DeBakey III; Stanford B)	
	Surgical	Medical	Surgical	Medical
In-hospital mortality	26%	58%	31%	11%
Average	35%		15%	

BIBLIOGRAPHY

1. Hagan PG, Nienaber CA, Isselbacher EM, et al: The international registry of acute aortic dissection (IRAD): New insights into an old disease. JAMA 283:897–903, 2000.

2. Januzzi J, Isselbacher EM, Fattori R, et al: Characterizing the young patient with aortic dissection: Results from the international registry of aortic dissection (IRAD). J Am Coll Cardiol 43:665–669, 2004.

3. Nienaber CA, von Kodolitsch Y, Nicolas V, et al: The diagnosis of thoracic aortic dissection by noninvasive imaging procedures. N Engl J Med 328:1–9, 1993.

4. Klompas M: Does this patient have an acute thoracic aortic dissection?. JAMA 287:2262–2272, 2002.

5. Von Kodolitsch Y, et al: Clinical prediction of acute aortic dissection. Arch Intern Med 160:2977–2982, 2000.

CHAPTER 29

HYPERTENSIVE CRISES

Yvette M. Cua, MD, and Nilesh Kalyanaraman, MD

1. **What is hypertension (HTN)?**
   The 7th report of the Joint National Committee on Detection, Evaluation, and Treatment of High Blood Pressure (JNC 7) defines *hypertension* as an elevated mean blood pressure (BP) based on ≥2 correctly taken seated BPs recorded on each of two separate days. The severity of BP elevation is categorized by the more severe of systolic (SBP) and diastolic (DBP) readings (Table 29-1).

TABLE 29-1. STAGES OF HYPERTENSION			
	SBP (mmHg)		**DBP (mmHg)**
Normal blood pressure	<120	*and*	<80
Prehypertension	120–139	*or*	80–89
Stage 1 hypertension	140–159	*or*	90–99
Stage 2 hypertension	≥160	*or*	≥100

2. **What is a hypertensive crisis?**
   Hypertensive crisis is defined as severely elevated BP requiring rapid lowering to prevent or halt progression of end-organ damage. There is no consensus for the exact BP level that defines a crisis, but SBP > 180 mmHg or DBP > 120 mmHg is commonly managed as a "crisis." Only 1% of patients with HTN ever go on to have a hypertensive crisis.

3. **How are hypertensive crises classified?**
   Severely elevated BP syndromes are termed *hypertensive emergencies* when associated with acute or progressive end-organ damage and *hypertensive urgencies* when no acute/progressive end-organ damage is present. This distinction is critical because emergencies require immediate BP lowering within 1–2 hours in a monitored setting with intravenous (IV) medicines, whereas urgencies require lowering over 24–48 hours, with oral therapy administered in an outpatient setting. No absolute BP cutoff separates emergencies and urgencies. The rate of BP increase is as important as the absolute level; modest but rapid increases in BP can also cause a crisis.

4. **What are *accelerated, malignant,* and *accelerated-malignant* HTN?**
   These terms, which have evolved over time, previously referred to stages of HTN-induced renal and ophthalmologic damage but currently lack accepted definitions. To avoid confusion, their use is not recommended.

5. **List the risk factors associated with hypertensive crises.**
   - Previous episode of hypertensive crisis
   - History of pregnancy-induced HTN
   - Lack of primary care physician

- Low socioeconomic status
- Elevated plasma renin, plasma adrenomedullin, or natriuretic peptides
- Genetic: Angiotensin-converting enzyme (ACE) DD genotype, G-protein β_3 subunit gene (GNβ3) polymorphism 825C→T

  Shea S, Misra D, Francis CK: Predisposing factors for severe, uncontrolled hypertension in an inner-city minority population. N Engl J Med 327:776–781, 1992.

6. **List the triggers/precipitants of a hypertensive crisis.**
   - **Noncompliance with anti-hypertensive medications:** No. 1 cause
   - **Sympathomimetic use:** Ephedrine, pseudoephedrine, dextromethorphan
   - **Illicit drug use:** Cocaine, phencyclidine (PCP), amphetamines
   - **Rebound HTN after abrupt discontinuation of a short-acting beta blocker or clonidine**
   - **Alcohol withdrawal**
   - **Herbal remedies:** St. John's Wort, yohimbine
   - **Tyramine ingestion while using monoamine oxidase inhibitors**

7. **List some examples of hypertensive emergencies.**
   See Table 29-2.

TABLE 29-2. EXAMPLES OF HYPERTENSIVE EMERGENCIES

Cardiopulmonary*	Acute aortic dissection
	Acute coronary syndromes: myocardial infarction or unstable angina
	Congestive heart failure, pulmonary edema
Renal*	Acute renal failure
Central nervous system*	Hypertensive encephalopathy
	Ischemic or hemorrhagic cerebrovascular accident
	Subarachnoid hemorrhage
Hematologic	Microangiopathic hemolytic anemia
	Postoperative bleeding from vascular suture lines
	Severe epistaxis
Pregnancy	Eclampsia

*The three most commonly affected organ systems.

8. **Which symptoms are suggestive of a hypertensive *emergency*?**
   The three most common symptoms with hypertensive emergency are chest pain, dyspnea, and focal neurologic deficits. Other symptoms include fatigue, irritability, faintness, orthopnea, cough, nausea, vomiting, headache, visual changes, confusion, somnolence, stupor, seizures, coma, oliguria, hematuria, epistaxis, and uncontrolled bleeding. An asymptomatic patient with normal physical examination can still have an emergency. The three most common symptoms associated with urgency are headache, epistaxis, and faintness.

9. **List the physical examination findings suggestive of a hypertensive emergency.**
   - **Vital signs:** Unequal BPs in the extremities
   - **Funduscopic:** Flare hemorrhages, exudates, papilledema
   - **Severe or prolonged epistaxis without other cause**

- **Cardiovascular:** Jugular venous distension, S_3 or S_4 heart sounds, widened/displaced point of maximum impulse
- **Pulmonary:** Rales
- **Neurologic:** Altered sensorium, visual field deficits, focal motor or sensory deficits
- **Extremity:** Edema, diminished or asymmetric pulses

10. **What is the main goal of the initial work-up of a patient with severely elevated BP?**

To determine whether you are dealing with an emergency or urgency based on evidence of acute or progressive end-organ damage in history, physical examination, and/or diagnostic studies. If at any point in the history, physical examination, or diagnostic work-up the evidence suggests an emergency, *immediately* initiate treatment while continuing your evaluation.

11. **Which diagnostic studies should be performed?**

All patients with hypertensive crisis should have a creatinine and urinalysis with microscopic analysis of sediment. Muddy brown casts or dysmorphic red blood cells indicate glomerular disease. In addition, patients with suspected hypertensive emergency should undergo the following tests:

- **Electrolytes (Na, K, Ca, Cl, HCO$_3$):** ↑K, ↓Ca, and metabolic acidosis may be seen with hemolysis. ↓K may suggest hyperaldosteronism.
- **Complete blood count with peripheral smear:** Microangiopathic hemolytic anemia, disseminated intravascular coagulation
- **Electrocardiography:** Evaluate for acute coronary syndrome
- **Chest x-ray:** May reveal pulmonary edema or widened mediastinum (may suggest aortic dissection)
- **Urine toxicology screen for cocaine and amphetamines:** May precipitate emergency and/or affect choice of BP-lowering agent

12. **What other studies may be needed based on history and physical examination findings?**

- **Creatine kinase, myocardial bound (CK-MB); troponin:** If acute coronary syndrome is suspected
- **Echocardiogram:** If congestive heart failure or aortic dissection is suspected
- **Computed tomography (CT) of the head without contrast:** If focal neurologic findings or altered mental status is present, to rule out intracranial hemorrhage; if CT has normal results, consider lumbar puncture for subarachnoid hemorrhage
- **Magnetic resonance imaging of the head with diffusion-weighted images:** If stroke is suspected
- **CT of the chest and abdomen:** If aortic dissection is suspected
- **Elevated liver enzymes (alanine aminotransferase and aspartate aminotransferase):** Elevated in eclampsia
- **Plasma renin activity and aldosterone concentration:** If renovascular disease or hypercortisolism is suspected; you need to draw blood *before* administering antihypertensives

13. **What are the general tenets of treatment of a hypertensive emergency?**

The patient must be admitted to a monitored bed to receive IV medications. Treat contributing factors such as pain, anxiety, bladder distention, hypoxia, and fluid overload; rarely, this will prevent the need for IV antihypertensive agents. Reduce *mean arterial pressure* (MAP) by no more than 25% in 1–2 hours, *and* to <160/100 mmHg within the first 6–24 hours. Lowering MAP too fast may cause cerebral or renal hypoperfusion. BP should slowly be normalized over the next 24–48 hours. Ensure BP is stable for 24–48 hours on oral medications before discharge. Treat complications of end-organ involvement with subspecialty assistance as needed (Table 29-3).

TABLE 29-3. HYPERTENSIVE EMERGENCIES. TREATMENT GOALS, AND RECOMMENDED MEDICATIONS

Disease	Blood Pressure Goals	Preferred Drug(s)
Aortic dissection	↓SBP < 120 mmHg within minutes to prevent further dissection. Goal to vasodilate.	Labetalol or (esmolol + nitroprusside) Avoid hydralazine and diazoxide—can ↑shear stress.
Unstable angina/ acute MI	↓MAP by 15–20% within 2 hours. Goal to vasodilate, ↓myocardial O₂ demand, and ↑cardiac perfusion.	(Labetalol or esmolol) + nitroglycerin Can add fenoldopam if BP not at goal. *Use caution* with nicardipine, hydralazine, and diazoxide—may cause reflex tachycardia.
Pulmonary edema	↓MAP by 10–15 % within 2 hours. Goal to ↓preload and afterload, ↑cardiac perfusion.	Loop diuretic + (enalaprilat or oral ACE-I) + (nitroprusside or nitroglycerin or fenoldopam)
Hypertensive encephalopathy	↓MAP by 25% within 2–3 hours.	Nitroprusside or labetalol
Ischemic CVA, intracranial hemorrhage	Need to maintain cerebral perfusion. Controversial to treat stroke in evolution. Consider treating if DBP > 120 mmHg. ↓DBP no more than 20% in first 24 hours. Stop meds if neurologic symptoms progress.	Avoid meds with central nervous system side effects: clonidine, methyldopa, and reserpine. Avoid diazoxide—can ↓CBF. Nicardipine or fenoldopam Use only short-acting meds. Avoid centrally acting meds. Nitroprusside controversial—may increase intracranial pressure.
Subarachnoid hemorrhage	Controversial to treat. Consider treating if SBP > 200 mmHg, DBP >120 mmHg.	Nimodipine. Do not use hydralazine—unpredictable effect and long half-life.

Continued

TABLE 29-3. HYPERTENSIVE EMERGENCIES, TREATMENT GOALS, AND RECOMMENDED MEDICATIONS—CONT'D

Disease	Blood Pressure Goals	Preferred Drug(s)
Acute renal failure/microangiopathic hemolytic anemia	↓MAP by 10–20% within 1–2 hours. Normalizing BP too quickly could worsen renal failure due to renal hypoperfusion.	Fenoldopam or nicardipine
Pheochromocytoma	Control paroxysms of BP.	Phentolamine
Cocaine-induced sympathetic crisis	↓MAP by 25% within 2–3 hours.	Phentolamine, nicardipine, or fenoldopam
Drug withdrawal, "rebound HTN"	↓MAP by 25% within 2 hours.	Give the drug withdrawn (e.g., clonidine, short-acting beta blocker), nicardipine, or fenoldopam.
Eclampsia	↓SBP < 180 mmHg and ↓DBP < 110 mmHg with goal of DBP = 90 mmHg to maintain placental perfusion.	First-line: magnesium sulfate + hydralazine Second-line: labetalol or nicardipine instead of hydralazine
Post-op HTN/bleeding	↓MAP by 25% within 2 hours.	Nicardipine
Uncontrolled epistaxis	↓MAP by 25% within 2 hours.	Nitroprusside. Any vasodilator, consider anxiolytic.

SBP = systolic blood pressure, MI = myocardial infarction, MAP = mean arterial pressure, ACE-I = angiotensin-converting enzyme inhibitor, meds = medications, CBF = cerebral blood flow, CVA = cerebrovascular accident, DBP = diastolic blood pressure, HTN = hypertension, Post-op = post-operative.

KEY POINTS: DEFINITION AND DIAGNOSIS OF HYPERTENSIVE CRISES

1. No absolute BP value defines hypertensive crises or differentiates hypertensive emergencies from hypertensive urgencies.

2. All patients with SBP > 180 mmHg or DBP > 120 mmHg should be screened, at least by means of a history and physical examination, for evidence of acute or progressive end-organ damage.

3. Although medication noncompliance is the most common trigger of a crisis, illicit drug use, herbal medicines, over-the-counter sympathomimetics, and alcohol withdrawal are not uncommon causes.

4. Hypertensive emergencies can affect any organ system, and in the face of a severely elevated BP, any symptom should be evaluated as a potential sign of an emergency.

14. **How is the MAP calculated?**

$$MAP = \frac{[SBP + 2(DBP)]}{3}$$

Example: if BP = 266/122, then MAP = [266 + (2 × 122)]/3 = 170

15. **Describe how to start and titrate medications in a hypertensive emergency.**
The ideal medicine has rapid onset, peak effect, and offset for safe and easy titration. Thus, IV medicines are most often used. Each drug has a standard starting dose—either a single bolus or a loading dose with continuous infusion. If the MAP goal is not met with the starting dose by the time of the drug's expected peak effect, increase the dose or re-bolus by the recommended increment and wait until this additional treatment achieves its peak effect. Repeat this process until the MAP goal is achieved, the maximum allowable dose is reached, or the patient experiences untoward side effects. If the maximum dose does not adequately control BP, switch to another IV agent (Table 29-4).

16. **When should oral medications be started?**
In *hypertensive emergency,* once initial MAP goals are met (generally within first 2–6 hours) start oral medications while weaning the patient off the IV medicine. If there is a delay in starting IV medicine, start an oral agent, such as clonidine 0.05–0.2 mg or labetalol 300 mg. Do not use short-acting nifedipine, which can precipitate a stroke or acute myocardial infarction.

In *hypertensive urgency,* there is no definitive data to support giving a dose of oral medication to immediately lower the BP. All patients with hypertensive crises should to be started on at least two antihypertensive agents. Selection of the agents is based on comorbidities (compelling indications), allergies, medication history, compliance, and response. Without compelling indications, patients should be started on a diuretic plus another agent: ACE inhibitor, angiotensin II receptor blocker, beta blocker, or calcium channel blocker (Table 29-5).

17. **What lifestyle modifications should be reviewed and implemented?**
    1. Educate oneself on Dietary Approaches to Stop Hypertension (DASH).
        - Limit Na^+ intake to <100 mmol/day (<2.4 gm Na^+ or 6.0 gm NaCl)
        - Maintain adequate intake of dietary K^+ (~90 mmol/day), Ca^{++}, and Mg^+

TABLE 29-4. IV MEDICATIONS FOR HYPERTENSIVE EMERGENCIES AND IMPORTANT/COMMON SIDE EFFECTS

Agent	Most Important and Common Side Effects
Diazoxide	Causes salt and water retention, ↑uric acid, hyperglycemia, flushing, and nausea.
Enalaprilat	Can cause precipitous drop in BP in high-renin states. Can cause angioedema.
Esmolol hydrochloride	Contraindicated in heart block and bronchospasm.
Fenoldopam mesylate	Use caution in hypokalemia and glaucoma (can cause ↑intraocular pressure).
Hydralazine hydrochloride	Difficult to use due to prolonged and unpredictable hypotensive effect. Causes reflex tachycardia.
Labetalol hydrochloride	Contraindicated in heart block and bronchospasm.
Nicardipine hydrochloride	Reduces cardiac and cerebral ischemia, but can cause tachycardia, so use caution when acute coronary syndromes are present. Causes local phlebitis.
Nitroglycerin	Causes tachycardia, flushing, and methemoglobinemia.
Phentolamine	Causes tachyarrhythmias, angina, flushing, and headache. Primarily used for sympathomimetic crises.
Sodium nitroprusside	Instant onset. Risk of toxicity at >2 μg/kg/min. Monitor thiocyanate levels if maintenance rate >3 μg/kg/min or if used >24 hours. Use caution in cases of liver and kidney disease.
Trimethaphan camsylate	Tachyphylaxis is a common side effect. Most useful in aortic dissection if unable to use esmolol/labetalol.

- Decrease intake of saturated fat, cholesterol, and total fat
- Increase fresh fruits, vegetables, and low-fat dairy products

2. Lose weight if body mass index (BMI) > 27.

$$BMI = \frac{Weight}{Height^2} \quad Metric\ units = \frac{kg}{m^2} \quad English\ units = \frac{704 \times lb}{[(ft \times 12) + in]^2}$$

For example, if weight = 192 lb and height = 5'4," then

$$BMI = \frac{(704 \times 192)}{[(5 \times 12) + 4]^2} = 33$$

3. Engage in aerobic exercise: ≥30 minutes most days of the week.
4. Stop smoking: classes, support groups, nicotine patch or gum.
5. Limit alcohol: ≤2 drinks/day; 1 drink = 1 oz (30 mL) ethanol ∼ 24 oz beer ∼ 10 oz wine ∼ 3 oz of 80-proof whiskey. Use half of above for woman or lightweight patient.
6. Limit caffeine.
7. Take stress reduction classes.

TABLE 29-5. COMPELLING INDICATIONS FOR SELECTION OF ANTIHYPERTENSIVE THERAPY

Compelling Indications	ACE Inhibitor	Angiotensin II Receptor Blocker	Beta blocker	Calcium Channel Blocker	Diuretic	Aldosterone Antagonist
Congestive heart failure:						
asymptomatic	X		Class II/III			
symptomatic	X	X	X		Loop	Class III/IV
Post–myocardial infarction	X		X			X
High-risk coronary artery disease	X		X	X	X	
Diabetes	X	X	X	X	Thiazide	
Chronic kidney disease	X	X				
Cerebrovascular accident	X				X	

KEY POINTS: MANAGEMENT OF HYPERTENSIVE EMERGENCY

1. Patients with hypertensive emergency often have labile BPs and should be admitted to a monitored bed and started on IV medications.

2. Once the initial MAP goal is met, aggressive treatment should be continued to maintain control and lower the BP to <160/100 mmHg over the next 6–24 hours.

3. Lowering the BP in a *stroke in evolution* is controversial and may extend the stroke: consult neurology before initiating therapy.

4. Although it is critical to start antihypertensive treatment in the short term, diet, weight loss, exercise, and other lifestyle modifications play an important role in lowering the BP over time.

18. **What discharge instructions, treatment interventions, and education are part of the management of hypertensive crises?**
Educate the patient on how to take medicines and what side effects may be experienced. Promote compliance through the use of pill boxes and other aids. Start aspirin at 81 mg/day (except with a hemorrhagic event or other contraindication). Recommend the patient avoid taking nonsteroidal anti-inflammatory drugs, over-the-counter sympathomimetics, and herbal remedies without consulting a physician. Offer information on drug rehabilitation programs, if indicated. Screen for and treat diabetes, hypercholesterolemia, and thyroid disease. Arrange follow-up **within 1 week**.

WEBSITE

National Heart, Lung, and Blood Institute DASH Eating Plan: http://www.nhlbi.nih.gov/health/public/heart/hbp/dash/

BIBLIOGRAPHY

1. Chobanian AV, Bakris GL, Black HR: The seventh report of the Joint National Committee on prevention, detection, evaluation, and treatment of high blood pressure: The JNC 7 report. JAMA 289:2560–2572, 2003.

2. Elliott WJ: Hypertensive emergencies. Crit Care Clin 17:435–451, 2001.

3. Kaplan NM: Hypertensive crises. In Kaplan NM Clinical Hypertension, 6th ed. Baltimore, MD, Williams & Wilkins, 1994, pp 281–297.

4. Shayne PH, Pitts SR: Severely increased blood pressure in the emergency department. Ann Emerg Med 41:513–529, 2003.

5. Varon J, Marik PE: The diagnosis and management of hypertensive crises. Chest 118:214–225, 2000.

6. Vaughn CJ, Delanty N: Hypertensive emergencies. Lancet 356:411–417, 2000.

7. Vidt DG: Emergency room management of hypertension urgencies and emergencies. J Clin Hypertens 3:158–164, 2001.

CHAPTER 30

HEART FAILURE

Wassim H. Fares, MD, and Franklin A. Michota, MD

1. **What is heart failure (HF), and how common is it?**
   Congestive heart failure (CHF), now referred to as *heart failure*, is a clinical syndrome
   characterized by a decreased ability of the heart to effectively pump blood out of the lungs and/
   or the venous system into the arterial system. There are approximately 5 million people with HF
   in the United States. There are approximately 550,000 new cases and 300,000 deaths annually,
   resulting in nearly one million hospital admissions at an estimated cost of $13.6 billion of direct
   hospital cost.

2. **What are the key features of the different types of HF?**
   HF is often described in terms of the type (i.e., systolic or diastolic) or ventricle (i.e., left or right)
   involved. In systolic HF there is a decreased ventricular ejection fraction (EF), whereas in
   diastolic HF there is decreased ventricular compliance. Left HF symptoms are mainly related to
   pulmonary congestion, with or without decreased cardiac output. Right HF leads to systemic
   venous congestion, manifesting as jugular venous distension, ascites, and lower extremity
   edema. The most common cause of right-sided HF is left-sided HF, and the separation of the
   symptoms between right- and left-sided HF is often artificial.

3. **What are the various classification schemes for HF?**
   The two commonly used classification schemes are the American College of Cardiology/American
   Heart Association (ACC/AHA) and the New York Heart Association (NYHA) systems (Table 30-1).

4. **What is the pathophysiology of HF?**
   Neurohormones are the cornerstone of the pathophysiology of HF. A failing heart stimulates
   a wide array of cytokines (e.g., prostacyclin), natriuretic peptides, sympathetic and

TABLE 30-1. CLASSIFICATIONS OF HEART FAILURE	
ACC/AHA Stages of HF	**NYHA Classification**
A: Patients have no symptoms ever and have no structural or functional abnormalities but are at high risk for developing HF	N/A
B: Patients have had no symptoms so far, but have developed structural heart disease	N/A
C: Patients have experienced symptoms of HF, whether currently or in the past	**I:** No symptoms from ordinary activities **II:** Mild limitation with ordinary activity **III:** Marked limitation with ordinary activity
D: Patients have advanced/end-stage HF	**IV:** Symptomatic even at rest

renin-angiotensin aldosterone systems, and other hormones (e.g., vasopressin, endothelin–1). Renal perfusion may also be compromised in view of the decreased arterial filing and vasoconstriction that results from stimulation of the above systems. These collectively lead to tachycardia, myocardial hypertrophy and pathologic remodeling, direct cardiotoxicity, and water and sodium retention, which are usually worsened by central stimulus for thirst. The result is a decreased myocardial contractility and functioning and further stimulation of all of the above, creating a vicious cycle (Fig. 30-1).

Failing heart	→ Increases BNP, ANP, PGE2, prostacyclin*	→ Tachycardia and myocardial hypertrophy/pathologic remodeling	→ Decreased mycocardial contractility
	→ Increases sympathetic system	→ Direct cardiotoxixity	
	→ Increases RAAS and release of endothelin-1 and vasopressin	→ Vasoconstriction and vascular hypertrophy Water and sodium retention	
	→ Renal perfusion may be compromised	→ Thirst	

Figure 30-1. Neurohormonal activation contributing to the pathophysiology of heart failure. *Counteracts sympathetic and RAA systems by causing diuresis and vasodilation. BNP = B-type natriuretic peptide, ANP = atrial natriuretic peptide, PGE2 = prostaglandin E2, RAAS = renin-angiotensin-aldosterone system.

5. **What are the common causes of cardiomyopathy?**
Cardiomyopathy is a heart disease that involves pathologic changes to the myocardium. It is commonly classified as either *dilated* or *hypertrophic*. Sixty percent of cardiomyopathy is due to coronary artery disease. Other causes include hypertension, valvular disease, myocarditis, infiltrating diseases, metabolic, alcohol, toxicity, pregnancy, connective disease, or familial causes. If no cause for the cardiomyopathy is elucidated after appropriate work-up, it is termed *idiopathic*. This group constitutes about 20% of all cardiomyopathies.

6. **What is meant by congestion and perfusion?**
A failing heart is equivalent to a failing pump, which has two main consequences: pooling of blood in the venous system, including the lungs (i.e., congestion), and inability to maintain the needs of the body through the arterial system (i.e., perfusion). In simple terms: "wet" or "dry" lungs describe the state of congestion. "Warm" or "cold" extremities describe the state of perfusion. Change in mental status and impaired kidney function may signify decreased perfusion.

7. **What is acutely decompensated HF (ADHF)?**
HF is a chronic remitting and relapsing illness. Most patients spend most of their time in a compensated phase. However, decompensations can be common. Patients in ADHF can present with one of three clinical presentations based on the presence or absence of congestion and perfusion abnormalities. Congested patients often present with pulmonary complaints such as shortness of breath (i.e., dyspnea) on exertion or at rest, difficulty breathing while laying flat (i.e., orthopnea), paroxysmal nocturnal dyspnea, or awakening from sleep with shortness of breath, and cough that is typically nonproductive or productive of pinkish-colored sputum. Additional congestive symptoms include lower extremity edema, abdominal extension (if ascites are present), and abdominal pain. Perfusion abnormalities do not tend to result in physical complaints and are more often detected on laboratory work-up and physical examination.

Patients with abnormal perfusion but no congestion are known as "cold and dry." Those with normal perfusion but evidence of congestion are referred to as "warm and wet." "Cold and wet" patients tend to be the sickest because they have poor perfusion and congestion.

8. **What are the common reasons why a patient may become decompensated?**
The most common reasons for decompensation include noncompliance with medications or diet, inadequate dose of medications, progression of disease, acute coronary syndrome (ACS), uncontrolled hypertension, arrhythmia, thyroid disease, valvular decompensation, and viral myocarditis. Certain medications, through various mechanisms, may increase the body's retention of fluids and electrolytes (e.g., nonsteroidal anti-inflammatory drugs, steroids, insulin sensitizers [e.g., rosiglitazone]) or directly compromise the heart's ability to adequately shift blood from the venous to the arterial system (e.g., calcium channel blockers, certain antiarrhythmics, chemotherapeutic agents [e.g., Adriamycin], and cardiotoxic drugs), and thus induce decompensation of HF.

9. **Describe the physical examination findings in a patient with ADHF**
Physical exam findings in ADHF depend on the type of HF and the severity of the ADHF. Most symptoms result from backup of blood flow (i.e., congestion). Findings in right-sided HF include jugular venous distention with or without a hepatojugular reflex, lower extremity edema, ascites, and right upper quadrant pain with palpation (due to congestion of the liver). Left-sided HF is associated with a cardiac gallop (i.e., S_3 heart sound) and congestion of the lungs manifest as crackles, tachypnea, and hypoxia.

10. **Which two physical exam findings are most specific for ADHF?**
An S_3 heart sound and a displaced point of maximal impulse (PMI) are the most specific findings for HF. An S_3 is a faint and soft sound that follows S_2 in early diastole and is caused by rapid influx of blood from the atrium to the ventricle. It may be physiologic in children, younger adults, and pregnant women; however, it is usually pathologic in older adults (e.g., those older than 40 years). The PMI is best detected by placing the patient in the left lateral decubitus position and feeling for the point on the chest with the most palpable lifting motion. The PMI is normally located within a 2-cm-square area at the midsternal line in the 4th or 5th left intercostal space. Displacement of the PMI laterally and inferiorly suggests left ventricular hypertrophy.

KEY POINTS: CRITICAL SIGNS ON PHYSICAL EXAMINATION

1. Hypotension, signifying hemodynamic instability

2. Cheyne-Stokes respiration: alteration of apnea and hyperventilation, signifying decreased cerebral perfusion, hypoxia, and elevated arterial CO_2 levels

3. New heart murmur or gallop, since a new valvular disease or arrhythmia may be causing the worsening of HF

4. Hypoxia or cold extremities, which signify decreased peripheral perfusion

11. **What is cardiogenic shock?**
Cardiogenic shock is a severe state of pump failure with decreased cardiac output (poor perfusion) and significant pooling in the lungs and venous system (congestion). A pulmonary artery catheter will confirm the diagnosis by showing an elevated wedge pressure, which is reflective of elevated left atrial pressure due to the heart's inability to pump the blood out of the heart. This condition most often requires intensive care because the patient may require vasopressors such as dobutamine.

12. **What other diseases can present with ADHF?**

ADHF may be the presentation of another underlying illness. Patients with myocardial ischemia (i.e., ACS) often present with symptoms of both ADHF and ACS. The onset of atrial fibrillation can also induce ADHF. Likewise, the presentation of pulmonary embolism, chronic obstructive pulmonary disease, asthma, and pneumonia can all be complicated by ADHF.

13. **Describe the initial evaluation of a patient with ADHF.**

After taking a thorough history, a complete physical exam should be done, evaluating for the common findings outlined above. Care should be taken to rule out diseases that can present with ADHF. Further work-up often includes an electrocardiogram, complete blood cell count, chemistry panel, chest x-ray (CXR), cardiac enzymes, and a brain-type natriuretic peptide (BNP).

14. **How does ADHF appear on CXR?**

- Patients who present with pulmonary congestion often have CXR findings of *Kerley B lines,* which are 1–3-cm lateral lines due to interstitial fluid within the pleural spaces, mainly in the interlobar septa (Fig. 30-2).

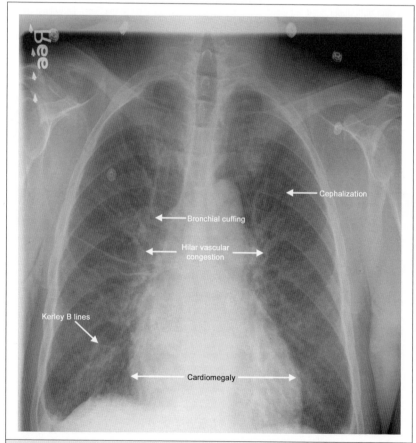

Figure 30-2. Chest x-ray of a patient who presented with ADHF.

- *Cephalization* is the term used to describe enlarged upper lung vessels, in contrast to lower lung vessels.
- *Cardiomegaly* (i.e., enlarged heart size) is demonstrated by a transverse cardiac dimension that is at least half the transthoracic dimension on a posteroanterior CXR.
- *Bronchial cuffing* describes the congested walls of the medium-sized bronchi when viewed in cross section.
- Bilateral *pleural effusions* may also be evident.

15. **What is BNP? How can it be used in the evaluation of HF?**

BNP is the B-type (or brain-) natriuretic peptide. It is a peptide that is mainly secreted by the cardiac ventricles and is believed to be responsible for natriuresis, diuresis, and vasodilation. BNP is highly associated with the diagnosis of ADHF, and some have suggested that it may be used to guide treatment and discharge planning. In patients with dyspnea, a very low BNP level (<100 pg/mL) practically rules out ADHF. Moderate levels of BNP (100–480 pg/mL) indicate that ADHF is likely contributing (alone or in concert with other illnesses) to the patient's symptoms. A very high BNP level (>480 pg/mL) almost always implicates HF as a cause of the patient's symptoms, indicating treatment aimed at reversing the ADHF.

16. **What are the limitations of BNP?**

Any process causing stretch of the ventricles, whether it is systolic or diastolic HF, valvular disease, or any pulmonary process that causes increased pressure or volume in the right ventricle (e.g., pulmonary embolism, pulmonary hypertension, emphysema) can elevate the BNP. Table 30-2 outlines other factors that influence the BNP level.

TABLE 30-2. CONDITIONS AFFECTING BNP LEVEL		
Condition		**BNP Change**
Age	Advanced age	Increase
Comorbidities	Renal failure	Increase
	Hypoalbuminemia	Increase
Pulmonary	Lung disease with right-sided failure	Increase
	Acute, large pulmonary embolism	Increase
Cardiac	Acute coronary syndrome	Increase
	Myocardial infarction	Increase
Site of cause of pulmonary edema	Left ventricle or downstream	Increase
	Upstream of left ventricle (e.g., mitral stenosis)	Decrease
Miscellaneous	Acute mitral regurgitation	Decrease
	Flash pulmonary edema	Decrease

17. **Describe the treatment options for ADHF.**

The treatment of patients with ADHF depends on their presentation, that is, the presence or absence of congestion and poor perfusion. Those who are congested are treated with oral or intravenous (IV) diuretics and vasodilators, such as angiotensin-converting enzyme inhibitors (ACEI), for afterload reduction. Patients with perfusion abnormalities often require inotropes.

18. **Discuss the role of diuretics in the care of patients with ADHF.**

Although loop diuretics (Table 30-3) have not been shown to improve survival, they are the most commonly used medication for patients with HF because they readily improve symptoms in congested patients. Intermittent metolazone, which is a thiazide-like diuretic that inhibits sodium reabsorption in the distal tubule, may be used in conjunction with loop diuretics to enhance diuresis. Thiazide drugs are weak diuretics and are not recommended as a sole diuretic in the setting of HF. The use of spironolactone, an aldosterone antagonist, in patients with NYHA class III and IV HF is associated with a survival benefit in addition to symptomatic relief. Despite a suggestion that there is decreased gut absorption of oral diuretics due to gut edema in HF requiring IV diuretic use, no convincing evidence for this phenomenon exists. The oral dose of furosemide is equivalent to half the IV dose (e.g., 40 mg of oral furosemide is equivalent to 20 mg of IV furosemide).

Pitt B, Zannad F, Remme WJ, et al: The effect of spironolactone on morbidity and mortality in patients with severe heart failure. Randomized Aldactone Evaluation Study Investigators. N Engl J Med 341:709–717, 1999.

19. **What are the indications for and risks of use for inotropic agents in the treatment of ADHF?**

Two commonly used inotropes are dobutamine and milrinone.

- **Dobutamine** is an adrenergic agonist, given IV for short periods of time for acute resuscitation for cardiac decompensation. Because of this beta-agonist activity, it usually increases heart rate, blood pressure, and ventricular response (e.g., ectopy or ventricular tachycardia), which in turn increases myocardial oxygen demand that might be detrimental to the heart compensatory mechanisms.
- **Milrinone,** on the other hand, is a phosphodiesterase enzyme inhibitor that is also given IV for short periods of time for ADHF. It increases the levels of cyclic adenosine monophosphate and thus increases calcium influx into myocardial cells, increasing contractility. It may also cause systemic arterial and venous dilation via inhibition of peripheral phosphodiesterase, and thus should be avoided in severe obstructive aortic and pulmonic valvular disease. Like dobutamine, arrhythmias and potentially increased mortality rate are the main risks of milrinone infusion.

20. **What are the indications for and risks of use for vasoactive agents in the treatment of ADHF?**

The three most commonly used are listed in Table 30-4. They all share the side effects of hypotension and headache.

- **Nitroglycerine:** Exerts its vasodilatory effect by dilating both the arterial and, more significantly, the venous system, thus reducing the preload. It is relatively cheap, but tolerance develops quickly.
- **Nitroprusside:** Causes vasodilation by directly relaxing the venous and arteriolar smooth muscles. Its main drawback is the potential for cyanide toxicity, especially when its use is prolonged or high doses are used.
- **Nesiritide:** A recombinant human B-type natriuretic peptide that causes an increase in intracellular cyclic guanylate monophosphate and thus causes relaxation of vascular smooth muscle and endothelial cells. Its association with worsening kidney function and increased mortality is controversial due to the lack of clinical trials primarily addressing these endpoints.

21. **What medications are associated with a survival benefit in patients with chronic HF?**

ACEIs, angiotensin receptor blockers (ARB), beta blockers, and spironolactone all improve morbidity and mortality in HF. A fixed dose of isosorbide dinitrate and hydralazine, added to standard therapy, has been shown to improve survival in African Americans with advanced HF.

TABLE 30-3. ORAL MEDICATIONS FOR HEART FAILURE						
Loop Diuretic (usual dose range)	Potassium-Sparing Diuretics (usual dose range)	Beta Blocker (starting/ target dose)	ACEI (starting/ target dose)	ARB (starting/ target dose)	Positive Inotropes (usual dose range)	Alternate to ACEI and ARB (starting/ maximum dose)
Furosemide (10–360 mg/day)	Spironolactone* (12.5–25 mg/day)	Metoprolol (12.5 mg/ 200 mg daily)	Captopril (6.25 mg/50 mg t.i.d.)	Losartan (25 mg/ 50–100 mg daily)	Digoxin (0.0625–0.25 mg/day)	Combination of hydralazine (10 mg t.i.d.-q.i.d./300 mg daily) and isosorbide dinitrate‡ (10 mg t.i.d./80 mg t.i.d.)
Bumetanide (0.5–20 mg/day)	Triamterene (100–300 mg/day)	Carvedilol (3.125 mg/ 25–50 mg b.i.d.)	Ramipril (2.5 mg/ 5 mg b.i.d.)	Candesartan (4 m/ 16–32 mg daily)	Digitoxin (0.05–0.3 mg daily)	
Torsemide (2.5–200 mg/day)	Amiloride (5–10 mg/day)	Bisoprolol† (1.25 mg/ 5 mg daily)	Enalapril (2.5 mg b.i.d/10 mg b.i.d.)	Irbesartan (75 mg/ 150 mg daily)		
Ethacrynic acid (50–200 mg/day)	Eplerenone* (25–50 mg/day)		Trandolapril (1 mg/1–2 mg daily) Lisinopril (5 mg/ 20 mg daily)	Valsartan (40 mg/ 80–160 mg b.i.d.)		

ACEI = angiotensin-converting enzyme inhibitor, ARB = angiotensin receptor blocker.
* Aldosterone antagonist.
† Not approved by the Food and Drug Administration for treatment of HF in the United States.
‡ Isosorbide dinitrate is an oral nitrate that proved to be beneficial in association with hydralazine, as an alternative for ACEI, or if other medical regimens could not control the HF.

TABLE 30-4.	IV VASOACTIVE MEDICATIONS	
Drug	**Half-Life($t_{1/2}$)**	**Effects**
Nitroglycerin	3–5 minutes	Can cause tachyphylaxis; no mortality benefit
Nesiritide	20 minutes	Improves central hemodynamics; effect on kidney function and mortality is controversial
Nitroprusside	4 hours	Contraindicated in severe renal insufficiency and for prolonged periods due to toxic metabolites

Additionally, digoxin and diuretics improve symptoms but do not have a mortality benefit. Table 30-3 outlines the important classes of medications used to treat HF.

22. **Which patients with HF should chronically use ACEIs?**
Studies have consistently shown that the neurohumoral effects of aldosterone can advance the progression of HF. ACEIs block the formation of aldosterone by inhibiting conversion of angiotensin I to angiotensin II. Therefore, unless contraindicated, all patients with left ventricular dysfunction or a history of myocardial infarction and those at high risk for cardiovascular disease (e.g., persons with diabetes mellitus, atherosclerotic vascular disease, or multiple cardiovascular risk factors) should be taking an ACEI. ACEIs, as a class, decrease mortality for patients with HF. Cough is a common adverse effect, and renal failure, hypotension, and angioedema are the most serious potential side effects.

Flather MD, Yusuf S, Kober L, et al: Long-term ACE-inhibitor therapy in patients with heart failure or left-ventricular dysfunction: A systemic overview of data from individual patients. Lancet 355:1575–1581, 2000.

Yusuf S, Sleight P, Pogue J, et al: Effects of an angiotensin-converting-enzyme inhibitor, ramipril, on cardiovascular events in high-risk patients. The Heart Outcomes Prevention Evaluation (HOPE) Study Investigators. N Engl J Med 342:145–153, 2000.

23. **What is the role of ARBs in the management of HF?**
An ARB may replace an ACEI if a patient is intolerant to the ACEI because of angioedema, cough, or rash because these side effects are due to elevated levels of bradykinin that occur from blockade of the conversion of kinins (by ACEI) to its inactive metabolites. Patients who develop renal failure, hyperkalemia, and hypotension with an ACEI are likely to develop the same with an ARB because these effects are secondary to decreased stimulation of the angiotensin II receptors, occurring directly with ARBs, and indirectly through decreased conversion of angiotensin I to angiotensin II, occurring with ACEIs.

24. **What is the role of digoxin in the management of chronic HF?**
Digoxin decreases morbidity, including improving HF symptoms and decreasing hospitalizations, especially in those with advanced HF (low EF and NYHA class III or IV), but it has no survival benefit.

The Digitalis Investigation Group: The effect of digoxin on mortality and morbidity in patients with heart failure. N Engl J Med 336:525–533, 1997.

25. **What is the role of beta blockers in the management of HF?**
The initiation of beta blockers in patients with ADHF is associated with poor outcomes due to its negative hemodynamic effects. However, in stable HF patients, multiple randomized controlled studies have shown that beta blockers reduce total mortality, cardiovascular mortality, cardiovascular or HF hospitalizations, HF symptoms, need for cardiac transplantation, and myocardial infarction in patients with NYHA class II–IV HF.

Cardiac Insufficiency Bisoprolol Study II (CIBIS-II): A randomised trial. Lancet 353:9–13, 1999.

Carvedilol Prospective Randomized Cumulative Survival (COPERNICUS) Study Group. Effects of initiating carvedilol in patients with severe chronic heart failure: Results from the COPERNICUS Study. JAMA 289:712–718, 2003.

Effects of controlled-release metoprolol on total mortality, hospitalizations, and well-being in patients with heart failure: The Metoprolol CR/XL Randomized Intervention Trial in congestive heart failure (MERIT-HF). MERIT-HF Study Group. JAMA 283:1295–1302, 2000.

26. **What nonpharmacologic management options are useful for patients with HF?**

Patients with HF should be instructed to monitor their weight frequently and report significant changes to their heath care providers. They should be counseled on the importance of a salt- and fluid-restricted diet, alcohol and smoking cessation, exercise and routine health maintenance. Elevating the legs and using compression stockings can cosmetically improve lower extremity edema.

27. **Which devices are beneficial in patients with chronic HF?**

Options for patients with end-stage HF include heart transplantation, automated implantable cardiac defibrillator, cardiac resynchronization therapy (CRT), intra-aortic balloon counterpulsation pump, left ventricular assist device, palliative care, and hospice. Patients with a peak oxygen consumption at maximal exercise of $<10–14$ mL/kg/min usually benefit from heart transplantation. Other indications for heart transplantation included inotrope dependence, recurrent HF hospitalizations despite maximal therapy, severe ischemic symptoms, and refractory cardiogenic shock. Defibrillators were shown to improve survival in patients with a history of surviving a sustained ventricular tachycardia/fibrillation event, or EF $< 35\%$ with a history of myocardial infarction or HF symptoms. CRT, also called *biventricular pacing,* is used for HF patients with interventricular conduction delay, low EF, and moderate to severe symptoms despite optimal medical therapy. The rationale for the use of CRT is primarily to avoid dyssynchrony of the ventricles and thus optimize cardiac pump function. Intra-aortic balloon counterpulsation pump and left ventricular assist device are mechanical devices that support the cardiopulmonary system until a more definitive therapy becomes available, such as heart transplantation or reversal of hemodynamic collapse. If the HF is advanced enough that it is deemed that extra intervention might have higher risks than potential benefits, referral to hospice care is appropriate.

28. **What is the typical outcome and prognosis of a patient with ADHF during hospitalization and after discharge?**

The in-hospital mortality rate may vary between 2% and 22%, depending on the patient's risk factors (the average is 4–5%). Kidney function and vital signs upon presentation are the most important prognostic factors of in-hospital mortality. After discharge, 50% of patients get readmitted within 6 months. Overall 5-year survival is 50%. Age, comorbidities, EF, NYHA class, BNP, hyponatremia, reason for decompensation, low exercise capacity, and presence of an audible S_3 heart sound or jugular venous distention all seem to be key prognostic factors.

29. **What considerations are important when discharging a patient with HF from the hospital?**

Unless contraindicated, patients should be prescribed an ACEI, a beta blocker (after attaining a euvolemic state), and a loop diuretic. The current Joint Commission on Accreditation of Healthcare Organizations quality indicators, including a documentation of the patient's EF, ACEI use, HF education, and smoking cessation counseling should be addressed. Follow-up with the primary care physician should be arranged, and the patient should know how to respond to significant changes in daily weight.

WEBSITES

1. Acute Decompensated HF National Registry (ADHERE): http://www.adhereregistry.com

2. American College of Cardiology HF guidelines: http://www.acc.org/clinical/guidelines/failure/index.pdf

BIBLIOGRAPHY

1. Braunwald E: Congestive heart failure cor pulmonale. In Kasper DL, Braunwald E, Fauci AS, et al (eds): Harrison's Online, 16th ed. New York, McGraw-Hill, 2005.

2. Fonarow GC, Adams KM, Abraham WT, et al: Risk stratification for in-hospital mortality in acutely decompensated heart failure. JAMA 39:572–580, 2005.

3. Jessup M, Brozena S: Medical progress: Heart failure. N Engl J Med 348:2007–2018, 2003.

CHAPTER 31

PERICARDIAL DISEASE

Ashish Aneja, MBBS, MD

1. **What is acute pericarditis? What are the common causes?**

   The heart is surrounded by visceral and parietal layers of fibrous tissue called the *pericardium* that, when inflamed, can result in acute pericarditis. The inflammation may be the result of local or systemic causes, which are listed in Table 31-1. The incidence of pericarditis in postmortem studies ranges from 1% to 6%. It is diagnosed antemortem in only 0.1% of hospitalized patients. The incidence is 5% in those presenting to the emergency department with chest pain without myocardial infarction.

TABLE 31-1.   CAUSES OF ACUTE PERICARDITIS

Infectious

   Viral: Coxsackie A and B, adenovirus, mumps, hepatitis B, varicella, HIV, echo virus, infectious mononucleosis

   Bacterial: *Streptococcus pneumoniae*, *Staphylococcus*, *Neisseria*, *Mycobacterium tuberculosis*, gram-negative bacilli, *Legionella pneumophila*

   Fungal: histoplasmosis, blastomyces, coccidioidomycosis

   Other: syphilitic, parasitic, protozoal

Autoimmune: acute rheumatic fever, SLE, scleroderma, mixed connective tissue disorder, Wegener's granulomatosis, polyarteritis nodosa, rheumatoid arthritis

Inflammatory/granulomatous disease: sarcoidosis, inflammatory bowel disease, amyloidosis

Drug-induced: procainamide, hydralazine, Dilantin, isoniazid, anticoagulants, methysergide, Adriamycin

Acute idiopathic

Neoplastic and post-radiation: lung, breast, lymphoma, leukemia, primary pericardial tumors

Post injury: acute MI, Dressler's syndrome (post-MI, post-cardiac surgery), post-penetrating trauma

Uremia

Myxedema

Familial Mediterranean fever

SLE = systemic lupus erythematosus, MI = myocardial infarction.
Adapted from Braunwald E, Zipes DP, Libby P: Heart Disease: A Textbook of Cardiovascular Medicine, 6th ed. Philadelphia, W. B. Saunders, 2001.

2. **How does acute pericarditis present?**

   Acute pericarditis is characterized by chest discomfort that classically gets worse upon lying down, radiates to the back or the trapezius ridge and often to the arm and neck; a pericardial rub; characteristic electrocardiographic (ECG) changes; and occasionally fever. The pathognomonic clinical sign of pericarditis, the pericardial rub, is often evanescent and of variable intensity. It is a scratchy sound, best heard at the lower left sternal border with the patient leaning forward, using the diaphragm, during expiration. It is classically triphasic (50% of patients), corresponding to the atrial systole, ventricular systole, and early ventricular diastole. It is biphasic in one-third of patients and monophasic in the remainder.

3. **What is the differential diagnoses of acute pericarditis?**

   Aortic dissection, pulmonary embolism, pneumothorax, or acute myocardial infarction (AMI) can mimic pericarditis. The clinical syndrome of acute pericarditis is often characterized by the presence of chest pain and slight elevations in troponin levels (seen in 35–50% of patients) and creatine kinase, myocardial bound. These other clinical conditions usually can be differentiated from acute pericarditis by history and physical examination, ECG, echocardiography, computed tomography, magnetic resonance imaging, or chest radiography.

4. **Describe the classic ECG findings of acute pericarditis.**

   The ECG changes of acute pericarditis typically evolve through four stages. Leads I, II, III, aVL, aVF, V_3–V_6 are often called *epicardial leads,* and leads aVR, V_1, and V_2 are referred to as *endocardial leads.*

   - **Stage 1 of acute pericarditis:** Typically characterized by ST-segment elevation, upright T waves, and depressed PR segments in the epicardial leads. Endocardial leads reveal ST-segment depression, T wave inversion, and PR-segment elevation.
   - **Stage 2:** Persistent PR-segment depression, gradual flattening and inversion of the T waves, and isoelectric ST segments in the epicardial leads.
   - **Stage 3:** Isoelectric PR and ST segments and fully inverted T waves in epicardial leads.
   - **Stage 4:** Findings revert back to normal in both epicardial and endocardial leads.

   These changes evolve over days to weeks, a process much slower than that observed in the ST-segment elevation myocardial infarction (STEMI). The ST elevations in acute pericarditis are characterized by an elevation of the J-point, which is defined as the junction of the QRS complex and the ST segment and are concave upward (Fig. 31-1). With the STEMI, ST-segment

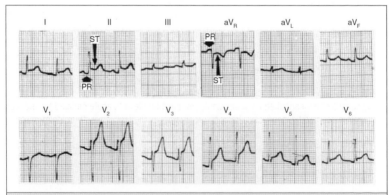

Figure 31-1. Acute pericarditis causing diffuse ST-segment elevations in leads I, II, aVF, and V_2–V_6, with reciprocal ST depressions in lead aVR. By contrast, a concomitant atrial current of injury causes PR-segment elevations in lead aVR with reciprocal PR depressions in the left chest leads and lead II. (From Goldberger AL: Myocardial Infarction: Electrocardiographic Differential Diagnosis, 4th ed. St. Louis, Mosby, 1991.)

elevations are often convex (i.e., dome-shaped) rather than concave in configuration, and they are localized to contiguous leads rather than widespread. In acute STEMI, T-wave inversions appear before the ST segments return to baseline; PR-segment depression isuncommon; and atrioventricular block or ventricular arrhythmias are more common.

5. **What is the initial and subsequent management of acute pericarditis?**
   Since most cases of acute pericarditis are self-limited, first-line treatment consists of nonsteroidal anti-inflammatory drugs (NSAIDs). Ibuprofen (1600–3200 mg in divided doses over 24 hours) or indomethacin (75–225 mg in divided doses over 24 hours) are the preferred agents, but aspirin (2–4 gm in divided doses over 24 hours) may be preferred in patients whose pericarditis is associated with an AMI. Indomethacin should be avoided in patients with AMI because of its potential to reduce coronary flow. Patients typically respond to NSAID therapy in a few days' time. Those with persistent symptoms after 2 weeks of therapy can be offered an alternative NSAID, colchicine, or a combination of the two. Those who fail to respond to NSAID and colchicine in combination or those with severe pericarditis of autoimmune etiology can be offered prednisone in doses of 1–1.5 mg/kg/day with a gradual taper over 3–4 weeks. Therapy with glucocorticoids should be reserved for patients who are unresponsive to combination therapy, since some studies suggest that the early use of these drugs may increase the risk of recurrence. Pericardiocentesis, which is an invasive procedure involving percutaneous aspiration of pericardial fluid, is not routinely recommended, although it should be performed in the presence of hemodynamic compromise, suspected purulent, or tuberculous pericarditis, or when fluid is required for diagnostic purposes.

6. **When should a patient with acute pericarditis be admitted to the hospital?**
   Most cases of pericarditis resolve with NSAID therapy and do not require admission. No specific criteria for admission exist, but patients with intractable pain, high fevers, evidence of myopericarditis (i.e., elevated cardiac markers), presence of a large pericardial effusion, immunosuppressed state, and those with reported recent use of anticoagulation should be considered for inpatient observation and treatment. Patients can be discharged home once their pain is adequately controlled and hemodynamic stability is ensured. Follow-up is required in patients with difficult-to-control pain, large effusions, immunosuppressed states, suspected autoimmune causes, frequent relapses, or when diagnostic dilemmas exist.

7. **What is the role of heparin in treating acute pericarditis?**
   Heparin use is relatively contraindicated in acute pericarditis because of the risk of pericardial hemorrhage and resultant tamponade. Since acute pericarditis often mimics AMI and can result in minor elevations in troponin levels, it must be excluded before heparin is used in suspected cases of acute coronary syndrome. In uremic patients with pericardial rub, heparin-free or low-dose heparin dialysis should be considered.

8. **What are the common causes of pericardial effusion?**
   The causes of pericardial effusion are similar to those that lead to acute pericarditis and include idiopathic pericarditis, congestive heart failure, uremia, malignancy, hypothyroidism/myxedema, nephrotic syndrome, cirrhosis, pregnancy, drugs, and postcardiac surgery. A diagnosis is often established based on the history and other blood test results including that of serologic tests. Sampling of pericardial fluid by pericardiocentesis is rarely necessary for establishing the diagnosis but may be performed in cases where tamponade is suspected or the diagnosis is elusive after extensive noninvasive testing. Table 31-2 lists some diagnostic modalities used in the differential diagnosis of pericardial effusions.

9. **What are the clinical findings in patients presenting with a pericardial effusion?**
   The spectrum of clinical symptoms and signs depends on the volume and rapidity of fluid accumulation. Slowly developing effusions that do not result in elevated pericardial pressure are

---

TABLE 31-2. IMAGING AND NONINVASIVE INVESTIGATIVE FINDINGS IN PERICARDIAL EFFUSIONS

ECG	Low-voltage complexes <5 mV in limb leads, <10 mV in chest leads.
	Electrical alternans
Chest radiography	Cardiomegaly (if >250 mL of fluid has accumulated)
	Prominent SVC and azygous vein
	Decreased pulmonary vascularity
	A pericardial line >2 mm from the lower heart border
Transthoracic echocardiography	Modality of choice
	Used quantitatively for estimation of effusion size
MRI	Effectively differentiates between loculated effusions, pericardial thickening, and fat
Electron beam CT	Can differentiate between blood, exudates, chyle, and serous fluid

SVC = superior vena cava, MRI = magnetic resonance imaging, CT = computerized tomography.

---

often asymptomatic. Large effusions can compress adjacent mediastinal structures and result in dysphagia, dyspnea, nausea, abdominal fullness, and hiccups. Physical examination with small effusions is normal. With larger effusions, heart sounds are muffled and Ewart's sign (i.e., left infrascapular egophony/bronchial breathing and dull percussion secondary to lung collapse) is sometimes noted. With the development of tamponade, an elevation in the jugular/systemic venous pressure is noted with prominent X and absent or diminished Y descent.

10. **How can pericardial effusion and tamponade be differentiated?**
   Symptoms of low cardiac output are often a harbinger of tamponade and consist of drowsiness, dyspnea, fatigue, restlessness, and oliguria. With the development of tamponade, an elevation in the jugular venous pressure is noted with prominent X and absent or diminished Y descents. In addition to a pericardial rub and diminished heart sounds, hypotension, tachycardia, tachypnea, and a pulsus paradoxus may develop. The paradox in pulsus paradoxus is the fall in systolic blood pressure of >10 mmHg with normal inspiration. The sign is not specific for tamponade and may be seen with severe chronic obstructive pulmonary disease exacerbation, acute severe asthma, right ventricular infarction, and pulmonary embolism. Pulsus paradoxus may be absent if tamponade is present concomitantly with severe left ventricular dysfunction, severe hypovolemia, atrial septal defect, or severe aortic regurgitation.

11. **What findings are noted on the echocardiogram in patients with cardiac tamponade?**
   Echocardiography often reveals a collapse of the right atrium in diastole. Right ventricular diastolic collapse can often be demonstrated in patients with medical causes of tamponade. A respiratory variation in the atrioventricular valve flow pattern with plethora of the inferior vena cava is also classically noted.

12. **How is cardiac tamponade managed?**
   Cardiac tamponade is a medical emergency and needs emergent drainage of pericardial fluid if significant hemodynamic compromise is present. Ideally, experienced personnel should

perform drainage in the catheterization laboratory under fluoroscopy. Surgical drainage is chosen if the effusion is likely to be recurrent, loculated, or if pericardial tissue is required for histopathologic or microbiologic purposes.

13. **What is constrictive pericarditis?**
Constrictive pericarditis is a fibrous thickening of the pericardium resulting from persistent pericardial inflammation. The physiology consists of rapid early filling of the ventricle in diastole with an abrupt cessation thereof due to a noncompliant pericardium, resulting in elevated and equalized diastolic pressures in all cardiac chambers. This results in elevated pulmonary and systemic venous pressures and signs of systemic venous congestion. Constrictive pericarditis often results from acute pericarditis and may not be preventable despite adequate initial treatment. Common causes include tuberculosis, radiation, infections, connective tissue disorders, and neoplastic processes.

KEY POINTS: PERICARDIAL DISEASE

1. Glucocorticoids have very little role in the treatment of early acute pericarditis.

2. Pulsus paradoxus is suggestive of cardiac tamponade in a patient with a pericardial effusion.

3. Pericardiocentesis is indicated in patients with pericardial tamponade who have evidence of hemodynamic instability.

4. Kussmaul's sign and pericardial knock are suggestive of the diagnosis of constrictive pericarditis.

14. **What clinical signs are particular to constrictive pericarditis?**
The symptoms are often insidious, and patients present with fatigability, poor exercise tolerance, and dyspnea on effort. Advanced disease may be clinically indistinguishable from liver cirrhosis owing to the presence of cachexia, ascites, hepatomegaly, splenomegaly, and lower extremity edema. Kussmaul's sign, which is a paradoxic elevation in jugular venous pressure with inspiration, is sensitive but not specific for constrictive pericarditis (present infrequently in tamponade). Jugular venous inspection may reveal a prominent Y descent and cardiac auscultation often reveals a pericardial knock, which is higher pitched and spaced closer to the S_2 heart sound than an S_3 (Fig. 31-2). The ECG may reveal low voltages and flattened T waves. Atrial fibrillation is the most common associated arrhythmia.

15. **How should constrictive pericarditis be managed?**
Constrictive pericarditis is treated definitively with surgical excision of the constricted pericardium. Every effort should be made to completely evacuate pus or blood from the pericardial cavity to prevent future constriction. Medical therapy with low-dose diuretics can be used to alleviate symptoms, but overdiuresis is a constant risk because of frequent intravascular volume contraction. Glucocorticoids have not been proved efficacious in the prevention of constriction.

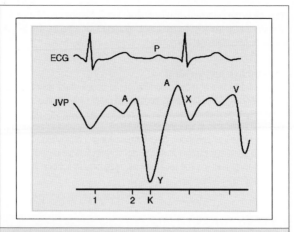

Figure 31-2. Constrictive pericarditis. In this condition, right ventricular diastolic pressure is greatly elevated. This elevation results in a prominent *Y* descent following tricuspid valve opening. The abrupt rise in venous pressure during right ventricular filling is due to the noncompliant right ventricular chamber encased in an unyielding pericardial shell. The venous pulse contour in constrictive pericarditis often takes on an M or W configuration. A pericardial knock (K), a high-frequency early diastolic filling sound, typically is present. (From Abrams J: Synopsis of Cardiac Physical Diagnosis, 2nd ed. Boston, Butterworth Heinemann, 2001, pp 23–35.)

BIBLIOGRAPHY

1. Adler Y, Finkelstein Y, Guindo J, et al: Colchicine treatment for recurrent pericarditis: A decade of experience. Circulation 97:2183–2185, 1998.

2. Imazio M, Demichelis B, Parrini I, et al: Day-hospital treatment of acute pericarditis: A management program for outpatient therapy. J Am Coll Cardiol 43:1042–1046, 2004.

3. LeWinter MM, Kabbani S: Pericardial diseases. In Zipes DP, Libby P, Bonow RO, Braunwald E (eds): Heart Disease: A Textbook of Cardiovascular Medicine, 7th ed. Philadelphia, Elsevier, 2005, pp 1757–1780.

4. Spodick DH: Diagnostic electrocardiographic sequences in acute pericarditis: Significance of PR segment and PR vector changes. Circulation 48:575–580, 1973.

5. Spodick DH: Pericardial rub: Prospective, multiple observer investigation of pericardial friction in 100 patients. Am J Cardiol 35:357–362, 1975.

6. Surawicz B, Lasseter KC: Electrocardiogram in pericarditis. Am J Cardiol 26:471–474, 1970.

CHAPTER 32

TACHYARRHYTHMIAS

Chong U. Kim, MD

1. **What is the definition of *tachycardia*?**
   Tachycardia is defined as pathophysiologic increase to a ventricular rate >100 beats/min (Table 32-1).

TABLE 32-1. TACHYARRHYTHMIAS AND USUAL RATES	
Sinus tachycardia	>100 beats/min
Atrial fibrillation	80–220 beats/min
Atrial flutter	100, 150, 300 beats/min
Junctional (supraventricular) tachycardia	100–220 beats/min
Ventricular tachycardia	100–160 beats/min

2. **What are the common causes of sinus tachycardia? How is it treated?**
   There are numerous causes of sinus tachycardia; most are due to reversible causes. Tachycardia arises from increased sympathetic stimulation to the sinus node. The most common cause of sinus tachycardia is activity. Listed below are various causes of sinus tachycardia:
   - **Drugs:** Amphetamines, caffeine, cocaine, thyroid replacement, beta agonists
   - **Central nervous system:** Fever, cerebrovascular accident, hemorrhage, increased central nervous system pressure, anxiety,
   - **Cardiovascular:** Hypotension, congestive heart failure (CHF), hypoxemia

   Sinus tachycardia is usually a physiologic response–driven mechanism and treatment should be directed toward treating the primary disorder. For example, if tachycardia is due to hypotension, you would give intravenous hydration to raise intravascular volume, and as a normal physiologic response, this will cause the heart to slow down (Fig. 32-1).

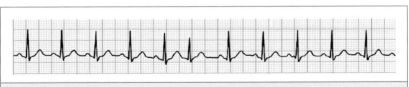

Figure 32-1. Sinus tachycardia.

3. **What is multifocal atrial tachycardia (MAT)? How does it look on electrocardiography (ECG)?**
   MAT presents with an irregularly irregular pulse due to impulses generated from different foci within the right atrium, along with electrical impulses from the sinus node. P waves are usually present in front of each QRS complex, but at irregular times. MAT is defined as having more

than three different P wave morphologies, with different P-P intervals. It differs from sinus tachycardia, which has the same P wave morphology, P-P intervals, and a regular rate (Fig. 32-2).

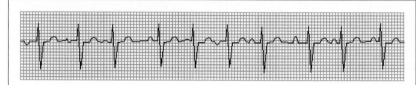

Figure 32-2. Multifocal atrial tachycardia.

4. What causes MAT? How is it managed?

MAT is associated with coronary artery disease, chronic obstructive pulmonary disease, hypoxemia, pulmonary embolism, CHF, and electrolyte abnormalities. Treatment is aimed at the underlying disease process. If MAT persists, medications such as beta blockers, calcium channel blockers, and magnesium have been known to be effective for treatment.

5. What is paroxysmal atrial tachycardia (PAT)? How is it treated?

PAT represents a supraventricular tachycardia with the same focus that is not sinus in origin. Consequently, the P waves are often inverted in the inferior leads as the atria depolarize from the bottom of the atria toward the top (opposite of sinus rhythm). The heart rate is usually 150–250 beats/min. There are many maneuvers, aimed at restoring vagal tone, for stopping PAT; these include the Valsalva maneuver, carotid sinus massage, and immersion of the head in cold water.

6. How does atrial fibrillation differ from atrial flutter?

Both are irregular tachycardias.
- **Atrial fibrillation:** (Fig. 32-3) Irregularly irregular, lacks discernable P waves, and has a faster atrial rate of >300–400 beats/min. Atrial fibrillation presents with an irregularly irregular pulse, a loss of *a* waves in the jugular venous pulse (due to the chaotic atrial activity, atrial filling time is disrupted), and a variable pulse pressure in the carotid pulse.
- **Atrial flutter:** (Fig. 32-4) Usually a regularly irregular rhythm with a saw-tooth wave pattern of P waves seen on ECGs. Atrial flutter usually demonstrates a slower atrial rate (~300 beats/min) and an atrioventricular (AV) block pattern of 2:1 or 4:1.

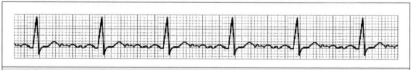

Figure 32-3. Atrial fibrillation.

7. List some of the causes of atrial fibrillation.

Atrial fibrillation may occur without inciting cause (lone atrial fibrillation) or in association with fever, stress, acute myocardial infarction, CHF, excessive alcohol intake or withdrawal, volume depletion, pericarditis, pulmonary embolism, mitral valve disease, or thyrotoxicosis.

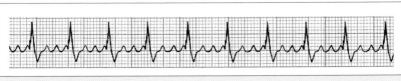

Figure 32-4. Atrial flutter.

8. **What is the estimated risk of stroke with atrial fibrillation?**
   Atrial fibrillation occurs in 2–4% of the population aged 60 years and older. The estimated annual risk of stroke in adults 60 years and older with atrial fibrillation is approximately 3.8% per patient per year. There is a higher risk of stroke in persons with comorbid conditions such as diabetes, hypertension, transient ischemic attacks, age greater 65 years, and recent CHF (Table 32-2).

TABLE 32-2. INCIDENCE OF STROKE PER YEAR WITH ATRIAL FIBRILLATION	
Age (years)	Rate (%/year)
50–59	1.3
60–69	2.2
70–79	4.2
80–89	5.1

9. **When are overdrive pacing and direct current (DC) cardioversion used in atrial fibrillation?**
   - **Overdrive pacing:** Requires external pacing at a rate faster than the rate of arrhythmia to prevent or terminate the tachycardia.
   - **DC cardioversion:** Primarily used in refractory or unstable atrial fibrillation, when pharmacologic treatment is unsuccessful. In DC cardioversion, an electric shock is applied via two paddles placed on the chest wall, one on the right second intercostal space and another placed on the midclavicular line in the left fifth intercostal space. Energy is delivered to the heart to "reset" the electrical activity. In atrial fibrillation, >100 joules are usually necessary to terminate the arrhythmia.

10. **What medications are typically used for rate control in atrial fibrillation?**
    The primary goal for initial treatment is rate control. Pharmacologic intervention is aimed at the AV node. Intravenous medications include digoxin, verapamil, diltiazem, and beta blockers, including metoprolol, esmolol, and propranolol.

11. **Discuss the different types of medications used for chemical cardioversion.**
    Cardioversion can be accomplished with electricity (see question 9) or medications. Type IA antiarrhythmic agents, such as procainamide and quinidine, and type IC antiarrhythmic agents, such as flecainide and propafenone, work by decreasing the excitation potential via sodium channel blockade. Type III antiarrhythmics include amiodarone, sotalol, and ibutilide. Amiodarone has been used in atrial fibrillation for chemical cardioversion, but it is more useful for rate control. Sotalol has not been shown to effectively terminate atrial fibrillation. Ibutilide, a newer type III antiarrhythmic drug, has been shown to terminate atrial fibrillation best in this class.

12. **What is the role of anticoagulation in atrial fibrillation?**

    The risk of long-term thromboembolic events is significant, unless anticoagulation is used. However, acutely, the risk of a cardioembolic event is low, so there is no need to urgently anticoagulate a patient. However, if a patient has been in atrial fibrillation for >48 hours, the risk of embolism with chemical or DC cardioversion is significant. As such, these patients should be anticoagulated for 3 weeks before cardioversion is attempted.

13. **How is AV reentry tachycardia distinguished from AV nodal reentry tachycardia on an ECG?**

    They are both classified as supraventricular tachycardias with regular rhythm and rate greater than 120 beats/min (Fig. 32-5). They are both tachycardias that originate above the ventricle; thus QRS complexes are usually narrow complex. AV reentry tachycardia (AVRT) uses an extranodal AV bypass tract and is distinguished from AV nodal reentry tachycardia (AVNRT) by the presence of retrograde P waves. AVNRT is associated with P waves that are commonly "buried" in the QRS complex. The treatment for both forms of SVT is intravenous adenosine or verapamil. Adenosine is very short acting drug that will terminate approximately 90% of AVNRT or AVRT.

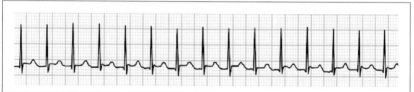

Figure 32-5. Supraventricular tachycardia.

14. **What is Wolff-Parkinson-White syndrome (WPW)?**

    WPW is a form of ventricular preexcitation syndrome (the ventricle is induced to depolarize early). It occurs when there is an accessory pathway, called the *bundle of Kent,* bypassing the AV node. On ECG, it is characterized by a short PR interval (<120 msec) as well as a delta wave, which is a "slurring" of the initial part of the QRS interval (Fig. 32-6). Activation of the accessory pathway leads to a supraventricular tachycardia. Atrial fibrillation is especially dangerous in WPW because the rapid atrial impulses may bypass the slowing effect of the AV node, resulting in ventricular fibrillation and death. Treatment involves radiofrequency ablation of the bypass tract, which is effective >95% of time.

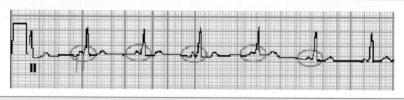

Figure 32-6. Wolff-Parkinson-White syndrome.

15. **What are premature ventricular contractions (PVCs)?**

    PVCs are characterized by wide QRS complexes that are different in morphology from sinus beats. The QRS complexes are >120 msec and are not preceded by a P wave. PVCs are seen in patients with or without underlying heart disease and are more concerning in patients with underlying cardiac disease. Other causes of PVCs are electrolyte disorders, such as hypokalemia, hypomagnesemia, and medication use (e.g., digoxin, tricyclic antidepressants). In young, healthy adults without underlying heart disease, no work-up is required.

16. **What are bigeminy and trigeminy?**
A repeating set of one (bigeminy) or two (trigeminy) normal sinus beats punctuated by a PAC (atrial) or PVC (ventricular). They are associated with cardiac causes such as ischemic heart disease, mitral valve prolapse, and cardiomyopathy but can also be associated with the use of medications (e.g., caffeine, cocaine, alcohol, and amphetamines) and electrolyte abnormalities (e.g., acidosis, hypokalemia, hypomagnesemia). Most cases are asymptomatically noticed as a regularly irregular pulse on physical examination and do not require treatment. If the patient has no heart disease, adjustment or removal of the cause usually treats the condition. If the patient has heart disease, antiarrhythmics can be considered.

17. **What is ventricular tachycardia (VT)?**
VT presents as a wide complex tachycardia (QRS > 120 msec), with a regular rate >100 beats/min that is dissociated from the atria (P waves are present but not associated with ventricular beats). VT, defined as three or more consecutive PVCs, can be sustained or nonsustained. VT that persists for more than 30 seconds is referred to as *sustained VT*. It often results in hemodynamic compromise and requires emergent treatment. *Nonsustained VT* persists for <30 seconds and is usually asymptomatic. The most common causes of VT are ischemic heart disease, dilated cardiomyopathy, hypertrophic cardiomyopathy, mitral valve prolapse, electrolyte abnormalities, medications, and myocarditis (Fig. 32-7).

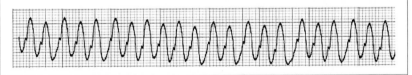

Figure 32-7. Ventricular tachycardia.

18. **What is torsades de pointes?**
Torsades de pointes is a French term meaning "twisting of the points." It is a form of VT with polymorphic QRS complexes. The term refers to the characteristic ECG finding of the tracing twisting around the baseline (Fig. 32–8). It is a life-threatening arrhythmia that is often seen in patients with prolonged QT intervals. Prolonged QT intervals can be seen in patients with long QT syndrome, electrolyte abnormalities, or medication use. There are over 40 medications that have been shown to cause QT prolongation, including tricyclic antidepressants, erythromycin, fluoroquinolones, and type IC antiarrhythmics.

19. **What are fusion and capture beats?**
Fusion beats and capture beats are seen in VT.
- **Fusion beats:** These result from simultaneous activation of the ventricle from a ventricular focus and a signal coming from the sinus node through the AV node. This results in a P wave (from the atrial contraction) that appears to conduct to a wide-complex QRS (from the ventricular focus).
- **Capture beats:** These are QRS complexes that are "captured" by a sinus impulse during a run of VT. This results in a narrow-complex QRS preceded by a P wave but surrounded by wide complexes associated with VT. It does not alter the tachycardia or affect the focus.

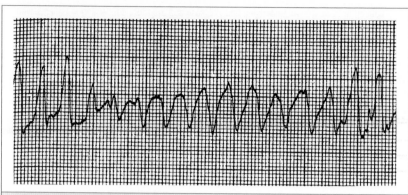

Figure 32-8. Torsades de pointes. (From Parsons PE, Wiener-Kronish JP [eds]: Critical Care Secrets, 2nd ed. Philadelphia, Hanley & Belfus, 1998, p 153.)

KEY POINTS: TACHYARRHYTHMIAS

1. In atrial fibrillation, the risk for stroke is higher in persons with comorbid conditions such as age greater than 65 years, diabetes, hypertension, and recent heart failure.

2. In patients undergoing cardioversion for atrial fibrillation, 3 weeks of anticoagulation at a therapeutic level is recommended before cardioversion.

3. Acute myocardial infarction is one of the more common causes of VT.

4. VT is identified on ECG with QRS duration >120 msec and rates >120 beats/min, with complete AV dissociation.

20. **How is VT treated?**

Treatment for VT is dependent on the clinical assessment of the patient. If the patient has stable vital signs without any symptoms of vascular compromise then the treatment can be more conservative, using pharmacologic intervention. However, if the patient is unstable, a more aggressive approach is warranted, involving DC cardioversion. First-line pharmacologic treatment is procainamide 20 mg/min IV followed by a constant infusion of 20–80 μg/kg/min. It functions by slowing the rate of VT, enabling the intrinsic sinus rhythm to correct the arrhythmia. Another treatment option is amiodarone 150 mg IV over 10 minutes followed by a slow infusion of 1 mg/min for 6 hours then a maintenance infusion of 0.5 mg/min. DC cardioversion applies a synchronized (at the top of the R wave to ensure proper depolarization to correct the rhythm) electrical shock of between 100–300 joules to the chest. Repletion of potassium levels to >4.0 mg/dL and magnesium to a level >2 mg/dL is also recommended.

21. **What is ventricular fibrillation (VF)?**

VF is a VT with a very rapid rate, usually more than 220 beats/min, associated with poor cardiac output. There are no P waves or T waves visible on ECG due to its rapid rate. It is highlighted by its monomorphic pattern and bizarre appearance of QRS complexes and is always considered a life-threatening arrhythmia that, if not immediately treated, will lead to death. VF is most commonly associated with acute cardiac ischemia but may be associated with electrolyte abnormalities or the use of antiarrhythmic medications that can prolong the QT interval. The most effective treatment of VF is external electrical defibrillation.

BIBLIOGRAPHY

1. Josephson M, Zimetbaum P: The tachyarrhythmias. In Harrison's Principles of Internal Medicine, 15th ed. New York, McGraw-Hill, 2001, pp 1292–1309.
2. McCord J, et al: Multifocal atrial tachycardia. Chest 113:203, 1998.
3. Prystowsky EN, Benson DW Jr, Wyse DG, et al: Management of patients with atrial fibrillation: A statement for healthcare professionals. Circulation 93:1262–1277, 1996.

CHAPTER 33

BRADYARRHYTHMIAS

Kevin Flemmons, MD, and Mitchell J. Wilson, MD

1. **How is the normal resting heart rate determined?**
   The normal heart rate is 60–100 beats/min. At night, the normal heart rate can be between 30–35 beats/min with 2–3-second pauses. Well-conditioned athletes can have heart rates <40 beats/min with 2-second pauses. The normal heart is innervated by the sympathetic and parasympathetic nervous systems. A balance between these two systems results in the baseline heart rate for any given individual. If both sympathetic and parasympathetic systems are removed, the heart rate would range from 85 to 105 beats/min inversely proportional to the person's age.

2. **How does the parasympathetic nervous system affect the heart rate?**
   Release of acetylcholine from the vagus nerve decreases sinus node automaticity (rate of contraction), slows atrioventricular (AV) nodal conduction, decreases the strength of contraction, and constricts coronary vessels. The parasympathetic activity is increased with vomiting, Valsalva maneuver, carotid massage, cough, and micturition.

3. **How does the sympathetic nervous system affect the heart rate?**
   Norepinephrine released from the cardiopulmonary splanchnic nerve increases sinus node automaticity, inhibits the effect of the parasympathetic nervous system, increases strength of contraction, and dilates coronary vessels.

4. **What is bradycardia?**
   Bradycardia is defined as a heart rate of <60 beats/min. It most commonly results from parasympathetic-induced sinus bradycardia. More pathologic causes of bradycardia include sinus arrest, sinus node dysfunction, and AV nodal blocks.

5. **Which bradyarrhythmias originate in the sinus node?**
   Sinus bradycardia is caused by decreased automaticity of the sinus node located in the right atrium. Sinus pause and sinus arrest occur when a sinus impulse fails to conduct out of the node to the atrium.

6. **What is the sick sinus syndrome?**
   Sick sinus syndrome, also referred to as *sinus node dysfunction,* can present with bradycardia, tachycardia, or tachycardia and bradycardia (i.e., tachy-brady syndrome). The latter manifests as episodes of tachycardia (most commonly sinus or atrial fibrillation) that are followed by periods of inappropriately slow heart rates (sinus bradycardia). Sinus node dysfunction may be due to intrinsic causes (i.e., related to the sinus node itself) or extrinsic causes. Intrinsic disease is caused by the replacement of the normal tissue of the node with fibrous tissue. Examples include infections such as endocarditis and Chagas' disease, infiltrative diseases such as sarcoidosis, connective tissue diseases, and trauma. Extrinsic causes include pharmacologic agents (e.g., β-adrenergic blockers, calcium channel blockers, digoxin, some antihypertensive agents, and antiarrhythmic drugs), electrolyte imbalances, hypothermia, hypothyroidism, increased intracranial pressure, and excessive vagal tone.

7. **What are the different types of AV nodal heart block?**

The various types of AV nodal heart block are broken down by the level of the block (Table 33-1). In general, first-degree AV block and type I second-degree AV block are asymptomatic and do not require treatment. A type II second-degree AV block may decompensate into third-degree AV block, which may result in unstable bradycardia and require placement of a cardiac pacemaker. (See Chapter 81 for more details.)

TABLE 33-1. CHARACTERISTICS OF THE MAIN TYPES OF AV BLOCKS

Type of AV Block	ECG Finding	Location of the Block
First-degree	PR interval >0.2 sec with QRS correlating with each P wave	Anywhere between sinus node and the ventricle
Second-degree type I (Wenckebach)	Progressively >PR interval until no QRS following P wave, normal QRS	Delay usually in AV node, occasionally in bundle of His
Second-degree type II (Mobitz II)	Intermittently blocked P wave; no progressively >PR, prolonged QRS	Between His bundle and Purkinje fibers
Third-degree (complete heart block)	Independent atrial and ventricular activity	If narrow QRS and rate 40–60 beats/min, usually AV node block; if wide QRS and rate <40 beats/min, block usually between bundle of His and Purkinje fibers

ECG = electrocardiography.

8. **Can myocardial ischemia cause sinus bradycardia?**

Yes. Ischemia of the right ventricle often involves the right coronary artery, which also supplies blood to the AV node. Loss of blood flow to the AV node can result in third-degree AV block.

9. **How does hypothyroidism affect the heart?**

Low thyroid hormone levels decrease the heart rate by lowering cardiac sensitivity to catecholamines. Hypothyroidism also decreases contractility by decreasing the production of myosin isoenzyme V1, which in turn decreases the rate of turnover of actin-myosin crossbridges in the ventricles.

10. **What are the key questions to ask in the evaluation of bradyarrhythmias?**

Questions should focus on symptoms such as syncope, dizziness, fatigue, weakness, chest pain, and heart failure. Questions regarding precipitating factors that increase vagal stimulus such as vomiting, Valsalva, cough, micturition, shaving, chest pain, fever, and infection are important. A history of use of medication that can cause bradycardia (e.g., beta blockers, calcium channel blockers, digoxin) should also be elicited.

11. **How should bradyarrhythmias be evaluated?**

Every patient with bradycardia should have an electrocardiogram (ECG) to determine whether he or she has an arrhythmia. Checking blood chemistries and thyroid-stimulating hormone is also important. If the ECG and laboratory test results are unrevealing then the patient can undergo a Holter monitor or a cardiac event monitor. Holter monitors are essentially telemetry monitors that the patient can wear at home for an extended period of time. These devices monitor every beat of the heart and generate reports that can reveal abnormal cardiac rhythms. An event monitor can be worn for longer periods of time but only records rhythms associated with "events" as indicated by a symptomatic patient pushing a button. More invasive testing with electrophysiology testing can also be done to determine the exact origin of the arrhythmia and the need for permanent pacing.

KEY POINTS: BRADYCARDIA

1. The balance between the parasympathetic and sympathetic tone on the sinus node determines the resting heart rate.

2. *Bradycardia* is defined as a heart rate <60 beats/min.

3. Sick sinus syndrome is the most common cause of symptomatic bradycardia.

4. The work-up of bradycardia includes a history and physical examination, ECG, laboratory testing, and cardiac monitoring.

5. Type II second-degree AV block and third-degree AV block often require permanent pacemaker placement.

12. **How does one manage patients with symptomatic bradycardia?**
If the patient has serious signs or symptoms (e.g., hypotension, loss of consciousness), the first step is to give the patient atropine 0.5–1.0 mg intravenously. This can be followed by dopamine, epinephrine, or isoproterenol as necessary. Transcutaneous pacing may temporarily stabilize the condition of a patient awaiting more definitive transvenous pacemaker placement.

13. **What are the indications for permanent pacemaker placement in patients with symptomatic bradyarrhythmias?**
Management of symptomatic bradycardia is determined by the severity of symptoms, the relationship between symptoms and confirmed bradycardia, and the presence of potentially reversible causes. Symptoms definitely related to confirmed bradycardia caused by intrinsic sinus node dysfunction or atrioventricular block should be treated with permanent pacing. The American College of Cardiology and American Heart Association guidelines for the implantation of pacemakers list the following as universally accepted (class I) indications in *asymptomatic* patients:
- Third-degree AV block with documented asystole lasting 3 or more seconds (in sinus rhythm) or escape rates <40 beats/min in patients while awake
- Third-degree AV block or type II second-degree AV block in patients with chronic bifascicular or trifascicular block
- Congenital third-degree AV block with a wide QRS escape rhythm, ventricular dysfunction, or bradycardia markedly inappropriate for age

Potential (class II) indications for pacing in asymptomatic patients include:
- Third-degree AV block with faster escape rates in patients who are awake
- Type II second-degree AV block in patients without bifascicular or trifascicular block
- Incidental finding on electrophysiologic study of block below or within the bundle of His.

BIBLIOGRAPHY

1. Gregoratos G, Cheitlin MD, Conill A, et al: ACC/AHA guidelines for implantation of cardiac pacemakers and antiarrhythmia devices: A report of the American College of Cardiology/ American Heart Association Task Force on Practice Guidelines (Committee on Pacemaker Implantation). J Am Coll Cardiol 31:1175–1209, 1998.
2. Mangrum JM, DiMarco JP: The evaluation and management of bradycardia. N Engl J Med 342:703–709, 2000.

CHAPTER 34

INFECTIVE ENDOCARDITIS

Hiren Shah, MD, MBA

1. **How common is infective endocarditis (IE)?**

   IE accounts for approximately 1 case per 1000 hospital admissions, and for an estimated incidence of 10,000–20,000 new cases annually. The mean age of patients with IE has gradually increased in the antibiotic era. In 1926, the mean age was <30 years. Currently, >50% of patients with IE are older than 50 years. Factors accounting for this shift in age distribution include the decreasing incidence of acute rheumatic fever and rheumatic heart disease, the increased prevalence of degenerative heart disease and prosthetic valve surgery in the elderly, and increased rates of nosocomial endocarditis (due to indwelling intravascular lines, implantable devices, and catheter-related infections). Men are more commonly affected than women.

2. **What conditions predispose persons to IE?**

   Almost any type of structural heart disease may predispose patients to IE, especially when the defect results in turbulence of blood flow. Rheumatic heart disease, especially affecting the mitral valve, was the most common structural abnormality in the past. Contemporary causes include congenital heart disease (e.g., patent ductus arteriosus, ventricular septal defect, coarctation of the aorta, bicuspid aortic valve, tetralogy of Fallot), degenerative heart disease (e.g., calcified lesions due to arteriosclerotic disease), prosthetic valve endocarditis, and intravenous (IV) drug use.

3. **What is the pathophysiology of IE?**
   - Endothelial disruption due to shear stress (predisposing conditions such as structural heart disease)
   - Formation of a sterile fibrin-platelet cardiac thrombus
   - Seeding of the thrombus due to transient bacteremia
   - Infected valvular vegetation increases in size due to bacterial proliferation leading to local tissue destruction, embolization of the infected mass, or formation of immune complexes
     See Fig. 34-1.

4. **What are the most common clinical symptoms, signs, and laboratory findings in patients with IE?**

   Fever is the most common presenting symptom, occurring in 90–95% of all cases. Other symptoms are noted in Table 34-1. Nonspecific physical examination findings are common, and laboratory findings often indicate evidence of systemic disease. Most patients with IE have a murmur (85–95%). However, only 5–10% of patients with IE have a change in an existing murmur, and only 3–5% of cases have the development of a new regurgitant murmur.

5. **What are the classic peripheral manifestations of IE?**

   Classic physical findings include petechiae (found on the palpebral conjunctiva, the buccal and palatal mucosa and the extremities), splinter or subungual hemorrhages (dark red, linear, or occasionally flame-shaped streaks in the nail bed of the fingers or toes), Osler's nodes (small, tender, bluish subcutaneous nodules on fingertips with erythematous base), Janeway lesions (nontender, small pink or hemorrhagic macular lesions on the palms and soles), and Roth's

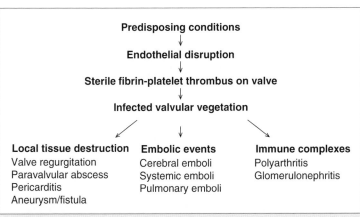

Figure 34-1. Pathophysiology of infective endocarditis. (Adapted from Otto C: Valvular Heart Disease, 2nd ed. Philadelphia, W.B. Saunders, 2004, p 483.)

TABLE 34-1. CLINICAL MANIFESTATIONS OF IE

Symptoms (Incidence)	Signs (% Affected)	Laboratory Findings (% Affected)
Fever (90–95%)	Preexisting unchanged murmur (85–95%)	Elevated ESR (90–100%): mean, 57 mm/h
Chills (42–75%)	Changing murmur (5–10%)	Anemia (50–80%)
Anorexia (25–55%)	New murmur (3–5%)	Leukocytosis (20–30% in acute cases)
Weight loss (25–35%)	Embolic event (20–40%)	Circulating immune complexes (95%)
Malaise (25–40%)	Splenomegaly (15–50%)	Microscopic hematuria (30–60%)
Myalgia/arthralgia (15–30%)	Clubbing (10–20%)	Positive rheumatoid factor (25–50%)
Neurologic changes (20–40%)	Osler's nodes (10–25%)	Low serum iron level (50–80%)
Headache (15–40%)	Splinter hemorrhages (5–15%)	Elevated cryoglobulins (20–50%)
Back pain (7–10%)	Petechiae (12–40%)	Proteinuria (50–65%)
Diaphoresis (25%)	Janeway lesions (3–5%)	Hypergammaglobulinemia (25–50%)
Cough (25%)	Roth spots (2–20%)	Thrombocytopenia (5–15%)

ESR = erythrocyte sedimentation rate.

spots (retinal hemorrhages with a central pale area seen on fundoscopic examination). It remains controversial whether these classic manifestations of endocarditis represent embolic events or immunologic phenomena.

KEY POINTS: PERIPHERAL MANIFESTATIONS OF IE

1. Petechiae

2. Splinter or subungual hemorrhages

3. Osler's nodes

4. Janeway lesions

5. Roth's spots

6. **What are the most common organisms that cause IE?**
Although almost any bacterium can cause IE, streptococci, enterococci, and staphylococci are responsible in a vast majority of cases. The most common causes of native valve endocarditis are *Streptococcus viridans* (25–40%). Coagulase-negative staphylococci (mainly *Staphylococcus epidermidis*) have emerged as an important pathogen in the setting of prosthetic valves, implanted devices, and hospitalization. In IV drug abusers, *Staphylococcus aureus* is the most common pathogen (>50%) followed by gram-negative bacilli, *Pseudomonas aeruginosa*, and fungi. Enterococcus is increasingly recognized as a cause of IE especially in IV drug abusers, older men undergoing genitourinary procedures, and women undergoing gynecologic procedures.

KEY POINTS: MOST COMMON ORGANISMS IN IE

1. Prosthetic valve (coagulase-negative staphylococci)

2. Native valve (*Streptococcus* species)

3. IV drug users (*S. aureus*)

7. **What are the HACEK organisms?**
The HACEK organisms account for 3–5% of all cases of IE and represent a group of slow-growing, fastidious, gram-negative bacilli that are part of the upper respiratory tract and oropharyngeal flora.
   - **H:** *Haemophilus* species *(H. parainfluenzae, H. aphrophilus,* and *H. paraphrophilus)*
   - **A:** *Actinobacillus actinomycetemcomitans*
   - **C:** *Cardiobacterium hominis*
   - **E:** *Eikenella corrodens*
   - **K:** *Kingella kingae*
   A prolonged blood culture incubation period (≥3 weeks) should be used to isolate these slow-growing organisms. Empiric therapy may safely be deferred—if patients are stable—until a more definite diagnosis is established. In patients with severe illness and cardiac compromise, initiation of empiric therapy after initial blood culture specimens remain sterile should be

targeted against the HACEK group organisms. Appropriate therapy includes ceftriaxone, ampicillin, or vancomycin and, in most cases, an aminoglycoside.

8. **Infection with _Streptococcus bovis_ has been associated with what type of malignancy?**
Infection with _S. bovis_, a nonenterococcal group D streptococcus, has been associated with the presence of coexistent colonic polyps or colonic neoplasia. Thus, it is important to perform diagnostic studies of the gastrointestinal tract in all patients diagnosed with systemic infection caused by this pathogen. One study in patients with _S. bovis_ endocarditis revealed polyps in 47% and colon cancer in 16% of patients. _S. bovis_ accounts for 2–6% of streptococcal bloodstream isolates in hospitalized patients and for 11–14% of streptococcal isolates associated with IE. _S. bovis_ is highly susceptible to penicillin.

9. **What are the Duke criteria?**
The Modified Duke Criteria for Infective Endocarditis incorporate risk factors, physical examination findings, microbiology, and imaging findings into a clinical prediction rule that aids in making the diagnosis of IE. Two major criteria, one major and three minor criteria, or five minor criteria are highly associated with IE. The Duke criteria are highly specific for the diagnosis of IE, with studies showing specificity rates of 99% (Table 34-2).

10. **What is the best method for obtaining blood culture specimens for the diagnosis of IE?**
A minimum of three blood culture specimens should be obtained, each from a separate venipuncture site to identify the causative organism and determine antibiotic sensitivities. If the patient is severely ill, these three specimens should be obtained over a 1-hour span before starting empiric therapy. If the patient is not critically ill, it is preferable to delay antibiotic therapy for 1 to 3 days while awaiting culture results. A minimum of 10 mL of blood per culture specimen should be obtained since many patients have low-grade bacteremia.

11. **What is "culture-negative" endocarditis?**
Negative blood culture results can be seen in 10–20% of all endocarditis cases. This may be due to several factors including prior antimicrobial therapy, fungal endocarditis, uremia, nonbacterial thrombotic endocarditis (_see_ question 18) or infection with organisms which are more difficult to isolate in culture. These organisms include _Coxiella burnetii_ (Q fever), _Tropheryma whipplei_, and _Brucella, Mycoplasma, Chlamydia, Histoplasma, Legionella,_ and _Bartonella_ species, which will not grow unless special media or microbiologic methods are used. The HACEK organisms may not be detected in culture unless incubated for 7–21 days.

12. **What is the recommended approach to the treatment of a patient with apparent culture-negative endocarditis?**
Incubate the cultures for a prolonged period (3 weeks) to allow for growth of fastidious organisms. Use special culture techniques for nutritionally variant streptococci, _Brucella_ species, fungi, and _Legionella_ species. Obtain serologic studies for Q fever (_C. burnetii_), _Brucella, Bartonella,_ and _Chlamydia_ species. Culture and use antibody stains for embolized valve tissue or vegetations if isolated. Repeat blood cultures with the patient off antibiotics for 2–4 days.

13. **How does echocardiography aid in the diagnosis of IE?**
Echocardiography is essential in the identification of valvular vegetations, the evaluation of the degree of valve destruction and consequent valve regurgitation, and the detection of possible complications of the disease. The reported sensitivity of transthoracic echocardiography (TTE) for the detection of valvular vegetations varies from 35 to 65% and depends on the patient's body habitus, operator experience, adequate exam time, and shadowing by prosthetic valves and conduits. The sensitivity of transesophageal echocardiography (TEE) has been reported to

TABLE 34-2. CLINICAL CRITERIA FOR DIAGNOSIS OF IE

Major Criteria	Minor Criteria
Positive blood cultures	**Predisposition:** Predisposing cardiac condition or IV drug use
Typical microorganism for IE from two separate blood cultures: *S. viridans,* *S. bovis,* HACEK group or community-acquired *S. aureus* or enterococci in the absence of a primary focus	**Fever:** Temperature > 100.4°F (38.0°C)
	Vascular phenomena: Major arterial emboli, septic pulmonary emboli, mycotic aneurysm, intracranial hemorrhage, conjunctival hemorrhages, Janeway lesions
or	**Immunologic phenomena:**
Persistently positive blood culture defined as: a microorganism consistent with IE from two blood cultures drawn more than 12 hours apart *or* all of three or the majority of four or more separate blood cultures (with first and last drawn at least 1 hour apart)	Glomerulonephritis, Osler's nodes, Roth's spots, rheumatoid factor
	Microbiologic finding: Positive blood culture not meeting major criteria as noted previously *or* serologic evidence of active infection (single isolate) with organism consistent with IE
or	
Single positive blood culture for *Coxiella burnetii* or phase I IgG Ab titer > 1:800	
Evidence of endocardial involvement	
Positive echocardiogram	
Oscillating intracardiac mass on valve or supporting structure	
or	
Abscess	
or	
New partial dehiscence of prosthetic valve	
or	
New valvular regurgitation	

IgA = Immunoglobulin A, Ab = antibody.

be 80–95% and is better for evaluation of prosthetic valves and posterior cardiac structures such as the mitral valve. Low-risk patients can first undergo TTE whereas high-risk patients (e.g., those with prosthetic valve, congenital heart disease, pervious endocarditis, congestive heart failure, new atrioventricular [AV] block, risk for intracardiac complications) and those with equivocal TTE evaluations should undergo TEE (Fig. 34-2).

14. **What is the empiric treatment of IE?**
In the absence of hemodynamic compromise, empiric therapy for native-valve IE should be held until after appropriate culture data has been collected. In treating IE, any empiric therapy should be bactericidal and tailored toward the most likely microbes. Native valve IE should be treated with a

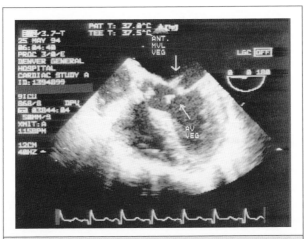

Figure 34-2. Infective endocarditis involving both aortic and mitral valves.

penicillin, a synthetic penicillin (e.g., nafcillin), or ceftriaxone in combination with an aminoglycoside. Injection drug users and patients with early prosthetic valve IE have a higher rate of methicillin-resistant staphylococci and should be treated with empiric vancomycin in place of penicillin.

15. **How is the effectiveness of antibiotic therapy monitored in IE?**
    Repeat blood cultures during and after the course of therapy, particularly with *S. aureus* endocarditis, are needed to ensure eradication of the infection. It is imperative that the minimal inhibiting concentration of the etiologic agent be determined and IV antibiotic be administered for 4–6 weeks.

16. **What is the role of anticoagulant and antiplatelet therapy in patients with IE?**
    Anticoagulant therapy has not been shown to prevent embolization in native valve IE and may contribute to intracerebral hemorrhage in patients with embolization to the central nervous system. Patients with prosthetic valve endocarditis involving devices that would usually warrant maintenance anticoagulation should continue to receive anticoagulant therapy except in cases of *S. aureus* IE, in which the risk of central nervous system hemorrhage is high.

17. **When is surgery indicated for IE?**
    See Table 34-3.

18. **What is nonbacterial thrombotic endocarditis (NBTE)? How is it managed?**
    Sterile valvular vegetations and a high risk of embolic events characterize NBTE. The vegetations represent the first portion of the endocarditis cascade, that is, sterile platelet-fibrin depositions. They often occur in patients with underlying malignancy (most commonly pancreatic, lung, or lymphoma) or with systemic lupus erythematosus (Libman-Sacks endocarditis). These vegetations are typically small (<10 mm diameter), broad based, and irregular in shape, occurring most often on the aortic or mitral valves. Blood cultures in NBTE are negative. The treatment of NBTE remains controversial. Anticoagulation with heparin to prevent embolic events when vegetations are detected and the use of long-term anticoagulation has not been examined in controlled studies. Individualized therapy based on the overall clinical situation, the occurrence of embolic events, and the risk of anticoagulation is suggested.

TABLE 34-3. INDICATIONS FOR SURGERY IN IE	
Absolute Indications	**Relative Indications**
Moderate to severe CHF due to valve dysfunction	Perivalvular extension of infection, intracardiac fistula
Unstable prosthesis	Poorly responsive *S. aureus* native valve IE
Uncontrolled infection despite optimal antimicrobial therapy	Relapse of native valve endocarditis after optimal antimicrobial therapy
Unavailable effective antimicrobial therapy	Culture-negative native valve IE or prosthetic valve endocarditis with persistent fever (>10 days)
Relapse of prosthetic valve endocarditis after optimal therapy	Large (>10-mm diameter) hypermobile vegetation
	IE due to antibiotic-resistant enterococci

CHF = congestive heart failure.

19. **Which group is at risk for right-sided endocarditis? What signs and symptoms do they manifest?**

    Endocarditis in IV drug abusers (IVDAs) is often right sided with a predilection to affect the tricuspid valve. Septic pulmonary emboli are common, occurring in up to 75% of patients with tricuspid involvement. *S. aureus* is the most common organism (>50%). Two thirds of these patients have *no* clinical evidence of underlying heart disease, and only 35% of IVDAs with IE have heart murmurs. Consequently, it is difficult to accurately predict the presence of IE in a febrile IVDA, warranting a high level of suspicion and liberal use of blood cultures.

20. **What types of patients are most susceptible to fungal endocarditis?**

    Immunocompromised patients, IVDAs, and patients with indwelling catheters or prosthetic valves are most susceptible to fungal endocarditis. *Candida albicans*, non-albicans *Candida* species, *Torulopsis glabrata*, and *Aspergillus* species are the most common causes. Blood culture results are negative in over 50% of the cases of fungal endocarditis and require the lysis-centrifugation method of blood culturing to detect. Vegetations due to fungi are frequently very large, have a high risk of embolization, and frequently cause paravalvular infection. Treatment often requires surgical intervention as well as prolonged therapy with amphotericin B or caspofungin.

21. **Does a patient with *S. aureus* bacteremia require an evaluation for IE?**

    Staphylococci are a common cause of IE and the proportion of IE due to *S. aureus* is increasing, with nearly half of the cases acquired nosocomially. Thus, nosocomially acquired *S. aureus* bacteremia should prompt a complete evaluation for underlying IE since the course is frequently fulminant and results in death in approximately 40% of patients.

22. **What are the renal complications of IE?**

    Patients can develop renal failure from immune complex-mediated glomerulonephritis (15% of patients with IE) due to deposition of immunoglobulins and complement in the glomerular membrane or acute interstitial nephritis. Septic emboli can result in renal abscesses and infarction.

23. **What are the effects of IE on the heart?**

    Infected valvular vegetations can lead to local tissue destruction and extension of the infective process into adjacent myocardial tissues. Local tissue destruction can impede valve closure, leading to valvular regurgitation and stenosis, and can lead to the formation of paravalvular abscess. New AV heart block suggests the possibility of paravalvular abscess. Extension of infection into adjacent tissue can lead to pericarditis or the development of a sinus of Valsalva aneurysm or intracardiac fistula formation. In addition, significant valvular regurgitation is the predominant cause of congestive heart failure in IE.

24. **What are the effects of embolization of vegetations in IE?**
Fragments or entire vegetations can embolize to the systemic vascular bed (in cases of left-sided endocarditis), the pulmonary vascular bed (in cases of right-sided endocarditis), or the cerebral circulation. Systemic vascular embolization can lead to ischemic bowel, peripheral arterial occlusion, or renal infarctions. Embolization to the cerebral circulation can lead to transient ischemic attacks, stroke, or mycotic aneurysms. The risk of embolization is highest before and during the first 2 weeks of antibiotic therapy and is more likely with large vegetations (>10 mm), mitral (versus aortic) valve vegetations, infection with *S. aureus*, increased mobility of the vegetations, and fungal causes.

25. **Describe the manifestations of immune complex-mediated tissue injury in IE.**
The predominant clinical manifestations of immune-mediated injury include polyarthritis and glomerulonephritis. Circulating immune complex levels are associated with disease duration and can be associated with hypocomplementemia. Immunoglobulin G and early complement components (C1q, C4, and C30) are deposited in the glomerular basement membrane, leading to glomerulonephritis.

26. **What are the recommendations for the prevention of bacterial endocarditis?**
Patients with underlying valvular defects should receive prophylaxis for some interventional procedures. Procedures for which IE prophylaxis is recommended are shown in Table 34-4.

TABLE 34-4. RECOMMENDATIONS FOR ANTIBIOTIC PROPHYLAXIS OF IE	
Prophylaxis Recommended	**Prophylaxis Not Recommended**
Dental extraction and dental procedures that induce gingival or mucosal bleeding such as cleaning	Dental procedures not likely to induce gingival or mucosal bleeding
Tonsillectomy or adenoidectomy	Endotracheal tube insertion
Surgery involving GI and upper respiratory mucosa	Transesophageal echocardiography, pacemaker insertion
Rigid bronchoscopy	Bronchoscopy with flexible bronchoscope with or without biopsy
Esophageal dilation and sclerotherapy for varices	Cardiac catheterization, coronary angiography
ERCP with biliary obstruction	GI endoscopy with or without biopsy
Cystoscopy, uretheral dilation	Cesarean section, vaginal delivery
Uretheral catheterization if UTI present; urinary tract surgery, including prostate surgery	Intraoral injections
Incision and drainage of infected tissue	

GI = gastrointestinal, UTI = urinary tract infection.

Regimens for chemoprophylaxis for IE for dental, respiratory tract, or esophageal procedures, include amoxicillin 2 gm orally 1 hour before the procedure. The recommendation for genitourinary and gastrointestinal (excluding esophageal) procedures is ampicillin 2 gm IV or IM plus gentamicin 1.5 mg/kg IM or IV within 30 minutes of starting the procedure and ampicillin 1 gm IV or IM 6 hours later.

WEBSITE

American Heart Association: http://www.americanheart.org

BIBLIOGRAPHY

1. Ballet M, Gevigney G, Gare JP, et al: Infective endocarditis due to *Streptococcus bovis*: A report of 53 cases. Eur Heart J 16:1975, 1995.

2. Bonow RO, Carabello D, de Leon AC Jr, et al: ACC/AHA guidelines for the management of patients with valvular heart disease: executive summary: A report of the American College of Cardiology/American Heart Association Task Force on Practice Guidelines (Committee on Management of Patients With Valvular Heart Disease). Circulation 98:1949–1984, 1998.

3. Crawford M, Durack D: Clinical presentation of infective endocarditis. Cardiol Clin 21:159–166, 2003.

4. Horstkotte D, Follath F, Gutschik E, et al: Guidelines on prevention, diagnosis, and treatment of infective endocarditis executive summary. The Task Force on Infective Endocarditis of the European Society of Cardiology. Eur Heart J 25:267–276, 2004.

5. Karchmer A: Infective endocarditis. In Braunwald E (ed): Heart Disease: A Textbook of Cardiovascular Medicine, 6th ed. Philadelphia, W.B. Saunders, 2001, pp 1724–1750.

6. Mylonakis E, Calderwood S: Infective endocarditis in adults. N Engl J Med 345:1318–1330, 2001.

7. Olaison L, Pettersson G: Current best practices and guidelines, indications for surgical intervention in infective endocarditis. Infect Dis Clin North Am 16:453–475, 2003.

8. Otto C: Infective endocarditis. In Otto C (ed): Valvular Heart Disease, 2nd ed. Philadelphia, W.B. Saunders, 2004, pp 482–521.

9. Petti C, Fowler V: *Staphylococcus aureus* bacteremia and endocarditis. Cardiol Clin 21:219–233, 2003.

10. Sachdev M, Peterson G, Jollis J: Imaging techniques for diagnosis of infective endocarditis. Cardiol Clin 21:185–195, 2003.

11. Sexton D, Spelman D: Current best practices and guidelines, assessment and management of complications in infective endocarditis. Infect Dis Clin North Am 16:507–521, 2002.

VI. GASTROENTEROLOGY

EVALUATION OF THE PATIENT WITH ABDOMINAL PAIN

David D.K. Rolston, MD

1. **How common is abdominal pain in patients who present to the emergency department?**

   Abdominal pain accounts for 5–10% (5–10 million visits) of all emergency department encounters annually. The percentage of patients admitted to the hospital from the emergency room varies from one medical center to another.

2. **What is the mechanism by which patients experience abdominal pain?**

   Pain is perceived by sensory neuroreceptors located in visceral organs, the peritoneum and mesentery. Afferent nerves A-δ (myelinated) and C fibers (unmyelinated) are responsible for transmitting pain sensation to the spinal nerves. Most intra-abdominal pain sensation is transmitted via the C fibers into the dorsal horn onto Lissauer's tract, ultimately ending in laminae I and V of the dorsal horn cells. Second-order neurons cross the anterior commissure and enter the contralateral spinothalamic tract to the reticular formation nuclei in the medulla, the pons, and the thalamic nuclei. The third-order neurons project to the sensory cortex.

3. **What is the approach to treatment of a patient with abdominal pain?**

   A systematic, detailed history and examination can help clinicians arrive at a diagnosis in the majority of patients. However, tests such as abdominal radiographs, computed tomography, or ultrasonography may be necessary to confirm the diagnosis. The finding of an "acute abdomen" does not necessarily imply the need for surgical intervention. Location and type of pain provide important clues to the clinical diagnosis. Table 35-1 summarizes the different causes of acute abdominal pain, the characteristics of the pain and the key physical examination, laboratory, and imaging findings.

4. **How can the location and type of pain help diagnose the cause of the pain?**

   Pain from the digestive tract is initially felt in the midline because of bilateral symmetric innervation. Only when the peritoneum over the affected organ is inflamed does the pain localize to that area.

   - **Epigastric pain:** Arises from structures derived from the foregut (esophagus, stomach, duodenum proximal to the entrance of the common bile duct, liver, gall bladder, and pancreas).
   - **Periumbilical pain:** Arises from midgut structures (distal duodenum, jejunum, ileum, cecum, appendix, and the proximal two-thirds of the transverse colon).
   - **Lower abdominal pain:** Arises from hindgut structures (distal one-third of transverse colon up to the upper anal canal).
   - **Generalized peritonitis:** Causes severe, diffuse abdominal pain. It results from a viscus perforation or when bacterial organisms translocate through a diseased viscus wall as in mesenteric ischemia and, in women, via the fallopian tube.

   Colicky abdominal pain generally arises from a hollow viscus such as the intestines, whereas pain from a solid organ (e.g., pancreas, liver) is generally continuous and unremitting. In the case of paired structures such as the kidneys, ureters, and ovaries, pain is ipsilateral and not felt in the midline.

TABLE 35-1. A SUMMARY OF THE CAUSES OF ACUTE ABDOMINAL PAIN. PRESENTATION. LABORATORY. AND IMAGING DATA

Etiology	Onset	Location	Character	Severity	Radiation	Relieving Factors	Exacerbating Factors	Cardinal Abdominal Findings	Laboratory Data	Diagnostic Imaging
Perforated peptic ulcer	Abrupt	Epigastrium initially, diffuse later	Burning, excruciating	+++	Shoulder	None	PO intake	Rigid, tender, rebound, silent, distended	Leukocytosis, elevated amylase	Erect plain film, upper GI series
Spontaneous esophageal perforation	Abrupt	Epigastrium, retrosternal	Excruciating	+++	Neck	None	PO intake	Epigastric tenderness, subcutaneous emphysema	Leukocytosis	Chest x-ray, contrast esophagogram, or spiral CT with contrast
Mesenteric infarction	Abrupt	Midabdominal initially, diffuse later	Excruciating	+++	None	None	None	Diffuse tenderness, peritoneal signs, distension—late	Leukocytosis, elevated amylase, lactic acidosis	CT, mesenteric angiogram
Ruptured ectopic pregnancy	Abrupt	Lower abdomen	Excruciating	+++	None	None	None	Lower abdominal and pouch of Douglas tenderness	Anemia, β-HCG, CBC	None
Intestinal obstruction	Gradual	Mid- or lower abdomen	Colicky	+ to ++	None	NPO, NG suction	PO intake	Distended abdomen, tinkling bowel sounds, clues to obstruction (e.g., surgical, scars, irreducible hernia)	Electrolyte imbalance	Plain x-ray, contrast radiography
Renal/ureteric colic	Gradual	Renal angle, flank and anteriorly to labium majorum or testicle	Colicky	+ to +++	Genitalia	None	None	Ill-defined tenderness	Urinalysis	CT of the kidneys and ureter, US, IVP, plain x-ray,
Biliary	Gradual	Right upper quadrant	Dull, continuous not colicky	+ to +++	Scapula angle	NPO	Fatty foods	RUQ tenderness, Murphy's sign	LFT	US, ERCP, MRCP

Continued

TABLE 35-1.   A SUMMARY OF THE CAUSES OF ACUTE ABDOMINAL PAIN. PRESENTATION. LABORATORY. AND IMAGING DATA—CONT'D

Etiology	Onset	Location	Character	Severity	Radiation	Relieving Factors	Exacerbating Factors	Cardinal Abdominal Findings	Laboratory Data	Diagnostic Imaging
Abdominal aneurysm rupture	Abrupt or gradual	Midline or lower quadrants	Throbbing before rupture, steady post-rupture	+ to +++	Testicles, groin, rectum, back	None	None	Mass ± bruit ± signs of intra-abdominal bleed	Anemia	CT, angiogram
Pancreatitis	Gradual	Epigastrium	Boring, severe, unremitting	+ to +++	Back and flanks	NPO	Alcohol, PO intake	Epigastric tenderness, Cullen's sign, Grey Turner's sign	Elevated amylase, lipase, abnormal LFT	CT, US
Appendicitis	Gradual	Periumbilical, RLQ—late	Ache, steady	++	None	Lying still	Movement	RLQ tenderness, guarding	Leukocytosis	CT, US
Diverticulitis	Gradual	LLQ or RLQ in Asians	Ache	++	None	Bowel movement	Food	LLQ or RLQ tenderness	Leukocytosis	CT
Pelvic inflammatory disease	Gradual	LLQ or RLQ, pelvic	Ache	+ to ++	Back, thighs	None	Jarring movement, coitus	Lower abdominal and cervical motion tenderness, vaginal discharge	Leukocytosis	Transvaginal US, endometrial biopsy, laparoscopy
Gastroenteritis	Gradual	Mid-abdomen	Colicky	++	None	Bowel movement	PO	Vague tenderness	CBC, stool, BMP	None
Infective colitis	Gradual	Lower abdomen	Colicky	++	None	Bowel movement	PO	Lower abdominal tenderness	CBC, stool, BMP	None

+ = mild pain, ++ = moderate pain, +++ = severe pain, PO = oral intake, GI = gastrointestinal, CT = computerized tomography, HCG = human chorionic gonadotropin, CBC = complete blood count, NG = nasogastric, NPO = no oral intake, US = ultrasonography, IVP = intravenous pyelogram, RUQ = right upper quadrant, LFT = liver function test, ERCP = endoscopic retrograde cholangiopancreatography, MRCP = magnetic resonance cholangiopancreatography, LLQ = left lower quadrant, RLQ = right lower quadrant, BMP = basal metabolic profile.

5. **Can the patient's past medical history provide clues to the etiology of abdominal pain?**

Intestinal obstruction, renal colic, biliary colic, and pelvic inflammatory disease are often recurrent. A history of previous abdominal surgery should raise suspicion of intestinal obstruction due to adhesions in a patient with colicky abdominal pain. A history of peptic ulcer disease may precede peptic ulcer perforation, whereas a history of alcohol intake, gallstones, or abdominal trauma may provide a clue to acute pancreatitis. Atrial fibrillation may cause mesenteric ischemia due to thromboemboli, and low output states, such as congestive heart failure and shock, may cause mesenteric ischemia from reduced perfusion. Evidence of vascular compromise elsewhere in the body (e.g., peripheral vascular disease) may also provide clues to mesenteric ischemia in a patient with abdominal pain. Systemic diseases such as sickle cell disease, porphyria, and the vasculitides can manifest with acute abdominal pain. Medication history may also provide clues to the etiology of abdominal pain (e.g., nonsteroidal anti-inflammatory drugs and peptic ulcer). When associated with weight loss, abdominal pain may be due to a malignancy or chronic mesenteric ischemia. Finally, diabetes mellitus with ketoacidosis can produce severe epigastric abdominal pain.

6. **What are the signs of peritonitis?**

Patients with peritonitis appear acutely ill. They are generally febrile, tachycardic, and diaphoretic. Abdominal tenderness is generally present, and patients will lie still in bed because movement exacerbates the pain. The tenderness may be localized, as in acute appendicitis without perforation, or diffuse as in intestinal gangrene resulting from mesenteric ischemia. Guarding (muscle spasm of the abdominal wall overlying the area of peritonitis), rebound tenderness (increase in pain when the palpating hand is abruptly removed from contact with the abdomen), abdominal distention, and absent bowel sounds are also prominent features of this condition.

7. **In what conditions may the signs of peritonitis be masked?**

The signs of peritonitis may be masked in the elderly, in patients with marked truncal obesity, in those taking immunosuppressives, especially glucocorticoids, and in patients in intensive care. It may be unrecognized in patients with thoracic and higher spinal cord injury. It may remain undetected in the presence of ascites, when sterile urine or blood leaks into the peritoneal cavity, when peritonitis is restricted to the pelvic peritoneum and in perforation associated with typhoid fever.

8. **What is the role of rectal and pelvic examinations in the evaluation of abdominal pain?**

Rectal and pelvic examinations should be done in all patients with abdominal pain. Rectal examination may reveal fecal impaction or a rectal mass that may explain intestinal obstruction, particularly in older patients; tenderness on the right side may be an important clue for retrocecal appendicitis; fecal occult blood may be due to peptic ulcer disease, intestinal malignancy, or bowel ischemia. Pelvic examination may reveal cervical motion tenderness or a vaginal discharge suggestive of pelvic inflammatory disease; vaginal bleeding may be seen in ectopic pregnancy.

9. **Which conditions can be associated with abdominal pain and shock?**
   - Acute pancreatitis
   - Mesenteric thrombosis or ischemia
   - Ruptured or dissecting abdominal aortic aneurysm
   - Ruptured ectopic pregnancy
   - Myocardial infarction (inferior wall)

10. **What is referred pain?**

Referred pain occurs when visceral afferent neurons and somatic afferent neurons from different body parts converge on second-order neurons in the spinal cord and stimulate the same spinothalamic pathways. There are two kinds of referred pain:

- Pain felt in one area of the abdomen may be pain referred either from affected organs in other areas of the abdomen or other parts of the body.
- Pain due to disease in the abdomen may be felt in an area remote from the abdomen.

Referred pain to the abdomen is often felt along a dermatomal segment and perceived as superficial and sharp. When pain due to abdominal disease is referred to another part of the body, it tends to be localized. Pain at the visceral site may be mild or forgotten, whereas the pain at the referred site can be severe. There may be associated hyperalgesia of the skin at the site of referred pain.

11. **List causes of pain due to intra-abdominal disease that is felt elsewhere in the body.**

Pain felt anteriorly

- Diaphragmatic inflammation can cause pain to be referred to the shoulder region.
- Ureteric pain can be referred to the testicle.

Pain felt posteriorly

- Splenic rupture or perforated peptic ulcer can cause pain to be felt at the left upper medial aspect of the trapezius and the shoulder region.
- Biliary colic can lead to pain in the angle of the left scapula.
- Renal pain can be felt at the renal angle.
- Pancreatic pain can be referred to the posterior lower thoracic region.
- Uterine pain can be referred to the low back in the midline.

12. **List causes of referred abdominal pain by disease outside the abdomen.**

Thoracic

- Myocardial infarction, particularly inferior wall infarction
- Pericarditis
- Pulmonary infarction, especially with pleural involvement
- Pneumonia affecting the lower lobe (can also cause shoulder pain)
- Esophageal disease (such as spasm, rupture)

When referred pain is due to pulmonary disease, there may be diminished chest excursion (splinting) on the side of the pulmonary involvement. The referred abdominal pain may be relieved by pressure over the site of pain.

Neurologic

- Herpes zoster: pain may precede, by several days, the appearance of vesicles
- Nerve impingement syndromes due to arthritis or tumors
- Diabetic neuropathy
- Tabes dorsalis
- Abdominal pain due to temporal lobe epilepsy

Neurogenic pain is typically lancing or burning in character. Hyperalgesia may be present.

13. **What are some of the metabolic and other rare causes of abdominal pain?**

- **Lead or arsenic poisoning:** Abdominal pain is often colicky in nature. The mechanism producing abdominal pain is unknown.
- **Uremia:** Abdominal pain is thought to be a result of uremia-induced gastritis, peptic ulcer disease, or mucosal ulcers anywhere in the gastrointestinal tract.
- **Diabetic ketoacidosis**
- **Acute intermittent porphyria**

- **Narcotic withdrawal:** Abdominal pain usually occurs 12–36 hours after abrupt narcotic cessation.
- **Abdominal vasculitides:** Including polyarteritis nodosa.
- **Hyperparathyroidism:** Can cause vague abdominal pain.
- **Hereditary angioneurotic edema:** Pain due to intestinal obstruction caused by mucosal and submucosal edema.
- **Sickle cell anemia:** Pain is secondary to veno-occlusion.
- **Familial Mediterranean fever:** Pain may range from a dull ache to severe pain with signs of peritonitis.
- **Black widow spider bites:** These can cause excruciating pain and are associated with marked rigidity of the abdominal wall.
- **Testicular torsion:** Also produce referred abdominal pain.

KEY POINTS: APPROACH TO ABDOMINAL PAIN

1. The finding of an "acute abdomen" does not necessarily imply the need for surgical intervention.

2. In the majority of patients, a careful history and physical examination will provide a clue to the etiology of the abdominal pain.

3. The signs of peritonitis may not be overt in some clinical settings.

4. Pain referred to the abdomen tends to be felt along dermatomal segments, is sharp, and is associated with hyperalgesia.

5. Elevated serum amylase and lipase levels are not pathognomonic of acute pancreatitis.

6. CT imaging of the abdomen with contrast is the imaging modality of choice for all causes of acute abdomen other than gallbladder and pelvic organ disease.

14. **What are the common laboratory tests that are helpful in differentiating among the various causes of abdominal pain?**
There is no laboratory test specific for any of the causes of abdominal pain. Tests may be ordered depending on the clinical presentation. An elevated white blood cell count, often with a shift to the left, indicates an inflammatory process such as peritonitis or bowel ischemia. In the latter condition, lactic acidosis may be present. A documented decrease in hemoglobin can result from the rupture of an abdominal aneurysm or a ruptured ectopic pregnancy. Elevated blood glucose levels in the presence of ketoacidosis may suggest diabetes as the cause of abdominal pain. Abnormalities in the levels of electrolytes, urea, and creatinine generally occur secondary to intravascular volume depletion, vomiting, diarrhea, or acidosis. Elevated serum transaminases, alkaline phosphatase, and bilirubin can be the result of biliary stones or acute cholangitis. Elevated serum amylase and lipase levels, though suggestive of acute pancreatitis, can be seen in several other conditions including perforated bowel, severe gastroenteritis, and acute cholecystitis. Urine microscopy may reveal hematuria in patients with renal colic. A pregnancy test should be done to exclude ectopic pregnancy in all women of childbearing age who present with lower abdominal pain. Stool examination for leukocytes may indicate inflammatory bowel disease. Positive blood and urine cultures are merely indicative of the presence of infection resulting from any of the several causes of abdominal pain. They are not specific for any one cause.

15. **What is the role of diagnostic imaging in determining the cause of abdominal pain?**
    - **Plain radiographs:** Radiographs of the abdomen (including upright or lateral decubitus) may demonstrate renal stones, gallstones, pancreatic calcification, dilated intestinal loops with air-fluid levels (intestinal obstruction), or free intra-peritoneal air (perforation). However, plain radiographs of the abdomen reveal a diagnostic abnormality only 10% of the time.
    - **Ultrasonography:** Ultrasound of the abdomen is useful in the evaluation of diseases of the gallbladder (e.g., gallstones, cholecystitis) and gynecologic conditions (e.g., ectopic pregnancy, tubo-ovarian abscess). It has limited utility in the evaluation of other diseases that present with acute abdominal pain.
    - **Computed tomography (CT) scanning:** CT of the abdomen is the imaging modality of choice for diverticulitis, appendicitis, pancreatitis, and mesenteric ischemia as well as pain after abdominal trauma. It is less useful than ultrasound for gallbladder and pelvic organ disease.
    - **Magnetic resonance imaging:** Magnetic resonance imaging is of limited value in the evaluation of acute abdominal pain. However, abdominal magnetic resonance angiography can visualize the abdominal vessels, and magnetic resonance cholangiopancreatography is useful in excluding common bile duct stones and stenosis.

BIBLIOGRAPHY

1. Fisher WE, Andersen DK, Bell RH, et al: Pancreas. In Brunicardi FC, Andersen DK, Billiar TR, Dunn DL, et al (eds): Schwartz's Principles of Surgery, 8th ed. New York, McGraw-Hill, 2005, pp 1221–1296.

2. Glasgow RE, Mulvihill SJ: Abdominal pain, including the acute abdomen. In Feldman M, Scharschmidt BF, Sleisenger MH (eds): Sleisenger Fordtran's Gastrointestinal and Liver Disease, 7th ed. Philadelphia, W.B. Saunders, 2002, pp 71–82.

3. Pasricha PJ: Approach to the patient with abdominal pain. In Yamada T, Alpers DH, Kaplowitz N, et al (eds): Textbook of Gastroenterology, 4th ed. Philadelphia, Lippincott Williams & Wilkins, 2003, pp 781–801.

4. Silen W: Abdominal pain. In Kasper DL, Braunwald E, Fauci AS, et al (eds): Harrison's Principles of Internal Medicine, 16th ed. New York, McGraw-Hill, 2005, pp 82–84.

5. Silen W: In Cope's Early Diagnosis of the Acute Abdomen, 10th ed. New York, Oxford University Press, 1996, pp 3–145, 150–197, 245–253.

CHAPTER 36

DIARRHEA IN THE HOSPITALIZED PATIENT

Jeffrey J. Glasheen, MD

1. **What is the general approach to diarrhea in a hospitalized patient?**

   Diarrhea, defined as loose voluminous stool, is a common complaint in hospitalized patients. Diarrhea can be categorized as acute (<4 weeks' duration) or chronic, community- or hospital-acquired, infectious or noninfectious, or inflammatory or noninflammatory. Most commonly it is acute, community-acquired, and infectious in nature. For example, it is estimated that there are >200 million cases of acute gastroenteritis annually in the United States, resulting in 900,000 hospitalizations and 6000 deaths. Overall, 32% of persons with diarrhea will seek medical attention in person or over the phone.

   Herikstad H, Yang S, Van Gilder TJ, et al: A population-based estimate of the burden of diarrheal illness in the United States: FoodNet, 1996–7. Epidemiol Infect 129:9–17, 2002.

   Mead PS, Slutsker L, Dietz V, et al: Food-related illness and death in the United States. Emerg Infect Dis 5:607–625, 1999.

2. **Why is it important to differentiate between hospital-acquired (HAD) and community-acquired diarrhea (CAD)?**

   Diarrhea that develops on or after the third hospital day is considered HAD. Like all nosocomial infections, this determination has important etiologic and diagnostic implications. Importantly, whereas CAD is most often infectious (Table 36-1) in nature, HAD is most frequently noninfectious. In fact, 85% of cases of HAD are noninfectious (see question 4).

3. **When should stool samples be sent for culture for enteric pathogens?**

   Less than 6% of stool samples sent for enteric pathogens such as *Campylobacter, Escherichia coli* 0157, *Salmonella,* or *Shigella* will return with positive results. This equates to approximately $1000 per positive stool culture and results from poor selection of specimens for testing. Nearly 50% of stool cultures for enteric pathogens are sent on inpatients. However, as noted above, only about 15% of inpatients will have infectious diarrhea, with *Clostridium difficile* being the only significant bacterial pathogen in hospitalized patients. Because it is rare to uncover enteric pathogens in patients with HAD, many hospitals have adopted a "3-day" rule that disallows enteric cultures in patients who develop diarrhea after 3 days in the hospital. Adherence to this policy is projected to save between $20 and $73 million annually (1996 dollars). Important exceptions to the 3-day rule include immunocompromised hosts and those older than 65 years with severe comorbidities, who may still present after day 3 with enteric pathogens.

   Guerrant RL, Van Gilder T, Steiner TS: Practice guidelines for the management of infectious diarrhea. Clin Infect Dis 32:331–351, 2001.

4. **What is the most common cause of HAD?**

   Antibiotics are responsible for the bulk of the cases of HAD, with up to 40% of antibiotic courses being complicated by diarrhea. Most commonly, antibiotics with high intestinal concentration induce an *osmotic* diarrhea by reductions in normal gut flora. This results in reduced bacterial carbohydrate metabolism, an increased osmotic load to the distal colon, and subsequent diarrhea. This is especially common in patients receiving enteral nutrition, which is often high in carbohydrates. Osmotic diarrhea improves when nutrition is withheld, thereby differentiating

TABLE 36-1. CAUSES OF ACUTE COMMUNITY-ACQUIRED DIARRHEA IN HEALTHY HOSTS IN DEVELOPED COUNTRIES

Bacterial Disease

Preformed toxin: *Staphylococcus aureus, Bacillus cereus, Clostridium perfringens*

Cytotoxin: *Clostridium difficile, Escherichia coli* O157:H7

Enterotoxin: Enterotoxigenic *E. coli, Vibrio cholera, Aeromonas* species

Invasive: *Salmonella, Shigella, Campylobacter, Listeria monocytogenes, Yersinia enterocolitica*

Medications (Partial List)*

Antibiotics: see question 4

Cardiovascular agents: digoxin, quinidine, hydralazine, beta blockers, angiotensin-converting enzyme inhibitors, diuretics

Gastrointestinal agents: laxatives, magnesium-containing antacids, misoprostol

Hyperlipidemia drugs: gemfibrozil, HMG-CoA reductase inhibitors

Others: thyroid hormones, colchicine, theophylline, alcohol

Medical conditions*

Celiac disease	Inflammatory bowel disease
Fecal impaction/constipation	Irritable bowel syndrome
Gastrointestinal bleed	Ischemic colitis
Hyperthyroidism	Lactose intolerance

Viral Agents

Rotavirus

Norwalk virus

Adenovirus

Parasitic/Protozoal Agents

Giardia lamblia

Entamoeba histolytica

Cryptosporidium

*Often presents with chronic symptoms.

itself from the other mechanisms of antibiotic-associated diarrhea. Other antibiotics, most commonly erythromycin and the β-lactamase inhibitor clavulanate, induce a *hypermotility* diarrhea by increasing gastrointestinal transit time. Finally, antibiotics can induce a toxin-mediated diarrhea thorough bacterial overgrowth of the colon with *C. difficile.*

5. **What is *C. difficile*? How does it induce diarrhea?**
   C. difficile is a spore-forming anaerobic gram-positive rod that induces disease through production of toxins A or B. Although its pathophysiology is intimately tied to two factors, *antibiotic use* and *hospitalization,* our understanding of how these two factors interact to cause disease has recently changed. Traditionally, it was assumed that *C. difficile* proliferated when asymptomatic carriers were given a course of antibiotics that altered the gut's bacterial homeostasis allowing *C. difficile* overgrowth. However, it has been shown that only about 1–3%

of adult patients harbor the bacterium, and that when those patients are admitted to the hospital, they are no more likely to develop diarrhea than noncolonized persons. As such, it is now recognized that acquisition of *C. difficile* requires three steps that must take place in a linear fashion. This "three-hit" hypothesis (Fig. 36-1) begins with a patient receiving an antibiotic that alters the gut flora and therefore the patient's innate immunity. The second hit involves the introduction of the bacterium to the altered gastrointestinal tract. This second step explains the role of hospitalization in the pathophysiology, i.e., the hospital acts a reservoir for *C. difficile* (its ability to form spores allows it to exist for extended periods of time in the hospital setting). Finally, the third hit requires some combination of high bacterial virulence or low host immune response. Clearly, some strains of *C. difficile* (e.g., toxin-forming strains) are more virulent, but many are kept in check by a robust host immune response. A lack of this third hit likely explains why so many patients remain asymptomatic despite acquiring the organism while in the hospital.

First Hit	**Second Hit**	**Third Hit**	***C. difficile* disease**
Antibiotics	*C. difficile* exposure	Virulence/immune response	Diarrhea/colitis

Figure 36-1. The three-hit hypothesis of *C. difficile* pathophysiology.

6. **Which antibiotics cause *C. difficile*?**
   Although clindamycin was the first antibiotic associated with *C. difficile*, all antibiotics, including those used to treat *C. difficile*, can induce the disease. However, based on the three-hit hypothesis, antibiotics that are more likely to alter the gastrointestinal flora (i.e., those with high gastrointestinal distribution and anaerobic/gram-negative coverage) are more likely to induce disease. Consequently, the use of clindamycin, second- and third-generation cephalosporins, quinolones, and aminopenicillins (e.g., amoxicillin) appear to be most highly associated with the acquisition of *C. difficile*.

7. **How common is *C. difficile*?**
   C. difficile can be isolated from upward of 25% of hospitalized patients, with 2–8% of all inpatients (or recently discharged patients) developing *C. difficile*–induced diarrhea. This makes *C. difficile* the fourth most common nosocomial infection. Because the first step in disease acquisition is antibiotic-induced gut alterations, it can even occur in patients receiving only perioperative prophylactic antibiotics.

8. **What are the clinical presentations of *C. difficile*?**
   - *C. difficile* most often results in an *asymptomatic carrier* state. In fact, nearly 85% of patients who become colonized as an inpatient will remain asymptomatic carriers. Furthermore, evidence suggests that colonization with *C. difficile* may impart a protective effect as colonized patients appear less likely to develop symptoms than noncolonized patients who acquire the organism. This likely reflects the effects of a robust immune system (i.e., a lack of the third hit) in keeping the organism in check and fending off new insults. Although these asymptomatic patients do well clinically, they do act as a significant reservoir for transmission of *C. difficile* throughout the hospital.
   - ***C. difficile*–associated diarrhea** (CDAD) most frequently presents within 1–2 weeks, but can present anytime from days to months after antibiotics are initiated. The diarrhea is usually semi-formed and foul smelling, with about 25% of patients having associated fever and mild abdominal pain. Patients commonly have an elevated serum white blood count. In fact,

unexplained leukocytosis (i.e., elevated white blood count that eludes diagnosis) is frequently later diagnosed as *C. difficile* infection.

- **Pseudomembranous colitis** (PMC) may present with diarrhea but often has a more toxic presentation with fever, leukocytosis, abdominal pain, and bloody diarrhea. This presentation is more common in the elderly, those who are profoundly debilitated, and those in the intensive care unit. Occasionally, PMC can present with constipation instead of diarrhea, requiring a high level of suspicion to make the diagnosis. These patients often have radiographic evidence of ileus and even toxic megacolon. Endoscopy will show the characteristic 1–5 mm yellowish-white plaques (i.e., pseudomembranes).

9. **What is the impact of CDAD?**
   CDAD is commonly believed to be little more than a "nuisance" diarrhea. However, as noted above, some patients will proceed to PMC, with up to 5% of patients developing an acute abdomen. Of those requiring surgical intervention, 30–50% will die. Furthermore, data suggest that patients with CDAD have a 3.6-day increase in hospital length of stay and nearly $4000 more in hospital costs. This results in an estimated $1.1 billion of cost per year.

   Kyne L, Hamel MB, Polavarm R, Kelly CP: Health care costs and mortality associated with nosocomial diarrhea due to *Clostridium difficile*. Clin Infect Dis 34:346–353, 2002.

10. **What tests are available for diagnosing *C. difficile*?**
    - **Fecal leukocytes:** These are present in only about one third to two thirds of patients with CDAD compared with about 40% of diarrheic patients without CDAD. Consequently, the test is neither sensitive nor specific enough to aid in diagnosis of *C. difficile* and should be avoided.
    - **Latex agglutination test:** This test assays for glutamate dehydrogenase, an enzyme seen in many different types of clostridial species as well as other bacteria. Furthermore, its presence does not differentiate between toxin and non–toxin-producing strains of *C. difficile*, further limiting its usefulness.
    - **Cytotoxin assay:** This test directly detects the *C. difficile* toxin and remains the gold standard for identifying toxigenic CDAD. However, the test is falling out of favor due to its time-consuming nature.
    - **Enzyme immunoassay (EIA):** This test is fast becoming the most used test because it combines a reasonable sensitivity (~70%) and specificity (~95%) with rapid turnaround. The test directly detects either toxin A or B (in many cases, laboratories will detect both) such that a positive test result in the appropriate setting is diagnostic for CDAD. The sensitivity can be increased to nearly 85% by sending two samples for testing.
    - **Stool culture:** A reasonable diagnostic approach is to send stool for EIA (specific test) along with a stool culture (sensitive test). The latter merely detects the bacterium without regard to toxin production such that it is sensitive for *C. difficile* but not specific for toxin-producing strains. Empiric treatment should be considered if there is a strong suspicion for *C. difficile* but two negative EIA and stool culture results.

11. **What is the general approach to treating diarrhea?**
    Patients with diarrhea from any cause need to be evaluated and treated for hypovolemia and electrolyte/acid–base abnormalities. Patients will commonly require repletion with normal saline (or preferably oral rehydration), potassium, and occasionally bicarbonate (secondary to bicarbonate loss in the stool). Patients should be encouraged to continue eating a soft, easily digestible diet. However, they often become acutely lactose intolerant and should avoid dairy products because this may worsen the diarrhea. Foods containing fiber, caffeine, and alcohol should also be avoided. Antidiarrheal medications (e.g., loperamide, bismuth subsalicylate) can be used in cases of mild diarrhea but should be avoided in cases of severe colitis (i.e., high fever, bloody stools, significant abdominal pain) for risk of worsening the illness. The vast majority of cases of acute diarrhea improve without antibiotics. Empiric antibiotics (e.g., quinolones,

trimethoprim/sulfamethoxazole) should be considered on presentation in severe cases (i.e., high fever, bloody stools, significant abdominal pain) and should be tailored to culture results for a course of 5–7 days. In general, antibiotics are not effective in reducing morbidity in cases of *E. coli* O157:H7, *Aeromonas* species, or nontyphoidal *Salmonella* species and are not recommended. Although not initially indicated, patients with *Yersinia* or *Campylobacter* infection may benefit from antibiotics in cases of persistent diarrhea. Patients who present with traveler's diarrhea, which is most commonly caused by bacterial pathogens, benefit from a 3-day course of a quinolone (or azithromycin if resistant) in combination with loperamide and/or bismuth.

12. How is *C. difficile*–associated disease treated?

C. difficile disease is most often a complication of antibiotic use, so the offending antibiotic should be discontinued if clinically appropriate. Although approximately 20% of mild cases of CDAD in relatively healthy patients will respond to this intervention alone, most patients will require additional antibiotic intervention. Oral metronidazole (250–500 mg every 6 hours for 10–14 days) is as effective as oral vancomycin (125 mg every 6 hours for 10–14 days) and has the added benefit of being cheaper and less likely to induce vancomycin-resistant organisms. Patients with adynamic ileus should be treated with intravenous metronidazole in addition to an oral agent because the slowing of the intestines results in proximal absorption (and decreased colonic concentrations) of either drug given via the oral route. Some data also support the use of adjunctive vancomycin administered via retention enema (500 mg in 500 mL of saline every 8 hours) in these patients.

13. When should a clinician get a follow-up stool sample to be sure a patient has cleared the *C. difficile* bacterium?

For most patients, symptoms begin to resolve by day 3 and are completely gone within 7–10 days. At the time of symptom resolution, about 30% of patients will continue to asymptomatically excrete the *C. difficile* bacterium. Although these patients remain a risk for transmission, they are not at a higher risk of recurrence and should not be seen as a treatment failure requiring another course of antibiotics. As such, stool samples sent to document resolution of *C. difficile*, so-called tests of cure, should be avoided because further treatment in an asymptomatic patient will only provide the first hit in the pathophysiology of CDAD (see Fig. 36-1), thereby increasing the likelihood of recurrence.

14. How common are recurrences?

Recurrences are very common, occurring in 7–20% of patients, and can be due to a relapse with the same strain or reinfection with a new strain.

- **Relapses:** These are often associated with shorter courses of metronidazole treatment and are due to reactivation of dormant spores after stopping the effective therapy.
- **Reinfection:** This is generally associated with longer courses of metronidazole treatment and results from the reintroduction of a new *C. difficile* strain to an altered gut flora (from the treatment metronidazole). In effect, reinfection results from the same three-hit hypothesis that led to the antecedent infection, with metronidazole acting as the first hit.

15. How should recurrences be treated?

It is important to note that neither relapses nor reinfection result from metronidazole resistance. Consequently, the treatment of choice for most recurrences is another course of metronidazole. Patients with multiple recurrences can be treated with an alternate antibiotic (vancomycin if metronidazole was the first choice, and vice versa), prolonged courses of metronidazole or vancomycin (4–6 weeks), pulse therapy with 7 days of antibiotic alternating with 7 days off antibiotic or combination therapy with vancomycin and rifampin (600 mg for 7–10 days). Additional treatment options aimed at reinstating colonic homeostasis—including the use of oral *Lactobacillus* or *Saccharomyces* species to repopulate the bowel flora, enemas with synthetic fecal material or administration of nontoxigenic *C. difficile*—may be effective but are not currently approved by the U.S. Food and Drug Administration.

KEY POINTS: DIARRHEA

1. Hospital-acquired diarrhea is most commonly due to antibiotic use, whereas community-acquired diarrhea is most commonly infectious in nature.

2. Antibiotics can induce diarrhea through three mechanisms: osmotic, hypermotility, and toxin.

3. Any antibiotic can cause *C. difficile*–associated disease.

4. The pathophysiology of *C. difficile* requires antibiotic use followed by bacterial exposure coupled with either a virulent strain or inadequate immune response.

5. Metronidazole is the preferred first-line agent for most cases of *C. difficile*–associated disease.

6. Recurrences are common and should generally be treated with a second course of metronidazole.

16. **How can *C. difficile* be prevented?**
    The mainstay of prevention is to ensure that at-risk patients do not come into contact with the bacterium. This includes isolating patients with the bacterium, cleaning hospital wards and instruments with sporicidal agents, using gloves and gowns while interacting with isolated patients, and adhering to strict handwashing policies (the use of alcohol based hand rubs does not kill the spores). Prudent use of antibiotics as well as programs aimed at reducing high-risk antibiotic use (e.g., clindamycin, cephalosporins and quinolones) are likely to be beneficial, especially in hospitals with high rates of *C. difficile* colonization.

17. **Does a patient with *Blastocystis hominis* require treatment?**
    Blastocystis species is a parasitic organism that often asymptomatically inhabits the intestine and is frequently found on routine stool samples in patients with diarrhea. It is generally not clear whether this organism is the true pathogen such that other causes of diarrhea should be sought before ascribing the symptoms to this microbe. Antibiotic treatment (metronidazole) is controversial and should be considered only after other causes of diarrhea (including noninfectious) are ruled out.

WEBSITES

1. Centers for Disease Control and Prevention: http://www.cdc.gov/travel/diseases.htm

2. Cleveland Clinic: http://www.clevelandclinicmeded.com/diseasemanagement/gastro/diarrhea/diarrhea.htm

BIBLIOGRAPHY

1. Apisarnthanarak A, Razavi B, Mundy LM: Adjunctive intracolonic vancomycin for severe *Clostridium difficile* colitis: Case series and review of the literature. Clin Infect Dis 35:690–696, 2002.

2. Bartlett JG: Antibiotic-associated diarrhea. N Engl J Med 346:334–339, 2002.

3. Climo MW, Israel DS, Wong ES, et al: Hospital-wide restriction of clindamycin: Effect on the incidence of *Clostridium difficile*–associated diarrhea and cost. Ann Intern Med 128:989–995, 1998.

4. Gerding DN, Johnson S, Peterson LR, et al: Society for Healthcare Epidemiology of America position paper on *Clostridium difficile*–associated diarrhea and colitis. Infect Control Hosp Epidemiol 16:459–477, 1995.

5. Glasheen JJ: *Clostridium difficile*–associated diseases. Prim Care Case Rev 6:2–11, 2003.

6. Guerrant RL, Van Gilder T, Steiner TS: Practice guidelines for the management of infectious diarrhea. Clin Infect Dis 32:331–351, 2001.

7. Herikstad H, Yang S, Van Gilder TJ, et al: A population-based estimate of the burden of diarrhoeal illness in the United States: FoodNet, 1996–7. Epidemiol Infect 129:9–17, 2002.

8. Johnson S, Gerding DN: *Clostridium difficile*–associated diarrhea. Clin Infect Dis 26:1027–1036, 1998.

9. Kyne L, Hamel MB, Polavarm R, Kelly CP: Health care costs and mortality associated with nosocomial diarrhea due to *Clostridium difficile*. Clin Infect Dis 34:346–353, 2002.

10. Kyne L, Warny M, Qamar A, et al: Asymptomatic carriage of *Clostridium difficile* and serum levels of IgG antibody against toxin A. N Engl J Med 342:390–397, 2000.

11. Mead PS, Slutsker L, Dietz V, et al: Food-related illness and death in the United States. Emerg Infect Dis 5:607–625, 1999.

12. Olson MM, Shanholtzer CJ, Lee JT, Gerding DN: Ten years of prospective *Clostridium difficile*–associated surveillance treatment at the Minneapolis VA Medical Center, 1982–1991. Infect Control Hosp Epidemiol 15:371–381, 1995.

13. Shim JK, Johnson S, Samore MH, et al: Primary symptomless colonisation by *Clostridium difficile* and decreased risk of subsequent diarrhoea. Lancet 351:633–636, 1998.

14. Starr J: *Clostridium difficile*–associated diarrhoea: Diagnosis and treatment. BMJ 331:498–501, 2005.

15. Wanahita A, Goldsmith EA, Marino BJ, Musher DM: *Clostridium difficile* infection in patients with unexplained leukocytosis. Am J Med 115:543–546, 2003.

CHAPTER 37

GASTROINTESTINAL BLEEDING

Chad T. Whelan, MD

1. **How common and problematic is gastrointestinal (GI) tract bleeding?**

   GI tract bleeding is among the most common reasons for admission to the hospital. The annual incidence of GI tract bleeding ranges from 20/100,000 adults for lower GI bleed to 100/100,000 for upper GI tract bleeds. The risk for bleeding as well as the associated morbidity and mortality increase significantly with age. Most patients admitted with GI tract bleeding require transfusions, and up to 5% may require surgical intervention to control the bleeding. Mortality rates range from 3% for lower GI tract bleed to approximately 10% for upper GI tract bleeds. When clinically significant bleeding occurs during a hospital stay, mortality rates climb to as high as 25%.

2. **What are the different types of GI tract bleeding?**

   The most common and clinically useful way of organizing GI tract bleeding is into upper and lower tract bleeding. This determination provides clues as to the etiology, prognosis, and management.

   - **Upper GI tract bleeding:** This includes bleeding proximal to the duodenum.
   - **Lower GI tract bleeding:** This occurs distal to this point.
   - **Obscure bleeding:** This refers to overt GI tract bleeding where initial evaluation (including diagnostic endoscopy) is unable to determine the source.
   - **Occult bleeding:** This type of bleeding is not overt but rather is discovered in the work-up for iron-deficiency anemia or during screening. Management of occult bleeding is fundamentally different than for acute GI tract bleeding.

3. **List the initial steps in the management of GI tract bleeding.**

   Just as in the management of any acutely ill patient, initial stabilization is critical:

   - **Airway:** Maintenance of the airway is primarily an issue with massive upper GI tract bleeding. In a patient who has an altered mental status or if the amount of bleeding is so massive that the airway is no longer protected intubation is indicated.
   - **Breathing:** Unless a patient is in shock or has aspirated, breathing in GI tract bleeding is usually not a major issue.
   - **Circulation:** Hemodynamic collapse can occur rapidly. Prevention and management requires rapid and aggressive volume resuscitation.
   - **Diagnosing upper versus lower GI tract bleeding:** The history and physical examination can provide essential clues in making this determination, which can be crucial in making future management decisions. A positive nasogastric tube aspirate will localize the bleed to the upper tract.
   - **Endoscopy:** Once you have determined the most likely source, endoscopy should be performed. Endoscopy can usually provide a diagnosis, additional prognostic information, and often therapeutic intervention.

4. **What are the key vital signs to monitor, and how can they aid in determining the degree of GI tract bleeding?**

   Although all vital signs are by definition important, the blood pressure and heart rate are of particular importance. Orthostatic vital sign measurements should be performed on all patients without hypotension on admission.

- **Orthostatic:** Patients who are orthostatic by blood pressure or pulse (>10 mmHg blood pressure drop, >30 beats/min increase in pulse) are likely to be significantly volume depleted and require fluid resuscitation.
- **Resting tachycardia:** This is suggestive of more significant volume loss.
- **Supine hypotension:** This suggests extreme volume loss and impending cardiovascular collapse. Repeated vital sign tests, including orthostatics, should be performed after initial fluid resuscitation.

5. **List important clues from the history and physical examination that suggest an upper versus a lower source.**
   The history is most important in determining the source of bleeding. For upper GI tract bleeding, patients are more likely to complain of frank hematemesis, coffee ground–like emesis, or melena (black tarry stools). Patients with a lower GI tract bleed will not complain of emesis associated with bleeding, but will more likely complain of hematochezia (passing bright red blood or maroon-colored stool from the rectum). Patients with a suspected GI tract bleeding should have a digital rectal examination to check the stool for occult blood as well as to inspect the color of stool. Although these clues are suggestive, only those associated with emesis are diagnostic. Slow proximal lower GI tract bleeding can cause melena, and massive upper GI tract bleeding can cause hematochezia.

6. **Describe the role of nasogastric tube placement and lavage.**
   Nasogastric tube placement can assist with the localization of bleeding. If you find a bloody return upon placement, you can diagnose upper GI tract bleeding. However, approximately 15% of upper GI tract bleeds will have negative nasogastric lavage results. Nasogastric lavage also provides prognostic information. Failure of the return to clear with saline lavage portends a higher-risk bleed. Additionally, lavage assists in the diagnostic yield of endoscopy. There is a theoretical risk of causing additional bleeding from variceal trauma. However, unless you are highly suspicious for a variceal bleed, most gastroenterologists recommend proceeding with nasogastric placement and lavage.

7. **Describe the initial laboratory orders, studies, and management of GI tract bleeding.**
   Patients should have a complete blood count, type and crossmatch for at least 2 units of packed red blood cells (PRBCs), coagulation laboratory tests, and an electrocardiogram (for most patients). The gastroenterologist should be notified early in the presentation to facilitate early endoscopy. Two large-bore (16G–18G) peripheral intravenous lines should be started immediately. Aggressive resuscitation is often required and, unless contraindicated, normal saline should be used as the initial fluid replacement.

8. **How can you tell whether your patient should be admitted, and if so, whether he or she will require care in the intensive care unit (ICU)?**
   Most patients with GI tract bleeding require admission to the hospital. However, some institutions are able to perform endoscopy in the emergency department and identify the lowest-risk GI tract bleeds that can be safely managed on an outpatient basis. The more common dilemma is whether to admit a patient to the ICU. Shock, orthostatic hypotension, or hemodynamic instability after initial resuscitation; requirement for large-volume transfusion (>2 units PRBC) on initial presentation; and vigorous ongoing bleeding are all indications for admission to an ICU.

9. **How do you decide when to transfuse someone with GI hemorrhage?**
   The deleterious effects of blood loss are usually the result of the loss of intravascular volume and not red blood cells. Consequently, the most important consideration is repletion of

intravascular volume. This is most successfully done with normal saline. High-risk patients (those with cardiopulmonary comorbidities or massive ongoing bleeding) require transfusions to maintain the hematocrit >30. Most other patients should generally be transfused to maintain a hematocrit of at least 20. Coagulopathies should be corrected with vitamin K, fresh frozen plasma, or platelets as appropriate.

10. **When is it safe to discharge the patient?**
The primary issues to consider are stability and likelihood of future bleeding. Once you have established that the patient is hemodynamically stable, close monitoring to ensure that bleeding has stopped is essential. Serial hemoglobin or hematocrit testing is used to assist with this. Close recording of stool output, including frequency and color, can also be helpful. Stool may remain Hemoccult positive for some time after the acute bleeding is stopped from residual blood in the colon, so it is not expected that Hemoccult test results will be negative before discharge. Once you have established that the patient is not currently bleeding, endoscopic findings can be very helpful in determining the chance of future bleeding in the immediate future. Endoscopic results should include guidance about the duration of observation required upon cessation of the bleeding.

11. **What are the common causes of upper GI tract bleeding and the risk factors associated with each?**
See Table 37-1.

TABLE 37-1. COMMON CAUSES OF UPPER GI TRACT BLEEDING		
Cause	**Factor**	**Treatment and Follow-up (If Indicated)**
Peptic ulcer disease	Aspirin, NSAIDs, *Helicobacter pylori* infection	Cessation of NSAIDs and use of PPIs until healing has occurred; treatment of *H. pylori* infection
Erosive disease	Aspirin, NSAIDs, EtOH	Cessation of NSAIDs and use of PPIs until healing has occurred; cessation of EtOH
Arteriovenous malformation	ESRD	
Mallory-Weiss tear	Traumatic emesis	
Variceal bleeding	Cirrhosis	Treatment of underlying cause, cessation of hepatotoxic exposures, somatostatin, or octreotide initially with addition of nonselective beta blockers after stabilization to prevent re-bleeding

NSAID = nonsteroidal anti-inflammatory drug, PPI = proton pump inhibitor, EtOH = ethanol, ESRD = end-stage renal disease.

12. **List other less common causes of upper GI tract bleeding.**
Malignancy, fistulas from the major blood vessels, epistaxis, duodenitis, and Dieulafoy's lesions (i.e., dilated aberrant submucosal vessels that erode to the surface in the absence of ulceration) are less common but important causes of upper GI bleeding.

13. **Describe the role of endoscopy in the diagnosis and management of upper GI tract bleeding.**
Endoscopy is the diagnostic study of choice. Additionally, a diagnostic endoscopy also provides information about the likelihood of re-bleeding. Risk stratification can guide discharge decisions. Many cases of upper GI tract bleeding are amenable to endoscopic treatment with epinephrine injection, thermal tamponade, or argon plasma coagulation. Finally, if endoscopic findings raise suspicion for malignancy, biopsy specimens may be taken or follow-up endoscopic examination arranged.

14. **What type of preparation does a patient need before an upper endoscopy?**
Upper endoscopy can be done on any patient who is hemodynamically stable. If possible, the patient should receive nothing by mouth (NPO) for at least 4 hours and preferably 8 hours before the endoscopy is performed.

15. **Discuss options that are available when initial management fails to control bleeding.**
Octreotide can be used in variceal or nonvariceal bleeds. Once medical and endoscopic therapy has failed, other invasive procedures can be tried. If the source of the bleeding can be identified, angiography can be very successful in controlling the bleeding by embolization of the affected vessel. Although rarely because of the increasing capabilities of less invasive procedures, surgical intervention can be required as a last resort.

16. **What are the common causes of, associated risk factors for, and treatments of lower GI tract bleeding?**
See Table 37-2.

TABLE 37-2. COMMON CAUSES OF LOWER GI TRACT BLEEDING		
Cause	Risk Factor	Treatment and Follow-up (If Indicated)
Hemorrhoids	Advancing age	If bleeding has stopped, addition of fiber to the diet. Surgical therapy may be required in refractory cases.
Diverticulosis	Advancing age, possibly traditional western diet	Recurrent diverticular bleeding may require partial colectomy
Arteriovenous malformation	Advancing age	If recurrent bleeding, consideration for estrogen-based hormonal treatment or surgical intervention is warranted.
Ischemic colitis	Any hypercoagulable state, advancing age, atrial fibrillation, dialysis, small vessel ischemic disease	Treatment of the underlying cause after stabilization of the bleeding.

TABLE 37-2. COMMON CAUSES OF LOWER GI TRACT BLEEDING—CONT'D

Cause	Risk Factor	Treatment and Follow-up (If Indicated)
Infectious	*Escherichia coli* O157:H7, *Shigella, Salmonella, Campylobacter, Clostridium difficile*	Consider empiric antibiotics, weighing potential risks of antibiotics in infections caused by enterohemorrhagic *E. coli* or *C. difficile* versus the potential benefits of treatment in other infections.
Neoplastic	Advancing age, family history or personal history of cancer or precancerous polyps	Medical and surgical oncology team evaluation and treatment.
Inflammatory	Peak incidence between 15–25 and 50–80 years of age; family history of IBD increases risk by 3–20 times	Depending on type and severity of IBD, multiple medical regimens of salicylic acid derivatives such as sulfasalazine are indicated.

IBD = inflammatory bowel disease.

KEY POINTS: GI TRACT BLEEDING

1. Hematemesis is diagnostic of an upper GI tract source, whereas melena is suggestive but not diagnostic of a lower source. Hematochezia is usually associated with a lower source but can occur in the setting of vigorous upper GI tract bleeding.

2. The initial evaluation of a GI tract bleed should include a complete blood count and coagulation laboratory tests, type and cross for at least two units of PRBCs, two large-bore peripheral intravenous lines, and fluid resuscitation with normal saline.

3. Endoscopy is the diagnostic test of choice for both upper and lower GI tract bleeds. Early endoscopy can provide risk stratification regarding the need for intensive monitoring and readiness for discharge as well as therapeutic options to control the bleeding.

17. Describe the role of endoscopy in the diagnosis and management of lower GI tract bleeding.

For most patients with lower GI bleeding, colonoscopy is the diagnostic test of choice. An experienced endoscopist can visualize the entire colon in the vast majority of cases. Pathologic and microbiologic specimens can be obtained when required. For many types of bleeds, therapeutic maneuvers can be performed to stop current bleeding and reduce the risk of future bleeding. Performing colonoscopy early in the hospitalization for lower GI tract bleeding can safely reduce the length of stay.

18. **What type of preparation does a patient undergoing a colonoscopy need?**
It is possible to perform a colonoscopy on an nonprepared patient, but this is often not useful because of difficulty with visualization of the colon. Consequently, most endoscopists prefer to prepare the patient with 4–6 L of polyethylene glycol.

19. **List therapeutic options available when initial management fails to control the bleeding.**
Like upper GI tract bleeding, most bleeding can be stopped with supportive and endoscopic interventions. However, there are patients in whom initial management fails. Angiography can be used to control the bleeding through intra-arterial embolization of the affected vessels. Surgical intervention also remains an option in lower GI tract bleeding, but localization of the bleeding is essential to minimize unnecessary colonic resection. A tagged red blood cell scan can be useful to noninvasively localize the site of bleeding.

20. **Describe the key features about the management of obscure GI tract bleeding.**
Obscure GI tract bleeding refers to a situation in which you are unable to identify the source of bleeding. Missed sources on upper or lower endoscopy account for some obscure bleeding, so repeated endoscopy should be considered. However, obscure bleeding can also occur in the distal portions of the small intestine that traditional endoscopy is unable to adequately visualize. Many diagnostic options are available to visualize the small intestine. These include capsule endoscopy, enteroclysis, angiography, and tagged red blood cell scanning. However, each of these modalities has significant limitations. Capsule endoscopy has the best diagnostic test characteristics (sensitivity and specificity) and so is often recommended as the diagnostic test of choice. However, there are no therapeutic options with capsule endoscopy. If a source of bleeding has not been found after endoscopy, then a decision about readiness for discharge hinges on patient stability. Once you have decided the patient is no longer bleeding and is stable for discharge, an appropriate plan to complete the diagnostic work-up must be in place.

WEBSITE

American Gastroenterological Association: http://www.gastro.org/

BIBLIOGRAPHY

1. Baradarian R, Ramdhaney S, Chapalamdugu R, et al: Early intensive resuscitation of patients with upper gastrointestinal bleeding decreases mortality. Am J Gastroenterol 99:619–622, 2004.

2. Barkun A, Bardou M, Marshall JK: Consensus recommendations for managing patients with nonvariceal upper gastrointestinal bleeding. Ann Intern Med 139:843–857, 2003.

3. Lau JY, Sung JJ, Lee KK, et al: Effect of intravenous omeprazole on recurrent bleeding after endoscopic treatment of bleeding peptic ulcers. N Engl J Med 343:310–316, 2000.

4. Saurin JC, Delvaux M, Bahedi K: Clinical impact of capsule endoscopy compared to push enteroscopy: 1-year follow-up study. Endoscopy 37:318–323, 2005.

5. Velayos FS, Williamson A, Sousa KH, et al: Early predictors of severe lower gastrointestinal bleeding and adverse outcomes: a prospective study. Clin Gastroenterol Hepatol 2:485, 2004.

CHAPTER 38

INFLAMMATORY BOWEL DISEASE

Ajay Kumar, MD, MRCP

1. **What are the types of inflammatory bowel disease (IBD)?**
   Ulcerative colitis (UC) and Crohn's disease (CD) constitute the two entities of IBD (Table 38-1). They must be distinguished from other inflammatory conditions affecting the intestinal tract, such as infectious colitis, ischemic colitis, or radiation- and drug-induced colitis. The clinical presentation during the early stages of IBD can be similar to other forms of colitis, and the histology may lack the chronic changes typically seen.

TABLE 38-1. COMPARISON OF UC AND CD		
Feature	**Ulcerative Colitis**	**Crohn's Disease**
History		
Tobacco use	Nonsmoker or former smoker	Commonly active smoker
Clinical Features		
Perianal exam	Normal perianal exam results	Perianal skin tags
Abdominal exam	No abdominal mass	Abdominal mass
Fistulas/abscesses	Absent	Present
Surgical outcome	Surgery curative	Recurs after surgery
Small bowel involvement	Only with backwash ileitis	Frequent
Endoscopic Features		
Rectal involvement	Always	Sparing common
Lesions	Continuous superficial inflammation	Skip lesions
Histology	Superficial ulcers with crypt abscesses	Transmural inflammation and noncaseating granulomas
Serology		
	Elevated p-ANCA (~60–80% of patients)	Elevated ASCA (~30% Patients)

p-ANCA = perinuclear antineutrophilic cytoplasmic antibody, ASCA = anti–*Saccharomyces cerevisiae* antibody.

2. **What are the incidence and prevalence of IBD in the United States?**
   The incidence of UC and CD in the United States is 7 per 100,000. The prevalence of UC and CD is 116 and 104 per 100,000, respectively. The incidence is higher among people of Ashkenazi

Jewish and Scandinavian descent and lower among people of Hispanic and African-American descent. The peak age of onset for both diseases is between 15 and 25 years with a second smaller peak between 50 and 80 years of age with equal distribution in both sexes.

3. **What causes IBD?**
   The etiology of IBD is best described as multifactorial. The current hypothesis postulates that the onset of disease occurs in genetically susceptible persons in a specific environment leading to sustained activation of mucosal immune response. Early childhood exposure to a variety of microorganisms may protect against future development of IBD. Patients with CD have been found to have an increased likelihood of developing antibodies to common brewer's yeast (*Saccharomyces cerevisiae*). Many cases of IBD are triggered by acute infections like traveler's diarrhea, suggesting that IBD may be initiated by environmental factors in susceptible persons. Nicotine is associated with an increased risk for CD and seems to have a protective effect in UC.

4. **How does the patient with UC present?**
   The presentation of UC is usually insidious, although occasionally patients present with an acute condition after an episode of infectious colitis. Rectal bleeding is the most consistent presenting feature. Diminished compliance of the rectum leads to tenesmus and rectal urgency, and diarrhea relates to the extent of colonic involvement. Constipation with interim passage of blood and mucus is seen in patients with proctitis. Abdominal pain or tenderness signifies progressive severe disease (Table 38-2), whereas abdominal cramps preceding bowel movements are common. In fulminant disease fever, night sweats, weight loss, and other constitutional symptoms can be present. Extraintestinal manifestations (Table 38-3) can include inflammation of the eyes, skin, liver, and joints.

TABLE 38-2. SEVERITY OF UC			
Criteria	**Mild Disease**	**Severe Disease**	**Fulminant Disease**
Stool frequency/day	<4	5–10	>10
Blood in stool	Infrequent	Frequent	Frequent
Temperature	Normal	>37.5°C	>37.5°C
Pulse	Normal	>90 beats/min	>90 beats/min
Hemoglobin	Normal	<75% normal	Requires transfusion
Sedimentation rate	<30 mm/h	>30 mm/h	>30 mm/h
Radiography	Normal gas pattern	Edematous colon wall, thumb printing	Dilated colon, edema, intramural air, free abdominal air

5. **Describe the clinical features of CD.**
   CD can involve the gastrointestinal tract from the mouth to the anus with focal asymmetric and transmural inflammation, strictures, and fistulas. CD is more heterogeneous in presentation, and the location and pattern of inflammation tends to remain constant for each individual. Diagnosis is often preceded by an extended period of nonspecific symptoms, such as decreased appetite, weight loss, or fever, but it can be acute with severe abdominal pain, intestinal obstruction, or hemorrhage. Abdominal cramps and postprandial pain are the most common symptoms in CD and are often associated with rectal bleeding, diarrhea, and constitutional symptoms. (For extraintestinal manifestations, see Table 38-3.)

TABLE 38-3. EXTRAINTESTINAL MANIFESTATIONS OF IBD	
System	Features
Ophthalmic	Episcleritis and scleritis
	Uveitis
Skin	Erythema nodosum
	Pyoderma gangrenosum
Musculoskeletal	Arthritis
	Metabolic bone disease due to steroid use and malabsorption
Hepatobiliary	Gallstones in patients with CD
	Sclerosing cholangitis with or without secondary biliary cirrhosis
	Hepatic steatosis
Genitourinary	Renal stones in patients with CD
Hematologic	Anemia
	Hypercoagulability

6. **Which serologic markers are associated with IBD?**

   The presence of anti–*Saccharomyces cerevisiae* antibody is highly specific for CD but has a poor sensitivity of 30%. Perinuclear antineutrophilic cytoplasmic antibodies are more frequently found in UC but have a high number of false-negative results.

7. **What is the initial therapy for patients diagnosed with UC?**

   Mild to moderate disease may be encountered in the inpatient setting and initially managed by mesalamine (5-aminosalicylic acid) for the induction and remission. The parent compound sulfasalazine is a cheaper alternative but induces side effects such as headache, nausea, vomiting, and abdominal pain more frequently because of the sulfapyridine moiety. Folic acid supplementation is recommended while sulfasalazine is being used because of the impaired folate absorption involved. Topical therapy, such as mesalamine suppositories and enemas or corticosteroid enemas, can effectively achieve remission in ulcerative proctitis. Oral prednisone at the starting dose of 40–60 mg daily is used in patients able to tolerate oral medication. Patients with fulminant UC are at increased risk for complications and are managed with intravenous steroids (e.g., methylprednisolone 20 mg q8h), strict bowel rest, and parenteral nutritional support.

8. **Does nicotine have any role in therapy for UC?**

   Nicotine has a protective effect and may be used as adjunctive therapy in a small subgroup of patients who develop UC after cessation of smoking. Nicotine patches, however, do not have any proven benefit over aminosalicylates at inducing or maintaining remissions.

9. **What are the indications for surgical treatment of UC?**

   A surgical consult should be considered for patients with fulminant disease refractory to medical therapy. Patients with toxic megacolon, severe bleeding, impending perforation, strictures, and high-grade dysplasia also require surgical evaluation.

KEY POINTS: ULCERATIVE COLITIS

1. Patients with UC nearly always have rectal involvement.

2. Small bowel involvement occurs only with backwash ileitis.

3. Surgery is curative except for the course of sclerosing cholangitis, which remains unchanged after surgery.

---

10. **What therapies are available for CD?**
    The management of mild inflammatory symptoms usually responds well to mesalamine, and the choice of dosage form depends on the target region. Mesalamine is available in different preparations that each target different portions of the gastrointestinal tract. The sustained-release granular formulation targets the upper gastrointestinal tract, ileum, and colon. The delayed-release, pH-sensitive preparation targets the ileum and colon, whereas sulfasalazine is active only in the colon. Ciprofloxacin and metronidazole are second-line agents. If patients are unresponsive to antibiotic therapy, they usually require steroids. Immunomodulators such as azathioprine and 6-mercaptopurine (6-MP) can also be used for patients with refractory disease and as an alternative to steroids.

11. **What is the role of the biologic agents?**
    Infliximab (chimeric monoclonal antibody targeting tumor necrosis factor α) is the first such agent approved by the U.S. Food and Drug Administration for treatment of fistulous CD as well as refractory inflammatory-type CD that is unresponsive to conventional therapy. Infliximab is administered as 5 mg/kg given intravenously at 0, 2, and 6 weeks and then subsequently given every 8 weeks. Tuberculosis and histoplasmosis reactivation, sepsis, and congestive heart failure are important concerns while using infliximab.

12. **What are the indications for surgical treatment of CD?**
    The most common indications are small bowel obstruction, perforation, massive hemorrhage, and high-grade dysplasia. CD usually recurs after surgery at a rate of 70% per year, and postoperative prophylaxis with mesalamine or metronidazole may reduce recurrence.

13. **What are the discharge issues for patients with UC and CD?**
    Patients with UC and CD should be discharged on a maintenance regimen with mesalamine to maintain remission. Prednisone should be tapered because it is ineffective in maintaining remission. Patients who respond to azathioprine and 6-MP should be maintained on these regimens. Both UC and CD predispose patients to colorectal cancer. The cancer risk is higher for UC, 0.5%–1% per year after 10 years. Patients should undergo an annual examination with colonoscopy for disease involving the colon for >8 years.

KEY POINTS: CROHN'S DISEASE

1. Nicotine use is associated with CD.

2. The histologic hallmark of CD is noncaseating granulomas; these are identified in only 30% of patients.

3. Patients may present with rectal sparing and perianal involvement.

4. Surgery is not curative.

14. **Highlight the importance of nutritional management in patients with IBD.**
    No specific dietary restriction is required for patients in remission. A low residual diet can provide symptomatic relief in patients with strictures and mild to moderate disease. Patients with an acute flare of CD may benefit from an elemental diet, although this can be unpalatable and poorly tolerated. Total parenteral nutrition and bowel rest may be required in patients with severe disease or while they are awaiting surgery.

15. **How should IBD be treated in pregnancy?**
    Women with active IBD are at increased risk of early miscarriage. The course and outcome of pregnancy does not differ from that of the general population if the disease is well controlled. Mesalamine, steroids, and immunomodulators are generally safe, and neither the maintenance nor acute treatment should be withdrawn in pregnant patients. The mother should be maintained in the best possible nutritional status during pregnancy and lactation.

WEBSITES

1. Crohn's & Colitis Foundation of America: http://www.ccfa.org

2. American College of Gastroenterology: http://www.acg.gi.org

BIBLIOGRAPHY

1. Steinlauf AF: Medical management of pregnant patient with inflammatory bowel disease. Gastroenterol Clin North Am 33:361–385, 2004.
2. Wood AJJ: Drug therapy; Inflammatory bowel disease. N Engl J Med 33:841–848, 1996.

CHAPTER 39

ACUTE LIVER DISEASE

Brian Harte, MD

1. **What is acute liver failure?**

   Acute liver failure describes liver injury with encephalopathy and coagulopathy in a patient who does not have a preceding history of liver disease. Although no formal definitions exist, acute liver failure is generally referred to as "fulminant" if it occurs within 8 weeks of initial liver injury, or "subfulminant" if it occurs within 6 months.

2. **What are the most common causes of fulminant liver failure?**

   Although the most common causes of fulminant liver failure differs worldwide, in the developed world the most frequent causes are viral hepatitis—specifically hepatitis B virus (HBV)—and drug toxicity. A recent prospective cohort study of 308 patients admitted to American hospitals with acute liver failure identified acetaminophen toxicity as the cause of liver failure in 39% of patients, followed by other drug reactions (13%) and viral hepatitis (12%). Other studies have generated different percentages, but viral hepatitis and drugs generally top the list. However, there are many other causes of acute liver failure (Table 39-1).

   Ostapowicz G, Fontana RJ, Schiodt FV, et al: Results of a prospective study of acute liver failure at 17 tertiary care centers in the United States. Ann Intern Med 137:947–954, 2002.

3. **What is the pathophysiology of acute liver failure due to HBV?**

   Less than 1% of all cases of hepatitis B present with acute liver failure, but the virus accounts for 50–70% of all cases of viral-induced fulminant hepatic failure. Acute liver failure is probably due to a massive immune response against HBV-infected liver cells. Acute coinfection with hepatitis D virus (the "delta agent"), which is dependent on the machinery of HBV for replication, is more likely to progress to acute liver failure.

4. **What other viruses are known to cause fulminant hepatic failure?**

   Hepatitis A can also cause acute liver failure, albeit rarely (0.1% of such infections). These patients generally have a good prognosis without transplant. Hepatitis E is a significant cause of liver disease in the developing world. Herpesviruses, including cytomegalovirus, the Epstein-Barr virus, and herpes simplex virus, have also been described as causing acute liver failure, particularly in immunosuppressed hosts.

5. **Which causes of acute liver failure are especially important to consider in pregnant women?**

   Hepatitis E, which is endemic in developing countries, causes acute liver failure more frequently during pregnancy and carries a mortality rate as high as 25%. Two entities unique to pregnancy are fatty liver of pregnancy, characterized by microvesicular fatty infiltration of liver cells, and the HELLP syndrome, which is marked by hemolysis, elevated liver enzyme levels, and low platelet count. Most cases occur late in pregnancy, and the treatment of both is usually delivery of the fetus after stabilizing the pregnant patient.

6. **How does acetaminophen cause liver toxicity?**

   Much of an ingested dose of acetaminophen is metabolized by the hepatic cytochrome P–450 system into a compound (*N*-acetyl-*p*-benzoquinoneimine [NAPQI]) that is toxic to hepatocytes. Ordinarily, NAPQI is quickly conjugated by glutathione into nontoxic metabolites. However, if the

TABLE 39-1. CAUSES OF ACUTE LIVER FAILURE

Infectious/Inflammatory	Hepatitis A, B, C, D, E, G
	Herpes simplex
	Cytomegalovirus
	Paramyxovirus
	Epstein-Barr virus
	Adenovirus
	Hemorrhagic fevers
	Autoimmune hepatitis
Ischemic injury	Hypotension
	Veno-occlusive disease
	Hepatic vein thrombosis
Drugs and toxins (partial list)	Alcohol
	Antibiotics
	Acetaminophen
	Halothane
	Amanita phalloides poisoning
	NSAIDs
	Isoniazid
	Monoamine oxidase inhibitors
	Valproic acid
	Phenytoin
	Troglitazone
	3,4-methylenedioxymethamphetamine (Ecstasy)
	Herbal preparations (e.g., comfrey, ginseng, chaparral, kava, black cohosh)
	Carbon tetrachloride
	Yellow phosphorus
Metabolic	Wilson's disease
	Reye's syndrome
Pregnancy-associated	Acute fatty liver of pregnancy
	HELLP syndrome

NSAIDs = nonsteroidal anti-inflammatory drugs, HELLP = hemolysis, elevated liver enzymes, and low platelet count.

liver's glutathione stores are depleted, the toxin accumulates and causes hepatocellular injury and necrosis. Administration of *N*-acetylcysteine (NAC) can restore the liver's glutathione reserves and prevent liver injury if given in time. Liver injury can occur at acetaminophen levels not usually considered toxic if the hepatic glutathione stores are already depleted (as in malnourished patients or alcohol users) and in patients who are taking medications that accelerate P–450 metabolism (e.g., phenytoin). When in doubt, treat the patient for presumed acetaminophen poisoning with NAC and call the local poison control center for further guidance. (See Chapter 71 for more details.)

7. **Aside from acetaminophen, which other common chemicals can cause fulminant liver failure?**
Drugs and other chemicals can cause liver injury either because they are known toxins or by idiosyncratic reactions. Some drugs, including oral contraceptives and chemotherapy agents, can cause hepatic veno-occlusive disease. Some common chemicals, including carbon tetrachloride and heavy metals, are direct hepatotoxins. Rarely, isoniazid, valproate, and phenytoin can cause liver failure. Isoniazid toxicity is treated with large doses of vitamin B_6. Clinicians may also encounter a number of hepatotoxic herbal remedies and should be aware of the "death cap mushroom," *Amanita phalloides*, which is an occasional cause of fulminant liver failure, particularly in the western United States. Even small amounts of the mushroom can cause massive liver injury.

8. **What is Wilson's disease?**
Wilson's disease is an autosomal recessive deficiency in copper metabolism and should be considered in cases of apparently cryptogenic liver failure in younger patients. Although Wilson's disease usually presents as chronic liver disease, it can occasionally present as acute liver failure requiring liver transplant. Slit-lamp examination may demonstrate *Kayser-Fleischer rings* (i.e., copper deposition on the inner surface of the cornea), though this is not a sensitive finding in younger patients who present with acute liver disease. Most patients with Wilson's disease will have a low serum ceruloplasmin level and liver biopsy demonstrating an elevated copper concentration.

9. **What is Budd-Chiari syndrome?**
Budd-Chiari syndrome refers to thrombosis of the hepatic veins and can present as acute liver failure. The disease can be associated with hypercoagulable states, malignancy, polycythemia vera, pregnancy, and use of oral contraceptive pills. The diagnosis is generally made with Doppler ultrasound to measure direction of flow through the hepatic veins. Anticoagulation may help relieve symptoms, but definitive treatment usually requires addressing the underlying cause, as well as liver transplant if necessary.

10. **What are the major clinical and laboratory manifestations of acute liver failure?**
The early clinical features of acute liver disease are nonspecific and include malaise, weakness, and nausea. However, jaundice and encephalopathy can occur quickly, progressing to coma and hypotension, mimicking sepsis. Laboratory evaluation generally demonstrates coagulopathy; elevations of aminotransferases, bilirubin, and alkaline phosphatase; hypoglycemia; and a mixed respiratory alkalosis and metabolic acidosis.

11. **What is the differential diagnosis for transaminase levels >1000 IU/L?**
Although elevations of hepatic transaminases do not clearly correlate with the extent of hepatocellular damage, the most striking elevations are caused by severe insults: hepatotoxic drugs or toxins (such as acetaminophen or *Amanita phalloides* poisoning), acute viral hepatitis, or an acute ischemic event or injury. Other illnesses such as infiltrative processes, alcoholic liver disease, chronic hepatitis, and most other drug-induced liver pathology generally do not cause such dramatic aminotransferase elevations.

12. **What are the critical initial management components for treatment of acute liver failure?**
Once the diagnosis of acute liver failure is considered likely, it is crucial to try to identify the cause, since some causes are medically treatable if initiated quickly. On physical examination, assessment of the patient's mental status and hemodynamic parameters should be performed, as should comprehensive chemistries, hepatitis serologies, measurement of acetaminophen levels, and assessment for infection and bleeding. Arrangements for airway protection, central

monitoring, and care in an intensive care unit or referral to a liver transplant center should be made as soon as possible.

13. **How is the coagulopathy of liver failure caused, monitored, and treated?**
The liver synthesizes most coagulation factors, including vitamin K–dependent factors II, VII, IX, and X, so liver dysfunction results in prolongation of the prothrombin and partial thromboplastin time. Additionally, thrombocytopenia may be present, as well as qualitative platelet dysfunction and rapid consumption of both platelets and clotting factors. Even in cases of dramatic coagulopathy, fresh-frozen plasma infusion is not beneficial unless active bleeding is present, and vitamin K will be ineffective if extensive hepatocellular necrosis has occurred.

14. **What are the causes and manifestations of hepatic encephalopathy? How is it categorized?**
Hepatic encephalopathy is one of the hallmarks of acute liver failure. The cause is not known precisely but is thought to be due in part to increased production of ammonia and changes in cerebral neurotransmitter and glucose metabolism. While classically presenting as lethargy, early hepatic encephalopathy can also be marked by agitation and delusions. Hepatic encephalopathy is graded as stage 0–IV; lesser degrees of encephalopathy are associated with better recovery of liver function and prognosis. Table 39-2 lists the various stages of hepatic encephalopathy. (See Chapter 40 for more details.)

TABLE 39-2. STAGES OF HEPATIC ENCEPHALOPATHY
Stage 0: Normal mental status but subtle changes in cognition
Stage I: Mild confusion and dysarthria, decreased ability to perform mental tasks; disordered sleep; asterixis may be present
Stage II: Lethargy, moderate confusion and personality changes; asterixis
Stage III: Incoherent, somnolent but arousable, disoriented and very confused; speech incomprehensible
Stage IV: Coma

15. **What causes cerebral edema? How can it be recognized and managed?**
Cerebral edema usually accompanies advanced encephalopathy of acute liver failure, and subsequent herniation is often the cause of death in such patients. Edema results from cellular permeability and disruption of the blood-brain barrier and may be manifested by the *Cushing's reflex* (i.e., hypertension and bradycardia), posturing, and *Cheyne-Stokes respirations,* an abnormal breathing pattern marked by alternating periods of deep and shallow breathing. However, these findings occur late in the course of edema, so direct monitoring via subdural or epidural catheters is preferred at some liver transplant centers. The goal of monitoring is to maintain cerebral perfusion pressure (the difference between the arterial and intracranial pressures) greater than about 40–50 mmHg. Mannitol is the primary treatment; modest head elevation (i.e., <20 degrees) may also be helpful.

16. **What is the differential diagnosis of renal failure in the setting of acute liver failure? What is the prognosis once renal failure has occurred?**
Approximately 50% of cases of acute liver failure are complicated by acute renal failure. Both prerenal physiology and acute tubular necrosis must be considered, but some drugs that cause hepatic injury can also cause renal damage (e.g., acetaminophen), and concomitant

administration of antibiotics and other medications can also cause renal injury. Hepatorenal syndrome is a poorly understood phenomenon of acute renal failure in the setting of liver disease, wherein the physiologic findings are similar to the prerenal state (i.e., the urinalysis is bland with low fractional excretion of sodium), but the condition does not respond to volume resuscitation. The prognosis for patients with hepatorenal syndrome is grim; the only certain treatment is liver transplant. Many other therapies have been studied and found to be ineffective, including dopamine. However, a number of uncontrolled studies have suggested that systemic vasoconstrictive agents such as vasopressin analogues or midodrine, combined with plasma expansion with albumin, may reverse the renal failure; these treatments require further study. (See Chapter 40 for more details.)

17. **What are the King's College criteria?**
Studies done at King's College Hospital in London on patients with liver failure who were treated medically led to the development of the King's College criteria. The prediction criteria are different depending on whether the injury was caused by acetaminophen because, in general, patients with acetaminophen toxicity have a better chance of recovery than those with other etiologies of liver failure. These criteria are listed in Table 39-3.

TABLE 39-3. KING'S COLLEGE CRITERIA FOR PREDICTING DEATH IN ACUTE LIVER FAILURE

Etiology	Criteria That Predict Death (Without Transplant)
Acetaminophen-induced liver failure	Arterial pH < 7.3 *or* Prothrombin time > 100 seconds *and* creatinine > 3.4 in a patient with grade III or IV encephalopathy
All other etiologies	Prothrombin time > 100 seconds *or* any three of the following: Prothrombin time > 50 seconds Age < 10 years or > 40 years Jaundice > 7 days prior to encephalopathy Bilirubin > 18 mg/dL Disease specifically due to non-A/non-B hepatitis, halothane, or idiosyncratic drug reaction

KEY POINTS: ACUTE LIVER FAILURE

1. Acute liver failure consists of an acute liver injury with rapid onset of encephalopathy and coagulopathy.

2. Early identification of treatable causes, especially acetaminophen poisoning, and prompt referral to a liver transplant center for further assessment and treatment is crucial.

3. End-organ complications and infections are common and must be managed aggressively.

4. Despite research advances in artificial liver systems, intensive monitoring and liver transplant remain the standard treatment.

18. **What role do artificial liver systems play in the treatment of acute liver disease?**
Several artificial liver systems have been developed to attempt to bridge the time to spontaneous recovery of liver function or transplant. These have included dialysis-type and adsorption systems to remove toxins and use of hepatocytes to replace the native liver's synthetic functions. However, a 2003 Cochrane Review concluded that there is no mortality benefit for any such available artificial liver support system.

   Kjaergard LL, Liu J, Als-Nielsen B, Gluud C: Artificial and bioartificial support systems for acute and acute-on-chronic liver failure: A systematic review. JAMA 289:217–222, 2003.

19. **What presenting features of acute liver disease suggest the diagnosis of alcoholic hepatitis?**
In addition to a history of heavy alcohol use and physical findings typical of chronic liver disease, the presence of moderate transaminase elevation (less than about 500 IU/L), with an aspartate aminotransferase/alanine aminotransferase ratio greater than 2 is characteristic of alcoholic hepatitis. Elevations of alkaline phosphatase and bilirubin levels and prothrombin time are also frequent, as is evidence of hepatic steatosis on imaging. Systemic symptoms such as fever, jaundice, and tender hepatomegaly are common, so infection, biliary disease, and intra-abdominal pathology must be ruled out before confirmation of the diagnosis. Liver biopsy is usually unnecessary but may help differentiate alcoholic hepatitis from viral disease or other causes of liver inflammation.

20. **What are the indications for therapy for alcoholic hepatitis? What treatments are available?**
All patients with signs of serious disease should be hospitalized for supportive care, including nutritional support and abstinence counseling. The "discriminant function" (DF) helps identify patients with a poor prognosis; it is calculated by the following formula, where PT = prothrombin time (in seconds):

$$DF = [4.6 \times (PT - control)] + bilirubin$$

Patients with DF > 32 have a short-term mortality rate of approximately 50%. Other findings associated with high mortality include encephalopathy, gastrointestinal tract bleeding, and neutrophil count < 5500/mm³. Prednisolone is considered the first-line treatment for patients with a DF > 32 or encephalopathy, although a mortality benefit has not been observed in all studies. Pentoxifylline, an inhibitor of tumor necrosis factor synthesis, reduced mortality in one study of patients with severe alcoholic hepatitis and could be used as an alternate agent. (A trial comparing pentoxifylline to corticosteroids is ongoing.)

   McCullough AJ, O'Connor JF: Alcoholic liver disease: Proposed recommendations for the American College of Gastroenterology. Am J Gastroenterol 93:2022–2036, 1998.

WEBSITE

1. Columbia University Gastroenterology Web: http://cpmcnet.columbia.edu/dept/gi/

BIBLIOGRAPHY

1. Hoofnagle JH, Carithers RL Jr, Shapiro C, Ascher N: Fulminant hepatic failure: Summary of a workshop. Hepatology 21:240–252, 1995.

2. Lee VM: Acute liver failure. N Engl J Med 329:1862–1872, 1993.

3. O'Grady JG, Alexander CJ, Hayllar KM, Williams R: Early indicators of prognosis in fulminant hepatic failure. Gastroenterology 97:439–445, 1989.

CHAPTER 40

CHRONIC LIVER DISEASE

Anna Loa Helgason, MD, PhD

1. **What is chronic liver disease?**

   Chronic liver disease represents a spectrum of disease ranging from mild liver injury to cirrhosis. The severity of disease may be measured by liver function tests, which can reflect inflammation, impairment of bile secretion, or diminished function, although normal liver function test results can be seen in patients with advanced disease. Liver biopsy is the best method to determine the extent of injury.

2. **What are the most common causes of chronic liver disease in the United States?**

   The two most common causes of chronic liver disease are alcoholic liver disease and chronic hepatitis C. Nonalcoholic steatohepatitis, autoimmune liver disease and inherited diseases such as hemochromatosis, Wilson's disease, and alpha$_1$ antitrypsin deficiency are other less common causes.

KEY POINTS: COMMON CAUSES OF CHRONIC LIVER DISEASE IN THE UNITED STATES

1. Chronic hepatitis C

2. Chronic alcoholism

3. Nonalcoholic steatohepatitis

4. Autoimmune disease

5. Inherited diseases (hemochromatosis, Wilson's disease, alpha$_1$ antitrypsin deficiency)

3. **What is cirrhosis? How is it classified?**

   Cirrhosis represents an advanced stage of chronic liver disease. On biopsy, the normal hepatic architecture is obscured by fibrosis and regenerative nodules. Destruction of the normal intrahepatic portal venous architecture may lead to portal hypertension. The Child-Pugh classification system (Table 40-1) for cirrhosis assigns points based on a number of parameters. The scoring system (Table 40-2) is based partly on subjective parameters that may be modified with medical therapy. Furthermore, its ability to discriminate patients with advanced liver disease (Child-Pugh class C) is limited.

4. **What does the Model for Endstage Liver Disease (MELD) score measure? How is it used?**

   The MELD score is a score between 6 and 40 that is calculated based on serum bilirubin, international normalized ratio (INR), and creatinine. Based on objective parameters, it is the primary model to predict transplant wait list mortality. The United Network for Organ Sharing allocates cadaveric livers for transplantation based on the MELD score.

TABLE 40-1. CHILD-PUGH CLASSIFICATION SYSTEM

Parameters	1 Point	2 Points	3 Points
Ascites	None	Slight	Moderate/severe
Bilirubin (mg/dL)	<2.0	2.0–3.0	>3.0
Encephalopathy*	None	Grade 1–2	Grade 3–4
Albumin (gm/L)	>3.5	2.8–3.5	<2.8
INR	<1.7	1.8–2.3	>2.3

*See Chapter 39 for grading of encephalopathy.
INR = international normalized ratio.

TABLE 40-2. PROGNOSTIC SIGNIFICANCE OF CHILD-PUGH SCORE

Numerical Score	Child-Pugh Class	Survival at 1 year
5–6	A	100%
7–9	B	80%
10–15	C	45%

$$MELD = 3.8[\log_e \text{ serum bilirubin(mg/dL)}] + 11.2[\log_e \text{ INR}]$$
$$+9.6[\log_e \text{ serum creatinine(mg/dL)}] + 6.4$$

MELD Calculator: http://www.unos.org/resources/MeldPeldCalculator.asp?index=98
Said A, Williams J, Holden J, et al: Model for end stage liver disease score predicts mortality across a broad spectrum of liver disease. J Hepatology 40:897–903, 2004.

5. **What are the common complications of cirrhosis?**
Portal hypertension can arise as a complication of cirrhosis, and this leads to the development of ascites and spontaneous bacterial peritonitis. High portal pressures can promote abnormal portosystemic venous shunts, including varices, which may bleed. Another complication of portosystemic shunting is the development of hepatic encephalopathy. The altered splanchnic hemodynamics seen in cirrhosis can lead to irreversible renal failure, known as *hepatorenal syndrome*. Finally, long-standing cirrhosis is a risk factor for hepatocellular carcinoma.

KEY POINTS: COMMON COMPLICATIONS OF CIRRHOSIS

1. Ascites

2. Spontaneous bacterial peritonitis

3. Variceal bleeding

4. Hepatic encephalopathy

5. Hepatorenal syndrome

6. Hepatocellular carcinoma

6. **How does ascites develop? How is it diagnosed?**
Alteration of the normal hepatic architecture by fibrosis promotes portal venous hypertension (PHTN), which in turn causes congested hepatic sinusoids and incomplete intrahepatic lymphatic drainage. PHTN also leads to high circulating levels of endogenous vasodilators, such as nitric oxide, which cause splanchnic vasodilation. Additionally, diminished hepatic albumin synthesis leads to low oncotic pressure and decreased effective circulating volume. The renin-angiotensin system attempts to compensate for decreased intravascular volume by increasing sodium and water retention. The end result of these processes is a pooling of fluid in the intra-abdominal cavity that manifests as bulging flanks, shifting dullness to percussion and a fluid wave over the abdomen. Ultrasonography is the best way to confirm the presence of ascites.

7. **Name some causes of new or worsening ascites in a patient with PHTN.**
Dietary and medication noncompliance can promote or worsen the formation of ascites. Ascites can also develop or worsen in the setting of portal vein thrombosis and hepatocellular carcinoma. Infection, gastrointestinal bleeding, or anything that diminishes glomerular filtration rate (e.g., volume depletion, overdiuresis) can cause the development or progression of ascites.

KEY POINTS: CAUSES OF NEW OR WORSENING ASCITES ✔ IN PATIENTS WITH PORTAL HYPERTENSION

1. Medication or dietary noncompliance

2. Portal vein thrombosis

3. Hepatocellular carcinoma

4. Gastrointestinal bleeding

5. Infection

6. Diminished glomerular filtration rate

8. **What is the SAAG? How is it useful?**
The serum-ascites-albumin gradient (SAAG) is determined by subtracting the ascitic fluid albumin from the serum albumin. The SAAG helps determine the etiology of ascites (Table 40-3).

9. **How is ascites resulting from portal hypertension treated?**
The mainstay of therapy is fluid and dietary sodium restriction (<2 gm daily). The use of diuretics like spironolactone dosed at 25–100 mg/day given orally can be augmented with furosemide use (starting dose at 20 mg orally twice daily). Patients with diuretic-resistant

TABLE 40-3. UTILIZATION OF THE SERUM-ASCITES-ALBUMIN GRADIENT (SAAG)	
SAAG > 1.1	SAAG < 1.1
Portal hypertension (from cardiac or liver disease)	Peritoneal carcinomatosis, tuberculosis, nephritic syndrome, connective tissue disorders

ascites may require large-volume paracentesis or transjugular intrahepatic portosystemic shunt (TIPS).

10. **What is a TIPS? What are the indications for its use?**
A TIPS is a percutaneous creation of a portocaval shunt through cannulation of the hepatic vein via the jugular vein. After the jugular vein is entered, a tunnel is created through the hepatic parenchyma into the portal vein, and a stent is placed to maintain patency. A TIPS may be more effective at treating ascites than serial large-volume paracentesis in diuretic-resistant patients, but may not confer better survival.

Saab S, Nieto JM, Ly D, et al: TIPS versus paracentesis for cirrhotic patients with refractory ascites. Cochrane Database Syst Rev 3:CD004889, 2004.

11. **What are the potential complications of TIPS placement?**
Hepatic encephalopathy occurs in up to 30% of patients, resulting from portosystemic shunting (i.e., bypassing liver clearance) of ammonia and other neuroactive compounds that arise from the gut. Lactulose is often started empirically to avoid this complication. Other complications include acute thrombosis or subacute stenosis with reaccumulation of ascites. Newer stents coated with polytetrafluoroethylene have much better patency rates. Bleeding is another potential complication. Finally, relative hepatic ischemia from shunting of portal blood systemically can lead to decompensated liver disease in patients with advanced cirrhosis.

Riggio O, Merlli M, Pedretti G, et al: Hepatic encephalopathy after transjugular intrahepatic portosystemic shunt: Incidence and risk factors. Dig Dis Sci 41:578–584, 1996.

KEY POINTS: POTENTIAL COMPLICATIONS OF TIPS PLACEMENT

1. Hepatic encephalopathy

2. Stent thrombosis and reaccumulation of ascites

3. Bleeding

4. Decompensated liver disease

12. **What is spontaneous bacterial peritonitis (SBP), and how is it diagnosed?**
SBP is an infection of the ascitic fluid. Signs and symptoms include fever, abdominal pain, altered mental status, leukocytosis, azotemia, metabolic acidosis, and unexplained gastrointestinal bleeding. A paracentesis establishes the diagnosis. A neutrophil count >250 per mm^3 of ascitic fluid confirms SBP. SBP is most commonly caused by *Escherichia coli*, *Klebsiella* species, and *Streptococcus* species. The route of infection is thought to arise from direct translocation of bacteria through an abnormally edematous and permeable intestinal wall, although hematogenous seeding of the ascitic fluid may also occur. Gram stain and culture of ascitic fluid may aid in the identification of the organism. Culture bottles should be inoculated at the bedside to optimize sensitivity.

13. **How is SBP treated? Who should receive prophylaxis?**
While awaiting culture results, begin empiric treatment with a third-generation cephalosporin or fluoroquinolone antibiotic. Aminoglycosides are contraindicated because of their potential for nephrotoxicity in patients who are already at risk for renal failure. Intravenous antibiotics, followed by oral therapy, should be continued for 10–14 days, depending on the clinical response. Intravenous albumin (1.5 gm/kg of body weight) given at the time of paracentesis

followed by 1.0 gm/kg of intravenous albumin on day 3 of treatment has been associated with a decreased incidence of hepatorenal syndrome, a dreaded complication of SBP. SBP prophylaxis is recommended for patients with a prior episode of SBP, an ascites albumin level of <1.0, and those with an intercurrent infection or active gastrointestinal bleeding. Fluoroquinolones or trimethoprim/sulfamethoxazole are most commonly used.

Sort P, Navasa M, Arroyo V, et al: Effect of intravenous albumin on renal impairment and mortality in patients with cirrhosis and spontaneous bacterial peritonitis. N Engl J Med 341:403–409, 1999.

14. **What are varices? How do they develop?**

Increased portal pressure promotes the development of large venous collaterals (varices) that bypass the liver and drain directly to the caval system. Varices are seen in the esophagus, stomach, and hemorrhoidal plexi where communication between the portal and caval system exist.

15. **How does one manage esophageal variceal hemorrhage?**

Variceal hemorrhage is an emergent situation that is treated with airway management, volume repletion with saline and blood, gastric decompression with a nasogastric tube, and reversal of coagulopathy with vitamin K, fresh frozen plasma, and platelets if needed.

Intravenous octreotide promotes splanchnic vasoconstriction and can temporarily reduce portal pressures, and thus bleeding. Emergent endoscopy to attempt band ligation or sclerotherapy is critical. In patients who fail endoscopic management, balloon tamponade with a Sengstaken-Blakemore tube is effective in temporarily controlling bleeding, but this may be complicated by aspiration or esophageal rupture, as well as a high rate of rebleeding after deflation of the balloon. Balloon tamponade followed by TIPS placement to decompress the high portal venous pressure is indicated in patients for whom endoscopic management is ineffective. Overzealous transfusion of blood or albumin can lead to volume overload and increases in portal venous pressure, which can exacerbate bleeding. A large percentage of patients who present with variceal bleeding have coexistent ascites and are at high risk for SBP. Therefore, antibiotic prophylaxis for SBP is warranted with either a third-generation cephalosporin or fluoroquinolone.

Sanyal AJ, Freedman AM, Luketic VA, et al: Transjugular intrahepatic portosystemic shunts for patients with active variceal hemorrhage unresponsive to sclerotherapy. Gastroenterology 111:138–146, 1996.
Soares-Weiser K, Brezis M, Tur-Kaspa R, et al: Antibiotic prophylaxis of bacterial infections in cirrhotic inpatients: A meta-analysis of randomized controlled trials. Scand J Gastroenterol 38:193–200, 2003.

KEY POINTS: KEYS TO MANAGEMENT OF VARICEAL HEMORRHAGE

1. Airway management

2. Volume resuscitation

3. Reversal of coagulopathy

4. Gastric decompression with nasogastric tube

5. Intravenous octreotide

6. Antibiotic prophylaxis

7. Emergent endoscopy to attempt band ligation or sclerotherapy

8. Temporary balloon tamponade if endoscopy fails

9. TIPS placement if endoscopic management fails

16. **What is the recommended long-term therapy for esophageal varices?**
Decreasing splanchnic blood flow and portal pressures with nonselective beta blockers will reduce the risk of rebleeding. The dose should be adjusted to reduce the resting heart rate by 25%. In patients who cannot tolerate beta blockers, short-term therapy with nitrates may be beneficial. Serial variceal banding may also reduce the risk of rebleeding. TIPS may be used as a salvage therapy for patients in whom medical therapy and serial banding is ineffective, but it has no role in the *primary* prophylaxis of esophageal variceal hemorrhage.

17. **What is hepatic encephalopathy?**
Ammonia, formed from the breakdown of glutamine and other nitrogenous waste in the gut, is normally reabsorbed through the portal system and used for amino acid synthesis within the liver. Impaired hepatic function results in portal-systemic shunting of blood allowing ammonia to circulate and enter the central nervous system, where it adversely affects neurotransmission through a variety of mechanisms. Common signs include tremor, asterixis (an inability to sustain a voluntary position), fetor hepaticus (musty breath odor), and altered mental status. The degree of alteration can range from a mild cognitive disturbance to lethargy, disorientation, and coma. A high serum ammonia level may confirm a clinical suspicion of encephalopathy, but it should not be used to track clinical progress. In patients with advanced liver disease, the blood-brain barrier is relatively permeable to ammonia. Therefore, ammonia levels correlate poorly with the degree of encephalopathy. (See Chapter 39 for more details.)

18. **List the precipitants and mechanisms of hepatic encephalopathy.**
Although hepatic encephalopathy can result from a major physiologic insult, more often than not it results from otherwise mild changes in a tenuous patient. For example:
- Constipation→increased ammonia generation by bacteria
- High dietary protein intake→high nitrogen load
- Infections of any cause→high protein catabolism
- Diuretic use→azotemia, hypokalemia, dehydration, metabolic alkalosis
- Gastrointestinal bleeding→high nitrogen load, hepatic hypoperfusion
- Metabolic alkalosis and hypokalemia→impaired renal secretion of ammonia
- Benzodiazepines, narcotics, and other sedatives→inhibition of neurotransmission
- Surgery→hepatic hypoperfusion from anesthesia
- Medication noncompliance or suboptimal dosing of lactulose

19. **How is hepatic encephalopathy treated?**
Lactulose is a nonabsorbable disaccharide that is the first-line agent for treatment of hepatic encephalopathy. It decreases the fecal pH and converts intestinal ammonia (NH_3) into the less absorbable ammonium (NH_4^+) ion. It is administered by mouth, nasogastric tube, or retention enema and should be titrated to effect, then to promote three to five bowel movements a day. Oral neomycin or metronidazole are second-line therapies that alter colonic flora and reduce ammonia production, but chronic treatment with these agents can cause adverse side effects such as renal toxicity and ototoxicity (neomycin) or neurotoxicity (metronidazole). Dietary protein restriction of 70 gm/day is important to prevent relapse.

20. **What is the hepatorenal syndrome (HRS)?**
HRS is a decline in renal function in patients with cirrhosis and PHTN. It is mediated by the nitric oxide–mediated splanchnic vasodilation seen with PHTN, leading to diminished renal perfusion despite renal vasoconstriction to maintain glomerular filtration. The diagnosis is made only after other causes of renal failure are excluded. Two types of HRS are recognized. Type 1 HRS is defined as a doubling of serum creatinine to greater than 2.5 mg/dL, or a 50% reduction in creatinine clearance to a level <20 mL/min over a period of <2 weeks. The urine sediment is bland and urinary sodium excretion is very low. Type 2 HRS involves a slow, progressive decline in renal function in the setting of diuretic-resistant ascites and an absence of other renal insults.

In both types, the kidneys are histologically normal and will function properly if the underlying physiologic abnormality is resolved.

21. **How is HRS treated?**
Ninety percent of patients with type 1 HRS die within 2 months of onset unless liver transplantation is performed. Treatment of concurrent illness, reversal of hepatic dysfunction if possible, and cessation of alcohol intake in patients with alcoholic cirrhosis are the mainstays of therapy. The combination of oral midodrine, (an alpha$_1$ adrenergic agent), subcutaneous octreotide (an inhibitor of endogenous vasodilators), and intravenous albumin is a safe and effective short-term treatment for HRS. Additional studies have suggested that certain patients who respond well to the above regimen may have more long-term benefit from TIPS placement.

Esrailian E, Pantangco ER, Kyulo N, et al: Octreotide/midodrine therapy significantly improves survival in type I hepatorenal syndrome: Analysis of 53 treated patients and 21 controls [abstract]. Gastroenterology 124:A718, 2003.

Wong F, Pantea L, Sniderman K: Midodrine, octreotide, albumin, and TIPS in selected patients with cirrhosis and type 1 hepatorenal syndrome. Hepatology 40:55–64, 2004.

22. **What are the indications and contraindications for liver transplant?**
- **Indications:** Cirrhosis and a MELD score >15, hepatocellular carcinoma (one lesion <5 cm or two to three lesions <3 cm)
- **Contraindications:** Active substance or alcohol use, active HIV infection, sepsis or fungemia, unresolved extrahepatic malignancy, advanced hepatobiliary malignancy, serious underlying medical illness

WEBSITES

1. American Association for the Study of Liver Diseases: http://www.aasld.org

2. Medline Plus, Cirrhosis: http://www.nlm.nih.gov/medlineplus/cirrhosis.html

3. UpToDate: http://www.uptodate.com

4. eMedicine: http://www.emedicine.com

BIBLIOGRAPHY

1. Friedman LS, Keefe EB: Handbook of Liver Disease, 2nd ed. Edinburgh, Churchill-Livingston, 2004.

CHAPTER 41

ACUTE AND CHRONIC PANCREATITIS

Joseph Michael Gergyes, MD

1. **What is pancreatitis?**
   Pancreatitis is inflammation of the pancreas. It is commonly classified as either being acute or chronic.
   - Patients with *acute pancreatitis* may develop abnormal exocrine and endocrine functions. Except in cases of severe or necrotizing pancreatitis, patients with bouts of acute pancreatitis usually regain their endocrine and exocrine functions.
   - A small percentage of patients with recurrent acute pancreatitis may develop *chronic pancreatitis*, also an inflammatory condition of the pancreas. In contrast to acute pancreatitis, there are permanent structural changes in the pancreas and chronic impairment of endocrine and exocrine functions.

2. **What are the symptoms and signs of acute and chronic pancreatitis?**
   - Patients with *acute pancreatitis* almost always experience upper quadrant abdominal pain that frequently radiates to the back. Many patients have associated nausea and vomiting. Fever, tachycardia, and tachypnea are other common symptoms. In patients with hemorrhagic complications, flank ecchymosis (Grey-Turner's sign), periumbilical hemorrhage (Cullen's sign), and retinal ischemia/hemorrhage (Purtscher's retinopathy) may be present.
   - Similarly, upper quadrant abdominal pain, nausea, and vomiting are the primary clinical manifestations of *chronic pancreatitis*. There is variability in pain patterns among patients with chronic pancreatitis. Some patients experience daily pain with intermittent exacerbations, whereas others have variable periods of pain-free intervals (days to years) with intermittent exacerbations. Unlike patients with acute pancreatitis, patients with chronic pancreatitis also have symptoms due to exocrine pancreatic insufficiency. Steatorrhea results from their inability to absorb fats and manifests as foul-smelling, greasy stools. Many patients experience glucose intolerance. Some will progress to overt diabetes mellitus as their disease progresses.

3. **What are the etiology and incidence of acute and chronic pancreatitis?**
   - Gallstone passage through the ampulla of Vater is responsible for over one-third of cases and is the primary cause of acute pancreatitis in the United States. Consumption of alcohol is the other major cause of acute pancreatitis. Less frequent causes include hypercalcemia, hypertriglyceridemia (serum levels typically >1000 mg/dL), trauma, infection (e.g., mumps), drugs (e.g., didanosine), and pancreatic divisum. Acute pancreatitis after an endoscopic retrograde cholangiopancreatography (ERCP) occurs in 3% of patients undergoing diagnostic studies and 5% in those who receive therapy.
   - In contrast, alcohol consumption accounts for over 70% of cases of chronic pancreatitis. Other causes of chronic pancreatitis include pancreatic ductal obstruction from strictures due to trauma and tumors, systemic diseases (e.g., cystic fibrosis), and hereditary pancreatitis. It is important to note that the majority of cases of chronic pancreatitis that are not due to alcohol consumption are due to idiopathic or unknown causes. In these cases, it is vitally important to rule out surreptitious alcohol use.

   Riela A, Zinsmeister AR, Melton JL, DiMagno EP: Etiology, incidence and survival of acute pancreatitis in Olmsted County, Minnesota. Gastroenterology 100:A296, 1991.

4. **What is the mortality rate of acute pancreatitis? Is there a way to predict which patients will do poorly?**

   There are approximately 200,000 cases of acute pancreatitis a year with a mortality rate of about 10%. However, in the subset of patients who develop severe necrotizing pancreatitis, the mortality rate may rise to 30%. Many scoring systems have been developed to predict which patients will develop severe pancreatitis. Ranson's criteria form one of many such scoring systems (Table 41-1). The APACHE II is a scoring system that can be updated continuously. Data suggest that, 24 hours after hospital admission, the APACHE II scoring system seems to be at least as accurate as Ranson's criteria at predicting disease severity. Therefore, the use of the APACHE II scoring system allows earlier identification of patients with severe pancreatitis. The drawback is that the APACHE II scoring system is more complex than the Ranson's criteria and other scoring systems.

   Sarles H: Revised classification of pancreatitis—Marseilles. Dig Dis Sci 30:573, 1985.

TABLE 41-1. RANSON'S CRITERIA

On Admission	Within 48 hours
Age > 55 years	$PaO_2 < 60$ mmHg
Glucose > 200 mg/dL	Albumin < 3.2 gm/L
WBC > 16,0000/μL	Increase in BUN > 5 mg/dL
LDH > 350 U/L	Decrease in Hct > 10%
AST > 250 U/L	Calcium < 8 mg/dL
	Estimate fluid sequestration > 4 L

Number of Criteria	Mortality Rate
<3	1%
3–4	15%
5–6	40%
7+	100%

WBC = whole blood cell count, BUN = blood urea nitrogen, LDH = lactate dehydrogenase, Hct = hematocrit, AST = aspartate aminotransferase.

5. **Describe the laboratory diagnosis of acute and chronic pancreatitis.**
   - Serum amylase and lipase are often elevated in *acute pancreatitis*. Their sensitivities are >85%, but neither test is highly specific for this disease. Other laboratory findings include leukocytosis, elevated liver enzyme levels, and hypocalcemia.
   - Patients with *chronic pancreatitis* often have normal or only slightly elevated amylase and lipase levels during their attacks. This is because the pancreas in these patients is often fibrotic with decreased concentrations of enzymes. In both acute and chronic pancreatitis, the level of amylase and lipase has no value in assessing the prognosis or clinical progress of the patient.

6. **What is the role of imaging in the diagnosis of acute and chronic pancreatitis?**
   An *abdominal radiograph* can often help exclude other causes of abdominal pain. In some patients with acute pancreatitis, there may be evidence of a localized intestinal ileus. This is known as a "sentinel loop" or a "colon cutoff sign." One third of patients with chronic pancreatitis have calcifications within the pancreatic duct. Up to one third of patients with acute pancreatitis have abnormalities on the *chest radiograph* (e.g., pleural effusions, pulmonary

infiltrates). An *ultrasound scan* can be helpful in detecting gallstones in the gallbladder and the biliary tree, but in up to one third of patients bowel gas obstructs the view of the pancreas. An abdominal *computed tomography (CT) scan* is a useful imaging study for acute pancreatitis. Aside from diagnosis of pancreatitis and its potential complications, the CT scan can also provide an assessment of the disease severity. A CT scan with oral and intravenous contrast should be considered for patients with acute pancreatitis who are deteriorating clinically or have severe pancreatitis as demonstrated by the APACHE II score. *Magnetic resonance imaging* is also a very effective modality to image the pancreas and has the advantage of using gadolinium, which is less toxic to the kidneys than CT contrast.

7. **How is acute pancreatitis treated?**
Treatment of pancreatitis should be aimed at removing any predisposing factors. For patients with gallstone pancreatitis, this may involve an ERCP with stone removal or cholecystectomy. Cessation of alcohol use is essential in patients with alcohol-induced pancreatitis. All patients should take nothing by mouth (to reduce pancreatic secretions) and receive supportive care including intravenous fluids and analgesics for pain control. Patients should be instructed not to take any food by mouth. The majority of patients with mild, acute pancreatitis will have symptom resolution within a few days. Antibiotics are generally not indicated unless the patient develops necrotizing pancreatitis or signs of sepsis. For patients with more severe acute pancreatitis, more intense supervision and care in the intensive care unit setting may be necessary. One cannot emphasize enough the importance of fluid resuscitation in patients with moderate to severe pancreatitis. These patients accumulate vast amounts of fluid in the inflamed pancreas. They frequently require 5–6 L of intravenous fluids daily. Inadequate fluid resuscitation leads to a poor outcome. Therefore, it is essential to monitor continuously for signs of adequate hydration and tissue perfusion.

8. **Comment on pain management in acute and chronic pancreatitis.**
Pain control is an important component of care for patients with acute and chronic pancreatitis. The use of a patient-controlled analgesia pump can be an effective way to administer narcotic analgesics. Meperidine has historically been used because morphine elevates sphincter of Oddi pressures, theoretically worsening the pancreatitis. However, there is no evidence that morphine worsens pancreatitis; meperidine has a narrow therapeutic window and its toxic metabolite, normeperidine, builds up in patients with renal or liver dysfunction. In patients with pain due to chronic pancreatitis, the use of long-acting narcotic analgesic products (e.g., sustained-release fentanyl patches) with as-needed use of short-acting agents (e.g., oxycodone) for breakthrough pain is recommended. (See Chapter 93 for more details.)

KEY POINTS: ACUTE AND CHRONIC PANCREATITIS

1. More than 80% of cases of acute pancreatitis are due to biliary or alcohol-related disease.

2. Chronic pancreatitis usually occurs after multiple acute episodes and is most often attributable to alcohol.

3. Most cases of acute pancreatitis will resolve with conservative therapy.

4. Complications of pancreatitis include pseudocyst and abscess formation, adult respiratory distress syndrome, disseminated intravascular coagulation, renal failure, and phlegmon.

9. **What are the potential complications of pancreatitis?**

Acute or chronic pancreatitis may be complicated by a phlegmon, which is an inflammatory mass caused by leakage of enzymes. It may progress to a pseudocyst or frank necrosis. Up to 10% of patients with chronic pancreatitis will develop pseudocysts, whose walls are formed by adjacent structures (e.g., stomach). Although most pseudocysts are asymptomatic, they can present as a failure of conservative therapy (i.e., continued pain and fever). Most pseudocysts communicate with the pancreatic duct and contain digestive enzymes. Occasionally, digestion of a nearby vessel can result in a pseudoaneurysm. The location of the splenic vein on the posterior surface of the pancreas makes it susceptible to not only pseudoaneurysm formation with pseudocysts but also splenic vein thrombosis due to pancreatic inflammation. Symptomatic pseudocysts require drainage, which can be done surgically or endoscopically. Asymptomatic pseudocysts can be monitored and drained as needed. Other complications of acute pancreatitis include intra-abdominal abscess formation, adult respiratory distress syndrome, disseminated intravascular coagulation, acute renal failure, and ascites. When the latter is hemorrhagic in nature, it carries a mortality of 30%.

Yeo CJ, Bastidas JA, Lynch-Nyan A, et al: The natural history of pancreatic pseudocysts documented by computed tomography. Surg Gyned Obstet 170:411–417, 1990.

BIBLIOGRAPHY

1. Banks PA: Practice guidelines in acute pancreatitis. Am J Gastoenterol 92:377–386, 1997.
2. Dervenis C, Johnson CD, Bassi C, et al: Diagnosis, objective assessment of severity and management of acute pancreatitis. Santorini Consensus Conference. Int J Pancreatol 25:195–210, 1999.
3. Ranson JH, Turner JW, Roses DF, et al: Respiratory complications in acute pancreatitis. Ann Surg 179:557–666, 1974.
4. Schmidt J, Hotz HG, Foitzik T, et al: Intravenous contrast medium aggravates the impairment of pancreatic microcirculation in necrotizing pancreatitis in the rat. Ann Surg 221:257–264, 1995.

BILIARY DISEASE

Edward J. Merrens, MD

1. **What are the components of the biliary system?**

   Bile, the breakdown product of heme metabolism, is produced mainly from red blood cell hemoglobin, but also comes from myoglobin, cytochromes, and enzymes. It is conjugated and excreted by hepatocytes. The hepatic biliary ductal system collects the bile from the hepatocytes, coalesces into larger hepatic ducts, and exits the liver into the common hepatic duct, cystic duct, and the gallbladder. From there, it travels through the common bile duct, which carries the bile to the duodenum, where is it is joined by the pancreatic duct. Bile and pancreatic secretions pass together through the distal portion of the common bile duct, through the sphincter of Oddi, and into the duodenum via the ampulla of Vater (Fig. 42-1).

2. **What are gallstones? How are they related to biliary disease?**

   Gallstones result from disrupted ratios of bile salts, cholesterol, and phospholipids. Most (85%) are cholesterol based, and 15% are related to bacterial processes. Pregnancy, oral contraceptive use, and estrogen therapy increase the risk of cholelithiasis by altering the cholesterol ratio and solubility. Progesterone may contribute to the formation of stones by slowing gallbladder motility. Postmenopausal hormone replacement increases the risk by three to four times. Oral contraceptives carry less risk than postmenopausal hormones; with lower-dose contraceptive preparations, the risk is even further reduced. Obesity, diabetes, cirrhosis, and age >40 years also contribute to gallstone risks. Although gallstones are common, 80% of persons with gallstones are asymptomatic.

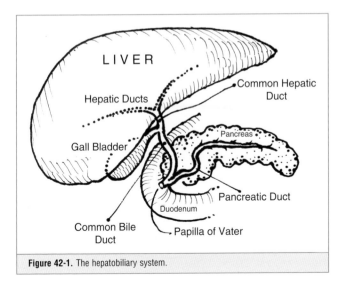

Figure 42-1. The hepatobiliary system.

3. **Describe the clinical presentation of biliary obstruction.**

The classic pattern of "biliary colic" involves right upper quadrant to epigastric pain that is deep and penetrating and may wax and wane, a phenomenon related to obstruction of the cystic or common bile duct. Referred pain from biliary obstruction may be felt in the posterior right scapula or shoulder as nociceptive input from the gallbladder enters the spinal cord at T5–T10, the cutaneous distribution affecting the right scapular area. Patients may experience anorexia, nausea and vomiting, jaundice (when serum bilirubin levels exceed 3 mg/dL), scleral icterus (in reality, it is the conjunctiva and not the sclera that is affected), and pruritus. Physical examination findings may include right upper quadrant fullness and pain on palpation. *Murphy's sign,* or inspiratory pause, can be elicited by placing the hands just below the right costal margin and asking the patient to take a deep breath. Taking the breath will cause pain and the associated inspiratory pause as the inflamed gallbladder contacts the examiner's hand.

4. **Name the mechanisms of biliary tract obstruction.**
   - **Calculous cholecystitis**: A stone obstructing the cystic duct of the gallbladder
   - **Choledocholithiasis:** A stone obstructing the common bile duct
   - **Acalculous cholecystitis**: Gallbladder stasis, ischemia, and necrosis in the absence of obstruction; seen in critical illness, major trauma, the postpartum period, total parenteral nutrition, burns, and diabetes
   - **Gallstone pancreatitis**: A stone obstructing the ampulla of Vater; patients often present with abdominal pain and acute pancreatitis

5. **What tests and studies can aid in the evaluation of the biliary tree?**

Serum tests include complete blood cell count; measurements of electrolytes, blood urea nitrogen, creatinine, bilirubin, alkaline phosphatase, aspartate aminotransferase, alanine aminotransferase, amylase, and lipase; blood cultures, and pregnancy testing in women. *Right upper quadrant ultrasound* is the study of choice to evaluate for cholelithiasis or cholecystitis. It is noninvasive and has no radiation risks. It detects ductal dilatation and gallbladder wall thickening and has a sensitivity and specificity of 97% for the detection of stones. A limitation is relatively poor visualization of the distal common bile duct and ampulla of Vater due to overlying bowel.

6. **What is the role of the computed tomography (CT) scan and the technetium-labeled hepato-iminodiacetic acid (HIDA) scan in biliary evaluation?**
   - **CT scan:** This is the most sensitive radiologic test for abdominal pain but may miss 20–25% of stones. It provides better imaging of the common bile duct and ampulla and is useful for suspected gallstone pancreatitis.
   - **HIDA scan:** This nuclear medicine study is used to assess for gallbladder obstruction after an inconclusive ultrasound study. HIDA is administered intravenously, taken up by hepatocytes, and excreted in the bile. A positive study is one in which the labeled contrast does not enter the gallbladder.

7. **Describe the basic management of patients with cholecystitis.**

Intravenous (IV) fluids and pain control. IV antibiotics have no proven benefit in uncomplicated cases but are commonly used in hospitalized patients to cover enterics, gram-negative rods, and enterococcus. Surgical consultation for cholecystectomy should be considered.

8. **How are choledocholithiasis and gallstone pancreatitis managed?**

IV fluids and pain control. IV antibiotics should be reserved for patients who are febrile or have evidence of necrotizing pancreatitis. Consider gastroenterology consult for an endoscopic retrograde cholangiopancreatography (ERCP), a diagnostic and therapeutic procedure in which an endoscope enters the ampulla of Vater to image and remove obstructions in the common bile duct, either by stone removal or sphincterotomy.

9. **What infections are associated with the biliary system?**
   - **Cholangitis:** Infection of the obstructed duct due to stone or neoplasm. Presents classically with fever, right upper quadrant pain, and jaundice (Charcot's triad) in 50–75% of cases. The added presence of confusion and hypotension (Reynolds' pentad) indicates a more fulminant process with nearly 50% mortality.
   - **Recurrent pyogenic cholangitis:** Also known as *Oriental cholangiohepatitis,* this rare infection is seen in Asians with chronic biliary ductal obstruction and stasis due to the biliary fluke *Opisthorchis sinensis.*

KEY POINTS: THE HEPATOBILIARY SYSTEM

1. The hepatobiliary system conjugates and carries bile to the hepatic ducts, gallbladder, and out through the bile duct, where it combines with the pancreatic duct in the duodenum.

2. Gallstones are primarily cholesterol concretions, resulting from alterations in bile salt composition.

3. The most important biliary diseases are obstructions from stones, variably causing pain, inflammation, pancreatitis, and infections.

---

10. **What is the hospital management of cholangitis?**
    Blood cultures, IV fluids, pain control, and IV antibiotics to cover enteric pathogens, anaerobes, gram-negative rods, and *Enterococcus*. Blood cultures as well as the culture of any drainage or aspirates from ERCP allow for more focused antimicrobial therapy. The conditions of a majority (80%) of patients resolve with antimicrobial therapy and can undergo elective ERCP, whereas the rest may require more urgent decompression or percutaneous drainage.

11. **What cancers are found in the biliary system?**
    - **Cholangiocarcinoma:** Adenocarcinoma of the bile ducts that represents 25% of biliary tract cancers; associated with primary sclerosing cholangitis, recurrent pyogenic cholangitis, and asbestos exposure
    - **Gallbladder:** Fifth most common gastrointestinal malignancy, representing 54% of biliary tract cancers; associated with a poor outcome
    - **Ampullary carcinoma:** 8% of biliary tract malignancies; presents with pancreatitis or jaundice

12. **What other diseases affect the biliary system?**
    - **Primary sclerosing cholangitis:** A chronic inflammatory disease causing fibrosis of the biliary ductal system; seen in patients with ulcerative and Crohn's colitis and other more rare autoimmune disorders
    - **Primary biliary cirrhosis:** A progressive and destructive autoimmune disease of the biliary ducts that leads to cirrhosis

---

WEBSITE

American Gastroenterological Association: http://www.gastro.org/

BIBLIOGRAPHY

1. Beckingham IJ, Ryder SD: ABC of diseases of liver, pancreas, and biliary system: Investigation of liver and biliary disease. BMJ 322:33–36, 2001.

2. Dreiling DA, Greenstein RJ: The sphincter of Oddi, sphincterotomy, and biliopancreatic disease. Am J Gastroenterol 72:665–670, 1979.

3. Johnston DE, Kaplan MM: Medical progress: Pathogenesis and treatment of gallstones. N Engl J Med 328:412–421, 1993.

4. Ransohoff DF, Gracie WA: Treatment of gallstones. Ann Intern Med 119:606–619, 1993.

5. Trowbridge RL, Rutkowski NK, Shojania KG: Does this patient have acute cholecystitis?. JAMA 289:80–86, 2003.

CHAPTER 43

ILEUS AND BOWEL OBSTRUCTION

Robert L. Matorin, MD, MS

1. **What are the leading causes of small bowel obstruction (SBO)?**

   SBO arises when the normal flow of intestinal contents through the small bowel is disrupted by means of a mechanical blockage. SBO can be caused by intrinsic, extrinsic, or luminal lesions. The most common cause, accounting for approximately 60% of cases, is postoperative adhesion. Malignancy and hernias are also frequently implicated. Some other causes are listed in Table 43-1.

TABLE 43-1. CAUSES OF SMALL BOWEL OBSTRUCTION		
Extrinsic Lesions (Outside the Bowel Wall)	**Intrinsic Lesions (Inside the Bowel Wall)**	**Luminal**
Congenital bands	Congenital atresia/stenosis	Gallstones
Postoperative adhesions	Inflammatory	Foreign bodies
Hernias (e.g., femoral, inguinal, umbilical, incisional, or internal abdominal)	Diverticulitis	Bezoars
	IBD (e.g., Crohn's disease)	Fecal impaction
	Ischemia	Meconium ileus
Volvulus	Radiation	
Carcinomatosis	Endometriosis	
Extraintestinal neoplasms (e.g., ovarian tumors, malignant melanoma, lymphomas, gastric or colonic carcinomas)	Postanastomotic	
	Infectious (e.g. tuberculosis, actinomycosis)	
Abscess	Intussusception	
	Polypoid neoplasms or neoplastic strictures	
IBD = inflammatory bowel disease.		

2. **What are the signs and symptoms associated with SBO?**

   Patients typically present with cramping abdominal pain and vomiting. If the obstruction is complete, no stool or flatus will be passed. On examination, the abdomen is often distended with high-pitched tinkling sounds and peristaltic rushes. Prior surgical scars may give a clue to etiology, such as adhesions. If a groin or abdominal hernia is present, consider possible bowel incarceration or strangulation as a cause. Hypotension and tachycardia may indicate intravascular volume depletion or sepsis, and the presence of fever may herald an intra-abdominal abscess or even bowel necrosis.

3. **How can the history and physical examination help identify the level of obstruction?**

Table 43-2 outlines how the intensity of pain, frequency and appearance of vomitus, and degree of distention may aid in identifying the level of obstruction.

TABLE 43-2.	DIAGNOSTIC CLUES TO THE LEVEL OF OBSTRUCTION			
Level of Blockage	Vomiting	Pain	Distention	Radiographic Appearance
Proximal small intestine	Early, violent, bilious	Great	Less prominent	Multiple air-fluid levels with distended loops of small bowel; cecum of normal caliber (≤ 4 cm)
Distal small intestine	Late, feculent (result of bacterial overgrowth)	Less severe than in proximal small intestine	Progresses over hours	
Large intestine	Late, infrequent	Less acute	Prominent from outset	Dilated large bowel; small bowel may be dilated if ileocecal valve is incompetent

4. **How does an SBO appear radiographically?**

Supine and upright abdominal plain radiographs will often show distension of the small bowel with associated air-fluid levels. Air-fluid levels are most prominent in the upright position. A complete obstruction is associated with a lack of air in the rectum on x-ray. An upright chest radiograph may reveal presence of free air under the diaphragm which, if identified, is worrisome for a perforated viscus. Computed tomography (CT) may provide additional information about the presence, level, severity, and cause of obstruction. A transition between disparate calibers of proximal and distal small bowel may be identified, signifying the point of obstruction.

5. **What is pneumatosis intestinalis?**

Pneumatosis intestinalis refers to gas in the bowel wall, identified on abdominal radiographs or CT scans. This finding often indicates bowel wall necrosis that may be seen with bowel strangulation, obstruction, trauma, or other causes of intestinal ischemia.

6. **Describe the initial management of partial bowel obstruction.**

The management can be summarized as "drip and suck." Patients are given nothing by mouth (NPO), are given intravenous fluids, and a nasogastric tube is placed if the patient is vomiting. Abdominal examinations should be performed multiple times per day, along with close monitoring of vital signs and fluid balance. Serial radiographs are obtained to assess for deterioration (partial obstruction may progress to complete obstruction) or improvement. Serum electrolyte levels and complete blood count should be monitored until the nasogastric tube is removed and bowel function returns.

7. **What are the indications for immediate surgery in partial bowel obstruction?**

Indications for surgery may include rising and unremitting pain; localized peritonitis, suggesting perforation or ischemia (lack of blood flow and oxygen to the involved bowel); development of a "closed loop," or segment of intestine obstructed in two locations (creating a segment with no proximal or distal outlet); obstruction occurring as a result of incarcerated hernia; deterioration of patient's condition; or failure to resolve within 48 hours with conservative treatment.

8. **What is the appropriate management of complete bowel obstruction?**
Complete bowel obstruction is highly associated with the development of intestinal strangulation. Consequently, complete intestinal obstruction represents a surgical emergency.

9. **What is intussusception?**
Intussusception is the telescoping of one portion of the intestine into another. Unlike children, in whom intussusception may occur in normal bowel, the process in adults is usually associated with an underlying pathologic lesion. Common causes include neoplasms, inflammatory lesions, and Meckel's diverticulum. The association of intestinal pathology in adults mandates primary resection of the bowel without an attempt at hydrostatic reduction by contrast enema, a technique that is often used in the pediatric population.

10. **What is a Richter's hernia?**
A Richter's hernia is a strangulated hernia (enterocele) in which only one wall of the viscus is involved. Recognizing a Richter's hernia may be difficult because bowel sounds may persist despite a worsening situation. The most common sites of Richter's hernias are laparoscopic ports that are inadequately closed. Suspicion for this complication is warranted in any case in which a patient develops nausea, vomiting, and evidence of SBO after laparoscopy.

11. **What is gallstone ileus?**
Gallstone ileus is an unusual complication of cholelithiasis, most often occurring in elderly women. Gallstones, often greater than 2 cm in diameter, enter the intestines through a cholecystoduodenal fistula and migrate through the gastrointestinal tract. A mechanical obstruction occurs most frequently in the terminal ileum or at the ileocecal valve, where the small intestine is the narrowest. Treatment is surgical.

12. **What are the most common causes of mechanical large bowel obstruction?**
Cancer of the colon is by far the most common cause. Volvulus or twisting of a coil of gut on its own axis and diverticulitis are other common causes.

13. **Describe the typical presenting features of colon cancer with respect to location.**
See Table 43-3.

TABLE 43-3. CLINICAL FEATURES OF COLON CANCER WITH RESPECT TO LOCATION	
Lesion Location	Clinical Features
Right-sided	Anemia from chronic occult blood loss
	Obstructive symptoms rare
Left-sided	"Apple core" or "napkin ring" obstructing masses
	Alteration in bowel habits, such as decreasing stool caliber, constipation, or obstipation
	Obstruction more typical
Rectum	Bright red blood per rectum
	Rectal pain and tenesmus

14. **What are the most common locations for volvulus?**

Volvulus occurs usually in one of two places—the sigmoid colon and the cecum. The sigmoid is by far the most common location, owing to a long and narrow attachment of the sigmoid mesocolon. Sigmoid volvulus occurs most commonly in elderly, constipated patients and occurs in men four times more frequently than in women.

The radiographic appearance is of a "bent inner-tube" or "inverted U." The erect film reveals large fluid levels within this loop. The proximal colon is distended, and no gas is seen in the lower pelvis and rectum. Cecal volvulus may appear as a "comma," with the distended cecum orienting itself away from the right iliac fossa. Barium enema in a patient with a volvulus shows a characteristic "bird's beak."

15. **How is a sigmoid volvulus managed?**

Sigmoidoscopy, with passage of a large-bore flatus tube into the volvulus, is the first-line therapy. Laparotomy may be required if sigmoidoscopy is unsuccessful or if gangrene is suspected from physical signs or the appearance of mucosa. As volvulus tends to recur, elective sigmoid colectomy may also be considered.

16. **Where is the most common site of perforation when the colon is obstructed?**

Perforation occurs most commonly in the cecum. Because the diameter of the cecum is greater than other portions of the large bowel, at any given intraluminal pressure, wall tension is greatest in the cecum (Laplace's law). When the ileocecal valve is competent, the cecum cannot decompress fluid and gas into the small bowel, and a radiographic cecal diameter of 12 cm or more suggests imminent danger of rupture.

17. **What is paralytic ileus?**

Paralytic, or adynamic, ileus is a functional (as opposed to mechanical) obstruction in intestinal flow resulting from impaired motility.

18. **List some of the major causes and clinical features of paralytic ileus.**

Unlike a mechanical obstruction wherein the bowel is functional and often hyperdynamic, the hallmark of an ileus is reduced activity of the intestines. Clinically, patients may present with abdominal distention but have an absence of bowel sounds. However, they may have little or no abdominal pain and lack of focal abdominal tenderness. Intermittent vomiting and failure to pass feces or flatus is typical. Radiographs usually show gas throughout small and large bowel, including the rectum, though this finding does not exclude partial mechanical obstruction. Table 43-4 outlines the most common causes of ileus.

19. **Describe the principles of management of paralytic ileus.**

Management is similar to the initial management phase in obstruction: drip and suck. This includes keeping the patient NPO, giving intravenous fluids, and correcting electrolyte disorders. Nasogastric suction is used if vomiting and gastric distention are present. Offending agents (e.g., opiates) or causative illnesses should be reversed, if possible.

20. **Does giving pain medication to patients with intestinal ileus or obstruction mask important changes in their course?**

No studies have demonstrated the concealment of abdominal findings with reasonably dosed pain medication. However, many experts remain concerned about the slowing of gut motility associated with the use of opioid analgesics, risking further prolongation of paralytic ileus. Use of opioid analgesics should therefore be used with caution. Still, the physician should not ignore the basic clinical imperative to relieve suffering. Some clinicians advocate the use of intravenous nonsteroidal analgesics, such as ketorolac, in selected patients.

TABLE 43-4. COMMON CAUSES OF ILEUS

Causes	Examples
Post-laparotomy	Bowel resection
	Appendectomy
	Gynecologic surgery
Electrolyte derangements	Hypokalemia
	Hypomagnesemia
Metabolic derangements	Uremia
	Diabetic ketoacidosis
	Hypothyroidism
Drugs	Opiates
	Anticholinergic agents
	Tricyclic antidepressants
	Anti-parkinsonian drugs
Intra-abdominal inflammation, systemic sepsis	Peritonitis
	Appendicitis
	Diverticulitis
	Perforated ulcer
Retroperitoneal hemorrhage or inflammation	Lumbar compression fracture
	Acute pancreatitis
	Pyelonephritis
Intestinal ischemia	Peripheral vascular disease
	Vasculitis
Thoracic processes	Lower rib fracture
	Lower lobe pneumonia
	Myocardial infarction

KEY POINTS: ILEUS AND BOWEL OBSTRUCTION

1. The most frequent causes of SBO include intra-abdominal adhesions following laparotomy (>60%), hernias (~10–20%) and neoplasms (~10–20%).

2. The absence of air in the rectum on plain radiographs makes a diagnosis of complete obstruction more likely.

3. The initial management of partial bowel obstruction may be summarized as "drip and suck."

4. Surgical intervention is imperative if the patient's condition deteriorates or if a complete bowel obstruction or peritoneal signs become apparent.

5. Cancer of the colon is the most common cause of large bowel obstruction.

6. The differential diagnosis for paralytic ileus is broad and often occurs after abdominal surgeries and the use of opiates.

21. **What are features of recovery from ileus?**

The patient may begin to pass flatus. Bowel sounds return, along with a return of appetite. Nasogastric tube output typically decreases, and urine output may increase as fluid is absorbed from the bowel.

22. **How can you distinguish colonic ileus from true large bowel mechanical obstruction?**

A barium enema or colonoscopy is the easiest way to distinguish between these entities. Colonoscopy can be both diagnostic and therapeutic but should be approached cautiously and even omitted in cases of colitis with marked distention, where risk of perforation is high.

23. **What are the common causes of acute colonic pseudo-obstruction (Ogilvie's syndrome)?**

Common causes of acute colonic pseudo-obstruction include malignant retroperitoneal infiltration, trauma to the lumbar spine or retroperitoneum, spinal anesthesia, or electrolyte imbalances, especially hypokalemia, hypocalcemia, or hypomagnesemia.

24. **List therapeutic options in the management of acute colonic pseudo-obstruction.**

Therapeutic options include supportive care and discontinuation of medications that inhibit gastrointestinal motility (e.g., narcotics, anticholinergics); use of pharmacologic agents (e.g., neostigmine) or enemas to increase colonic motility; decompression via colonoscopy or placement of a percutaneous cecostomy tube; or surgery, in patients who develop signs and symptoms of peritonitis, ischemia, or perforation.

BIBLIOGRAPHY

1. Silen W: Cope's Early Diagnosis of the Acute Abdomen, 20th ed. New York, Oxford University Press, 2000, pp 150–187.
2. Townsend CM, Beauchamp RD, Evers BM, et al: Sebastian Textbook of Surgery: The Biological Basis of Modern Surgical Practice, 17th ed. Philadelphia, W.B. Saunders, 2004, pp 318–320, 1334–1342, 1424–1441.

URINARY TRACT INFECTIONS
Martin C. Were, MD

1. **What is the difference between an uncomplicated and a complicated urinary tract infection (UTI)?**
   - An *uncomplicated UTI* is defined as cystitis in a healthy nonpregnant woman without any structural or neurologic disease.
   - *Complicated UTI* includes everything else: infection in the upper tract, or infection in a pregnant woman, a man, or a patient with underlying anatomic or neurologic disease.

2. **Describe the microbiology of the following UTIs.**
   - **Uncomplicated UTI:** *Escherichia coli* (70–95%), *Staphylococcus saprophyticus, Proteus, Klebsiella, Enterococcus* species
   - **Complicated UTI:** Broader spectrum of organisms, including *E. coli, Proteus, Klebsiella, Pseudomonas, Serratia, Providencia,* enterococci, staphylococci, and fungi; *S. saprophyticus* is uncommon
   - **Catheter-associated UTI:** *E. coli* (25%), yeast (30%), other gram-negative rods, *Staphylococcus epidermidis,* enterococci
   - **Lower tract UTI in men:** Same organisms as in uncomplicated UTI in women
   - **Urethritis:** *Neisseria gonorrhoeae, Chlamydia trachomatis*

3. **What is asymptomatic bacteriuria? When should it be treated?**
   Asymptomatic bacteriuria refers to the presence of a positive urine culture (i.e., $>10^5$ cfu/mL of a urinary tract pathogen on a single midstream clean-catch specimen) in an asymptomatic patient. It does not need to be treated except in patients who are pregnant (treatment is usually initiated when cultures have $\geq 10^4$ cfu/mL) or have recently undergone urologic instrumentation or surgery.

4. **How are lower and upper UTIs differentiated anatomically?**
   - **Lower:** Urethritis, cystitis (superficial infection of the bladder), prostatitis
   - **Upper:** Pyelonephritis (inflammation of the renal parenchyma), perinephric abscess (involvement of the perirenal fat), renal abscess

5. **How do lower UTIs present?**
   - **Urethritis:** Dysuria, urethral discharge.
   - **Cystitis:** Dysuria, increased frequency, urgency, suprapubic pain, and/or hematuria.
   - **Prostatitis:** Presents like cystitis with signs of outlet obstruction, including weak stream and hesitancy. Patients can have fevers, malaise, and myalgias.

6. **Which urinalysis findings suggest that a patient has UTI?**
   There are variable methods (and levels of certainty) to diagnose a UTI. The gold standard is the growth of bacteria in urine culture. Short of culture data, the presence of white blood cells implies the presence of bacteria and is a relatively sensitive marker of UTI in a symptomatic patient. The finding of leukocyte esterase implies the presence of white blood cells, which implies the presence of bacteria. The nitrite test is a surrogate for the presence of bacteria (Enterobacteriaceae) that convert urinary nitrate to nitrite.

7. **What is the role of urine cultures and blood cultures in evaluating a patient with lower tract UTI?**

It is not necessary to obtain urine or blood culture specimens in women with uncomplicated cystitis, but these should be obtained in pregnant women, immunocompromised patients, catheterized patients, and men, especially those suspected to have prostatitis, to help guide therapy.

8. **What is the treatment for the following infections?**
   - **Acute uncomplicated cystitis:** Trimethoprim/sulfamethoxazole, trimethoprim, a fluoroquinolone, cefpodoxime proxetil for 3 days, or nitrofurantoin for 7 days.
   - **Acute complicated cystitis:** Oral fluoroquinolone for 7–14 days if patient can tolerate oral medications. More acutely ill patients may benefit from intravenous fluoroquinolone, ceftriaxone, or aminoglycoside. Patients with suspected enterococci (gram-positive cocci in chains) might also need ampicillin or amoxicillin.
   - **Cystitis in men:** Treat for 7 days instead of 3 days, preferably with a fluoroquinolone (which has the best prostatic penetration) or trimethoprim/sulfamethoxazole.
   - **Acute prostatitis:** Treat for 4–6 weeks guided by cultures. For empiric treatment and for gram-negative rods, use a fluoroquinolone or trimethoprim/sulfamethoxazole. For enterococci, use ampicillin or amoxicillin. Gram-positive cocci in clusters (*Staphylococcus aureus* or *S. epidermidis*) are treated with a cephalosporin or penicillinase-resistant penicillin (e.g., dicloxacillin), and methicillin-resistant *S. aureus* requires vancomycin. If obstruction develops, suprapubic catheterization is recommended, not Foley catheterization.
   - **Chronic prostatitis:** Administer fluoroquinolones or trimethoprim/sulfamethoxazole for 6–12 weeks. Consider *C. trachomatis* when routine urine and prostatic secretion cultures are negative.
   - **Urethritis:** Give azithromycin or doxycycline for *C. trachomatis*, and ceftriaxone or ofloxacin for *N. gonorrhoeae*.

9. **When and for how long should you use urinary analgesia?**

Urinary analgesia (phenazopyridine 200 mg orally t.i.d.) can be offered to patients with severe dysuria, but only for 1–2 days. A longer duration of therapy provides no added benefit but may cause adverse effects. Nonsteroidal anti-inflammatory drugs are useful in the treatment of prostatitis.

10. **Describe the clinical presentation of pyelonephritis.**

In addition to dysuria, patients may present with flank or back pain, fever and chills, nausea/vomiting, and occasionally diarrhea.

11. **Which clinical features suggest that a patient has renal or perinephric abscess?**
   - **Renal abscess:** This often presents like pyelonephritis with fever, pain, and leukocytosis, but the signs and symptoms usually persist >5 days despite antimicrobial therapy, whereas patients with pyelonephritis usually defervesce within 3–4 days of therapy.
   - **Perinephric abscess:** The onset of pain, fever, and leukocytosis is more progressive. Flank and abdominal tenderness are more superficial, and inflammation of the skin may be observed around the flank. Computed tomography (CT) scan detects 96% of abscesses, and ultrasonography detects approximately 92%.

12. **What additional studies are recommended in a patient with acute pyelonephritis?**

All patients with acute pyelonephritis require urine culture and antimicrobial susceptibility testing. Blood cultures can be limited to only those patients who require hospitalization. An imaging study is not necessary to diagnose acute pyelonephritis but should be considered if the patient does not defervesce after 3 days of antibiotic therapy.

KEY POINTS: DIAGNOSIS OF URINARY TRACT INFECTIONS

1. Suspect pyelonephritis in a patient who presents with dysuria but also has flank and/or back pain, fever, chills, and nausea and vomiting.

2. An imaging study is not necessary to diagnose acute pyelonephritis, but should be considered if the patient does not defervesce after 3 days of antibiotic therapy.

3. Suspect renal abscess in a patient who has symptoms of pyelonephritis and whose fever persists for >5 days with appropriate antimicrobial therapy.

4. CT scans detect 96% of abscesses, and ultrasonography detects approximately 92%.

13. **What factors increase the probability of having acute pyelonephritis as opposed to simple cystitis in adults?**
Obstruction, diverticula, fistulae, ileal conduits and other urinary diversions, neurogenic bladder, vesicoureteral reflux, indwelling catheter, nephrostomy tube, pregnancy, diabetes, renal failure, renal transplantation, immunosuppression, multidrug-resistant uropathogens, and hospital-acquired infections.

14. **What are the indications for hospitalization in a patient with upper UTI?**
    - Inability to maintain oral intake or take oral medications
    - Severe illness with high fevers, pain, and severely impaired functional status
    - Acute renal failure
    - Renal or perinephric abscess
    - Uncertainty about the diagnosis
    - Significant comorbid states (e.g., immunosuppression and possibly cancer or diabetes)

15. **Describe the antibiotic treatment of acute pyelonephritis.**
Similar to that described above for acute complicated cystitis, but length of therapy is usually extended for 14 days. Patients with bacteremia do not necessarily need a longer course of antibiotics. If initial therapy is intravenous, it can be changed to oral once the patient is afebrile and improving for 24–48 hours.

16. **What post-treatment follow-up is recommended in a patient with acute pyelonephritis?**
Routine post-treatment cultures are not indicated. In women, if symptoms resolve and recur within weeks, a repeat urine culture and susceptibility testing are recommended. If the initial organism is isolated again, renal ultrasound or CT scan is recommended and 14 days of treatment with another agent should be considered. Recurrence of symptoms after 2 weeks should be managed like other sporadic episodes of pyelonephritis.

17. **Describe the medical and surgical treatment of renal abscess.**
Abscesses >3 cm require catheter-drainage. Abscesses >5 cm require more than one percutaneous drainage procedure or open surgical intervention, especially if staghorn calculi are present. Consider surgical drainage if there is an anatomic abnormality and rescue nephrectomy for large abscesses in immunocompromised hosts, especially in diabetics. Prolonged antibiotic courses are often required.

18. **How can catheter-associated infections be prevented?**
    - Use urinary catheters only when medically indicated, not simply for convenience.
    - Insert the catheter in a sterile fashion.
    - Wash hands, secure the catheter properly, maintain unobstructed flow, and keep the urine collection bag below the patient at all times to decrease urine backflow.
    - Maintain a closed drainage system.
    - Minimize the duration of use of the indwelling catheter.
    - Condom catheters still pose a risk of catheter-related UTI, but less so than with indwelling catheters.
    - Consider using silver alloy–coated catheters.
    - Prophylactic antibiotics are generally not recommended for prevention of catheter-associated UTIs. (See Chapter 55 for more details.)

19. **Describe the treatment of bacterial catheter-associated infections.**
    Asymptomatic bacteriuria in patients with long-term bladder catheters should not be treated. Symptomatic patients without yeast or gram-positive cocci on urine culture should be treated for 10–14 days with a third-generation cephalosporin or fluoroquinolone. If the presence of *Pseudomonas* organisms is suspected, an anti-pseudomonal cephalosporin (e.g., ceftazidime) or penicillin (e.g., piperacillin), and/or aminoglycoside should be used. Enterococcal infections are treated with ampicillin or vancomycin. *Staphylococcus* infection is initially treated with vancomycin, with antibiotics subsequently tailored according to sensitivities.

20. **What are the strategies for managing candiduria associated with an indwelling catheter?**
    In all patients (whether catheterized or not) there is no need to treat asymptomatic candiduria, except in settings of kidney transplantation, neutropenia, low-birth-weight neonates, or urinary tract manipulation. Instead, it is recommended that the catheter be removed or replaced, or intermittent bladder catheterization used. Patients with symptomatic candiduria need treatment. Options include an antifungal azole (e.g., fluconazole), amphotericin B, or flucytosine. Persistent candiduria should prompt radiologic imaging of the kidneys.

KEY POINTS: TREATMENT OF URINARY TRACT INFECTIONS

1. Acute complicated cystitis should be treated with a fluoroquinolone, cephalosporin, or aminoglycoside.

2. Pyelonephritis usually requires 2 weeks of antibiotic therapy.

3. Treat acute prostatitis for 4–6 weeks guided by culture data.

4. The decision to medically or surgically manage renal abscess is governed by the size of the abscess, the presence of anatomic abnormalities, and the immunologic status of the host.

5. In all patients, whether catheterized or not, there is no need to treat asymptomatic candiduria, except in settings of kidney transplantation, neutropenia, or urinary tract manipulation.

BIBLIOGRAPHY

1. Dembry LM, Andriole VT: Renal and perirenal abscesses. Infect Dis Clin North Am 11:663, 1997.
2. Fihn SD: Acute uncomplicated urinary tract infection in women. N Engl J Med 349:259–266, 2003.

3. Foxman B: Epidemiology of urinary tract infections: incidence, morbidity, and economic costs. Am J Med 113 (Suppl 1A):5S–13S, 2002.

4. Hooton TM, Besser R, Foxman B, et al: Acute uncomplicated cystitis in an era of increasing antibiotic resistance: a proposed approach to empirical therapy. Clin Infect Dis 39:75–80, 2004.

5. Nicolle LE: A practical guide to the management of complicated urinary tract infection. Drugs 53:583, 1997.

6. Nicolle LE, Bradley S, Colgan R, et al: Infectious Diseases Society of America guidelines for the diagnosis and treatment of asymptomatic bacteriuria in adults. Clin Infect Dis 40:643, 2005.

7. Pappas PG, Rex JH, Sobel JD, et al: Infectious Diseases Society of America. Guidelines for treatment of candidiasis. Clin Infect Dis 38:161, 2004.

8. Wilson ML, Gaido L: Laboratory diagnosis of urinary tract infections in adult patients. Clin Infect Dis 38:1150–1158, 2004.

CHAPTER 45

ACUTE RENAL FAILURE

Margaret McLees, MD

1. How is renal function determined?

The glomerular filtration rate (GFR), which measures the amount of plasma filtered across the capillary bed, is a useful marker of renal function. GFR can be estimated indirectly by the Cockcroft-Gault equation or from the Modification of Diet in Renal Disease Study (MDRD) equation.

$$\text{Cockcroft-Gault: GFR} = \text{CrCl(mL/min)} = [(140 - \text{age}) \times \text{IBM}]/(72 \times \text{Scr}) \times 0.85$$
$$(\text{if female})$$

where CrCl = creatinine clearance, IBW = ideal body weight, and Scr = serum creatinine.

$$\text{MDRD: GFR} = 170 \times [S_{cr}]^{-0.999} \times [\text{age}]^{-0.176} \times [0.762 \text{ if patient is female}] \times$$
$$[1.180 \text{ if patient is African-American}] \times [\text{SUN}]^{-0.170} \times [\text{Alb}]^{+0.318}$$

where SUN = serum urea nitrogen and Alb = albumin. The MDRD equation takes into account age, sex, ethnicity, and serum albumin and serum creatinine levels and is thought to be the most accurate estimation of GFR.

2. What is acute renal failure (ARF)?

ARF is a rapid decline in renal function occurring over the period of days that results in a decreased excretion of nitrogen waste products, acid–base abnormalities, and decreased ability to regulate electrolyte and fluid balance.

3. What are common signs and symptoms of ARF?

Presentation may be variable depending on the cause. Common symptoms include nausea, vomiting, confusion, anorexia due to uremia, and decreased urine output or change in urine color due to decreased filtration. Additionally, they may have edema, shortness of breath, and pulmonary rales due to volume overload. Less commonly, the physical examination may reveal a cardiac rub indicative of uremic pericarditis. Patients with urinary obstructive causes may have flank pain and lower abdominal fullness, whereas those with glomerulonephritis may present with hematuria.

4. What are common electrolyte abnormalities seen in ARF?

Initially, elevated blood urea nitrogen (BUN) and creatinine levels are seen, then hyperkalemia, metabolic acidosis, hyperphosphatemia, Hyponatremia, and hypocalcemia. If BUN and creatinine levels are elevated but there are no other abnormalities such as hyperkalemia or hyperphosphatemia, the renal failure is likely to be subacute or chronic in nature. Elevated BUN (uremia) will cause an anion gap metabolic acidosis, whether acute or chronic.

5. What are the types and common causes of ARF in a hospitalized patient?

ARF is classified by the location of the injury with reference to the kidney:

- *Prerenal disease* accounts for about one fifth of the cases of ARF in hospitalized patients and is most often due to reduced renal perfusion from volume depletion or medications that reduce renal blood flow (e.g., angiotensin-converting enzyme [ACE] inhibitors).

- As much as 70% of ARF in the hospitalized patient is caused by *intrinsic renal failure*. Intrinsic renal failure is further classified by the type of cell that is injured: tubular, interstitial or glomerular.
- *Postrenal disease*, accounting for 10% of ARF in hospitalized patients, is most commonly due to obstruction of urinary flow out of the urinary system.

Overall, the most common causes of ARF in the hospital are acute tubular necrosis (ATN) (45%), nephrotoxic dye, and medication. ARF confers a mortality rate of 45%; when ARF is associated with sepsis, mortality rises to 70%.

Note: The incidences quoted above refer to the development of ARF while the patient is hospitalized, not on presentation.

6. **What is prerenal azotemia?**
   Prerenal azotemia results from insults that decrease renal perfusion and reverses quickly with restoration of renal blood flow and filtration pressure. There is usually no damage to the renal parenchyma with mild to moderate hypoperfusion, but if the insult is severe and/or prolonged, prerenal azotemia can lead to renal ischemia and ATN (Table 45-1).

TABLE 45-1. CAUSES, EXAM FINDINGS AND TREATMENT OF PRERENAL AZOTEMIA

Causes	Exam Findings	Treatment
Volume loss: dehydration, hemorrhage, overdiuresis	Dry mucous membrane, tenting skin, tachycardia, hypotension, orthostasis, cool extremities, concentrated urine	Resuscitate as appropriate: crystalloids or packed red blood cells (PRBCs) if due to hemorrhage
Third spacing: sepsis, burns, pancreatitis, liver disease	Ascites, pleural effusions, septic shock (warm extremities), anasarca, burns	Burns: fluids Sepsis: fluids, antibiotics +/− drotrecogin Liver: **gentle** diuresis
Low cardiac output: heart failure, valvular disease, severe pulmonary hypertension	Jugular venous distention, rales, pleural effusions, S4 gallop, tachycardia, edema, cool extremities	Improve Starling curve: afterload reduction, diuresis, inotropic agents if necessary
Medications: ACEI, ARB, diuretics, cyclosporine, amphotericin B		Stop the offending medication

ACEI = angiotensin converting enzyme inhibitor; ARB = angiotensin receptor blockers.

7. **How can liver disease lead to prerenal azotemia?**

   In advanced liver disease, there is systemic vasodilatation with decreased effective blood flow to the kidneys that can lead to ARF with a very low fractional excretion of sodium (FeNa) refractory to fluid challenge. Known as *hepatorenal syndrome,* it is often incited by dramatic fluid shifts like bleeding, aggressive diuresis, or large volume paracentesis. See Chapter 40 for more details.

8. **What are the major causes of hyperviscosity that can cause prerenal azotemia?**

   Hyperviscosity causes sludging and decreased blood flow to the kidneys, resulting in prerenal azotemia. Multiple myeloma, macroglobulinemia, and polycythemia all increase serum viscosity, leading to sludging and ARF.

9. **How does postrenal azotemia occur?**

   Postrenal azotemia is caused by blockage or cessation of urinary flow at any point between the renal pelvises and the urethra. It can be caused internally by blood clot, kidney stones, sloughed papilla, tumor, fungus ball, uric acid or sulfonamide crystals in the ureter, abnormal ureterovesicular sphincter or neurogenic bladder. Extrinsic causes include compression from tumor, adhesions, or prostatic hypertrophy. Medications with anticholinergic effects (e.g., tricyclic antidepressants, diphenhydramine) commonly induce postrenal kidney disease by inhibiting bladder emptying.

10. **What electrolyte abnormalities can follow relief of postobstructive ARF?**

    Relieving an obstruction can lead to rapid diuresis, hypovolemia, and sodium imbalance.

11. **Describe the clinical features and causes of acute interstitial nephritis (AIN).**

    AIN may be due to drugs, infection, autoimmune process, or idiopathic causes. Clinically, there is a rapid decline in renal function and usually fevers and symptoms localizing infection, or if due to a drug, maculopapular rash, urine eosinophils, and fever. Less than 35% of patients with drug-induced AIN have all three features.

12. **Describe the clinical features and causes of acute glomerulonephritis.**

    Glomerulonephritis can cause chronic, rapidly progressive, or acute renal failure. Patients present with hypertension, renal failure, oliguria or anuria, hematuria, proteinuria, and red blood cell casts, due to inflammatory injury to the glomerulus. ARF due to poststreptococcal glomerulonephritis is seen most often in children. In adults, glomerulonephritis may be associated with a wide range of autoimmune diseases and vasculitides, such as Henoch-Schönlein purpura disease, systemic lupus erythematosus, and antineutrophil cytoplasmic antibody (ANCA)-associated disease. Initial evaluation includes complement levels and antiglomerular basement membrane, P-ANCA, C-ANCA, and anti–streptolysin-O antibodies. Histologically, rapidly progressive glomerulonephritis is defined by immune complex deposition patterns: pauci-immune, immune complex, or antiglomerular basement membrane patterns. Renal biopsy is usually required to make a final diagnosis and to determine prognosis and treatment.

13. **What medications can induce ATN?**
    - **Antibiotics:** Acyclovir, amphotericin B, aminoglycosides, foscarnet, cidofovir, indinavir, pentamidine
    - **Chemotherapeutic agents:** Cisplatin, ifosfamide
    - **Radiocontrast agents**
    - **Nonsteroidal anti-inflammatory drugs and cyclooxygenase-2 inhibitors**
    - **Immunosuppressants:** Cyclosporine, tacrolimus
    - **Antihypertensives:** ACE inhibitors, angiotensin receptor blockers, diuretics (severe prerenal disease)

14. **What are some endogenous substances that can cause ATN?**
Myoglobin (rhabdomyolysis), hemoglobin, myeloma light chains, uric acid, and tumor lysis syndrome can all cause ATN through tubular deposition, obstruction, and subsequent ischemia or, in the case of myeloma light chains, direct tubular toxicity.

15. **Which patients are at greatest risk of injury from radiocontrast dye-induced ATN? What methods have been used to decrease the risk?**
Elderly patients, patients with underlying chronic renal insufficiency, patients with diabetes, and hypovolemic patients are at highest risk for dye-induced nephropathy. Currently, both N-acetyl cysteine and bicarbonate drips are used to prevent dye injury. Although both may increase the filtration of BUN and reduce the rate of small rises in serum creatinine, neither affect the incidence of clinically significant nephropathy requiring dialysis. However, both interventions are relatively inexpensive and nontoxic such that any potential nephro-protection may be worthwhile. Still, the most important prophylactic intervention appears to be adequate volume resuscitation, when appropriate, to ensure euvolemia prior to the dye load.

16. **What are the initial laboratory studies used in the diagnosis of ARF?**
The work-up of ARF should be tailored to the likely causes based on history and physical examination. All patients should have a basic metabolic panel and urinalysis with microscopic evaluation of urinary sediment. If prerenal azotemia is suggested, urine sodium and creatinine, urine osmolality, and urine urea nitrogen measurements to evaluate tubular concentrating ability should be preformed. Postrenal causes can be evaluated with a post-void residual to evaluate for urinary retention (normal < 50 mL) and a renal ultrasound or computed tomography angiography if obstruction from kidney stones is a possibility. Renal ultrasound will also help distinguish acute versus chronic renal disease by evaluating kidney size (large globular kidneys suggest an infiltrative disease such as myeloma, amyloid, or polycystic kidney disease; normal size suggests ARF; small kidneys with thinning renal cortices are suggestive of chronic medicorenal disease such as hypertension). Intrarenal disease, such as acute tubular, interstitial, or glomerular processes will most often reveal useful sediment on urinalysis.

17. **Describe the urine sediment of the various causes of ARF.**
See Table 45-2.

TABLE 45-2. URINE SEDIMENT IN ACUTE RENAL FAILURE	
Prerenal	No sediment or hyaline casts
Postrenal	Normal or pyuria, RBC, casts
Acute tubular necrosis	Granular casts, muddy brown casts, epithelial cells
Interstitial nephritis	RBCs, white blood cells, eosinophils, casts
Glomerulonephritis	RBCs and RBC casts, proteinuria
Vascular disease	Normal or RBCs and proteinuria

RBC = red blood cells.
Adapted from Toto R: Approaches to the patient with kidney disease. In Brenner BM, Levine, SA (eds.): Brenner & Rector's The Kidney, 7th ed., Philadelphia, Elsevier, 2004, p 1083.

18. **What is the FeNa?**
FeNa reflects the ability of the renal tubules to resorb sodium, one indicator of intrinsic renal function. FeNa is the most sensitive test to distinguish prerenal azotemia from intrinsic

TABLE 45-3. USE OF FENA TO DIFFERENTIATE THE CAUSES OF ACUTE RENAL FAILURE

FeNa	Cause of Acute Renal Failure
<1%	Pre-renal azotemia*
1–2%	Indeterminate
>2%	Acute tubular necrosis/intrinsic renal failure

FeNa = fractional excretion of sodium.
*Glomerulonephritis, urinary tract obstruction, and vasculitis may also have FeNa < 1% but are not ruled out with a FeNa > 1%.

renal failure (Table 45-3) but is unreliable in patients taking diuretics and those with glucosuria, chronic renal disease, or adrenal insufficiency.

$$FeNa = (U_{Na} \times S_{Cr}/S_{Na} \times U_{Cr}) \times 100$$

where U_{Na} = urine sodium, S_{Cr} = serum creatinine, S_{Na} = serum sodium, U_{Cr} = urine creatinine. A useful mnemonic for numerator is **U** k**N**ow **A** Se**Cr**et.

19. **How do complement levels contribute to the evaluation of intrinsic ARF?**
Decreased complement levels are suggestive of an ongoing immune complex-deposition process that is consuming C3 and C4, such as a glomerulonephritis or antiglomerular basement membrane disease.

20. **What are the indications for renal biopsy in ARF?**
Biopsy is used to diagnose the cause of ARF when results of the above studies are inconclusive, especially in patients presenting with evidence of rapidly progressive glomerulonephritis. Biopsy is also used for prognosis and direction of therapy. Contraindications include uncontrolled hypertension, coagulopathy, and ultrasound evidence of a small, shrunken kidney. Relative contraindications include use of aspirin, nonsteroidal anti-inflammatory drugs, or heparin.

KEY POINTS: ACUTE RENAL FAILURE

1. The most common cause of renal failure in a hospitalized patient is intrinsic renal failure due to ATN.

2. ARF is categorized as prerenal, intrinsic, and postrenal disease.

3. All ARF work-ups should start with a basic metabolic panel and a urinalysis with microscopic evaluation.

4. The development of ARF in a hospitalized patient confers a mortality risk of 45%—up to 70% when associated with sepsis.

21. **What are the potential complications of renal biopsy?**
The most common complication is hematuria. Nearly all patients will develop microscopic hematuria but less than 10% will have gross hematuria, both resolving within 48–72 hours.

Other complications include perinephric hematoma, intrarenal arteriovenous fistula, aneurysm, infection, ileus, laceration of abdominal organs, pneumothorax, and ureteral obstruction.

22. **What are the major complications of ARF?**
Complications of ARF are multisystemic.
- **Neurologic:** Confusion and altered mental status due to uremia, asterixis, seizures
- **Cardiopulmonary:** Pulmonary edema, arrhythmias, pericarditis, pericardial effusions, pulmonary embolism, hypertension, myocardial infarction
- **Gastrointestinal:** Nausea, vomiting, malnutrition, gastrointestinal hemorrhage
- **Metabolic:** Hyperkalemia, metabolic acidosis, hyponatremia, hypocalcemia, hyperphosphatemia, hypermagnesemia, hyperuricemia
- **Hematologic:** Anemia and bleeding

23. **What are the indications for hemodialysis?**
The major indications for hemodialysis are volume overload, symptomatic uremia, refractory acidosis, refractory hyperkalemia, and toxic ingestions.

BIBLIOGRAPHY

1. Brady HR, Clarkson MR, Leiberthal W: Etiologies of acute renal failure. In Brenner BM, Levine SA (eds): Brenner & Rector's The Kidney, 7th ed. Philadelphia, Elsevier, 2004, pp 1215–1270.

2. Levey AS, Bosch JP, Lewis JB, et al: A more accurate method to measure glomerular filtration rate from serum creatinine: A new prediction equation. Ann Intern Med 130:461–470, 1999.

3. Nally JV: Acute renal failure in hospitalized patients. Cleve Clin J Medicine 69:569–574, 2002.

4. Pannu N, Manns B, Lee H, Tonelli M: Systematic review of the impact of N-acetylcysteine on contrast nephropathy. Kidney Int 65:1366–1374, 2004.

5. Schrier RW, Wang W: Acute renal failure and sepsis. N Engl J Med 351:159–169, 2004.

6. Sesso R, Roque A, Vicioso B, Stella A: Prognosis of ARF in hospitalized elderly patients. Am J Kidney Dis 44:410–419, 2004.

CHAPTER 46

ELECTROLYTE DERANGEMENTS

David Krakow, MD

1. **Define *hypercalcemia*.**
   Hypercalcemia is defined as calcium levels persistently above the normal range (total serum calcium = 8.1–10.5 mg/dL or 2.0–2.6 mmol/dL). However, more than one half of the measured serum calcium is protein bound, so low protein levels (mainly albumin) will yield a low serum calcium level that does not correlate with the physiologically important ionized calcium. In these cases, it is prudent to measure the ionized or unbound free calcium (normal range, 1.1–1.3 mmol/dL).

2. **How is the calcium level corrected for a low serum albumin level?**

   Corrected serum calcium = measured calcium + [0.8 × (normal albumin−
   measured albumin)]

   Example : Measured calcium = 6.5 mg/dL
   Measured albumin = 2.0 gm/dL
   Corrected serum calcium = 6.5 mg/dL + [0.8 × (4.5 gm/dL − 2.0 gm/dL)] = 8.5 mg/dL

3. **What are the common causes of hypercalcemia?**
   Approximately 90% of the time, hypercalcemia is due to increased bone resorption from primary hyperparathyroidism or malignancy (e.g., multiple myeloma, lymphoma, carcinomas). Less common causes include the milk alkali syndrome, granulomatous diseases, (e.g., sarcoidosis, tuberculosis, fungal infections), hyperthyroidism, Addison's disease, immobilization, acromegaly, Paget's disease and familial hypercalcemic hypocalciuria. Commonly used drugs, such as thiazide diuretics, lithium, theophylline, and vitamin A and its analogs, can also cause mild hypercalcemia.

4. **How does cancer induce hypercalcemia?**
   Malignancy can induce hypercalcemia via four mechanisms: osteolytic metastases, humoral hypercalcemia (parathyroid hormone–related peptide [PTH-rP]), stimulation of calcitriol production or osteoclast-activating factor. Many squamous cell cancers (e.g., lung cancer) produce PTH-rP. (See Chapter 61 for more details.)

5. **What are the common signs and symptoms of hypercalcemia?**
   The common symptoms, usually nonspecific, include fatigue, nausea, anorexia, constipation, muscle weakness, bone pain, renal stones, vague abdominal pain, depression, and delirium. The latter symptoms are represented in the mnemonic device "bones, stones, abdominal groans, and psychiatric moans." Hypercalcemia is also associated with peptic ulcer disease, pancreatitis, and renal failure. Electrocardiographic changes include PR interval prolongation, QT interval shortening, and T-wave abnormalities.

6. **Describe the work-up of hypercalcemia.**
   A thorough history and physical examination is important. For example, a history of calcium carbonate ingestion might suggest milk-alkali syndrome as the cause of hypercalcemia.

Laboratory evaluation of hypercalcemia includes measurements of serum calcium, phosphorus, PTH, and PTH-rP levels and serum and urine protein electrophoresis for multiple myeloma, 25-hydroxyvitamin D (calcidiol), and 1,25-hydroxyvitamin D (calcitriol). An elevated serum PTH level suggests primary hyperparathyroidism, lithium use, or familial hypercalcemic hypocalciuria. All other causes of hypercalcemia are associated with a low (i.e., suppressed) serum PTH level. A clue to primary hyperparathyroidism is hypophosphatemia from PTH-induced renal phosphate wasting. The combination of a low serum PTH level and an elevated calcitriol level suggests granulomatous disease, lymphoma, or excess calcitriol ingestion as a cause for the hypercalcemia. Elevated calcidiol levels are only very rarely associated with hypercalcemia.

7. **Does a normal plasma PTH level rule out primary hyperparathyroidism?**
   No. Approximately 10–20% of patients with primary hyperparathyroidism have a plasma PTH level within the normal reference range, usually close to the upper limit of normal.

8. **What is the mechanism of hypercalcemia in granulomatous diseases?**
   In normal subjects, the conversion of calcidiol to calcitriol occurs via 1-hydroxylase in the kidney and is regulated by PTH. Hypercalcemia suppresses the release of PTH and therefore the production of calcitriol. The lack of suppression of calcitriol production in granulomatous diseases is due to PTH-independent production of calcitriol from calcidiol by activated mononuclear cells in granulomas.

9. **Describe the treatment of hypercalcemia.**
   Start with a saline infusion to expand volume and increase urinary calcium excretion. Once the patient is euvolemic, add a loop diuretic (e.g., furosemide) to further excrete calcium in the urine. Concurrently, administer a bisphosphonate (e.g., pamidronate 90 mg IV × one dose) to inhibit osteoclasts and calcitonin to stimulate osteoblasts. The calcitonin takes effect immediately, lasting 48 hours but with only a modest calcium-lowering effect. The bisphosphonate effect requires approximately 48 hours. Steroids may be used for hypercalcemia due to overproduction of calcitriol (e.g., lymphomas, granulomatous diseases).

10. **What are the signs, symptoms, and causes of acute hypocalcemia?**
    Ionized hypocalcemia is quite common in critically ill patients. Patients with hypocalcemia can experience tetany, carpopedal spasm, paresthesias, and seizures. Chvostek's sign, ipsilateral facial twitching elicited by tapping at the point anterior to the ear and inferior to the zygomatic bone, and Trousseau's sign, flexion of the wrist and hyperextension of the fingers after inflation of a blood pressure cuff for several minutes, are common physical findings in hypocalcemia. Acute alkalosis induces calcium to bind more vigorously to albumin (in exchange for protons), thereby lowering the ionized but not the total calcium level. It is therefore wise to measure ionized calcium in acutely alkalotic patients. A similar situation can occur when calcium binds to bicarbonate during a sodium bicarbonate infusion. Large quantities of blood transfusion can result in hypocalcemia as the banked blood's preservative (citrate) binds serum calcium. This often resolves quickly as the citrate is metabolized. Renal failure causes hypocalcemia due to impaired conversion of vitamin D to its active metabolite in the kidney. Rhabdomyolysis, tumor lysis, or massive hemolysis also results in hypocalcemia. Severe pancreatitis can lead to acute precipitation of calcium soaps in the abdominal cavity with resultant hypocalcemia.

11. **Name the causes of hyperkalemia.**
    Hyperkalemia may result from increased potassium load (e.g., tissue destruction due to rhabdomyolysis, hemolysis, gastrointestinal bleeding), decreased excretion of potassium (e.g., renal failure) or transcellular shift of potassium from inside cells to the extracellular matrix (e.g., lack of insulin, acidosis). Other important causes of hyperkalemia include blood

transfusions (red cell breakdown leads to hyperkalemia in stored banked blood) and medications (e.g., angiotensin-converting enzyme [ACE] inhibitors, beta blockers, digitalis, potassium-sparing diuretics).

12. **What is pseudohyperkalemia?**
Pseudohyperkalemia is an elevated measured serum potassium level with a normal, in vivo, plasma potassium concentration. Most commonly it results from traumatic hemolysis, with associated potassium leak, during venipuncture. Additionally, the prolonged use of a tourniquet and vigorous opening and closing of the hand prior to the blood draw can falsely elevate the measured potassium. All unexpected reports of hyperkalemia should prompt a repeat serum potassium measurement on a fresh blood draw. Patients with severely elevated white blood cell ($>50,000/mm^3$) or platelet counts ($>1,000,000/mm^3$) can have an artificially elevated potassium level due to cellular potassium release during clotting of the specimen. In these situations, a plasma potassium level should be measured from an unclotted blood specimen, such as with an arterial blood gas measurement.

13. **How can beta-blocker therapy contribute to hyperkalemia?**
Potassium enters cells via stimulation of the $beta_2$ receptor. $Beta_2$ blockade with a nonselective beta blocker, such as propranolol, blunts this defense to a potassium load.
Selective $beta_1$ receptor blockers, such as metoprolol, are much less likely to have this effect.

14. **Describe the treatment of hyperkalemia.**
Acute elevation of potassium to levels >5.5 mEq/L should be treated as a medical urgency. Chronic elevations of potassium levels, such as those seen in patients with end-stage renal failure before hemodialysis, are better tolerated and can be treated less urgently. Immediate steps to treat hyperkalemia should include close cardiac monitoring; stabilization of the cardiac conduction system with calcium gluconate or calcium chloride given intravenously; transcellular shift of potassium into cells with sodium bicarbonate and regular insulin given intravenously; and use of nebulized beta agonists (e.g., albuterol). The use of intravenous insulin should be administered with 50% dextrose (1–2 ampules) to avoid hypoglycemia. After initially stabilizing the patient by using transcellular shifts, steps are taken to remove potassium from the body. Potassium excretion can occur through the gut (i.e., Kayexylate [sodium polystyrene sulfonate]), via the kidney (e.g., furosemide), or with the use of hemodialysis. (See Chapter 48 for more details.)

15. **What are the signs, symptoms, and causes of hypokalemia?**
Hypokalemia, which can cause diffuse weakness, can result from decreased intake, increased losses, or transcellular shift of potassium. Potassium is most commonly lost from the gastrointestinal tract or through the kidney. Measurement of a urinary potassium level (>30 mEq/L favors urinary loss, assuming the patient is not on diuretic therapy) can help augment your clinical suspicion. Diarrhea is the most common cause of extrarenal potassium loss, whereas diuretic therapy is the most common cause of renal potassium loss. Increased insulin levels, the use of $beta_2$ agonists, and alkalosis all promote potassium entry into cells, resulting in hypokalemia. Hypomagnesemia is seen in 40% of patients with hypokalemia. Hypokalemia cannot be corrected if magnesium levels are not repleted.

16. **How much potassium does it take to correct a low potassium level?**
Serum potassium is a rough estimate of total body potassium stores. Hundreds of milliequivalents (mEq) are often necessary to correct serum potassium levels of <3.0 mEq/L. Frequent monitoring of the serum potassium level may be required during the repletion process.

17. **What are the most common causes of hypernatremia?**
Hypernatremia results from having more intravascular sodium than water. It is caused by either free water loss (e.g., osmotic diarrhea, diabetes insipidus) or administration of hypertonic saline (e.g., 3% NaCl solution). Hypernatremia leads to increased plasma osmolality, which stimulates antidiuretic hormone (ADH) release and thirst. Patients with an intact thirst drive and access to water dilute their plasma sodium concentrations with increased water intake. Patients with altered mental status or defects in their thirst drive due to hypothalamic lesions are at risk for hypernatremia. The most common cause of hypernatremia in a hospitalized patient is osmotic-induced (e.g., hyperglycemic) or diuretic-induced urinary water loss and gastrointestinal tract losses (e.g., vomiting, diarrhea). Additional causes include diabetes insipidus, hypertonic saline use, and sodium bicarbonate infusions.

18. **Describe the work-up of hypernatremia.**
The kidney responds to hypernatremia by conserving water. Thus, one would expect very concentrated urine in the face of hypernatremia. A urine osmolality >700 mEq/L is considered normal in the face of hypernatremia. If the urine osmolality is less than this, one should consider diabetes insipidus. Most patients with frank diabetes insipidus have urine osmolalities <300 mEq/L in the face of hypernatremia.

19. **Differentiate between central and nephrogenic diabetes insipidus.**
Diabetes insipidus results from a lack of ADH secretion (central) or a lack of kidney response to ADH (nephrogenic). Exogenous administration of ADH (desmopressin; DDAVP) will result in an appropriate increase in urine concentration in patients with central diabetes insipidus but not in those with nephrogenic diabetes insipidus. The chronic use of lithium can cause nephrogenic diabetes insipidus. The degree of free water wasting in nephrogenic diabetes insipidus can paradoxically be blunted by the use of thiazide diuretics.

20. **How is the free water deficit estimated in a patient with hypernatremia?**
$$\text{Free water deficit} = \text{total body water} \times [(\text{plasma Na} \div 140) - 1].$$

Total body water is approximately 50% of body weight.

Example : 80 kg man
Serum sodium = 168 mEq/L
Free water deficit = 40 L × [(168 mEq/L ÷ 140 mEq/L) − 1] = 8 L

KEY POINTS: ELECTROLYTE DERANGEMENTS

1. Hydrochlorothiazide use is a common cause of hyponatremia in the elderly.

2. In the work-up of hyponatremia, a low serum uric acid level suggests SIADH.

3. In the treatment of hyponatremia, the serum sodium level should never be increased >12 mEq/day and preferably <8 mEq/day, to lessen the risk of developing central pontine myelinolysis.

4. Thiazide diuretics can be used in the treatment of nephrogenic diabetes insipidus.

5. The combined finding of hypercalcemia and increased serum PTH level is seen only with primary and tertiary hyperparathyroidism, chronic lithium use, and familial hypercalcemic hypocalciuria.

21. **What is the maximal rate at which hypernatremia should be corrected?**

Rapid correction of hypernatremia can lead to cerebral edema, seizures, and permanent neurologic damage (see question 26). In general, the correction should occur no faster than a rate of 0.5 mEq/h or no more than 12 mEq/day. Patients with a rapid increase in serum sodium, however, can be corrected more rapidly if the clinical scenario warrants (e.g., recalcitrant seizures).

22. **What is the first step in the work-up of hyponatremia?**

The first step is to assess the serum osmolality. This can be estimated by the equation below but to properly classify hyponatremia, one must use the measured and not the calculated osmolarity. A measured serum osmolality less than normal is classified as hypotonic hyponatremia; higher than normal is hypertonic; and normal is termed isotonic. Example:

- Calculated serum osmolality $= 2\text{Na} + \{\text{glucose}/18\} + \{\text{blood urea nitrogen(BUN)}/2.8\}$

$$\text{Na} = 140 \text{ mEq/L}$$
$$\text{BUN} = 14$$
$$\text{Glucose} = 90$$

- Calculated serum osmolality $= 2(140) + 90/18 + 14/2.8 = 290 \text{ mEq/L}$

Normal serum tonicity is 290 mEq/L. Isotonic hyponatremia (i.e., pseudo-hyponatremia) is due to either hyperlipidemia or hyperproteinemia interfering with the laboratory test that measures serum sodium. Hypertonic hyponatremia is due to hyperglycemia or the administration of mannitol. For patients with hypotonic hyponatremia, one needs to evaluate their volume status to help them understand the nature of their hyponatremia.

23. **Describe the work-up of hypotonic hyponatremia.**

After confirmation of a low serum osmolality, check the urine osmolarity. Dilute urine (i.e., a urine osmolarity <100 mEq/L) confirms either psychogenic polydipsia or beer potomania. Once psychogenic polydipsia and beer potomania are ruled out, evaluate the patient's volume status by history and examination as well as blood and urine testing. Evaluate for signs of hypervolemia (e.g., pulmonary and lower extremity edema). The four causes of hypotonic *hypervolemic* hyponatremia are heart failure, chronic kidney disease, nephrotic syndrome, and cirrhosis.

If the patient is not hypervolemic, determine whether he or she is euvolemic or hypovolemic. Physical examination and lab findings, such as dry mucous membranes, orthostasis, urine sodium <20 mEq/L, serum BUN/creatinine ratio >20:1, and a normal or elevated serum uric acid level all support the diagnosis of hypovolemia. Hypotonic *hypovolemic* hyponatremia is caused by volume loss that is replaced with excess free water but not sodium. Measurement of urinary sodium excretion can help make a diagnosis. Patients with extrarenal losses (e.g., volume depletion from diarrhea or vomiting) have <20 mEq/L of urine sodium. Patients with renal sodium loss (e.g., due to diuretics, ACE inhibitors, mineralocorticoid deficiency, nephropathies or cerebral sodium wasting syndrome) have >20 mEq/L of urine sodium.

Urine sodium testing is often invalid in the presence of diuretic therapy. A normal serum BUN/creatinine ratio of 10:1, a urine sodium >40 mEq/L and a low serum uric acid level would support a euvolemic state. Most cases of hypotonic *euvolemic* hyponatremia are caused by the syndrome of inappropriate antidiuretic hormone (SIADH). Causes of SIADH include malignancy, lung pathology (e.g., tuberculosis, pneumonia), medications (e.g., carbamazepine, opiates), nausea, and central nervous system disease (e.g., meningitis). Severe hypothyroidism and frank adrenal insufficiency can, by laboratory parameters, also appear to be consistent with SIADH. The rare syndrome of cerebral salt wasting can have laboratory parameters that suggest euvolemia (i.e., low serum uric acid and urine sodium >40 mEq/L) and thus SIADH. However, these patients are hypovolemic and require saline therapy, not fluid restriction as one would use in SIADH.

24. **Describe the correction of serum sodium levels in the presence of hyperglycemia.**

For every 100 mg/dL the glucose is above 100 mg/dL, add 1.6 mEq/L to the measured serum sodium. For example, the corrected serum sodium for a patient with a glucose measurement of 600 mg/dL and measured serum sodium of 130 mEq/L is 138 mEq/L.

25. **How is hypotonic hyponatremia treated?**

The treatment of cases of hypotonic hyponatremia can be inferred from an understanding of the type of sodium/water imbalance present.

■ **Hypovolemic hypotonic hyponatremia:** This imbalance results from a loss of more sodium than water. For example, diarrheic patients lose more sodium than water in their stool. Consequently, they need repletion with both sodium and water, in the form of normal saline (0.9% NaCl in water).

■ **Euvolemic hypotonic hyponatremia:** This results from a gain of water with no change in sodium. For example, SIADH results in retention of water without an effect on sodium. Consequently, the treatment is water restriction.

■ **Hypervolemic hypotonic hyponatremia:** This imbalance results from a gain of more water than sodium. For example, edematous states like congestive heart failure are associated with retention of water (ADH) and water and sodium (aldosterone) resulting in a total net gain of more water than sodium. Consequently, the treatment is water and sodium restriction plus sodium wasting from a loop diuretic.

26. **How is symptomatic hyponatremia treated? What is central pontine myelinolysis?**

Symptomatic hyponatremia usually refers to a state involving active delirium or seizures and requires treatment with hypertonic saline (3% saline). Furosemide, which dilutes urine, can be used in conjunction with hypertonic saline infusion to raise the serum sodium level acutely. By diluting the urine, the kidney is able to excrete more free water and thus more rapidly increase the serum sodium level. The patient's serum sodium should initially be corrected rapidly over a few hours, usually no more than 4 mEq/L. However, the total serum sodium correction should still not exceed a total of 8–12 mEq/day to decrease the risk of developing central pontine myelinolysis, a severe, commonly fatal, neurologic disease that is characterized by symmetric demyelination of the central pons. It classically presents several days to weeks after rapid correction of serum sodium and is seen most frequently in malnourished, alcoholic patients with liver disease. Clinical features include flaccid quadriplegia, respiratory paralysis, and coma. Magnetic resonance imaging is diagnostic and therapy is supportive. Measures to avoid central pontine myelinolysis include frequent assessment of serum sodium during correction and raising the serum sodium <12 mEq/L/day (preferably <8 mEq/L/day).

27. **Predict the serum sodium correction from hypertonic saline.**

One liter of intravenous fluid will raise the serum sodium concentration as follows:

$$[(\text{Na} + \text{K concentration of intravenous fluid}) - \text{present serum sodium concentration}] / (\text{total body water} + 1)$$

Example:

■ Serum sodium = 113 mEq/L

■ Patient weight = 78 kg, therefore total body water = 78 × 0.5 = 39 L

■ Hypertonic saline (3% saline) has a sodium concentration of 513 mEq /L and a potassium concentration of zero

■ One liter of hypertonic saline will increase this patient's serum sodium by: [(513 + 0) − 113]/ 39 + 1 = 400/40 = 10 mEq per liter given

■ Therefore, 1 L of hypertonic saline would increase this patient's serum sodium to 123 mEq/L; 500 cc would increase it to 118 mEq/L; every 100 cc would increase it 1 mEq/L.

CHAPTER 47

ACID–BASE DISORDERS

Cynthia A. Korzelius, MD, MSc

1. **How is the body's daily acid load eliminated?**
   Approximately 15,000 mmol of acid (H^+) are produced in the body each day. The kidneys eliminate 50–100 mmol of H^+ through combination with titratable acids (e.g., phosphate) or ammonia (NH_3). The lungs rid the body of 15,000 mmol of carbon dioxide (CO_2), 150 times the amount of acid removed by the kidneys. (Since CO_2 combines with water to form carbonic acid, H_2CO_3, it can be considered an acid.)

2. **What are the important ways the body minimizes pH changes?**
   The body has several mechanisms to correct pH toward normal (7.4). In the acute phase (minutes to hours), extracellular and intracellular buffer systems minimize pH changes. In the subacute phase (hours to days), renal or respiratory compensation restores pH toward normal. In the chronic phase, bone becomes a significant source of buffer. The most important buffer system for acute changes in acid–base balance is the bicarbonate (HCO_3^-) system:

$$H^+ + HCO_3^- \rightarrow H_2CO_3 \rightarrow CO_2 + H_2O$$

3. **Define acidemia, acidosis, alkalemia, and alkalosis, both metabolic and respiratory.**
   - **Acidemia:** A blood pH below the normal range of 7.35–7.45
   - **Acidosis:** A process that tends to lower blood pH
   - **Alkalemia:** A blood pH above the normal range of 7.35–7.45
   - **Alkalosis:** A process that tends to increase blood pH
   - **Metabolic disorder:** A disorder resulting from a primary alteration in H^+ or HCO_3^-
   - **Respiratory disorder:** A disorder resulting from a primary alteration in CO_2 elimination

4. **What are some signs and symptoms of an acid–base imbalance?**
   See Table 47-1.

TABLE 47-1. SIGNS AND SYMPTOMS OF SEVERE ACID–BASE IMBALANCE		
	Acidemia	**Alkalemia**
Cardiovascular	Impaired cardiac perfusion	Increased myocardial contractility
	Impaired cardiac output	Coronary vasospasm
	Hypotension	
	Arrhythmias	
Cerebral	Altered mental status	Altered mental status
		Myoclonus
		Asterixis
		Loss of consciousness

TABLE 47-1. SIGNS AND SYMPTOMS OF SEVERE ACID–BASE IMBALANCE—CONT'D

	Acidemia	Alkalemia
Respiratory	Hyperventilation	
	Muscle fatigue and	
	respiratory failure	
Metabolic	Hyperkalemia	Hyponatremia, hypokalemia,
		hypophosphatemia
	Death	Decreased ionized calcium
		Death

5. **What causes metabolic acidosis?**

   Metabolic acidosis results from either loss of HCO_3^- or addition of H^+. It is characterized by a primary decrease in the $[HCO_3^-]$ and a compensatory decrease in the pCO_2.

6. **What is the anion gap?**

   The body must always remain electrically neutral. In other words, the positive charges (cations) must equal the negative charges (anions). However, we do not usually measure all of these charges. The anion gap is the difference between *measured* cations and *measured* anions, and it is used to differentiate the two broad categories of acidosis: "gap" and "non-gap." It is calculated by the equation:

$$\text{Anion gap} = [Na^+] - [Cl^-] - [HCO_3^-]$$

   When the anion gap is larger than expected (usually because the concentration of measured anions decreases) we can assume there must be an equal amount of unmeasured anions offsetting this drop in measured anions. An increased anion gap acidosis occurs when the anion replacing the HCO_3^- is not one that is routinely measured. A normal or non-gap acidosis occurs when Cl^- replaces the HCO_3^- lost in buffering $H.^+$ A decreased anion gap may result either when there is an excess of unmeasured cations or a reduction in unmeasured anions (most commonly hypoalbuminemia). After finding an altered anion gap, the challenge becomes determining which unmeasured anion or cation accounts for the change from the predicted gap (Table 47-2).

TABLE 47-2. CAUSES OF INCREASED OR DECREASED ANION GAP

Increased Anion Gap	Decreased Anion Gap
Decreased unmeasured cations	Increased unmeasured cations
■ Hypocalcemia	■ Lithium toxicity
■ Hypokalemia	■ Hypermagnesemia
■ Hypomagnesemia	■ Cationic paraproteinemia (multiple myeloma)
Increased unmeasured anions	Decreased unmeasured anions
■ Hyperalbuminemia (hemoconcentration)	■ Hypoalbuminemia
■ Bromide intoxication	
■ Anion gap acidosis (see Table 47-3)	

KEY POINTS: FEATURES OF SIMPLE METABOLIC ACIDOSIS

1. pH < 7.4

2. $[HCO_3^-] < 24$ mmol/L due to loss of HCO_3^- or gain of H^+

3. $pCO_2 < 40$ mmHg due to respiratory compensation

4. Possible anion gap

5. Variable clinical presentation depending on etiology and severity

7. **Why is the serum albumin concentration important in interpretation of the anion gap?**
The anion gap is typically three times the albumin concentration (in milligrams per deciliter) or about 12 mEq/L. Because the negative charges on albumin result in much of the usual anion gap, hypoalbuminemic patients have a lower baseline anion gap, which could mask a gap acidosis. For example, if a patient has a serum albumin of 2 mg/dL, his usual anion gap would be approximately 6 mEq/L. Thus, an anion gap of 12 mEq/L in this patient would be elevated and should prompt a search for an unmeasured anion.

8. **What is the differential diagnosis for anion gap acidosis, and what is the unmeasured anion in each condition?**
MUDPILES (Table 47-3) is a useful mnemonic for the differential diagnosis of anion gap acidosis.

TABLE 47-3. DIFFERENTIAL DIAGNOSIS FOR ANION GAP ACIDOSIS	
Cause	**Unmeasured Anion**
Methanol intoxication	Formate
Uremia	Sulfates, phosphates, urates, hippurate
Diabetic ketoacidosis	β-hydroxybutyrate, acetoacetate
Paraldehyde intoxication	Organic anions
Iron, isoniazid	Lactate
Lactic acidosis	Lactate
Ethylene glycol intoxication	Oxalate, glycolate
Salicylates	Lactate

9. **What is the differential diagnosis for a non–anion gap acidosis? What is the pathogenesis of each cause?**
In general, non–anion gap acidosis is due to either the loss of HCO_3^- from the kidney or gut, an impaired ability to excrete H^+, or the addition of H^+ (Table 47-4).

TABLE 47-4. DIFFERENTIAL DIAGNOSIS FOR NON–ANION GAP ACIDOSIS	
Diagnosis	**Pathogenesis of Acidosis**
Diarrhea	Gastrointestinal loss of HCO_3^-
Biliary or pancreatic drainage	Gastrointestinal loss of HCO_3^-
Renal tubular acidosis	Renal loss of HCO_3^- or inability to excrete H^+
Renal failure	Impaired ammoniagenesis or inability to excrete H^+
Carbonic anhydrase inhibitors	Renal loss of HCO_3^- from the proximal tubule
Urinary diversion to gut	Exchange of urinary Cl^- for HCO_3^- in colon, absorption of urinary ammonium (NH_4^+)
Acid load	Addition of acid such as HCl, lysine HCl, arginine HCl, NH_4Cl

10. **What is the urine anion gap, and how is it used clinically?**

$$\text{Urine anion gap} = \text{urinary } ([Na^+] + [K^+]) - \text{urinary } [Cl^-]$$

The urine anion gap may be helpful in distinguishing between renal and nonrenal etiologies of a non–anion gap acidosis because it is a surrogate measure of urinary ammonium (NH_4^+). Usually NH_4^+ (the major unmeasured urinary cation) is accompanied by the measured anion Cl^-, and the urine anion gap is slightly positive. In metabolic acidosis, due to gastrointestinal HCO_3^- loss, urinary NH_4^+ and accompanying Cl^- increase substantially, resulting in a negative urine anion gap. However, in cases of impaired renal ammoniagenesis, as in types 1 and 4 renal tubular acidosis (RTA), there is less urinary NH_4^+, and thus less chloride, and the gap remains slightly positive in the setting of a non–anion gap acidosis. The urine anion gap should not be used in a patient with serum anion gap acidosis or severe volume depletion.

11. **What is renal tubular acidosis (RTA)?**
RTA describes either a renal defect of proximal tubular bicarbonate reclamation or a defect in acid excretion due to impaired ammoniagenesis or excretion of H^+. A tiny amount of acid is excreted as free protons and is measured as the urine pH; however, most acid is excreted as NH_4^+. Urine pH may provide a clue to the nature or location of the tubular defect but provides no information regarding the magnitude of the problem.

12. **What features distinguish the types of RTA?**
- **Type 1 (distal) RTA:** Characterized by a defect in H^+ excretion in the distal tubule, type 1 RTA results in elevated urine pH, an inability to excrete the daily acid load, and systemic acidosis that may be severe as acid accumulates over time. Type 1 RTA results from one of three possible defects in distal hydrogen ion secretion: decreased proton pump activity (H^+-adenosinetriphosphatase), back leak of H^+ due to increased membrane permeability, or diminished distal tubular sodium resorption that reduces the electric gradient for proton secretion. There is often significant potassium loss in the urine, resulting in hypokalemia.
- **Type 2 (proximal) RTA:** This type of RTA results from defective proximal tubular HCO_3^- resorption from one of several mechanisms leading to urinary HCO_3^- wasting. It may be

associated with Fanconi syndrome with concurrent proximal tubular wasting of glucose, phosphate, amino acid, and uric acid. The acidosis tends to be mild because once a sufficient decrease in filtered bicarbonate occurs, all of the filtered bicarbonate can then be resorbed. Also, the distal nephron may resorb bicarbonate. Because H^+ excretion in the distal tubule is preserved, the urine pH may be low. Potassium wasting and hypokalemia are variable in type 2 RTA and may be worsened by bicarbonate treatment.

- **Type 4 (distal) RTA:** Commonly seen in diabetic patients, type 4 RTA is usually mild and results from hypoaldosteronism. Hyperkalemia, resulting from decreased aldosterone effect in the distal tubule, helps to distinguish type 4 from types 1 and 2 RTA, which are usually associated with hypokalemia.

Features of RTA in untreated patients in the presence of acidosis are summarized in Table 47-5.

13. **What are some clinical consequences of chronic metabolic acidosis?**
   Chronic acidosis causes bone loss due to marked bone buffering of unexcreted acid and may cause hyperkalemia due to transcellular shift. Additionally, chronic acidosis leads to a diminished capacity to handle an additional acid load (decreased reserves).

14. **What are the risks of treatment with sodium bicarbonate?**
   The risks include volume overload from the sodium load, hypokalemia, increased pCO_2 from H^+ buffering, tissue hypoxia (via leftward shift of hemoglobin-oxygen dissociation curve), stimulation of organic acidosis (lactate), decreased ionized calcium, and postrecovery alkalosis.

15. **What clinical entities cause metabolic alkalosis? How is it treated?**
   Metabolic alkalosis is most commonly initiated by volume depletion (contraction alkalosis), loss of gastric secretions (loss of hydrogen ion), or ingestion of alkali (retention of bicarbonate) (Table 47-6). Once present, alkalosis is often sustained by circulating volume and chloride depletion, increased aldosterone secretion, and hypokalemia. In volume- and chloride-depleted states, HCO_3^- resorption will accompany Na^+ resorption to maintain systemic electric neutrality. Therefore, the treatment of metabolic alkalosis in volume-depleted states requires correction of chloride and volume depletion to enable the kidney to excrete excess bicarbonate. Treatment of hypokalemia is also essential. In severe cases where volume expansion is contraindicated, renal excretion of bicarbonate may be facilitated by the use of carbonic anhydrase inhibitors. Hyperaldosteronism (as in Cushing's and Conn's syndromes) causes a non–chloride responsive metabolic alkalosis. Excess aldosterone causes increased sodium reclamation in the distal tubule, generating an electronegative tubular lumen favoring H^+ and K^+ excretion in the urine.

KEY POINTS: FEATURES OF SIMPLE METABOLIC ALKALOSIS

1. pH > 7.4

2. $[HCO_3^-]$ > 24 mmol/L due to gain of HCO_3^- or loss of H^+

3. pCO_2 > 40 mmHg due to respiratory compensation

4. Variable clinical presentation depending on etiology and severity

TABLE 47-5. FEATURES OF RENAL TUBULAR ACIDOSIS IN UNTREATED PATIENTS IN THE PRESENCE OF ACIDOSIS

Type	Urine pH	Serum K+	Serum [HCO3−]	Mechanism	Causes
Type 1 (distal)	>5.5	Low	May be <10 mmol/L	Impaired distal acidification	Familial, Sjögren's syndrome, rheumatoid arthritis
Type 2 (proximal)	Variable, <5.5 in steady state	Low or high	12–20 mmol/L	Decreased proximal HCO3− resorption	Cystinosis, Wilson's disease, multiple myeloma, carbonic anhydrase inhibitors, exposure to heavy metals
Type 4 (distal)	<5.5	High	Mildly decreased, usually >17 mmol/L	Hypoaldosteronism	Adrenal insufficiency, diabetic nephropathy, drugs

K+ = potassium, HCO3− = bicarbonate.

TABLE 47-6.	CAUSES OF METABOLIC ALKALOSIS
Chloride Responsive	Vomiting or nasogastric drainage
	Diuretics (loop and thiazide)
	Posthypercapnic states
Chloride Unresponsive	Severe magnesium or potassium depletion
	Hypermineralocorticoidism (Cushing's syndrome, primary hyperaldosteronism, renal artery stenosis)
	Glycyrrhetinic acid (chewing tobacco, licorice)
	Inherited renal disorders (Bartter and Gitelman's syndromes)

16. **What is the differential diagnosis for respiratory acidosis?**
    Respiratory acidosis is caused by alveolar hypoventilation with retention of CO_2. Table 47-7 lists some causes of this disorder.

TABLE 47-7.	CAUSES OF RESPIRATORY ACIDOSIS
Acute	Central nervous system depression
	Paralysis of respiratory muscles
	Airway obstruction
	Respiratory failure
Chronic	Chronic obstructive pulmonary disease
	Extreme obesity
	Chest wall deformity

KEY POINTS: FEATURES OF SIMPLE RESPIRATORY ACIDOSIS

1. pH < 7.4

2. pCO_2 > 40 mmHg due to primary hypoventilation

3. $[HCO_3^-]$ > 24 mmol/L due to renal compensation

4. Magnitude of renal compensation depends on whether acute or chronic

17. **What is the differential diagnosis for respiratory alkalosis?**
    Respiratory alkalosis is caused by alveolar hyperventilation with loss of CO_2. Table 47-8 lists some causes of this disorder.

TABLE 47-8. CAUSES OF RESPIRATORY ALKALOSIS

Category	Specific Causes
Central nervous system	Pain, hyperventilation, anxiety, psychosis, fever, stroke, infection, tumor, trauma
Hypoxemia	High altitude, anemia, right-to-left shunt
Drugs	Progesterone, methylxanthines, salicylates, catecholamines, nicotine
Endocrine	Pregnancy, hyperthyroidism
Stimulation of chest receptors	Pneumothorax, hemothorax, pulmonary edema, pulmonary embolism, aspiration, interstitial lung disease
Miscellaneous	Sepsis, hepatic failure, mechanical ventilation

KEY POINTS: FEATURES OF SIMPLE RESPIRATORY ALKALOSIS

1. pH > 7.4

2. pCO_2 < 40 mmHg due to primary hyperventilation

3. $[HCO_3^-]$ < 24 mmol/L due to renal compensation

4. Magnitude of renal compensation depends on whether acute or chronic

18. **How should one analyze the acid–base status of a patient?**
    The acid–base status can be determined using the following seven-step process:
    - **Step 1:** Gather relevant data: arterial or venous blood gas (for pH and pCO_2), $[Na^+]$, $[Cl^-]$, $[HCO_3^-]$, serum albumin. Calculate the anion gap, accounting for hypoalbuminemia if present.
    - **Step 2:** Determine whether the pH is acidemic (<7.4) or alkalemic (>7.4).
    - **Step 3:** Determine whether the primary disturbance is respiratory or metabolic by checking the pCO_2 and $[HCO_3^-]$ (Table 47-9).
    - **Step 4:** If there is a respiratory disturbance, is it acute or chronic? Use compensation formulas to estimate expected $[HCO_3^-]$ change and compare with the measured $[HCO_3^-]$ (Table 47-10).
    - **Step 5:** If there is a metabolic disturbance, is there an increased anion gap? If the anion gap is elevated, a metabolic acidosis is almost certainly present regardless of the pH or $[HCO_3^-]$.
    - **Step 6:** Are there other metabolic processes concurrent with the anion gap acidosis? Determine whether the anion gap acidosis alone accounts for the decrease in $[HCO_3^-]$ by calculating the $[HCO_3^-]$ "corrected" for decline due to anion gap acidosis alone.
      1. Subtract 12 (the average anion gap) from calculated anion gap to estimate the increase in anion gap due to the gap acidosis alone.
      2. Add this difference to the measured $[HCO_3^-]$ to estimate what $[HCO_3^-]$ "would be" without the gap acidosis, i.e., the "corrected" $[HCO_3^-]$.

3. If the corrected $[HCO_3^-] > 26$ mmol/L, then a metabolic alkalosis coexists.
4. If the corrected $[HCO_3^-]$ is 22–26 mmol/L, then no other metabolic disturbance coexists.
5. If the corrected $[HCO_3^-] < 22$ mmol/L, then a non-gap metabolic acidosis coexists.
- **Step 7:** Is the respiratory system compensating adequately for a metabolic disturbance? Use compensation formulas to determine the expected pCO_2 changes (Table 47-11).
  1. If the measured $pCO_2 >$ expected pCO_2, then a respiratory acidosis coexists.
  2. If the measured $pCO_2 <$ expected pCO_2, then a respiratory alkalosis coexists.

TABLE 47-9. IS THE PRIMARY DISTURBANCE RESPIRATORY OR METABOLIC?

Disorder	pH	pCO₂ (mmHg)	[HCO₃⁻] (mmol/L)
Metabolic acidosis	<7.4		<24
Metabolic alkalosis	>7.4		>24
Respiratory acidosis	<7.4	>40	
Respiratory alkalosis	>7.4	<40	

TABLE 47-10. IS THE RESPIRATORY DISTURBANCE ACUTE OR CHRONIC?

	Acute	Chronic
Respiratory Acidosis	$[HCO_3^-]$ increases 0.10 mmol/L for each 1 mmHg increase in pCO_2	$[HCO_3^-]$ increases 0.35 mmol/L for each 1 mmHg increase in pCO_2
Respiratory Alkalosis	$[HCO_3^-]$ decreases 0.22 mmol/L for each 1 mmHg decrease in pCO_2	$[HCO_3^-]$ decreases 0.5 mmol/L for each 1 mmHg decrease in pCO_2

TABLE 47-11. COMPENSATION FORMULAS FOR EXPECTED CHANGE IN PCO₂ IN METABOLIC DISTURBANCE

Metabolic Disturbance	Expected Change in pCO₂
Metabolic Acidosis	pCO_2 decreases 1.2 for each 1 mmol/L decrease in $[HCO_3^-]$ or $pCO_2 = 1.5[HCO_3^-] + 8$ (Winter's formula) (Shortcut: pCO_2 = last two digits of pH)
Metabolic Alkalosis	pCO_2 increases 0.6 for each 1 mmol/L increase in $[HCO_3^-]$

KEY POINTS: GENERAL FEATURES OF ACID–BASE BALANCE

1. Decreased [HCO_3^-] may represent either an acidosis or compensation for respiratory alkalosis, thus interpretation of a patient's acid–base balance requires a blood gas.

2. Regardless of the [HCO_3^-], the presence of an anion gap suggests an anion gap acidosis.

3. It is important to understand that compensatory mechanisms do not represent another metabolic disorder.

4. The urine anion gap can help to distinguish between renal and nonrenal causes of a non–anion gap acidosis.

5. RTA may result from either proximal loss of bicarbonate, inability to excrete protons, impaired ammoniagenesis, or hypoaldosteronism.

CHAPTER 48

CARE OF THE INPATIENT DIALYSIS PATIENT

Mark B. Reid, MD, and Scott E. Clemens, MD

1. **How many Americans receive hemodialysis?**
   In the year 2002 (when the most recent data was published by the United States Renal Data System), approximately 91,000 Americans began hemodialysis. Of the 431,000 total patients who required renal replacement therapies, including all forms of dialysis and transplants, approximately 282,000 were receiving hemodialysis.

2. **When did we first start to use chronic dialysis for patients with end-stage renal disease (ESRD)?**
   Although it has been possible to get hemodialysis for acute renal failure since the 1940s, chronic hemodialysis was not offered as a treatment for ESRD until the 1960s. The spread of chronic dialysis centers in the United States followed a 1972 law that required Medicare payment of 80% of the cost of dialysis.

3. **Is hemodialysis a permanent solution for treating ESRD?**
   Although chronic dialysis keeps many people alive who would otherwise have died from renal failure, it is far from an ideal form of treatment. Hemodialysis requires thrice weekly visits to the dialysis center for about 4 hours. It results in imperfect management of volume and electrolytes, requiring patients to adhere to a low-potassium and fluid-restricted diet. Many patients feel exhausted immediately after their dialysis treatments and tired for the remainder of that day.

4. **What is the most common cause of death in patients on chronic hemodialysis? What is the life expectancy of a patient on dialysis?**
   The most common cause of death of patients receiving chronic hemodialysis treatment is coronary artery disease, followed by infection. Patients on hemodialysis, irrespective of the cause of their chronic renal failure, are 10–20 times more likely to die from coronary artery disease than age-matched control subjects. More than half of patients started on chronic dialysis will die within the first 5 years (Fig. 48-1).

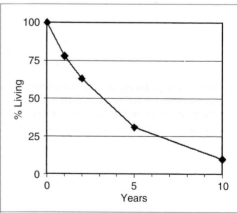

Figure 48-1. Unadjusted survival rates of patients on hemodialysis. Data from http://www.usrds.org/reference.htm.

5. **What is a "renal diet"?**
   A renal diet is a general set of guidelines to minimize buildup of excess volume and certain

electrolytes. It limits sodium to <2 gm/day and the total volume of fluid consumed to <6 cups/day. It is also low in potassium and phosphorus. Foods high in potassium that should be limited include salt substitute (which is often potassium chloride), oranges, bananas, watermelon, potatoes, milk, raisins, tomatoes, and cantaloupe. Foods high in phosphorus include milk, nuts, and colas. Patients on dialysis are recommended to maintain their intake of high-quality protein such as meat, fish, poultry, and egg whites.

National Kidney and Urologic Diseases Information Clearinghouse: Eat right to feel right on hemodialysis. Available at: http://kidney.niddk.nih.gov/kudiseases/pubs/eatright/index.htm.

6. **Why is it important to control hyperphosphatemia in hemodialysis patients?**
Hyperphosphatemia is common in patients receiving hemodialysis because phosphorus is excreted by the kidney. Treatment of hyperphosphatemia with calcium carbonate or phosphate binders helps halt secondary hyperparathyroidism, a disease that results in bone loss. Elevated levels of phosphorous, albumin-corrected calcium, calcium-phosphorus product ($Ca \times PO_4 > 60$), and parathyroid hormone are associated with increased all-cause and cardiovascular mortality.

Young EW, Akiba T, Albert JM, et al: Magnitude and impact of abnormal mineral metabolism in hemodialysis patients in the Dialysis Outcomes and Practice Patterns Study (DOPPS). Am J Kidney Dis 44 (5 Suppl 2):34–38, 2004.

7. **What blood pressure goals are reasonable in patients receiving hemodialysis?**
The majority of patients receiving hemodialysis have significant hypertension, and many have diabetes. Patients with ESRD are at high risk for myocardial infarction and stroke, which necessitates aggressive blood pressure control. However, in practice, *overly* aggressive blood pressure control may cause some patients to become significantly hypotensive at the end of dialysis and thereby limit the amount of volume that can be removed. Hypotension is also a potential risk factor for mortality in patients receiving hemodialysis. In the end, good clinical judgment must be used when administering antihypertensive medications to this patient population. The physician must sometimes tolerate less-than-ideal blood pressure in patients who are known to become hypotensive during dialysis, and the practicing hospitalist becomes accustomed to observing this behavior among nephrologists.

8. **What is the difference between an arteriovenous (AV) fistula and an AV graft?**
Both are surgical AV connections used to access a patient's blood for hemodialysis. An AV fistula is created by connecting an artery directly to a vein—commonly the radial artery and the cephalic vein in the forearm or the brachial artery and the cephalic vein above the elbow. A graft involves connecting the artery to the vein via a polytetrafluoroethylene (GoreTex) tube. Both fistulas and grafts require a period of "maturation" before they can be used for hemodialysis. Grafts can be used sooner after creation than fistulas, although they tend not to be as durable over time and are more prone to infection.

9. **Which drugs are either contraindicated or require significant dose adjustments for patients receiving hemodialysis?**
Many medications require dose adjustment in ESRD (Table 48-1). It is always valuable to refer to a respected reference (such as *Physicians' Desk Reference* or *The Sanford Guide to Antimicrobial Therapy*) or to consult an inpatient pharmacist when questions arise regarding medication use or dose adjustments for patients with renal failure.

10. **Which blood tests are affected by ESRD and/or hemodialysis?**
   - **D-dimer test:** The results of this test tend to be elevated in hemodialysis patients without thromboembolism, but a negative test result retains its powerful value in ruling out venous thromboembolism.
   - **Lipase test:** Results of this test can be elevated up to five times the normal level in patients with chronic renal failure who are receiving hemodialysis and do not have pancreatitis.

TABLE 48-1. PARTIAL REVIEW OF MEDICATION USE IN RENAL FAILURE

Contraindicated	Require Significant Dose Adjustments	Usually Safe Without Dose Adjustment
Low-molecular-weight heparins*	Digoxin	NSAIDs
Metformin increases risk of lactic acidosis	In general, all antibiotics except macrolides	
Magnesium citrate	Lithium	Glucocorticoids
Meperidine can cause seizures	Insulin	Warfarin
	Sulfonylureas can cause significant hypoglycemia	Macrolides
	KCl	
	K-Phos	
	H₂ blockers	
	IV fluids due to volume overload	
	Allopurinol	

NSAIDs = nonsteroidal anti-inflammatory drugs, IV = intravenous, KCl = potassium chloride, K-Phos = potassium phosphate.
* Can be used if dose is adjusted according to factor Xa levels.

- **Troponin I test:** This test for cardiac muscle injury is *not* significantly affected by chronic renal failure or hemodialysis. It is not appropriate to dismiss positive or indeterminate troponin I test results due to "renal failure."

11. **What are the indications for emergent hemodialysis?**
    - Severe hyperkalemia with electrocardiographic (ECG) changes; changes may include peaked T waves, flat P waves, prolonged PR interval, and wide QRS complex
    - Volume overload with significant compromise of ventilation or oxygenation
    - Severe uremia with symptoms or signs including uremic encephalopathy (altered level of consciousness) or uremic pericarditis (pericardial friction rub)
    - Bleeding diathesis due to qualitative platelet abnormalities (due to uremia) not resolved by conventional means including administration of DDAVP (desmopressin)
    - Severe metabolic acidosis ($HCO_3 < 10$).

KEY POINTS: INDICATIONS FOR EMERGENT DIALYSIS

1. Severe hyperkalemia with ECG changes

2. Severe volume overload with compromise of ventilation or oxygenation

3. Severe uremia with symptoms or signs including uremic encephalopathy or uremic pericarditis

4. Bleeding diathesis not resolved by conventional means

5. Severe metabolic acidosis

12. **What are the classic physical findings associated with hyperkalemia?**
Although patients with hyperkalemia may occasionally experience weakness or flaccid paralysis, most patients with elevated potassium levels have neither signs nor symptoms of their electrolyte imbalance. This remains true even up to deadly levels of hyperkalemia and is especially true of patients who develop hyperkalemia slowly, as is often the case with patients receiving hemodialysis. Patients who gradually develop hyperkalemia typically can tolerate higher potassium levels and will not show characteristic ECG changes until the level is significantly higher than their baseline.

13. **Describe the treatment of hyperkalemia.**
See Table 48-2.

14. **For a patient on chronic hemodialysis, what laboratory test do you need to check *before* giving calcium for elevated potassium?**
Patients receiving hemodialysis often have chronically elevated phosphorus and low calcium levels. The elevated phosphorus may make these patients susceptible to precipitation of calcium-phosphorus complexes (e.g., calciphylaxis, *see below*) if their serum calcium concentration is raised acutely through intravenous administration. The physician must weigh the risks of calciphylaxis with the benefits of cardiac myocyte membrane stabilization that come from administration of calcium. Using other maneuvers to lower the patient's potassium level is often preferable to administration of intravenous calcium in patients with ESRD.

15. **What is calciphylaxis? How is it different from metastatic calcification?**
Metastatic calcification is a chronic condition common in patients with ESRD resulting in deposition of calcium in soft tissues. Calciphylaxis is a rare, acute, and severe form of metastatic calcification characterized by abrupt onset of skin ischemia and necrosis after a minor trauma. It results in nonhealing skin wounds that frequently become infected. Although you may hear on rounds that you can easily identify patients at risk based upon their "calcium-phosphorus product" ($Ca \times PO_4 > 60$), it is clear from the recent literature that the calcium-phosphorus product is not a discriminating diagnostic test. Patients with a high product frequently do not get calciphylaxis, whereas patients with a product under 60 can still develop this entity. There are multiple other risk factors for the development of calciphylaxis including a low albumin level, female sex, and an elevated alkaline phosphatase level.

Mazhar AR, Johnson RJ, Gillen D, et al: Risk factors and mortality associated with calciphylaxis in end-stage renal disease. Kidney Int 60:324–332, 2001.

16. **How does uremia affect hemostasis?**
The true reason why uremic patients bleed more easily continues to be a point of debate, although the fact that they bleed more easily is well established. Candidate causes include abnormal platelet-vessel interaction caused by altered von Willebrand factor and abnormal production of nitric oxide caused by increased guanidinosuccinic acid, among others. The bleeding tendency in uremic patients can be temporarily corrected through the administration of desmopressin (DDAVP), which causes release of factor VIII:vWF multimers from the endothelium, although this drug is usually only effective with the first dose. Dialysis is the only true way to correct the physiologic abnormalities leading to bleeding in uremia. Transfusion of platelets has not been shown to be effective.

DeLoughery TG: Management of bleeding with uremia and liver disease. Curr Opin Hematol 6:329–333, 1999.

17. **How are vascular access infections managed?**
Central venous catheters get infected much more commonly than grafts and fistulas. It is very uncommon for fistulas to get infected. Bacteria may adhere to the inner lumen of the catheter or infect the soft tissues surrounding the catheter. The latter are known as *tunneled infections* and

TABLE 48-2. TREATMENT OF HYPERKALEMIA: RANKED BY USUAL ORDER OF CONSIDERATION

Intervention	Effect on K$^+$	Mechanism	Time Course
1. IV calcium gluconate (1 amp)	None	Stabilization of the cardiac myocyte membrane	Onset: minutes Duration: minutes
2. Insulin 10 units IV plus glucose (1 amp of D50 IV)	Redistribute	Increased uptake of K$^+$ into cells through the Na-K-ATPase pump in skeletal muscle	Onset: 15 minutes Peak: 60 minutes Duration: hours
3. Oral sodium polystyrene sulfonate (Kayexalate)	Remove	Binds K$^+$ in the gut while releasing Na$^+$, also induces diarrhea	Onset: variable based on gut transit time; typically, potassium is not lowered until patient develops diarrhea Duration: hours to days
4. Hemodialysis	Remove	Concentration gradient	Onset: minutes (but requires IV access, a dialysis machine, a nephrologist, and a tech) Duration: variable (generally hours to days)
5. IV sodium bicarbonate (in severe metabolic acidosis)	Redistribute	Alkalinization of blood resulting in exchange of protons in cells for potassium in serum	Onset: 30–60 minutes Duration: hours
6. Furosemide (if the patient is still making urine)	Remove	Impaired K$^+$, Na$^+$, Cl$^-$ reabsorption in the loop of Henle	Onset: hours Duration: hours to days
7. Beta agonists (in true emergency situations or when IV access is not available)	Redistribute	Increased uptake of K$^+$ into cells through Na-K-ATPase	Peak: IV epinephrine, 30 minutes; nebulized albuterol, 90 minutes Duration: minutes to hours

IV = intravenous, D50 = 50% dextrose solution, Na = sodium, K = potassium, ATPase = adenosine triphosphatase, Cl = chloride.

exit-site infections. Gram-positive organisms predominate, but gram-negative infection can also occur. It is essential to draw cultures from the dialysis catheter as well as peripheral sites before antibiotics are given. Empiric antibiotics must include coverage of methicillin-resistant *Staphylococcus aureus* due to its high incidence in this patient population. It is always prudent to discuss removal of the dialysis catheter with the nephrologist before removing lines unless the patient is hypotensive and septic. Treatment of dialysis catheter infections without removal of the line is only successful about one-third of the time, but it presents a low risk of complications and is therefore often the initial approach.

BIBLIOGRAPHY

1. Levey AS: Clinical practice: Nondiabetic kidney disease. N Engl J Med 347:1505–1511, 2002.
2. Rahman M, Smith MC: Chronic renal insufficiency: A diagnostic and therapeutic approach. Arch Intern Med 158:1743–1752, 1998.
3. Yu HT: Progression of chronic renal failure. Arch Intern Med 163:1417–1429, 2003.

CHAPTER 49

FLUID MANAGEMENT

Bradley A. Sharpe, MD

1. **What percentage of your body weight is water?**
   Water makes up approximately 60% of the total body weight in men and 50% in women.

2. **How is water distributed in the body?**
   The total body water in humans is distributed between the intracellular fluid (ICF) and extracellular fluid (ECF) compartments (Fig. 49-1). Approximately two thirds of the total body water is intracellular and one third is extracellular. Within the extracellular space, approximately 20–30% of the water is intravascular (within the blood vessels of the body) and 70–80% is extravascular (in the interstitium).

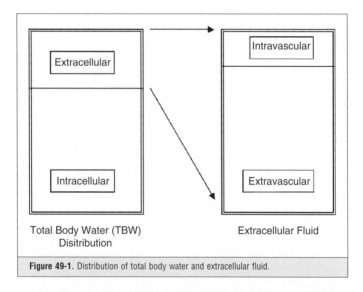

Figure 49-1. Distribution of total body water and extracellular fluid.

3. **What is the volume of blood in the average 70-kg man?**
   There is approximately 5 L of total blood volume in the average 70-kg man.

4. **Describe the different avenues by which water is lost from the body.**
   Water is lost from the body by sensible and insensible pathways.
   - **Sensible losses:** Those that can be *sensed* and measured (e.g., the volume of water that is lost in urine output).
   - **Insensible losses:** Those that are not measured, consisting of skin (sweat and convective loss), respiratory (evaporation), and gastrointestinal (fecal) losses.

5. **How much fluid does the average human need in a day?**
Humans must take in a volume of water equivalent to their sensible and insensible losses to maintain homeostasis. An average healthy human taking part in normal daily activities will require approximately 2–3 L of fluid intake daily.

6. **Describe the components and costs of the standard intravenous solutions.**
See Tables 49-1 and 49-2.

TABLE 49-1.   COMPOSITION OF COMMON INTRAVENOUS SOLUTIONS

Solution	Na$^+$	K$^+$	Cl$^-$	Ca^{2+}	Lactate	Glucose	Albumin
NS	154	0	154	0	0	0	0
LR	130	4	109	3	28	0	0
½ NS	77	0	77	0	0	0	0
3% NS	513	0	513	0	0	0	0
D$_5$W	0	0	0	0	0	50	0
D$_5$½NS	77	0	77	0	0	50	0
5% Albumin	130–160	0	130–160	0	0	0	50

Note: [ ] of glucose and albumin is gm/L; others are mEq/L.
NS = normal saline (0.9% concentration of NaCl), LR = lactated Ringer's solution, ½ NS = one half normal saline (0.45% concentration of NaCl), 3%NS = hypertonic saline (3% concentration of NaCl), D$_5$W = 5% dextrose in water, D$_5$½NS = 5% dextrose in half-normal saline, 5% albumin = 5% concentration of albumin in normal saline.

TABLE 49-2.   COSTS OF COMMON INTRAVENOUS SOLUTIONS*

Solution	Cost per Liter
NS	$0.87
LR	$1.03
5% albumin	$67.40

NS = normal saline, LR = lactated Ringer's solution 5% albumin = 5% concentration of human albumin in normal saline.
*Costs are representative and presented for comparison only. Actual costs may vary.

7. **Why do we not give patients pure water intravenously?**
The normal osmolarity of body fluid is approximately 280 mOsm/L. Administration of pure water, with an osmolarity of 0 mOsm/L, would result in rapid diffusion of water across cell membranes to equalize the osmolarity. The fluid influx would result in hemolysis and death of vascular endothelial and other cells. All intravenous fluids must contain a solute in addition to water (e.g., sodium chloride, dextrose).

8. **Why add 5% dextrose to standard intravenous solutions (rather than 10% or 20%)?**
   Five percent dextrose provides most of the carbohydrate needs of the average human to prevent cellular catabolism and muscle breakdown.

9. **How much fluid remains intravascularly when we administer 1 L of normal saline (NS) or lactated Ringer's solution (LR)?**
   Both NS and LR are approximately iso-osmotic with the blood (osmolarity $\cong$ 280–300 mOsm/L). Therefore, when NS or LR is administered intravascularly, the fluid volume is distributed like all ECF. The ECF is 20–30% intravascular and 70–80% extravascular. Therefore, with 1 L of NS or LR, only 200–300 mL of fluid remains intravascularly.

10. **How much fluid remains intravascularly when we administer 1 L of 5% dextrose in water (D_5W)?**
    D_5W is composed of dextrose and water, which are distributed by cellular uptake and diffusion in the ICF and the ECF. Total body water is divided into two thirds ICF and one third ECF. In 1 L of D_5W, approximately 330 mL will be extracellular. And yet the ECF is divided between the intravascular (20–30%) and extravascular (70–80%) space. Thus, only 65–100 mL of 1 L of D_5W will remain intravascular (20–30% of 330 mL).

11. **Describe the difference between crystalloid and colloid.**
    Crystalloids are fluids that contain only water and electrolytes. Examples include NS and LR. Colloid solutions contain macromolecules in addition to water and electrolytes. Examples of colloid solutions include albumin, hydroxyethyl starch, and dextran.

12. **Theoretically, why would albumin be better than crystalloid solutions for intravascular volume repletion?**
    As a macromolecule, albumin should remain intravascular and thus increase the intravascular oncotic pressure, resulting in retention of fluid in the intravascular space.

13. **In practice, why is albumin not better than crystalloid solutions for intravascular volume repletion?**
    In states of increased vascular permeability (e.g., surgery, sepsis), albumin can diffuse into the extravascular space, reducing the intravascular oncotic pressure. A Cochrane meta-analysis examined 30 randomized controlled trials of albumin versus crystalloid solution in critically ill patients and found an *increased* mortality in those given albumin. As well, a recent randomized controlled trial of albumin infusion for fluid resuscitation in patients in the intensive care unit showed no mortality or other clinical benefit. In general, albumin should not be used for volume resuscitation.

    Albumin Reviewers: Human albumin solution for resuscitation and volume expansion in critically ill patients. Cochrane Database of Systematic Reviews 4:CD001208.pub2, 2004.

    SAFE Study Investigators: A comparison of albumin and saline for fluid resuscitation in the intensive care unit. N Engl J Med 350:2247–2256, 2004.

14. **What happens to the lactate in LR ("I thought lactate was bad")?**
    The *lactate* in LR is in a basic form (as opposed to *lactic acid*), is equivalent to bicarbonate, and acts as a buffer in the blood. It is metabolized in the liver into pyruvate, which can be converted into glucose.

15. **What is the difference between dehydration and volume depletion?**
    These often interchanged terms are not synonyms. *Dehydration* refers to loss of water, whereas *volume depletion* describes the net loss of total body sodium (and subsequently, water). By definition, dehydration should result in hypernatremia and not necessarily a reduction in intravascular volume. The loss of salt and water in volume depletion will result in a decrease in intravascular volume.

16. **Describe the signs and symptoms of a volume-depleted patient.**
A volume-depleted patient will likely complain of thirst, fatigue, light-headedness, dizziness upon standing (orthostatic hypotension), and even syncope. On physical examination, the patient may have orthostatic heart rate and blood pressure changes, dry mucous membranes, a low jugular venous pressure, dry axilla, and decreased skin turgor.

17. **Define orthostatic hypotension and state how it is measured.**
Orthostatic hypotension is defined as a drop in blood pressure that is precipitated by changes in body position. To measure "orthostatics," blood pressure should be measured while the patient is lying flat and 1 minute after he or she rises to a standing position. Classically, a patient is defined as "orthostatic" if her heart rate increases by more than 10 beats/min and the systolic blood pressure drops by 10 mmHg or more upon standing. A recent systematic review revealed that the most helpful physical findings to diagnose hypovolemia are a postural pulse increase of >30 beats/min and severe postural dizziness upon standing.

McGhee S, Abernethy WB, Simel DL: Is this patient hypovolemic? JAMA 281:1022–1029, 1999.

18. **What laboratory abnormalities might you find in a volume-depleted patient?**
Hypovolemic patients might have an elevated blood urea nitrogen (BUN) and creatinine level with the ratio of BUN to creatinine exceeding 20. They may also have a fractional excretion of sodium of <1%. Volume-depleted patients also commonly have a contraction alkalosis as evidenced by an increased bicarbonate level.

Toto RD: Approach to the patient with kidney disease. In Brenner BM (ed): Brenner and Rector's The Kidney, 7th ed. Philadelphia, Elsevier, 2004, p 1084.

19. **Name four physical examination findings in a patient who is volume overloaded.**
Elevated jugular venous pressure, S_3 cardiac gallop, basilar crackles on pulmonary auscultation, and lower extremity edema. The presence of lower extremity edema (secondary to volume overload) implies an excess total body water level of ≥ 3 L.

20. **What is the most effective and accurate measurement of a patient's day-to-day change in volume status?**
Daily weights (same scale, same clothing) provide the most accurate assessment of volume status. Recorded "ins" and "outs" can be estimates and are often inaccurate.

21. **For a 70-kg man who is hospitalized and has had no food or drink by mouth (NPO), what is the standard order you should write for maintenance fluid?**
$D_5(\frac{1}{2})NS$ with 20 mEq of K at 125 mL/h. The volume at 125 mL/h will provide 3 L of fluid over 24 hours, equivalent to average fluid losses for a 70-kg man. The 5% dextrose provides the calories to prevent catabolic muscle breakdown. Half-normal saline provides the 1.0–1.5-gm/day sodium requirement, and 20 mEq of potassium supplies the basal potassium requirement in 3 L of fluid. Volumes should be adjusted for weight and gender. A 50-kg woman may only require 75 ml/h of $D_5\frac{1}{2}NS$ with 20 mEq of K^+.

KEY POINTS: CLINICAL FLUID THERAPY

1. NS or LR should be the intravenous fluid given to patients in shock.

2. The order for maintenance fluid in a 70-kg man who is NPO is $D_5(\frac{1}{2})NS$ with 20 mEq K^+ at 125 mL/h.

3. Three liters of NS or LR must be given to replace 1 L of blood loss.

22. **What is the appropriate initial intravenous fluid choice for a patient in shock?**
Patients in shock should be resuscitated with NS or LR. Both are iso-osmotic with blood, which will maximize fluid in the intravascular space.

23. **How much NS or LR must be given to replace each liter of blood loss?**
For each liter of NS or LR given to a patient, only 200–300 mL remain intravascular (see question 9). Therefore, 3 L of NS or LR must be given for each liter of blood lost.

24. **Define the order "TKO."**
TKO means "to keep open" and orders a minimal amount of fluid that will keep the intravenous line patent, typically approximately 30 mL/h. Therefore, a patient who is "TKO'd," will receive approximately 700 mL over 24 hours. Although this is not enough replacement fluid, it can be a substantial volume in a patient with congestive heart failure or volume overload from renal failure.

25. **What laboratory data must you know before you add potassium to the intravenous solution?**
Intravenous fluids can be ordered with potassium added to the solution. Before ordering potassium as an additive, be sure you know the patient's potassium and creatinine levels. Elevated creatinine may indicate renal failure and patients with renal failure may not be able to clear the potassium; this could result in life-threatening hyperkalemia. Remember that lactated Ringer's solution has potassium in it.

26. **Describe a simple technique to prevent hospitalized patients from becoming volume overloaded.**
Intravenous fluid orders are often ordered and forgotten about even as patients improve or are no longer NPO. To avoid iatrogenic volume overload, always write fluid orders with stop parameters after a certain time frame or total volume. For example, you could write, "D_5 {½} NS @ 100 mL/h $\times$ 2 L then TKO."

BIBLIOGRAPHY

1. Rose BD, Post T (eds): Clinical Physiology of Acid-Base and Electrolyte Disorders, 5th ed. New York, McGraw-Hill, 2001.

CHAPTER 50

RENAL STONES

Gregory Busse, DO

1. **What are renal stones?**

   Renal stones are crystallized aggregates of urine or salts. Their formation is not completely understood, but it involves a disruption in the balance of one or more of three parts:
   - High levels of excreted crystalloid (i.e., calcium salts)
   - Promoters (i.e., high/low urine pH)
   - Decreased inhibitor activity (i.e., low urine citrate level)

2. **What is the prevalence of renal stones?**

   Studies show an average lifetime prevalence of approximately 10% in white men, followed by (in order of frequency) white women, Hispanic and Asian populations, black women, and black men.

3. **What are the signs and symptoms of nephrolithiasis?**

   Kidney stones commonly present with nausea, vomiting, fever, and gross hematuria. Additionally, patients most often have acute, unilateral, colicky flank pain. The location of the pain is often reflective of a stone's position in the ureter:
   - **Flank pain:** Upper ureter
   - **Flank pain with radiation to testicle/labia:** Lower third of ureter
   - **Lower quadrant pain with radiation to tip of urethra (dysuria):** Ureterovesical junction

4. **What imaging studies are used to diagnose suspected renal stones?**

   A non-contrast helical computed tomography (CT) scan is the test of choice and is the current gold standard (sensitivity ~96 %). Almost all modern CT scans use helical imaging. CT scans to investigate abdominal pathology are performed with oral and intravenous contrast that can obscure stones. Therefore, a dedicated noncontrast scan or scanning performed before contrast is given is needed to evaluate renal stones. Intravenous urography (sensitivity ~87%) can be used if CT scanning is unavailable. Plain abdominal radiograph can identify stones that are radiopaque. Pregnant women may undergo ultrasonography to avoid radiation.

5. **What are the types of renal stones? What are their radiographic and microscopic characteristics?**

   See Table 50-1 and Figs. 50-1 and 50-2.

TABLE 50-1. RENAL STONE FREQUENCY AND CHARACTERISTICS			
Stone	**Frequency (%)**	**Microscopic Character**	**Radiopaque?**
Calcium (oxalate and phosphate)	80%	Envelope	Yes
Struvite	10–20%	Coffin-lid	Yes
Uric acid	10%	Diamond	No
Cysteine	1%	Hexagon	Intermediate

6. **What are indications for hospitalization?**
   Patients with radiographic evidence of obstruction, signs or symptoms of infection (i.e., fever, chills, pyuria), acute renal failure (>0.5–1 mg/dL increase above baseline serum creatinine concentration), intractable pain, nausea, vomiting, or stones >5 mm should be admitted for monitoring, antibiotics, analgesics, antiemetics, or urology consultation.

7. **When should a urologist be involved in the care of hospitalized patients with nephrolithiasis?**
   Inpatient urologic consultation should be obtained for patients with renal stones >5 mm (stones ≤4 mm have a 80–98% chance of passage within 1 year compared to stones >8 mm, which have only a 10% chance of passage) or in cases involving obstructive signs on CT/ultrasonography or signs of renal failure or pyelonephritis. Struvite stones are a nidus for infection and should be removed regardless of size.

8. **Describe the medical treatments for nephrolithiasis.**
   Hydration and supportive care are the mainstays of therapy. Unless contraindicated, patients should receive 2 L of fluid per day. This is most often administered via an intravenous line because of nausea and vomiting. Antiemetics are commonly required. Narcotics should be used for severe pain when nonsteroidal anti-inflammatory drugs (NSAIDs) are contraindicated. NSAIDs should not be used in patients with acute renal failure or those with a planned procedure because of the increased risk of bleeding.

   Empiric antibiotics should be started if the patient has signs and symptoms

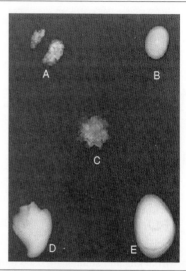

Figure 50-1. Radiodensities in air (to improve contrast) of five human calculi: **A,** Calcium oxalate; **B,** calcium phosphate; **C,** uric acid; **D,** cystine; **E,** magnesium ammonium phosphate (struvite). Note that only the uric acid calculus is truly radiolucent. (From Walsh C: Campbell's Urology, 8th ed. Philadelphia, Elsevier, p 3268.)

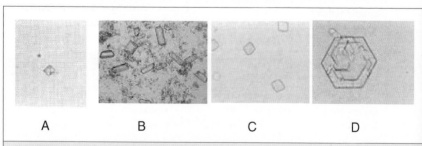

Figure 50-2. Microscopic appearance of renal stones. **A,** Calcium (oxalate and phosphate). **B,** Struvite. **C,** Uric acid. **D,** Cysteine. (From Henry J: Clinical Diagnosis and Management by Laboratory Methods, 20th ed. Philadelphia, Elsevier, 2001.)

of infection. Empiric antibiotic coverage should be directed at gram-negative rods and enterococci. Common regimens include a fluoroquinolone, ampicillin plus an aminoglycoside, or a broad-spectrum antipseudomonal penicillin.

9. **What urologic procedures can be used to treat nephrolithiasis?**
   - **Extracorporeal shock wave lithotripsy:** Acoustic shock waves are used to fracture larger stones for ureteral passage. A temporary ureteral stent is often inserted to facilitate passage of stone debris.
   - **Percutaneous nephrolithotomy (PNL):** A nephrostomy tube inserted into the renal pelvis is used to directly extract stones up to 1 cm. Larger stones can be fragmented using laser or ultrasound lithotripsy via an ureteroscope. The larger fragments can be removed by a stone basket inserted through the ureteroscope.
   - **Open lithotomy:** This procedure consists of direct surgical exploration of ureter with stone removal (rarely needed).

10. **Describe the evaluation of a patient with nephrolithiasis.**
    Begin by straining the patient's urine for stones and analyzing a 24-hour urine collection to include volume, pH, creatinine, calcium, oxalate, uric acid, phosphate, sodium, citrate, and cystine measurements. Serum metabolic profile including calcium and uric acid concentrations should be done, along with an intact parathyroid hormone and 1,25-dihydroxyvitamin D (calcitriol) survey if the calcium level is elevated.

11. **How can renal stones be prevented?**
    The most important preventive method for all types of stones is adequate hydration (>2 L/day). Thiazide diuretics (e.g., hydrochlorothiazide) inhibit calcium excretion and are first-line agents for treating stones due to hypercalciuria. Other preventive measures are outlined in Table 50-2.

TABLE 50-2. PREVENTIVE MEASURES FOR RENAL STONES	
Type of Renal Stone	**Treatment**
Calcium stone	Thiazide diuretic; dietary restrictions (i.e., low sodium, limited protein/red meat)
Oxalate stone	Dietary restriction of oxalate (e.g., tea, cola, chocolate, peanuts), limited protein/red meat; adequate calcium intake.
Hypocitrauria	Potassium citrate (if increased potassium load a concern, 4 oz of lemon juice/day is adequate)
Uric acid stone	Urine alkalinization (potassium citrate/bicarbonate); allopurinol
Struvite stone	Stone removal; treatment of infection (antibiotics); acetohydroxamic acid
Cystine stone	Maintain urine output > 3 L/day; captopril, penicillamine

12. **What are the risk factors for calcium stones?**
    Recurrent stone formation in previous stone formers approximates 40% if the patient's risk factors are not treated. Risk factors include hypercalciuria (>4 mg/kg in 24-hour sample), increased oxalate excretion, decreased citrate excretion, and elevated uric acid secretion (matrix surface for calcium stone formation). Dietary risks include poor fluid intake, high sodium (which

causes increases calcium excretion and decreases citrate excretion), and high protein (which causes increased calcium and oxalate excretion as well as lowering the urine pH). Limiting dietary calcium actually has shown to increase the incidence of stones, possibly due to the inability to bind dietary oxalate in the gastrointestinal tract, therefore raising urine oxalate levels and increasing the risk of calcium oxalate stones.

KEY POINTS: RENAL STONES

1. Eighty percent of stones are calcium oxalate or phosphate.

2. Stones >5 mm in diameter should be evaluated by an urologist because the likelihood of spontaneous passage is lower.

3. Limiting oral calcium intake actually results in a *higher* likelihood of calcium stone formation because low-calcium diets stimulate intestinal oxalate absorption and hyperoxaluria.

4. Hydration is the mainstay of all stone treatment and prophylaxis.

13. **What are drug-induced stones?**
Renal stones can be generated through metabolic alterations from medications (most common) or from actual precipitation of the drug itself (1% of all stones). The most common mechanism of inducing stones is through dehydration (e.g., diuretics). Table 50-3 outlines medications that most commonly precipitate as kidney stones.

TABLE 50-3. COMMON STONE-FORMING DRUGS
Protease inhibitors (e.g., indinavir, nelfinavir)
Acyclovir
Sulfonamides
Triamterene
Methotrexate

14. **What causes struvite stones? How are they treated?**
Recurrent urinary infections with urease-positive bacteria (e.g., *Proteus, Klebsiella* species) cause struvite stones. Urease cleaves urea to ammonia and raises urinary pH. Both the elevated ammonia level and elevated pH cause a decrease in the solubility of phosphate, thus precipitating stone formation. Struvite (triple phosphate) stones consist of a matrix of magnesium ammonium phosphate and calcium phosphate (apatite). Large collections of struvite stones are commonly called *staghorn calculi*. Struvite stones are difficult to treat because the infected stones serve as a nidus for infection. Complete surgical stone removal via PNL is the primary treatment option with concomitant antibiotic administration until stone clearance. Without operative stone clearance, almost all will have renal failure, sepsis, or both. Recurrence rates even after stone removal by PNL are approximately 23% at 40.5 months. The use of long-term suppressive antibiotic therapy is a clinical option in those patients who are

unable to undergo surgical removal or in those harboring retained stones. A urease inhibitor such as acetohydroxamic acid can be considered in patients at highest risk (e.g., neurogenic bladder or bladder diversion).

Streem SB, Yost A, Dolmatch B: Combination sandwich therapy for extensive renal calculi in 100 consecutive patients: Immediate, long-term and stratified results from a 10-year experience. J Urol 158:342, 1997

15. **What causes cystine stones?**

Cystine stones are caused by rare inherited tubular reabsorptive disorder of cysteine, arginine, ornithine, and lysine (COAL). Two cysteine molecules form the insoluble cystine via a double sulfide bond. Treatment options include therapy with penicillamine or captopril as both agents can form a disulfide bond with cysteine that increases its solubility. Captopril is often the treatment of choice because it is three times as soluble as penicillamine when joined with cysteine and is better tolerated.

BIBLIOGRAPHY

1. Borghi L, Meschi T, Amato F, et al: Urinary volume, water and recurrences in idiopathic calcium nephrolithiasis: A 5-year randomized prospective study. J Urol 155:839, 1996.

2. Soucie JM: Demographics and geographic variability of kidney stones in the US. Kidney Int 46:893–989, 1994.

3. Teichman JM: Acute renal colic from ureteral calculi. N Engl J Med 350:684–689, 2004.

APPROACH TO THE FEBRILE INPATIENT

Vincent Barba, MD

CHAPTER 51

1. **Describe the diurnal fluctuation in body temperature.**
   Most patients' morning oral temperature is between 96.8°F and 99.3°F. There is a normal variation of body temperature throughout the day, with most patients exhibiting their lowest readings in the morning and highest readings at night. The normal range is 1.8°F.

2. **Does it matter how the temperature is measured?**
   Yes. The rectal temperature is 0.9°F > oral temperature, which is 0.9°F > axillary temperature. Oral temperature may not be accurate if the patient is hyperventilating or mouth breathing or has drunk a hot or cold liquid just before his or her temperature was taken. Rectal temperature measurement in neutropenic or immunocompromised patients is not recommended given the risk of inducing bacteremia secondary to anal mucosal injury.

3. **Define *fever*.**
   A fever is an elevation of body temperature above 100.4°F. Fever occurs when the hypothalamic "thermostat" is adjusted to a higher set-point and the body responds by increasing the temperature. Temperatures >105.8°F may be fatal in adults due to protein denaturation. Drugs like acetaminophen lower the hypothalamic thermostat and thereby treat fever.

4. **How does the body raise the hypothalamic set-point?**
   Monocytes and macrophages elaborate cytokines via cyclooxygenase-mediated mechanisms that act on the hypothalamus to raise the set-point and give rise to fever. Interleukin-1, interleukin-6, tumor necrosis factor, and interferon-gamma have all been implicated in the pyrogenic pathway. Patients develop rigors as their body tries to generate heat to reach the new hypothalamic set-point. As the set-point returns to normal, patients are left "too warm" and sweat as a mechanism to dissipate heat and return to the original set-point.

5. **What is hyperthermia? How does it differ from fever?**
   Hyperthermia occurs when the body either uncontrollably produces heat or loses the ability to dissipate heat. The most common example of hyperthermia is "heat stroke." Less common causes include neuroleptic malignant syndrome and malignant hyperthermia of anesthesia. Unlike fever, the body temperature may rise to 105.8°F or higher in hyperthermia. The cyclooxygenase/cytokine pathway does not mediate hyperthermia. Therefore, acetaminophen and other anti-inflammatory agents are ineffective in reducing the temperature in hyperthermia.

6. **Should fever be treated?**
   Fever is likely a protective response against infection or inflammation, and as such it may be harmful to lower a patient's temperature. To this effect, patients with hypothermia appear to have a worse outcome than those with a more robust fever response. Still, it is unclear whether treating fever has a deleterious effect on a patient's outcome. Unless the patient is uncomfortable or the temperature is approaching 105°F, it is reasonable to allow fever to go untreated. Of course, the underlying cause of the fever (e.g., infection) needs to be treated aggressively. Table 51-1 summarizes the effect of body temperature on mortality.

TABLE 51-1. EFFECT OF BODY TEMPERATURE ON MORTALITY

Body Temperature (°F)	Number of Patients	Mortality Rate
95–100.9	24	71%
101–102.9	70	31%
>103	124	27%

Data from Bryant RE, Hood AF, Hood CE, Koenig MG: Factors affecting mortality of gram-negative rod bacteremia. Arch Intern Med 127:120–128, 1971.

7. **What is fever of unknown origin (FUO)?**

In 1961, FUO was originally defined as a temperature >101°F of >3 weeks' duration with a failure to reach a diagnosis despite 1 week of inpatient evaluation. The FUO definition has changed over time. The new definition of FUO is divided into four categories:

- Classic FUO
- Nosocomial FUO
- Neutropenic FUO
- Human immunodeficiency virus (HIV)-associated FUO

Classic FUO is no different than the original definition except the duration is limited to 3 days in the hospital or three outpatient visits instead of 1 week of inpatient evaluation. Hospitalized patients with a fever of 101°F who did not manifest a fever until after hospitalization are said to have a nosocomial FUO. Three days of investigation, including 2 days of cultures, are required for the diagnosis. Neutropenic FUO and HIV-associated FUO are FUOs associated with their namesake disease states.

8. **What are the most common causes of FUO?**

Up to 30% of all FUO cases remain undiagnosed. Infection, cancer, and noninfectious inflammatory diseases are the main causes of diagnosable FUOs. The widespread use of antibiotics and improving diagnostic technologies have decreased the incidence of infection as a cause of FUO, but it still remains the most common cause. Extrapulmonary tuberculosis-prolonged mononucleosis syndromes, endocarditis with slow-growing organisms, and fungal diseases are common causes of FUOs due to infection. Improving diagnostic technology is also responsible for the decreasing incidence of neoplasm as a cause of FUO, but it still remains the second most common cause of FUO. The most common causes of diagnosed classic FUO at U.S. community hospitals (in decreasing incidence) include lymphoma, collagen vascular disease, abscess, solid tumor, thrombosis, nonmycobacterial granulomatous disease, endocarditis, mycobacterial disease, and viral disease.

9. **Describe the work-up of a classic FUO.**

After a thorough history and physical examination, the following laboratory studies should be considered: complete blood count with differential and smear, test of erythrocyte sedimentation rate, C-reactive protein measurement, urinalysis, liver function tests, measurements of muscle enzymes, venereal disease research laboratory test, skin testing for tuberculosis with controls, rheumatoid factor test, anti-nuclear antibodies test, chemistry panel, calcium measurement, iron studies, test of vitamin B_{12} level, and serologies against HIV, cytomegalovirus, and Epstein-Barr virus. Cultures should be taken of blood, urine, sputum, and other fluids as appropriate. Serum should be set aside for testing of acute and convalescent antibodies. Any potentially diagnostic clue should be pursued. In cases without clues, consider proceeding with torso imaging as well as colonoscopy. If the work-up continues to have negative results, consider a gallium or tagged white blood cell scan. Consider watchful waiting versus empiric therapy (e.g., anti-microbials, anti-inflammatory medications, or steroids) for patients with persistent fever despite this level of evaluation.

10. **Describe the work-up of a nosocomial fever.**
More than 50% of patients who develop a fever in the hospital (i.e., nosocomial) are infected. The most common nosocomial infectious sources of fever are urinary tract infections, pneumonia, and bloodstream infections. Therefore, urinary catheters, vascular lines, phlebitis, and prostheses are primary suspects. Think of occult infections (e.g., sinusitis in intubated patients). *Clostridium difficile* infection can present with fever and leukocytosis *before* any evidence of diarrhea. Many patients with nosocomial fever have a noninfectious cause. Deep vein thrombosis, pulmonary embolism, drug fever, transfusion reaction, gout, pseudogout, and drug withdrawal are common causes of noninfectious nosocomial fever. Table 51-2 summarizes potential interventions for work-up of nosocomial fever.

Arbo M, Fine MJ, Hanusa BH, et al: Fever of nosocomial origin: Etiology, risk factors, and outcomes. Am J Med 95:505–512, 1993.

TABLE 51-2. POTENTIAL INTERVENTIONS FOR WORK-UP OF NOSOCOMIAL FEVER

Perform imaging to rule out DVT or PE.

Send stool for *C difficile* toxin.

Change or discontinue Foley catheter and send urine for culture.

Remove central lines and send catheter tip for culture.

Image sinuses if patient is intubated or has nasogastric tube in place.

Examine and/or image prosthetic devices.

Review the medication list for causes of drug fever.

DVT = deep vein thrombosis, PE = pulmonary embolism.

---

11. **What is the clinical utility of chest radiographs and blood and urine cultures in the evaluation of nosocomial fever?**
In general, the utility of these tests is limited and should be discouraged. Only 20% of chest radiographs will demonstrate a new infiltrate; 10% of blood cultures and 40% of urine cultures will grow an organism. Consequently, these tests should not be ordered in all hospitalized patients with fever but should be a part of a focused evaluation of a history and/or physical finding (e.g., cough, new crackles, dysuria).

Arbo M, Fine MJ, Hanusa BH, et al: Fever of nosocomial origin: Etiology, risk factors, and outcomes. Am J Med 95:505–512, 1993.

12. **Does atelectasis cause fever?**
There is very little objective evidence to support or dispute the relationship between fever and atelectasis. A study of postoperative cardiac surgery patients in 1995 failed to demonstrate a relationship between fever and atelectasis. (See Chapter 78 for more details.)

13. **How should febrile neutropenic patients be treated?**

Neutropenic patients, those with an absolute neutrophil count (ANC) <1000, are at high risk for infections. Up to 60% of febrile neutropenic patients are infected, and up to 20% are bacteremic. Therefore, all febrile neutropenic patients should receive empiric antibiotic therapy. Gram-positive bacteria account for up to 70% of microbiologically documented infections and must be accounted for in the antibiotic regimen. Treatment with oral antibiotics (ciprofloxacin + amoxicillin/clavulanate) may be appropriate for patients considered to be at low risk for complications (i.e., ANC >100 cells/mm^3, monocyte count >100 cells/mm^3, duration of neutropenia <7 days, malignancy in remission, normal chest radiograph, normal renal function and liver function test results, and no mental status changes). However, most patients are treated with intravenous antibiotics. Monotherapy with a carbapenem or ceftazidime is reasonable. Depending on suspicion, many include double antipseudomonal or methicillin-resistant *Streptococcus aureus* coverage by adding an aminoglycoside or vancomycin, respectively.

Hughes WT, Armstrong D, Bodey GP, et al: 2002 Guidelines for the Use of Antimicrobial Agents in Neutropenic Patients with Cancer. Clin Infect Dis 34:730–751, 2002.

KEY POINTS: FEVER IN THE HOSPITALIZED PATIENT

1. Fever is an elevation of body temperature above 100.4°F.

2. More than 50% of patients who develop a fever in the hospital are infected.

3. The most common nosocomial infectious sources of fever are urinary tract infections, pneumonia, and bloodstream infections.

4. Very little objective evidence supports the relationship between fever and atelectasis.

5. The work-up of fever in a hospitalized patient should include focused testing as opposed to routine laboratory and imaging studies.

14. **How long should a febrile neutropenic patient be treated with antibiotics?**

Empiric antibiotic therapy should be broad but rapidly tailored to culture results. After 3 days of therapy, reassess therapy. If the cultures are negative and the patient has been afebrile with an ANC >500 cells/mm^3 for more than 48 hours it is reasonable to stop antibiotics. If, however, the patient remains febrile and the ANC remains <500 cells/mm^3, antibiotics should be continued for a minimum of 2 more weeks. At day 3, if the patient remains febrile but the ANC is >500 cells/mm^3, stop antibiotics 5 days after the ANC rose above 500 cells/mm^3. Consider addition of anti-fungal therapy (e.g., amphotericin-b) with or without change of antibiotic therapy in all febrile neutropenic patients who remain febrile after 5 days of appropriate empiric antibiotic therapy.

Hughes, WT, Armstrong D, Bodey GP, et al: 2002 Guidelines for the Use of Antimicrobial Agents in Neutropenic Patients with Cancer. Clin Infect Dis 34:730–751, 2002.

WEBSITE

Infectious Diseases Society of America: http://www.idsociety.org

BIBLIOGRAPHY

1. Arbo M, Fine MJ, Hanusa BH, et al: Fever of nosocomial origin: Etiology, risk factors, and outcomes. Am J Med 95:505–512, 1993.
2. Bryant RE, Hood AF, Hood CE, Koenig MG: Factors affecting mortality of gram-negative rod bacteremia. Arch Intern Med 127:120–128, 1971.
3. Engoren M: Lack of association between atelectasis and fever. Chest 107:81–84, 1995.
4. Hughes WT, Armstrong D, Bodey GP, et al: 2002 Guidelines for the Use of Antimicrobial Agents in Neutropenic Patients with Cancer. Clin Infect Dis 34:730–751, 2002.

CHAPTER 52

ANTIBIOTIC RESISTANCE AND SELECTION

James Joyner, MD

1. **How do bacteria become resistant to antibiotics?**

   Bacteria can undergo chromosomal mutations, express a latent resistance gene, or exchange DNA with other bacteria. These changes allow development of resistance via three mechanisms: production of an enzyme that inactivates the antibiotic, alteration of the antibiotic target site, or prevention of access of the antibiotic to the target site.

2. **How do patients become colonized with resistant bacteria?**

   With rare exception, for gram-positive organisms the modality is *transmission* from other colonized people (usually health care personnel) or equipment followed by *selection* pressure in the form of antibiotics that leads to multiplication of the resistant bacteria in preference to other bacteria. Resistant gram-negative organisms are also transmitted and selected in this fashion but infection can occur *de novo* by expression of latent resistance genes or development of chromosomal mutations. This *de novo* emergence of resistance is especially frequent with *Pseudomonas* species.

3. **What factors increase the risk that a patient has a resistant organism?**

   Recent or current stay in a hospital or extended care facility, time spent in an intensive care unit, ongoing hemodialysis, organ transplantation, and recent antimicrobial use are all associated with the presence of resistant organisms.

KEY POINTS: HOW PATIENTS BECOME COLONIZED WITH RESISTANT BACTERIA

1. Transmission, usually via the hands of hospital personnel

2. Selection via pressure with antibiotics that favor the growth of resistant bacteria

4. **What are some commonly encountered resistant bacteria?**

   The most common resistant gram-positive organisms are vancomycin-resistant enterococci (VRE) and methicillin-resistant *Staphylococcus aureus* (MRSA). Commonly encountered resistant gram-negative organisms are *Pseudomonas aeruginosa*, *Acinetobacter baumannii*, *Stenotrophomonas maltophilia*, *Enterobacter cloacae*, and extended-spectrum β-lactamase (ESBL)–producing *Klebsiella* species and *Escherichia coli*.

5. **How common is MRSA? How can it be treated?**

   The prevalence of colonization with this organism varies widely. Countries like Denmark have essentially eliminated MRSA from health care institutions by aggressive infection control measures. In contrast, in many institutions in the United States, MRSA accounts for more than half of the *S. aureus* isolates. Treatment of asymptomatic colonization is controversial.

Vancomycin has long been the gold standard for treatment of infections with MRSA. New antibiotics such as linezolid (Zyvox), quinupristin-dalfopristin (Synercid), and daptomycin (Cubicin) offer useful alternatives to vancomycin.

6. **How common is VRE? How can it be treated?**
Similarly to MRSA, the prevalence of VRE varies widely. In many institutions in the United States, nearly 10% of the *Enterococcus faecalis* and more than half of the *Enterococcus faecium* isolates are now resistant to vancomycin. These organisms are frequently isolated as asymptomatic stool colonizers and in this scenario should not be treated. Infections with VRE can be treated with linezolid and quinupristin-dalfopristin (this drug is only effective against *E. faecium*). Emerging data also supports the efficacy of daptomycin in VRE infections. Importantly, cases of VRE resistance to all of these new agents have already been noted.

7. **How common are resistant gram-negative infections? How can they be treated?**
ESBL-producing *E. coli, Klebsiella* species, and similarly resistant *Enterobacter* species frequently represent 10% of hospital isolates in the United States. The treatment of choice for infections with these pathogens is a carbapenem (e.g., imipenem, meropenem, ertapenem). Multidrug-resistant *Pseudomonas, Acinetobacter,* and *Stenotrophomonas* species are frequently isolated in the context of long-term broad-spectrum antibiotic use in medically or surgically complex institutionalized patients. Resistant versions of these organisms are the rule rather than the exception, and they are especially common in intensive care units. Treatment of infections with these organisms is individualized based on susceptibility results. Treatment options for *Pseudomonas* infections are discussed below. Drug-resistant *Acinetobacter* is frequently only susceptible to imipenem. Although *Stenotrophomonas* is resistant to nearly all typical gram-negative antimicrobials, it is usually susceptible to trimethoprim-sulfamethoxazole (Bactrim).

8. **How do resistant organisms lead to clinically significant infections?**
After transmission from health care workers, MRSA colonizes the skin. Likewise, fecal incontinence leads to colonization of the skin with VRE and resistant gram-negative organisms. Central venous and peripheral catheters, Foley catheters, decubitus ulcers, and invasive procedures subsequently allow skin colonizers access to normally sterile sites where infection ensues in the form of bloodstream infection, urinary tract infection, or wound infection. Similarly, use of proton pump inhibitors reduces stomach acidity, allowing colonization of the upper gastrointestinal tract and mouth with enteric gram-negative bacteria. Subsequent aspiration via altered mental status, nasogastric tube, or endotracheal tube allows oropharyngeal colonizers access to the lower airway, causing nosocomial pneumonia.

KEY POINTS: FACTORS TO CONSIDER IN PREDICTING INFECTING ORGANISM

1. Nosocomial versus community-acquired infection

2. Anatomic location of infection

3. Origin of the infecting organism

4. Previous culture results

5. Previous antimicrobial exposure

9. **Do infections with resistant organisms result in worse outcomes?**
   The cost of care associated with infections due to resistant organisms clearly increases in comparison to infections with similar susceptible organisms. The annual national cost of hospital-acquired infections due to resistant organisms was estimated to be over $4 billion in 1990. Clinical outcomes are also negatively affected; patients with septic shock, febrile neutropenia, or nosocomial pneumonia have an increased likelihood of morbidity and mortality if the initial empiric antibiotic choice does not cover the organism that is subsequently isolated. The chance of this greatly increases in the presence of resistant organisms. For less critical infections, the delay in effective therapy results in a longer hospital stay.

10. **What can be done to prevent infections with resistant bacteria?**
    The key is prevention of transmission and selection. Transmission is prevented by the use of strict handwashing before and after contact with every patient and by the use of gowns, gloves, and masks when appropriate. Current guidelines from both the Centers of Disease Control and Prevention (CDC) and the Society for Healthcare Epidemiology of America (SHEA) recommend contact isolation of patients found to harbor MRSA and VRE, especially if the organisms are being actively excreted into the environment (e.g., an incontinent patient with diarrhea containing VRE). Isolation should be considered for patients with resistant gram-negative bacteria if there is evidence of ongoing transmission. An excellent summary of the CDC and SHEA guidelines is included in the bibliography. Selection of resistant organisms is prevented by judicious antimicrobial use. This involves initiation of treatment with antimicrobials only in association with clinical diagnoses that call for their use, narrowing antimicrobial regimens once culture results become available, and discontinuing therapy as soon as the required treatment duration is complete.

11. **Before culture results are final, how does one predict the most likely causative organism?**
    It is useful to first decide whether the infection is community-acquired or hospital-acquired (i.e., nosocomial). Altered flora and resistant bacteria are far more likely in nosocomial infections (see question 3). Next, define the likely location(s) of infection and postulate how the bacteria may have arrived. Bacteria may originate at or near the site of infection (e.g., cholecystitis) or may be introduced there via hematogenous spread (e.g., splenic abscess), percutaneous introduction (e.g., catheter-related infections), aspiration (e.g., nosocomial pneumonia), or some combination of these. This allows one to generate a list of potential pathogens. The final step is to use knowledge of previous culture results and antibiotic exposure to refine this list of potential pathogens. Infecting organisms are likely to be resistant to recently used antimicrobial agents.

KEY POINTS: FACTORS DEFINING THE *IN VIVO* ACTIVITY OF AN ANTIBIOTIC

1. The *in vitro* minimum inhibitory concentration (MIC) of the antibiotic versus the organism

2. The ability of the antibiotic to be delivered to the organism *in vivo* in concentrations that exceed the MIC in a time-dependent or concentration-dependent fashion

12. **What is an antibiogram?**
    An antibiogram is a listing of susceptibility patterns for a given hospital. Susceptibility patterns vary from country to country and from institution to institution. Clinical syndromes such as

septic shock, febrile neutropenia, and nosocomial pneumonia require administration of effective antibiotics before the results of susceptibility testing are known (see question 9). An antibiogram should guide antibiotic decision making in these scenarios. For example, *P. aeruginosa* infection is the most common cause of nosocomial pneumonia in most hospitals. In a hospital with 50% of *Pseudomonas* isolates resistant to fluoroquinolones, ciprofloxacin is not a good empiric choice for a patient who develops nosocomial pneumonia.

13. **In addition to the hospital antibiogram, what other factors should be considered in selecting an antibiotic?**
    These can be divided into organism factors, host factors, and drug factors (Table 52-1).

TABLE 52-1. FACTORS TO CONSIDER WHEN SELECTING AN ANTIBIOTIC

Organism Factors	Host Factors	Drug Factors
Identity	Anatomic location of infection	Side effects
Susceptibility	Involvement of prosthetic	Drug interactions
Potential for resistance	Systemic immune competence	Bactericidal/bacteriostatic
	Local immune competence	Pharmacokinetics
	Severity of illness	Pharmacodynamics
	Drug allergies	Clinical efficacy data
	Renal/hepatic dysfunction	Spectrum of coverage
		Cost

14. **How can the site of infection alter the effectiveness of antimicrobial therapy?**
    Antibiotic efficacy requires adequate concentrations at the site of infection. This is difficult to achieve in areas such as the central nervous system (meningitis), the vitreous of the eye (endophthalmitis), a cardiac valve vegetation (endocarditis), biofilm (prosthetic hip infection), endobronchial secretions (pneumonia), bone (osteomyelitis), and abscesses. Antibiotics work best in conjunction with an effective local immune response. Ironically, this is also a problem in many of the areas mentioned above.

15. **What does it mean when an antibiotic is bactericidal? When is it important to use such an antimicrobial?**
    - *Bacteriostatic* antibiotics inhibit the growth of the organism, but when removed the organism is free to grow again. Bacteriostatic antibiotics are clinically effective in conjunction with an effective systemic and local immune system.
    - *Bactericidal* antibiotics kill the organism outright. Their use is preferred when there is systemic immune impairment (e.g., febrile neutropenia, patients on immunosuppressive medication) or when the immune system cannot effectively access the site of infection (e.g., meningitis, endophthalmitis, endocarditis, osteomyelitis, biofilms).
    Technically, the bactericidal or bacteriostatic property of an antimicrobial is concentration and organism dependent and can only be defined by very complex *in vitro* testing against the organism in question. However, in general, some antibiotics have a bacteristatic mode of action whereas others have a bactericidal mode of action (Table 52-2).

TABLE 52-2. SELECTED PHARMACOKINETIC PROPERTIES FOR ANTIBIOTICS

	Bacteriostatic	Bacteriocidal
Time-dependent	Clindamycin	β-lactams
	Linezolid	Penicillins
	Macrolides (except azithromycin)	Cephalosporins
		Carbapenems
		Aztreonam
Concentration-dependent		Aminoglycosides
		Daptomycin
		Fluoroquinolones
		Metronidazole
AUC/MIC-dependent	Azithromycin	Vancomycin
	Tetracyclines	

AUC = area under the curve, MIC = minimum inhibitory concentration.

16. **What is the minimum inhibitory concentration (MIC)? How does it relate to the efficacy of an antibiotic against a particular organism?**

MIC is the minimum inhibitory concentration required to inhibit the growth of 90% of isolates of a particular species *in vitro*. Drugs with lower MICs are more potent *in vitro*. For some antibiotics to work it is only important that the concentration of the drug stay just above the MIC for most of the time (time-dependent antibiotics). For other antibiotics, it is only important that the peak concentration of the drug is many times the MIC (concentration-dependent antibiotics). For these drugs, studies have shown that high peak plasma concentration (Cmax)/MIC ratios correlate with clinical efficacy, microbiologic cure, and prevent emergence of resistance on therapy. Finally, some antibiotics exhibit a mixture of concentration and time dependency. For these antibiotics, the ratio of the area under the concentration curve and the MIC best predicts clinical and microbiologic outcome.

17. **Why does *P. aeruginosa* require specialized dosing of many antimicrobials?**

Pseudomonas is the most complex bacterial pathogen in humans, with nearly 10% of its genome devoted to regulation of protein expression. It possesses a wide array of latent resistance mechanisms that it may activate in response to antimicrobial pressure. Its outer membrane is intrinsically 100-fold less permeable to antimicrobials than that of *E. coli*. To achieve proper concentrations of time-dependent drugs like piperacillin, larger doses (at least 16 gm/day) are required. Likewise, the doses of concentration-dependent drugs such as ciprofloxacin must be increased to achieve proper levels. Without proper attention to pharmacodynamic factors and associated dosing requirements, emergence of resistance occurs during therapy in 10–50% of pseudomonal infections. Table 52-3 summarizes dosing recommendations for antipseudomonal drugs in patients with normal renal function.

18. **When should combination therapy be used?**

This remains very uncertain for a good portion of infectious diseases. Most of the studies addressing this question are seriously flawed or are now so old that they may no longer be valid with our current antimicrobials. For example, studies demonstrating superiority of combination therapy in neutropenic patients with gram-negative bacteremia were performed in the 1970s before the availability of cefepime, imipenem, and piperacillin/tazobactam, which all have monotherapy indications for febrile neutropenia. There are only a few diagnoses for which combination therapy has been shown to improve clinical outcome or to shorten necessary antibiotic course. Table 52-4 lists situations in which combination therapy is commonly used and indicates which uses are supported by good clinical data.

TABLE 52-3. ANTIBIOTIC DOSING FOR *P. AERUGINOSA**

- Piperacillin 4–6 gm IV every 6–8 hours (piperacillin/tazobactam equivalent is 4.5 gm IV every 6 hours)
- Ticarcillin 3–4 gm IV every 4–6 hours (Note that the clavulanic acid in ticarcillin/clavulanate [Timentin] has been associated with induction of beta-lactamase production in multiple studies.)
- Ceftazidime 2 gm IV every 6–8 hours
- Cefepime 2 gm IV every 6–8 hours
- Aztreonam 2–3 gm IV every 8 hours
- Imipenem 1 gm IV every 6–8 hours
- Meropenem 1–2 gm IV every 8 hours
- Ciprofloxacin 400 mg IV every 8 hours or 750 mg PO every 12 hours
- Levofloxacin 750 mg IV or PO every 24 hours

* These doses assume normal renal function.

TABLE 52-4. CONSIDERATIONS FOR COMBINATION THERAPY

Clinically Proven Useful	Unproven but Accepted
Enterococcal endocarditis	*Pseudomonas* infections
Ampicillin + gentamicin	β-lactam + aminoglycoside
Vancomycin + gentamicin	Necrotizing fasciitis (group A
Streptococcal endocarditis	*Streptococcus*)
Penicillin + gentamicin	Penicillin + clindamycin
Gram-negative bacteremia in neutropenic hosts	*S. aureus* endocarditis
β-lactam + aminoglycoside	Nafcillin + gentamicin
	Refractory bacteremia

BIBLIOGRAPHY

1. Giamarellou H, Antoniadou A: Antipseudomonal antibiotics. Med Clin North Am 85:19–42, 2001.
2. Jackson M, Jarvis WR, Scheckler WE: HICPAC/SHEA—conflicting guidelines: What is the standard of care? Am J Infect Control 32:504–511, 2004.
3. Moellering RC, Eliopoulos GM: Principles of anti-infective therapy. In Mandell, Bennet, Dolin (eds): Principles and Practice of Infectious Diseases, 6th ed. Philadelphia, Elsevier Science, 2000, pp 223–235.
4. Shlaes DM, Gerding DN, John JF Jr, et al: Society for Healthcare Epidemiology of America and Infectious Diseases Society of America Joint Committee on the Prevention of Antimicrobial Resistance: Guidelines for the prevention of antimicrobial resistance in hospitals. Clin Infect Dis 25:584–599, 1997.

CHAPTER 53

APPROACH TO THE IMMUNOCOMPROMISED PATIENT

Robin K. Avery, MD

1. **What are the different kinds of immunocompromise seen in hospitalized patients?**

   The most common causes of immunocompromise are neutropenia (most commonly chemotherapy induced), rheumatologic diseases, bone marrow or solid organ transplantation, HIV, and congenital or acquired immunodeficiencies.

2. **What are the most important factors in risk stratifying a neutropenic patient?**

   The total white blood cell (WBC) count and absolute neutrophil count (ANC), especially if below 100 cells/mm^3, are useful risk predictors. The Infectious Disease Society of America's 2002 guidelines define *neutropenia* as an ANC <500 cells/mm^3, or <1000 cells/mm^3 with predicted decrease to <500 cells/mm^3. Longer durations (>10 days) of sustained neutropenia are associated with increased risk of infection.

   Hughes WT, Armstrong D, Bodey GP, et al: 2002 guidelines for the use of antimicrobial agents in neutropenic patients with cancer. Clin Infect Dis 34:730–751, 2002.

3. **What are the most important factors in risk stratifying nonneutropenic immunocompromised patients?**

   The type, degree, and duration of immunocompromise are important, for example, humoral immune function (immunoglobulin levels), cellular immune function (lymphocyte subsets in HIV and in transplant recipients), and WBC function (chronic granulomatous disease). The type and dose of immunosuppressive agents (e.g., steroids, cyclophosphamide, cyclosporine, and mycophenolate) are all important.

4. **What are the most urgent issues involved in evaluating a febrile neutropenic patient?**

   This represents a medical emergency because of the risk of mortality from fulminant sepsis, particularly from gram-negative organisms. A rapid history and examination should be performed and empiric antibiotic therapy begun promptly. Patients should be checked for signs of infection related to the eye, ear, nose, or central nervous system (CNS) because these may represent rapidly progressive fungal infections that may require urgent computed tomography (CT), magnetic resonance imaging (MRI), and subspecialty consultation.

5. **What features of the history and physical examination are important in a febrile neutropenic patient? How might these differ from those with a normal WBC count?**

   Classic signs of inflammation are often absent. Abdominal pain without peritoneal signs may indicate acute appendicitis, diverticulitis, or even a perforated viscus. Signs of pulmonary consolidation, such as egophony, are usually absent; cough is dry rather than purulent. Impending sepsis may be heralded by tachycardia, tachypnea, or both without specific findings. Special attention should be paid to signs and symptoms relating to head, sinuses, eye, ear, lungs, abdomen, skin lesions or rashes, catheters, and focal neurologic complaints.

6. **What organisms are most likely to cause infection in a febrile neutropenic patient?**

   Twenty years ago, gram-negative infections (including *E. coli, Klebsiella,* and *Pseudomonas*) predominated, often from the patient's own intestinal flora. More recently, due to indwelling intravenous catheters, oral mucositis from chemotherapy, and use of quinolone prophylaxis, gram-positive infections have become more prominent; these include coagulase-negative staphylococci, *S. aureus*, and viridans streptococci. Fungal infections commonly occur after several days to a week of neutropenia and broad-spectrum antibacterial therapy. Viral infections are occasional causes of fever in this population. Emerging infections (e.g., *Corynebacterium jeikeium, Leuconostoc* species) or multiresistant organisms (e.g., *Stenotrophomonas, Acinetobacter*) may be the consequence of widespread antibiotic use.

7. **Describe the ideal characteristics of an empirical antibiotic regimen for febrile neutropenia.**

   Given the threat of gram-negative sepsis, the empiric regimen should always cover gram-negative bacilli, including *Pseudomonas* species, taking into account antimicrobial susceptibilities at each institution. The inclusion of vancomycin in the initial regimen is controversial and center specific (e.g., centers with high rates of MRSA). The literature supports both dual therapy (such as a β-lactam and aminoglycoside combination, e.g., piperacillin-tazobactam plus gentamicin) and monotherapy (such as ceftazidime or imipenem). Many clinicians reserve monotherapy for lower-risk patients.

8. **When should antifungal therapy be started in a febrile neutropenic patient?**

   Most experts recommend empiric antifungal therapy after >5 days of fever despite broad-spectrum antibiotic therapy. Traditionally amphotericin B was used, but newer antifungal agents are gaining popularity. Nodular infiltrates on chest radiograph or dark skin lesions can be clues to the presence of fungal infection.

9. **Outline the timeline of possible major infections after solid organ transplant.**

   Solid organ transplant recipients usually receive at least two immunosuppressive drugs. Those with multiple episodes of rejection and additional immunosuppression are at highest risk of infection. In the first month after transplant, infections are generally related to surgery (e.g., wound, lung, urine, catheter) or preexisting infections in donor or recipient. Between the second and sixth months after transplant, opportunistic infections become more common (e.g., cytomegalovirus [CMV], *Aspergillus, Pneumocystis,* and *Nocardia* infection, toxoplasmosis, EBV-related lymphoproliferative disease). After 6 months, the patient generally falls into one of three categories:

   - Those with minimal immunosuppression (who become more like the general population, susceptible to respiratory viruses, pneumococcal pneumonia, and urinary tract infections)
   - Those with poor transplant function and heavy immunosuppression (who remain susceptible to opportunistic infections)
   - Those who did well initially but develop late disease due to slow-onset infections such as hepatitis B or C or BK virus

10. **Outline the timeline of major infections after bone marrow transplant.**

   The course of infection during the neutropenic period right after bone marrow or stem cell transplant (lasting usually 10 days to 3 weeks) is similar to that of the neutropenic leukemic patient. The second period, after engraftment (recovery of WBC count), is often characterized by acute graft-versus-host disease (GVHD) of the skin, liver, and gastrointestinal tract. GVHD requires immunosuppressive therapy and is associated with increased risk for infections. In the late posttransplant period, patients may have chronic GVHD of the skin, mucous membranes, lungs, eyes, and sinuses that is more like an autoimmune disease.

11. **Name the most common drug interactions that may arise between antibiotics and transplant-related medications.**

    Cyclosporine, tacrolimus, and sirolimus interact with other drugs, especially antibiotics. Macrolides (especially clarithromycin and erythromycin) will raise levels of the above medications and may precipitate toxicity; azithromycin is generally safe and preferred. Azole antifungal agents will also raise the levels of the above medications but can be initiated with close monitoring of levels. Nephrotoxic antibiotics (e.g., aminoglycosides) should be avoided whenever possible. The transplant team should be consulted whenever a new medication is started.

12. **What are some of the infections seen in steroid-treated patients?**

    Staphylococcal infections, including pneumonia, cellulitis, septic arthritis, and osteomyelitis, are more common in steroid-treated patients. Pneumonias may be due to conventional organisms like *Streptococcus pneumoniae* but may also be due to gram-negative bacteria and *Legionella* species. Be on the alert for reactivation of past infections such as tuberculosis, histoplasmosis, and strongyloidiasis. Pneumocystis pneumonia rarely occurs in patients treated with steroids alone, but is more common in conjunction with Wegener's granulomatosis and in persons treated with two or more immunosuppressive drugs.

13. **What infections may occur in patients who have received tumor necrosis factor (TNF) inhibitors such as infliximab?**

    TNF inhibitors have been associated with an increased incidence of tuberculosis reactivation, granulomatous diseases such as disseminated histoplasmosis, and other infections. A PPD skin test (purified protein derivative skin test for tuberculosis) should be performed before initiation of therapy, and the physician should assess for prior granulomatous infections (e.g., presence of calcified nodes or splenic granulomas on chest radiograph).

14. **What are the most important causes of fever in hospitalized HIV-positive patients?**

    With the advent of highly active antiretroviral therapy, severe immunocompromise is much less common than in the past. However, patients may still have low CD4 counts and high viral loads due to noncompliance or multidrug-resistant HIV. Patients with CD4 counts <200 cells/μL are much more susceptible to *Pneumocystis* infection, cryptococcal meningitis, *Mycobacterium avium* complex, CMV retinitis and colitis, and infections from other opportunistic pathogens. Patients with any CD4 count may have bacterial pneumonia, tuberculosis, bacteremia, endocarditis, sexually transmitted diseases, and diarrheal illnesses. Fever and pancytopenia in an HIV-positive patient should raise suspicion for disseminated fungal or mycobacterial disease or CMV infection.

15. **What are the most appropriate diagnostic tests in a patient with severe respiratory infection?**

    Immunocompromised patients are subject to a wide variety of infections and should not be assumed to have "usual" community-acquired pathogens. If there are only subtle abnormalities on chest radiograph, a chest CT scan can clarify whether nodules or cavities are present. Unless clearly purulent sputum is produced in a non-neutropenic patient, rapid bronchoalveolar lavage (BAL) is helpful. Whenever possible, transbronchial biopsy specimen should also be obtained since tissue involvement is important in diagnosis (e.g., CMV growing in BAL cultures may not signify the presence of CMV pneumonitis unless viral inclusions are seen on pathology).

16. **What cultures should be obtained when an immunocompromised patient undergoes bronchoscopy?**

    Many centers have a set panel of tests for an immunocompromised BAL. These include bacterial, fungal, nocardial, and acid-fast stains and cultures; stain for *Pneumocystis*; direct fluorescent assay and culture for *Legionella*; viral culture for herpes simplex virus (HSV), CMV, and respiratory viruses.

17. **What are the most likely pathogens in a patient with HIV and pulmonary infiltrates?**
For a patient with CD4 < 200 cells/μL, consider *Pneumocystis* (especially if not receiving prophylaxis), fungal infection (e.g., *Cryptococcus*, histoplasmosis), CMV, and mycobacterial infection. For a patient with a higher CD4 count, bacterial pneumonias and respiratory viruses would be more common. *Pneumocystis* pneumonia can occur with hypoxemia out of proportion to early chest radiograph findings. For a patient with suspected *Pneumocystis carinii* pneumonia (PCP), trimethoprim-sulfamethoxazole should be started at a dose of 15–20 mg/kg/day (divided q6h). In sulfa-allergic patients, options include intravenous pentamidine or trimetrexate; for less severe disease, dapsone-trimethoprim, atovaquone, or clindamycin-primaquine may be used. Adjunctive steroids have been shown to be life-saving in cases of severe PCP.

18. **What is the role of open lung biopsy in the management of these infections?**
Open lung biopsy should be considered in a patient with severe, progressive infiltrates and hypoxemia without response to empiric therapy and without a microbiologic diagnosis on bronchoscopy. The open lung biopsy allows a larger piece of tissue to reveal other diagnostic clues such as diffuse alveolar damage, granulomas, or other conditions.

19. **Name some of the major causes of impaired consciousness in immunocompromised patients.**
Mental status changes can be due to medications, sepsis, fever, or focal lesions such as cerebrovascular accident, brain abscess, progressive multifocal leukoencephalopathy, or meningitis (bacterial, viral, fungal, or noninfectious). Mental status changes should prompt a detailed neurologic examination and rapid diagnostic evaluation.

20. **What is the role of CT, MRI, and lumbar puncture (LP) in this group of patients (see question 19)?**
The noncontrast brain CT scan is rapidly available to rule out cerebral hemorrhage. The MRI with gadolinium is the imaging method of choice for suspected brain abscess or septic emboli. The MR angiogram is also useful in excluding mycotic aneurysms. LP is not recommended as an empiric procedure in a febrile neutropenic patient without CNS signs or symptoms. However, sampling of cerebrospinal fluid (CSF) should be considered in patients with CNS signs and symptoms, particularly in the presence of devices such as Ommaya reservoirs and CNS shunts. When the LP is performed, include routine analysis (i.e., cell count and differential, protein and glucose); Gram stain and culture; fungal smear, cryptococcal antigen, and culture; acid-fast bacilli stain and culture; cytology; and consider a rapid plasma reagin test for syphilis and CSF polymerase chain reaction (PCR) for viruses such as HSV, CMV, varicella-zoster virus (VZV), human herpesvirus 6, Jakob-Creutzfeldt virus, and others (more common in bone marrow transplant recipients). Viral cultures on CSF are very low-yield, but viral PCRs are helpful.

KEY POINTS: TESTS TO ORDER WHEN AN IMMUNOCOMPROMISED PATIENT UNDERGOES BRONCHOSCOPY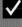

1. Gram stain, fungal, acid-fast, and *Nocardia* stains and cultures

2. Stain for *Pneumocystis* species

3. Viral cultures for CMV, HSV, and respiratory viruses

4. Direct fluorescent assay and culture for *Legionella* species

5. Cytology

6. Transbronchial biopsy, if possible

21. **What empiric antibiotic therapy should be initiated in the case of a suspected CNS infection?**

    For gram-negative coverage in a febrile neutropenic patient with suspected CNS infection, choose antibiotics that cross the blood-brain barrier (e.g., ceftazidime). Include vancomycin in a patient with brain abscess, septic emboli, suspected infection related to CNS devices, or suspected bacterial meningitis. In cases of suspected meningitis, ampicillin for *Listeria* coverage should also be added in an immunocompromised patient. Antifungal agents should be used for focal CNS lesions or suspected cryptococcal meningitis. Consider acyclovir if HSV or VZV encephalitis is a possibility (i.e., presence of impaired consciousness, pleocytosis, and fever, particularly with temporal lobe involvement).

22. **What are some of the causes of mental status changes in the HIV-positive patient?**

    The rapidity of onset and CD4 count are important to consider. Acute-onset conditions include bacterial meningitis, brain abscess, cryptococcal or mycobacterial meningitis, and CMV, HSV, or VZV encephalitis (although some of these may have insidious onset). Slower-onset conditions include CNS toxoplasmosis, lymphoma, and progressive multifocal leukoencephalopathy as well as dementia due to HIV itself.

23. **Name the most common organisms that can cause catheter-related infections in immunocompromised patients.**

    Gram-positive organisms, including coagulase-negative staphylococci, *S. aureus,* and other skin flora, are most common. Gram-negative organisms such as *E. coli, Klebsiella* species, and yeast may also be seen. Emerging pathogens such as *C. jeikeium* or multiantibiotic-resistant pathogens such as *Stenotrophomonas* species may also be involved.

24. **Which situations should lead to the removal of an indwelling intravenous catheter?**

    - Tunnel infections (in a subcutaneously tunneled catheter) with pain, swelling, or erythema of the tunnel (not merely the exit site) mandate catheter removal.
    - Septic thrombophlebitis (where the infected clot is associated with an infected catheter) should prompt catheter removal, but some specialists advise anticoagulation before removal, if feasible.
    - Exit-site infections with mild cellulitis or drainage without positive blood culture results may be treated with appropriate antibiotics.
    - Bacteremia without tunnel infection may or may not require catheter removal.
    - Uncomplicated coagulase-negative staphylococcal infections may often be treated with the catheter in place.
    - Many clinicians will remove any catheter in the setting of *S. aureus*, vancomycin-resistant *Enterococcus* species, or candidal infection.
    - Sometimes catheter removal can be postponed in the setting of pancytopenia and ongoing need for multilumen access if the infection can be otherwise controlled.

BIBLIOGRAPHY

1. Gomez L, Martino R, Rolston KV: Neutropenic enterocolitis: Spectrum of the disease and comparison of definite and possible cases. Clin Infect Dis 27:695–699, 1998.

2. Mermel LA, Farr BM, Sherertz RA, et al: Guidelines for the management of intravascular catheter-related infections. Clin Infect Dis 32:1249–1272, 2001.

3. Rolston KV: Challenges in the treatment of infections caused by gram-positive and gram-negative bacteria in patients with cancer and neutropenia. Clin Infect Dis 40(Suppl 4):S246–S252, 2005.

4. Rolston KV: The spectrum of pulmonary infections in cancer patients. Curr Opin Oncol 13:218–223, 2001.

5. Shlaes DM, Binczewski B, Rice LB: Emerging antibiotic resistance and the immunocompromised host. Clin Infect Dis 17(Suppl 2):S527–S536, 1993.

CHAPTER 54

SEPSIS

Steven B. Deitelzweig, MD, and Jeffrey J. Glasheen, MD

1. **What is the difference between systemic inflammatory response syndrome (SIRS) and sepsis?**

   SIRS is a board category of generalized inflammation with subsets that include sepsis, severe sepsis, and septic shock.

   - **SIRS:** A syndrome defined by the presence of two or more markers of inflammation: body temperature, heart rate, respiratory rate, and leukocyte (white blood cell) count (Table 54-1). Many noninfectious conditions can cause SIRS, such as pulmonary embolism and acute myocardial infarction.
   - **Sepsis:** SIRS that is caused by infection. It is diagnosed through a documented (e.g., positive culture or Gram stain) or presumed infection.
   - **Severe sepsis:** The addition of organ hypoperfusion or dysfunction to the diagnosis of sepsis.

TABLE 54-1. DEFINITION OF SEPSIS

Systemic inflammatory response syndrome (SIRS)

Two or more of the following:

- Temperature $<36°C$ or $>38.5°C$
- HR > 90 beats/min (unless using a drug that affects chronotropy)
- RR > 20 breaths/min or $PaCO_2 < 32$ mmHg or mechanical ventilation
- WBC count $< 4000/\mu L$ or $> 12,000/\mu L$

Sepsis

SIRS + documented or presumed infection

Severe sepsis

Sepsis + at least one sign of organ hypoperfusion or dysfunction

- Increased blood lactate levels
- Oliguria or acute renal failure
- Poor capillary refill (≥ 3 sec) or mottled skin
- Altered mental status
- Thrombocytopenia/disseminated intravascular coagulation
- Acute lung injury or adult respiratory distress syndrome
- Hepatic dysfunction (e.g., elevated bilirubin)
- Cardiac dysfunction (e.g., reduced ejection fraction)

Septic shock

Severe sepsis + refractory hypotension ($<90/65$ mmHg) or vasopressor need

HR = heart rate, RR = respiratory rate, WBC = white blood cell.

■ **Septic shock:** The further presence of refractory hypotension (i.e., not responsive to fluid resuscitation).

2. **How common is sepsis?**
Sepsis affects approximately 750,000 Americans annually, resulting in 225,000 deaths. This is roughly equivalent to the number of deaths from myocardial infarction. Severe sepsis and septic shock account for 2–3% of all hospital admissions and 10% of admissions to the intensive care unit, where it is the most common noncardiac cause of death. The mortality rate for severe sepsis and septic shock exceeds 30%, making it the 11th most common cause of death in the United States. Although the mortality rates have improved in recent years, the overall number of deaths has increased owing to a 9% annual increase in the rate of severe sepsis.

3. **What are the common causes of sepsis?**
Sepsis most commonly results from infections of the pulmonary, abdominal, bloodstream, or urinary systems. Lower respiratory tract and intra-abdominal infections as well as those without a documented source are associated with the highest rate of mortality. Gram-positive organisms are now more common than their gram-negative counterparts with *Staphylococcus aureus* and *Escherichia coli* accounting for the most cases. Less commonly fungi, parasites, and viruses can be implicated. Up to one third of cultures are negative, most commonly secondary to antibiotics being given before the cultures are drawn. Sepsis caused by *Enterococcus* and *Candida* species seems to be associated with the highest rate of mortality (Table 54-2).

TABLE 54-2. MOST COMMON PATHOGENS IN SEPTIC SHOCK	
Organism	Frequency
Gram-positive bacteria	
Staphylococcus aureus	19–35%
Streptococcus pneumoniae	9–12%
Enterococcus species	3–13%
Anaerobes	1–2%
Other gram-positive bacteria	8–19%
Gram-negative bacteria	
E. coli	9–27%
Pseudomonas aeruginosa	8–15%
Klebsiella pneumoniae	2–7%
Haemophilus influenzae	2–10%
Anaerobes	3–7%
Other gram-negative bacteria	9–28%
Fungus	
Candida albicans	1–3%
Other Candida species	1–2%
Yeast	1%
Parasites and viruses	3–7%

Adapted from Annane D, Bellissant E, Cavaillon JM: Septic shock. Lancet 365:63–78, 2005.

4. **What is the pathophysiology of sepsis?**
   Septic pathophysiology is complex and involves the interaction between the bacterium and the hosts' humoral, cellular, and neuroendocrine systems. This interaction results in release of numerous cytokines and inflammatory mediators. These inflammatory effects are heightened by the activation of the complement and coagulation cascades, which affects the endothelium and ultimately the microcirculation and its ability to supply adequate tissue oxygenation. This, in turn, leads to tissue damage and eventually organ dysfunction.

5. **What is the general approach to treating sepsis?**
   The first step in treating sepsis is early recognition. This requires an understanding of the diagnostic criteria and vigilance in identifying patients at risk of developing sepsis. Several scoring systems, such as the Acute Physiology and Chronic Health Score (APACHE) II, can aid in determining the severity of the illness and provide prognostic data. Rapid initiation of broad-spectrum antibiotics (preferably within 1 hour of presentation and later tailored to culture results) and early hemodynamic resuscitation should be augmented by the use of as-needed vasopressors, ventilatory support, activated protein C (APC), tight glycemic control, and adjuvant corticosteroids (Fig. 54-1).

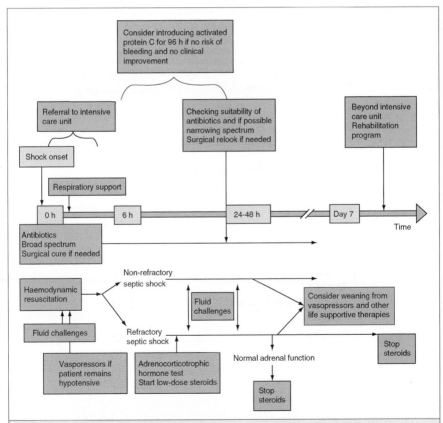

Figure 54-1. Principles of treatment in septic shock. (From Annane D, Bellissant E, Cavaillon JM: Septic shock. Lancet 365:63–78, 2005, with permission.)

6. **What is early goal-directed therapy (EGDT)?**

   EGDT is an aggressive treatment protocol aimed at rapidly (within 6 hours of presentation) achieving hemodynamic resuscitation. It involves an algorithmic approach to improving tissue oxygenation through enhancement of preload (intravascular volume), cardiac contractility, afterload (systemic blood pressure), and oxygen-carrying capacity (erythrocyte transfusion to keep hematocrit >30% if central venous oxygen saturation [$ScvO_2$] is low). The cornerstone of EGDT is the ability to accurately and rapidly monitor hemodynamic changes. This involves monitoring the central venous pressure (CVP), systemic blood pressure (commonly through an arterial line), and $ScvO_2$, which are all commonly low in sepsis. Goals include:
   - CVP > 8–12 mmHg
   - Mean arterial blood pressure (MAP) > 65–90 mmHg
   - $ScvO_2$ > 70%

     Interventions to achieve the goals include:
   - Crystalloid infusions for low CVP
   - Vasopressors for low MAP
   - Erythrocyte transfusions and inotropes until the goal $ScvO_2$ is achieved

     Achieving and sustaining EGDT parameters is associated with significant improvements in mortality rates (Fig. 54-2).

7. **Which vasopressors can be used in sepsis?**

   Vasopressors should be used in all patients who do not respond adequately to aggressive volume resuscitation. They are also indicated in severely hypotensive patients undergoing volume resuscitation and patients with severely reduced cardiac output. First-line agents include dopamine (5–20 μg/min) and norepinephrine (2–20 μg/min). Other options include phenylephrine (40–300 μg/min) and vasopressin (0.01–0.04 units/min). Dobutamine (titrated to effect in 2.5-μg/kg/min increments) can be considered in patients with low cardiac output. Unlike other vasoactive agents, vasopressin acts to replace endogenous stores of vasopressin that are deficient in severe sepsis. It has a synergistic effect with other vasopressors and should not be titrated beyond the physiologic doses of 0.04 units/min. All patients taking vasopressors should be monitored for deleterious effects such as tachycardia and coronary, digital, and intra-abdominal ischemia.

8. **Should all septic patients receive corticosteroids?**

   Sepsis negatively affects the hypothalamic-pituitary-adrenal axis via poorly understood mechanisms resulting in relative adrenal insufficiency (RAI). Unlike absolute adrenal insufficiency, RAI is transient and responds to treatment of the underlying sepsis such that steroid replacement can be discontinued after 7 days without a dose taper. RAI is present in patients with a <9 μg/dL rise in serum cortisol 60 minutes after a 250 μg dose of corticotropin. Studies have shown that hydrocortisone 50 μg given intravenously every 6 hours along with fludrocortisone 50 μg daily by mouth in patients with RAI reduces both vasopressor needs and mortality. (See Chapter 63 for more information on diagnosing adrenal insufficiency.)

9. **Is tight glycemic control beneficial in treating sepsis?**

   Aggressive control of hyperglycemia in patients with diabetes has been shown to markedly reduce mortality in critically ill surgical patients, many of whom had a septic focus. Intensive treatment of hyperglycemia, which is initiated by intravenous insulin infusion if the glucose is >110 mg/dL and adjusted to maintain a target of 80–110 mg/dL, reduces morbidity and mortality in comparison to conventionally treated patients maintained in a glucose range of 180–200 mg/dL. Additionally, intensive insulin therapy is associated with reductions in the incidence of dialysis, bacteremia, and neuropathy.

10. **When is drotrecogin alpha indicated?**

    Drotrecogin alpha (Xigris), or recombinant human APC, has anticoagulant, profibrinolytic and anti-inflammatory properties. As an inhibitor of the coagulation pathway, APC counteracts the

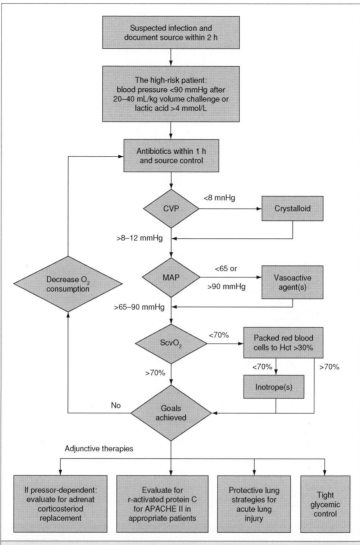

Figure 54-2. Early goal-directed therapy. (From Rivers E, McIntyre L, Morro D, Rivers K: Early and innovative interventions for severe sepsis and septic shock: Taking advantage of a window of opportunity. CMAJ 173:1054–1065, 2005, with permission.)

pathophysiologic effects of sepsis at the microcirculatory level, thereby improving tissue perfusion and organ function. Its role appears to be limited to the sickest patients (i.e., APACHE II score ≥25) with severe sepsis or septic shock and should be started as early in the course as possible, and generally before 24 hours. Used appropriately, it has been shown to significantly decrease the progression to multiorgan system dysfunction and death in septic patients (5% absolute reduction in hospital mortality and a 6% reduction at 28 days). Additionally, APC was associated with faster resolution of respiratory and cardiovascular dysfunction over the first week. There is a trend toward higher risk of bleeding with APC therapy.

KEY POINTS: EVIDENCE-BASED THERAPY TO REDUCE SEPSIS MORTALITY IN THE INTENSIVE CARE UNIT

1. EGDT for sepsis

2. Stress dose steroids for septic patients with RAI

3. Intensive glycemic control for critically ill patients

4. APC for severe sepsis or septic shock

5. Daily hemodialysis for acute renal failure

6. Low tidal volume ventilation for acute respiratory distress syndrome

11. **In critically ill patients with acute renal failure, does daily hemodialysis affect mortality?**
The high mortality rate among critically ill patients with acute renal failure who require renal replacement therapy is related to both coexisting conditions and uremic damage to other organ systems. Intensive or daily hemodialysis results in a mortality of 28% versus 46% with alternate day dialysis.

12. **What is the role of low tidal volume ventilation in acute respiratory distress syndrome (ARDS)?**
Sepsis is the most common cause of ARDS. Low tidal volume (V_T) ventilation is a method aimed at reducing pulmonary barotrauma and the inflammatory response that leads to acute lung injury. The use of low V_T (6 mL/kg of estimated body weight) versus traditional V_T (12 mL/kg), and plateau pressures <30 cm H_2O is associated with improved outcomes in patients with ARDS or acute lung injury. (See Chapter 10, Conventional and Noninvasive Ventilation, for more details.)

WEBSITES

1. Surviving Sepsis Campaign: http://www.survivingsepsis.com

2. Society of Critical Care Medicine: http://www.sccm.org

BIBLIOGRAPHY

1. Annane D, Bellissant E, Cavaillon JM: Septic shock. Lancet 365:63–78, 2005.

2. Annane D, Sebille V, Charpentier C, et al: Effect of treatment with low doses of hydrocortisone and fludrocortisone on mortality in patients with septic shock. JAMA 288:862–871, 2002.

3. Bernard GR, Vincent JL, Laterre PF, et al: Efficacy and safety of recombinant human activated protein C for severe sepsis. N Engl J Med 344:699–709, 2001.

4. Hebert PC, Wells G, Blajchman MA, et al: A multicenter, randomized, controlled clinical trial of transfusion requirements in critical care. Transfusion Requirements in Critical Care Investigators, Canadian Critical Care Trials Group. N Engl J Med 340:409–417, 1999.

5. Levy MM, Fink MP, Marshall JC, et al: 2001 SCCM/ESICM/ACCP/ATS/SIS International Sepsis Definitions Conference. Crit Care Med 31:1250–1256, 2003.

6. Rivers E, McIntyre L, Morro D, Rivers K: Early and innovative interventions for severe sepsis and septic shock: taking advantage of a window of opportunity. CMAJ 173:1054–1065, 2005.

7. Rivers E, Nguyen B, Havstad S, et al: Early goal-directed therapy in the treatment of severe sepsis and septic shock. N Engl J Med 345:1368–1377, 2001.

8. Van den Berghe G, Wouters P, Weekers F, et al: Intensive insulin therapy in the critically ill patients. N Engl J Med 345:1359–1367, 2001.

9. Ventilation with lower tidal volumes as compared with traditional tidal volumes for acute lung injury and the acute respiratory distress syndrome. The Acute Respiratory Distress Syndrome Network. N Engl J Med 342:1301–1308, 2000.

CHAPTER 55

NOSOCOMIAL INFECTIONS

Robert Dexter, MD, and Joseph Ming Wah Li, MD

1. **What are nosocomial infections?**
   Nosocomial infections are those that are acquired >48–72 hours after admission to a health care facility, such as a hospital or rehabilitation center. Any infection that develops within the first 48 hours of admission was likely acquired in the community. Identifying the site where the infection was acquired is essential in determining the most likely infecting organisms and the appropriate empiric therapy.

2. **Which nosocomial infections are the leading cause of morbidity and mortality?**
   Urinary tract infection is the most common, accounting for up to 40% of all nosocomial infections. Hospital-acquired pneumonia is the leading cause of death due to nosocomial infections, with a mortality rate estimated at up to 50%. Other common nosocomial infections include intravenous catheter–associated infections and *Clostridium difficile* colitis.

KEY POINTS: MOST COMMON NOSOCOMIAL INFECTIONS RANKED BY INCIDENCE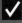

1. Urinary tract infection

2. Pneumonia

3. Catheter-related bloodstream infection

4. *C. difficile*–associated diarrhea

5. Surgical site infections

3. **Which organisms are of greatest concern for infection control in institutional settings?**
   As antimicrobial resistance increases, multidrug-resistant gram-negative rods, especially *Pseudomonas aeruginosa*, and other bacteria such as methicillin-resistant *Staphylococcus aureus* (MRSA), and vancomycin-resistant *Enterococcus* have become prevalent in hospitals throughout the United States.

4. **Describe the prevention of nosocomial infections.**
   The major methods of infection control include surveillance, isolation precautions, hand hygiene, and sterilization. For physicians, hand hygiene is the single most important measure to prevent the transmission of nosocomial infections. The use of alcohol-containing hand disinfection products is likely to be superior to simple handwashing with plain soap, but it does not eliminate the spores of *C. difficile*.

5. **Differentiate between primary and secondary bloodstream infections.**
   Primary bloodstream infections are infections unrelated to an infection at another site, such as lung, urinary tract, or skin; those related to infection at another site are termed *secondary*. The majority of nosocomial bloodstream infections are primary infections, and most of these are related to the use of central venous catheters. Approximately 250,000 primary bloodstream infections occur each year in the United States, making it the third most common nosocomial infection.

6. **Which pathogens commonly cause nosocomial primary bloodstream infections (NPBIs)?**
   - Coagulase-negative staphylococci (31%)
   - *S. aureus* (20%)
   - *Enterococci* (9%)
   - *Candida* species (9%)
   - *Escherichia coli* (6%)
   - *Klebsiella* species (5%)
   - *Pseudomonas* (4%)
   - *Enterobacter* species (4%)
   - *Serratia* species (2%)
   - *Acinetobacter baumannii* (1%)

7. **What patient factors contribute to susceptibility to NPBIs?**
   Factors include the severity of the underlying illness, immunocompromised states (especially neutropenia), malnutrition, extremes of age, and severe burns or disruption of skin integrity.

8. **Describe extrinsic factors associated with NPBIs.**
   As the majority of NPBIs occur in relation to venous catheterization, the type of catheter used, location of catheterization, and method used to insert the catheter directly affect the development of NPBIs. The site of catheter insertion is associated with the risk of infection, with the following sites listed in decreasing order of risk of infection: femoral vein > internal jugular vein > subclavian vein. Non-tunneled catheters impart a greater risk of infection than tunneled catheters. Tunneled catheters, implanted entirely beneath the skin, have the lowest risk of infection. Antimicrobial and antiseptic impregnated catheters carry a lower risk of infection than nonimpregnated catheters, and catheters with attachable silver-impregnated cuffs also lower the risk of infection. The skill of the physician inserting the catheter is inversely related to the risk of infection. Other measures important to lowering the risk of infection include the use of cutaneous antiseptics (alcohol and povidone iodine are better than chlorhexidine) and keeping the skin dry under the dressing. (See Chapter 86 for more information.)

9. **How prevalent is hospital-acquired pneumonia? What is its significance?**
   There are approximately 300,000 cases of hospital-acquired pneumonia annually in the United States, making it the second most common nosocomial infection. It accounts for approximately 60% of all deaths in patients with nosocomial infections, making it the leading cause of mortality from nosocomial infections.

10. **Which organisms are most frequently implicated in hospital-acquired pneumonia?**
    - *P. aeruginosa* (17%)
    - *S. aureus* (16%)
    - *Klebsiella* species (7%)
    - *E. coli* (6%)
    - *Haemophilus influenzae* (6%)

- *Serratia marcescens* (5%)
- Other Enterobacteriaceae species (11%)

Individual organisms most commonly associated with ventilator-associated pneumonia in decreasing order of frequency include *S. aureus* (18.1%), *P. aeruginosa* (17.0%), and *Enterobacter* species (11.2%). Polymicrobial infections are responsible for up to 50% of all cases of ventilator-associated pneumonia.

11. **What factors increase the risk for hospital-acquired pneumonia?**

Mechanical ventilation is the single greatest risk factor for hospital-acquired pneumonia. Other risk factors include advanced age, chronic lung disease, altered consciousness, intrathoracic surgery, large-volume aspiration, ventilator circuit changes, presence of nasogastric tube or intracranial pressure monitor, antacid therapy, and reintubation.

12. **How is hospital-acquired pneumonia diagnosed?**

The diagnosis of hospital-acquired pneumonia may be difficult and is often obscured by concurrent infections and microbial colonization in critically ill patients. The following constellation of findings is associated with hospital-acquired pneumonia: a new and persistent infiltrate (present for >48 hours) on chest imaging, together with:

- Isolation of the same organism in pleural fluid or blood culture as in respiratory secretions, *or*
- Radiographic evidence of pulmonary cavitation or necrosis, *or*
- Two of the following: temperature > 38.3°C, peripheral leukocytosis, and purulent sputum

13. **Describe measures to prevent hospital-acquired and ventilator-associated pneumonia.**

Endotracheal intubation is the major risk for developing nosocomial pneumonia; therefore, the use of alternative therapies such as noninvasive ventilation, when clinically appropriate, decreases the risk of ventilator-associated pneumonia. Noninvasive ventilation has been studied and should be considered in patients with chronic obstructive pulmonary disease, pulmonary edema, community-acquired pneumonia, and hypoxemic respiratory failure. When patients are receiving invasive ventilation, measures such as semi-recumbent positioning, continuous subglottic suctioning, lateral rotation of the patient in their hospital beds, less frequent ventilator circuit changes, and strict adherence to handwashing, universal precautions, and barrier precautions can reduce the risk of ventilator-associated pneumonia. A number of other factors may decrease the risk of ventilator-associated pneumonia. These include limiting oversedation, limiting the use of paralytic agents, maintaining persistent endotracheal intracuff pressure >20 cmH$_2$O, use of orotracheal rather than nasotracheal intubation, use of a closed suctioning system, and treatment with sucralfate rather than H$_2$-receptor antagonists for stress ulcer prophylaxis. Selective decontamination of the digestive tract has been studied, but available data do not justify its routine use.

14. **Describe the treatment for hospital-acquired pneumonia.**

The treatment of hospital-acquired pneumonia should follow three guidelines:

- Select initial empiric antimicrobial regimen that is active against the suspected pathogens.
- Limit the unnecessary use of antibiotics.
- Tailor antibiotic therapy after culture results are returned.

In the majority of patients with nosocomial pneumonia, a specific pathogen is not identified. Empiric antimicrobial therapy should target the most common bacterial causes of nosocomial pneumonia, namely *Staphylococcus* and *Pseudomonas* species, paying attention to local hospital flora and antibiotic resistance patterns. Empiric broad-spectrum gram-negative coverage should include one of the following: antipseudomonal penicillins (e.g., Piperacillin), third- or fourth-generation cephalosporins with antipseudomonal activity (e.g., Ceftazidime or Cefepime, respectively), aminoglycosides (e.g., Gentamicin), Imipenem-Cilastin, Piperacillin-Tazobactam, Ticarcillin-Clavulanate, or Aztreonam. The use of combination therapy with antipseudomonal agents is controversial. If MRSA is a possible pathogen, Vancomycin should be used initially and discontinued later if MRSA is not isolated in cultures.

15. **Why are catheter-associated urinary tract infections (CAUTIs) important?**
CAUTIs are the most common nosocomial infection in the United States. Although <5% of catheter-associated bacteriuric patients will become bacteremic, the large numbers of patients with urinary catheters result in CAUTIs accounting for nearly 15% of nosocomial bloodstream infections. CAUTIs are responsible for approximately 900,000 additional hospital days annually and directly cause almost 1000 deaths.

16. **What patient-specific factors are associated with CAUTIs?**
The longer a patient has a urinary catheter, the more likely he or she is to develop a urinary tract infection. Patient-specific factors that increase the risk of CAUTIs include female sex, immunocompromised conditions such as diabetes mellitus, malnutrition, prolonged hospitalization, abnormal serum creatinine concentration, prolonged hospitalization, and presence of ureteral stents.

17. **How can CAUTIs be prevented?**
The best prevention is to avoid or minimize the duration of indwelling urinary catheters. Aseptic technique should be used for placing the catheter, and while the patient is catheterized, it is important to maintain a closed drainage system. The collection tubing and bag should always be kept lower than the patient, and the tubing should be higher than the bag to prevent urine reflux. For men with urinary incontinence, some have suggested that condom catheters (i.e., condom is applied about the penis and empties through a collection tube into a drainage bag) may lower the incidence of bacteriuria compared with placement of an indwelling urinary catheter. However, urine within the condom itself may lead to colonization of the urethra and skin, and bladder bacteriuria may develop. Intermittent catheterization and placement of a suprapubic catheter, alternative methods for patients who require long-term catheterization, are beneficial in lowering the incidence of bacteriuria.

18. **What is the role of prophylactic antimicrobial therapy in the prevention of CAUTIs?**
Prophylactic systemic antimicrobial therapy can decrease the incidence of bacteriuria. However, the increased risk of antimicrobial resistance outweighs the benefits derived from such therapy. For this reason, the use of prophylactic systemic antibiotic therapy is typically not recommended. The application of topical antimicrobial agents between the catheter and the urethra, irrigation of the bladder with antibacterial solutions, and placement of antimicrobials in the collection bag have not been shown to prevent CAUTIs.

19. **Describe the cause, risk factors, and treatment of funguria.**
Funguria is commonly associated with hospitalized patients with an indwelling urinary catheter. Antimicrobial therapy, increased age, and the presence of diabetes mellitus are common risk factors. *Candida* species are the most common cause of funguria. Funguria usually represents colonization rather than true infection. The presence of pyuria is not helpful in distinguishing colonization from infection. Only 1.3% of patients with candiduria develop candidemia. Asymptomatic candiduria often responds to removal of the urinary catheter, urologic stents, or discontinuation of antibiotics. Asymptomatic candiduria rarely requires antifungal therapy. Patients with symptomatic candiduria should always receive antifungal treatment after identification of the *Candida* species. Most *Candida* species respond to Fluconazole therapy for 7–14 days. Azole-resistant candida should be treated with intravenous Amphotericin B 0.3–0.7 mg/kg/day for up to 7 days. Oral Flucytosine 100 mg/kg/day in four divided doses for 5–7 days is an alternative for non-*albicans* species of candida. Amphotericin B bladder irrigation clears

funguria only transiently, so it is not recommended. Persistent candiduria is an indication for radiologic imaging to evaluate for renal involvement.

KEY POINTS: OVERVIEW OF NOSOCOMIAL INFECTIONS

1. Nosocomial infections are a vast problem in the care of hospitalized patients and lead to significant morbidity and mortality.

2. The majority of nosocomial infections are due to invasion of the patient's barriers to infection with urinary and intravascular catheters, endotracheal intubation, and surgical procedures, as well as the use of inadequate infection control methods.

3. Procedures should be performed with sterile technique, and invasive catheters should be removed at the earliest time when their use is no longer required.

4. The prevalence of multidrug-resistant infectious organisms is rapidly increasing in hospitals and intensive care units, and antibiotics should be used judiciously to prevent the unnecessary development of antimicrobial resistance.

20. **What is antibiotic-associated colitis? What is the etiologic agent?**
Antibiotic-associated colitis is caused by *C. difficile*, which has a broad range of clinical manifestations, from asymptomatic carrier to severe colitis and toxic megacolon. It is an important cause of morbidity and mortality in elderly hospitalized patients. (See Chapter 36 for more details.)

21. **When does nosocomial sinusitis most commonly occur?**
Nosocomial sinusitis is associated with both nasal and oral intubation. Additional predisposing factors include nasogastric tubes, facial and cranial trauma, nasal packing, corticosteroid use, and prior antibiotic use.

22. **How are surgical wound infections diagnosed?**
The diagnosis of a surgical wound infection is made based on the clinical manifestations of fever, erythema, induration, pain, and warmth at the incision site. Necrotizing fasciitis is the most serious wound infection and is a surgical emergency. The cornerstone of treatment of surgical wound infections is opening and exploring the wound, followed by irrigation, drainage, and debridement if necessary. Mild superficial wound infections may be managed without antimicrobial therapy, but if there are signs of local invasion of infection or systemic symptoms, antimicrobial therapy should be directed at gram-positive cocci from the skin as well as the expected flora at the surgical site.

BIBLIOGRAPHY

1. Craven DE, Steger KA: Epidemiology of nosocomial pneumonia: New perspectives on an old disease. Chest 108(Suppl):1S, 1995.

2. Enright MC, Robinson DA, Randle G, et al: The evolutionary history of methicillin-resistant *Staphylococcus aureus* (MRSA). Proc Natl Acad Sci U S A 99:7687, 2002.

3. Garner JS, Jarvis WR, Emori TG, et al: CDC definitions for nosocomial infections, 1988. Am J Infect Control 16:128, 1988.

4. Guidelines for the management of adults with hospital-acquired, ventilator-associated, and healthcare-associated pneumonia. Am J Respir Crit Care Med 171:388, 2005.

5. Kauffman CA, Vazquez JA, Sobel JD, et al: Prospective multicenter surveillance study of funguria in hospitalized patients. The National Institute for Allergy and Infectious Diseases (NIAID) Mycoses Study Group. Clin Infect Dis 30:14, 2000.

6. Kollef MH: Prevention of hospital-associated pneumonia and ventilator-associated pneumonia. Crit Care Med 32:1396, 2004.

7. Prod'hom G, Leuenberger P, Koerfer J, et al: Nosocomial pneumonia in mechanically ventilated patients receiving antacid, ranitidine, or sucralfate. Ann Intern Med 120:653, 1994.

8. Raad II, Bodey GP: Infectious complications of indwelling vascular catheters. Clin Infect Dis 15:197, 1992.

9. Whitehouse JD, Sexton DJ, Kirkland KB: Infection control: Past, present, and future issues. Compr Ther 24:71, 1998.

CHAPTER 56

BONE, JOINT, AND PROSTHETIC JOINT INFECTIONS

Patrick Cawley, MD

1. **What is osteomyelitis (OM)?**
   OM is inflammation and destruction of bone caused by infection. OM is best categorized based on its source: hematogenous spread, contiguous spread from a local infection, local inoculation after trauma or surgery, or secondary to vascular insufficiency.

2. **Who is susceptible to OM from hematogenous spread?**
   Children are especially prone to hematogenous spread to the metaphysis of long bones due to the rich blood supply in this area. Hospitalized patients, especially those older than 50 years, are also susceptible due to the increased presence of risk factors such as diabetes mellitus, urinary tract infections, and intravenous and urinary catheter use.

3. **Which organisms commonly cause OM?**
   Staphylococcus aureus is the most frequent causative organism. Various other bacteria, including coagulase-negative staphylococci, streptococci, Enterobacteriaceae, enterococci, *Propionobacterium* species, anaerobic species, *Salmonella* species, *Bartonella henselae*, *Pasturella multocida*, *Eikenella corrodens*, and *Coxiella burnetii*, can also cause OM. Mycobacteria, including *Mycobacterium avium* and *Mycobacterium tuberculosis*, and fungal pathogens such as *Aspergillus* and *Candida* species are also occasionally implicated.

4. **How is OM diagnosed?**
   Classically, patients present with localized bone pain, fever, tenderness, and swelling; however, approximately 50% of patients present with vague or subacute symptoms.
   A firm diagnosis requires two of the following conditions:
   - Clinical suspicion
   - Abnormal diagnostic study
   - Microbiologic growth

5. **Which studies can be used to diagnose OM?**
   Plain radiographs may reveal soft tissue edema within the first 5 days of infection, but bony abnormalities, periosteal lifting, and cortical lucencies are not usually evident for 2–3 weeks. Other useful studies include a nuclear imaging with technetium (bone scan) or indium (white blood cell scan) showing increased bone uptake and magnetic resonance imaging or computed tomography showing bony changes consistent with OM. The magnetic resonance imaging of the bone is the most sensitive and specific for the diagnosis of OM. Elevated serum markers of inflammation such as sedimentation rate and C-reactive protein in conjunction with an abnormal study can confirm the diagnosis of OM.

6. **What is a bone scan? What are its limitations?**
   A bone scan is a nuclear medicine study that uses a technetium tracer, which is taken up by areas of high bone activity (e.g., fractures, infection, neoplasm). The three phases of a bone scan are described in Table 56-1. The bone scan is limited in patients with diabetic foot ulcers (since all three phases will have increased tracer activity), vascular insufficiency (because the

tracer is unable to reach the area of concern), and areas of increased bone turnover such as neoplasm, injury, Paget's disease, and recent surgery.

TABLE 56-1. THREE PHASES OF A BONE SCAN

Phase	Name	Timing	Tracer Activity	
			Soft Tissue Infection	Bone Infection
First	Angiographic	Immediate	Increased	Increased
Second	Blood pool	15 minutes	Increased	Increased
Third	Bone	3–6 hours	Normal or diffuse mild	Increased and often focal

7. **What is the general treatment of OM?**
   Resolution of OM requires a prolonged course of antibiotics because eradication of bacteria from bone is difficult. The typical antibiotic course is 4–6 weeks of parenteral therapy with a synthetic penicillin (e.g., nafcillin, oxacillin) to cover *Staphylococcus* in healthy adults. Diabetic patients are usually treated with ampicillin/sulbactam to cover gram-negative and anaerobic organisms as well. Patients at risk for methicillin-resistant *S. aureus* (MRSA) infection should be treated with vancomycin or another antibiotic that has MRSA activity (e.g., linezolid, daptomycin, quinupristin/dalfopristin). The role of surgery is both diagnostic and therapeutic, with debridement being an important adjunct in long-standing or severe disease. Cultures of adjacent abscesses, bone biopsy specimens, and blood cultures help tailor the antibiotic treatment. Cultures of draining sinus tracts are perilous in that they may simply reflect overlying skin flora.

8. **What conditions predispose to OM?**
   Diabetes mellitus, sickle cell disease, acquired immunodeficiency syndrome, intravenous drug abuse, alcoholism, chronic steroid use, immunosuppression, chronic joint disease, trauma, hemodialysis, asplenia, and tobacco use all increase one's risk of developing OM.

9. **What is the differential diagnosis of an acutely swollen joint?**
   See Table 56-2.

TABLE 56-2. DIFFERENTIAL DIAGNOSIS OF AN ACUTE SWOLLEN JOINT

Infectious arthritis	Bacterial, viral, rickettsial, and fungal causes
Inflammatory arthritis	Rheumatoid arthritis, psoriatic arthritis, arthritis associated with inflammatory bowel disease
Crystal arthropathies	Gout, pseudogout
Reactive arthritis	Reiter's syndrome
Trauma	Fractures, dislocations, ligament tears

10. **What is the initial management of an acutely swollen joint?**
    Acutely swollen joints require immediate joint aspiration and synovial fluid analysis. Most joints are easily accessed directly with a needle, whereas some, such as the hip or sacroiliac joints,

require imaging to guide placement of the needle. Synovial fluid should be examined with Gram stain, culture and sensitivity, white blood cell count with differential, and crystals via polarized microscopy. (See Chapter 64 for more details.)

11. **Describe the various categories of synovial fluid based on the white blood cell count.**
Using cell counts to separate these groups is done with caution because of significant overlap. Low cell counts never exclude infection (Table 56-3).

TABLE 56-3. CLASSIFICATION OF ARTHRITIS BY SYNOVIAL FLUID				
	Normal	**Noninflammatory**	**Inflammatory**	**Septic**
WBC (cells/mm)^3	<180	200–2000	2000–100,000	>100,000
% of PMNs	<25	<25	>50	>75

WBC = white blood cell, PMN = polymorphonuclear leukocyte.

12. **Which conditions predispose to joint infections?**
Joint infections, or septic arthritis, are associated with bacteremia, intravenous drug use, indwelling catheters, trauma, bites, HIV infection, immunocompromised state, previous joint infection, recent joint surgery or injection, diabetes mellitus, and underlying chronic joint disease.

13. **What organisms can cause septic arthritis?**
S. aureus is the most common organism. Others are noted in Table 56-4.

TABLE 56-4. ORGANISMS THAT CAN CAUSE SEPTIC ARTHRITIS	
Bacteria	*Staphylococcus aureus*, streptococci, *Neisseria gonorrhoeae*, *Borrelia burgdorferi*, Enterobacteriaceae, and *Salmonella* species
Mycobacteria	*M. tuberculosis*
Fungi	*Candida* species, sporotrichosis, cryptococcus, coccidioidomycosis
Viruses	Rubella, parvovirus B19, mumps

14. **When should cultures be sent for unusual organisms?**
Unusual organisms should be suspected in immunosuppressed patients; patients with a history of travel, animal bite, or tuberculosis exposure; and in cases of monoarthritis refractory to therapy.

15. **How commonly does septic arthritis present with monoarticular versus polyarticular involvement?**
Ninety percent have a monoarticular septic joint. Ten percent have polyarticular involvement. Viral arthritis and disseminated gonococcal infections are more often polyarticular in nature.

16. **How is septic arthritis managed?**

    Unless a less commonly encountered organism is suspected, empiric therapy usually begins with oxacillin to cover the most common organism, staphylococcus. If the patient has risk factors for MRSA, then empiric vancomycin should be initiated. Adequate serial drainage is often necessary to decrease the inflammatory component of the joint effusion. Drainage is accomplished by needle aspiration in small joints and arthroscopy in larger joints.

17. **How do disseminated gonococcal infections present?**

    Patients usually present with tenosynovitis, dermatitis, and migratory polyarthralgia or purulent arthritis without skin lesions.

18. **What laboratory tests are useful in the diagnosis of gonococcal arthritis?**

    Blood cultures are useful if results are positive, but a negative result does not rule out the diagnosis. Growth of *Neisseria gonorrhoeae* often requires a special growth media such as Thayer-Martin plates. Samples from the synovium, skin, urethra, cervix, pharynx, or rectum can be tested for *N. gonorrhoeae* using a DNA probe.

19. **How common are prosthetic joint infections (PJIs)?**

    Prosthetic joints are about 10–15-fold more likely to become infected than nonprosthetic joints. However, improved surgical techniques, laminar airflow in the surgical environment, and the use of perioperative antibiotics have led to much lower infections rates. The rate of infection by prosthetic location is as follows:

    - **Hip:** 0.5–1.0 %
    - **Knee:** 0.5–2%
    - **Shoulder:** 1%

20. **Why are prosthetic joints prone to infection?**

    The prosthetic joint lacks a functional microcirculation to deliver immune cells, thus lowering the inoculum of bacteria required to cause an infection by a factor of 100,000. Another critical concept is that of the bacterial biofilm. Certain bacteria are capable of growing in highly differentiated, complex communities of cells adherent to prosthetic material. They erect barriers to antibiotic entry and are less susceptible to many antibiotics because the bacteria are not actively dividing.

KEY POINTS: OSTEOMYELITIS, SEPTIC ARTHRITIS, AND PROSTHETIC JOINT INFECTIONS

1. OM is categorized based on its source: hematogenous spread, contiguous spread from a local infection, local inoculation after trauma or surgery, or secondary to vascular insufficiency.

2. OM requires prolonged antibiotics (e.g., 4–6 weeks) directed at the most likely culprits.

3. Septic arthritis is most commonly caused by *S. aureus*.

4. Prosthetic joints are 10–15 times more likely to become infected than nonprosthetic joints.

5. Infected prosthetic joints require both surgical (device removal) and medical therapy (antibiotics).

21. **What are risk factors for PJI?**

    Rheumatoid arthritis or other systemic illnesses, perioperative nonarticular infections (e.g., urinary tract infection, cellulitis), prior infection of the joint or adjacent bone, and prior surgery on the joint all increase the risk of PJI. Additionally, prolonged duration of surgery, higher number of operating room personnel, postoperative bleeding or hematoma formation, advanced age, diabetes, steroid use, and absence of perioperative antibiotics all increase the risk of infection.

22. **What organisms cause PJI?**

    The most common causative organism is coagulase-negative staphylococcus, causing up to 40% of cases. *S. aureus* is responsible for 20% of infections, with the remaining cases resulting from streptococci, enterococci, gram-negative bacilli, and anaerobes.

23. **What organism is associated with shoulder PJI but not hip or knee?**

    Propionibacterium acnes accounts for up to 16% of infections in prosthetic shoulder joints.

24. **How does the time after arthroplasty help differentiate the causes of PJI?**

    See Table 56-5.

TABLE 56-5.   CHARACTERISTICS OF PROSTHETIC JOINT INFECTIONS BY TIME AFTER ARTHROPLASTY

Category	Time Course	Percent of Total	Typical Pathogens	Presentation	Infection Origin
Early	<3 months	29%	*S. aureus*, gram-negative organisms	Acutely ill; fever, erythema, tenderness over the surgical site	Intraoperative wound contamination
Delayed	3–12 months	41%	Coagulase-negative staph., viridans strep, diphtheroids	Subacutely ill; pain without overlying swelling or systemic signs of illness	Intraoperative wound contamination
Late	>12 months	30%	Skin flora such as staphylococcus and streptococcus	Acutely or subacutely ill; may have symptoms from primary sites of infection	Bacteremia and hematogenous seeding

25. **How is the diagnosis of PJI made?**

    Although there is no consensus on the diagnosis of PJI, a diagnosis generally requires two of the following:
    - Clinical suspicion
    - Microbiologic confirmation via joint aspiration
    - Operative examination noting purulence at the implant site or presence of a sinus tract

Other factors that support a diagnosis of PJI include growth in more than one specimen (e.g., blood, bone, joint fluid), a short time to culture positivity, a positive Gram stain result, and the presence of acute inflammation on histopathologic examination.

26. What is the general treatment for PJI?
Treatment is divided into initial medical and surgical treatment, management of treatment failures, and long-term suppressive or preventive treatment. Initial treatment typically consists of intravenous antibiotics and debridement, with device removal in most cases. Device removal can be a one- or two-stage exchange. The latter involves initial removal of the infected prosthesis, interval placement of an internal or external joint spacer for several weeks, and eventual reimplantation of a new prosthesis. The joint spacer maintains the potential space for future reimplantation of a new hip prosthesis and is usually impregnated with antibiotics that slowly leak out of the material into the surrounding area. Management of treatment failures is complex and varied. Arthrodesis is joint fusion typically for pain relief and limited mobility when reimplantation of another joint is not possible. Long-term suppressive antibiotics are occasionally used in the case of chronic infection.

BIBLIOGRAPHY

1. Costerton JW, Stewart PS, et al: Bacterial biofilms: A common cause of persistent infections. Science 284:1318–1322, 1999.
2. Giulieri SG, Ochsner PE, Zimmerli W: Management of infection associated with total hip arthroplasty according to a treatment algorithm. Infection 32:222–228, 2004.
3. Mandell GB, Dolin R (eds): Principles and Practice of Infectious Disease. Philadelphia, Churchill Livingstone, 2000.
4. Zimmerli WT, Ochsner P: Current concepts: Prosthetic joint infections. N Engl J Med 351:1645–1654, 2004.

VENOUS THROMBOEMBOLISM

Val Akopov, MD, and Alpesh N. Amin, MD, MBA

CHAPTER 57

1. **What is venous thromboembolism (VTE)?**

   Venous thromboembolism is a cumulative term describing the presence of thrombus in the deep vein (DVT) or thrombus dislodged and embolized to the pulmonary circulation (PE). Clinical presentation ranges from minimally symptomatic calf thrombosis to fatal PE.

2. **How common is VTE?**

   An estimated 2 million cases of DVT and 600,000 cases of symptomatic PE occur annually in the United States. PE accounts for 200,000 deaths and 30,000 cases of pulmonary hypertension. Another 1 million cases of silent PE are estimated to occur annually. Furthermore, approximately 40% of the annual 2 million cases of DVT (800,000 cases) develop post-thrombotic syndrome.

3. **What conditions predispose to VTE?**

   Two centuries ago an Austrian physician, Rudolph Virchow, postulated that three conditions must be present for a blood clot to form: venous stasis, blood vessel damage, and blood hypercoagulability. His brilliant theory proved to be true, and we refer to it as a *Virchow's triad*. (See Chapter 77 for more details.)

4. **Name the risk factors for VTE.**

   Some risk factors for VTE are acquired, whereas other are inherited.
   - **Acquired risk factors:** Age, surgery, and estrogen therapy
   - **Inherited risk factors:** Thrombophilias, cancer, and surgery

   All clinical risk factors for VTE are linked to the Virchow's triad. For instance, surgery is associated with vessel wall damage, as well as immobilization (i.e., venous stasis) and hypercoagulability due to massive release of procoagulation tissue factors triggering the coagulation cascade. These risk factors are generally cumulative; thus, the more risk factors present in an individual patient, the higher likelihood of VTE (Table 57-1).

5. **How do patients with DVT present?**

   Diagnosis of DVT is not easy to make at the bedside. DVT of the iliac, femoral, or popliteal veins is suggested by unilateral swelling, warmth, and erythema. The most common complaint is calf pain. Physical examination may reveal posterior calf tenderness, increased tissue turgor, modest swelling, and occasionally a cord. Homan's sign, increased resistance or pain during dorsiflexion of the foot, is an unreliable diagnostic sign. Sensitivity has been estimated to be 50%.

6. **What is the differential diagnosis of DVT?**

   The differential diagnosis of DVT includes a ruptured popliteal cyst (Baker's cyst), muscle rupture or hemorrhage, arterial occlusive disorders, cellulitis, tendonitis, and nerve compression syndromes.

TABLE 57-1. RISK FACTORS FOR VTE
Inherited risk factors
Antithrombin III deficiency
Dysfibrinogenemia
Protein C deficiency
Protein S deficiency
Factor V Leiden
Prothrombin 20210A
Acquired risk factors
Trauma (major or lower extremity)
Surgery
Immobility or paresis
Malignancy
Cancer therapy (hormonal, chemotherapy or radiotherapy)
Previous VTE
Increasing age (65 years and older)
Pregnancy and postpartum state
Hormone replacement therapy or estrogen-containing oral contraception
Acute medical illness
Heart or respiratory failure
Inflammatory bowel disease
Nephrotic syndrome
Myeloproliferative disorders
Paroxysmal nocturnal hemoglobinuria
Obesity
Tobacco use
Varicose veins
Central venous catheterization
Acquired hypercoagulable states (antiphospholipid syndrome)

7. **What are the Wells' criteria?**
   Wells' clinical prediction rule is a validated tool for assessing the likelihood of DVT in an individual patient. Based on the scoring system, a patient's likelihood of having DVT can be determined to be low, intermediate, or high. Wells' scoring system helps to interpret the results of commonly used diagnostic tests. For instance, a combination of low or intermediate likelihood of DVT by Wells' criteria combined with the negative D-dimer test safely eliminates need for any further diagnostic testing, such as ultrasonography (Table 57-2).

8. **What is the role of Doppler or compression ultrasound in the diagnosis of DVT?**
   Doppler ultrasound measures the velocity of blood flow in veins with flow abnormalities occurring when deep venous obstruction is present. Compression ultrasound detects thrombus

TABLE 57-2. PRETEST PROBABILITY OF DEEP VEIN THROMBOSIS USING WELLS' CRITERIA

Clinical Feature	Score
Active cancer (treatment ongoing, within the previous 6 months, or palliative)	1
Paralysis, paresis, or recent plaster immobilization of the lower extremities	1
Recently bedridden for more than 3 days or major surgery, within 4 weeks	1
Localized tenderness along the distribution of the deep venous system	1
Entire leg swollen	1
Calf swelling by more than 3 cm compared with the asymptomatic leg (measured below tibial tuberosity)	1
Pitting edema (greater in the symptomatic leg)	1
Collateral superficial veins (nonvaricose)	1
Alternative diagnosis as likely or more likely than that of deep vein thrombosis	−2

Probability

High probability = 3 or greater

Moderate probability = 1 or 2

Low probability = 0 or less

Adapted from Wells PS, Anderson DR, Bormanis J, et al: Value of assessment of pretest probability of deep-vein thrombosis in clinical management. Lancet 350:1795–1798, 1997, and Wells PS, Anderson DR, Rodger M, et al: Evaluation of D-dimer in the diagnosis of suspected deep-vein thrombosis. N Engl J Med 349:1227–1235, 2003.

when the vein does not collapse on compressive maneuvers. Both sensitivity and specificity of venous ultrasonography approach 95%.

9. **What is the role of magnetic resonance imaging in diagnosing DVT?**
The diagnostic accuracy of magnetic resonance imaging is similar to that of ultrasound. It is useful in patients with suspected superior or inferior venae cavae or pelvic vein clots.

10. **What are D-dimers?**
D-Dimers are by-products of degradation of fibrin, resulting from activation of endogenous thrombolysis. D-Dimers can be measured quantitatively via enzyme-linked immunosorbent assay (ELISA) or latex agglutination tests, or qualitatively. The ELISA tests are the most sensitive.

11. **What is the utility of D-dimer tests in the diagnosis of DVT?**
D-Dimer tests are in general highly sensitive (95–99%) but very nonspecific (40–60%). The main utility of the D-dimer test is to rule out DVT because its high sensitivity translates into a high negative predictive value. In another words, if the D-dimer test result is negative, the patient has a very low likelihood of having a DVT. However, a positive D-dimer test result is less helpful because there are multiple conditions that may lead to elevated D-dimer titers including advanced age, recent surgery, infection, inflammatory states, and elevated liver enzyme levels.

12. **What is the role of venography in diagnosing DVT?**

Venography remains the gold standard for diagnosing DVT. It offers a high sensitivity (90%) and specificity (95%). The disadvantage of venography is that it is an invasive test requiring injection of contrast medium into the superficial vein of the foot.

13. **How do patients with PE present?**

A careful history and thorough physical examination can be immensely helpful in diagnosing PE. The most common symptoms (with associated sensitivity) are dyspnea (73%), pleuritic chest pain (66%), cough (37%), and hemoptysis (13%). The most common signs are tachypnea (70%), rales (51%), tachycardia (30%), and S_4 gallop (24%). Because of the broad range of presenting symptoms and signs PE is often called the "great mimicker."

14. **How is PE diagnosed?**

- **Pretest probability:** The first step is to determine the pretest probability of PE based on history and physical examination. The major predictors of PE (from the modified Well's criteria) include a clinical syndrome consistent with DVT and a lack of an alternative diagnoses for the patient's symptoms. Additional testing can help confirm the diagnoses.
- **D-dimer test:** Similar to the work-up of DVT, a negative D-dimer test result virtually rules out the diagnosis of PE.
- **Pulmonary angiography:** This remains the gold standard for diagnosing PE but is rarely used because of its invasive nature and risk of contrast-induced nephropathy.
- **Chest x-ray:** Chest radiographs commonly show atelectasis (69%) and pleural effusion (47%). Other radiographic abnormalities include Westermark's sign (focal oligemia, noted as lack of vascularity), Hampton's hump (peripheral wedge-shaped density above the diaphragm), and Palla's sign (enlarged right descending pulmonary artery).
- **Spiral computed tomography scan:** This test has a sensitivity approaching 75–80%. At the present time, a negative computed tomography result does not rule out PE in patients with a high clinical suspicion for PE.
- **Ventilation/perfusion (V/Q) scan:** This scan is very helpful when the result is reported as normal or high probability (which occurs in only ~15% of cases). When the V/Q scan is reported as low or intermediate probability, the results should be interpreted in light of the clinical suspicion (pretest probability) for PE using Well's criteria.
- **Electrocardiography (ECG):** ECG results are often abnormal, but the findings lack sensitivity and specificity. The most common ECG abnormality is sinus tachycardia. However, rhythm disturbances and signs of right-sided heart failure from pulmonary hypertension, including right bundle branch block and an s1q3t3 pattern, may be seen. The s1q3t3 pattern indicates a prominent s wave in lead 1, a q wave in lead 3, and t wave inversion or flattening in lead 3. Table 57-3 summarizes the modified Well's criteria for clinical assessment for PE.

15. **What are the initial treatment options for VTE?**

There are two initial treatment options for VTE:

- Intravenous *unfractionated heparin* (at a dose of 80-U/kg bolus followed by 18-U/kg infusion with close monitoring of PTT), *or*
- Subcutaneous *low-molecular-weight heparin* (LMWH) injections administered once or twice daily depending on the type of LMWH. The advantage of LMWH is that no routine monitoring is required in most patients. LMWH is relatively contraindicated in obese patients and those with renal insufficiency but may be used if anti-Xa levels are measured periodically to ensure therapeutic levels of anticoagulation.

Coumadin (warfarin) should be started simultaneously with heparin and continued for approximately 5 days to ensure adequate anticoagulation before stopping the heparin.

TABLE 57-3. MODIFIED WELLS' CRITERIA: CLINICAL ASSESSMENT FOR PE	
Clinical Feature	**Score**
Clinical symptoms of DVT	3
Other diagnosis less likely than pulmonary embolism	3
Heart rate > 100	1
Immobilization or surgery in the previous 4 weeks	1
Previous DVT/PE	1
Hemoptysis	1
Malignancy	1
Probability	**Score**
High	>6
Moderate	2–6
Low	<2

Adapted from Wells PS, Anderson DR, Rodger M, et al: Excluding pulmonary embolism at the bedside without diagnostic imaging: Management of patients with suspected pulmonary embolism presenting to the emergency department by using a simple clinical model and D-dimer. Ann Intern Med 135:98–107, 2001.

16. **What is the role of outpatient treatment for DVT and PE?**
Outpatient treatment of DVT with LMWH and warfarin has become the standard of care in selected patients. Outpatient treatment of uncomplicated PE with LMWH (patients who are hemodynamically stable, not hypoxic, and without significant comorbid conditions) is an accepted and safe alternative to the inpatient treatment. This should only be considered in patients with good follow-up and social support structures.

17. **What is the role of thrombolytic therapy in the initial treatment of VTE?**
In patients with acute DVT of the lower or upper extremity, thrombolytic therapy is generally reserved for limb-salvaging situations. However, young, otherwise healthy patients with a significantly large clot burden should also be considered for thrombolytic therapy to help avoid the risks of postphlebitic syndrome. Postphlebitic syndrome occurs in about 40% of patients with DVT and is a significant cause of morbidity (i.e., chronic pain, swelling, and recurrent dermatitis), recurrent DVT, and cost. In patients with acute PE, thrombolytic therapy is reserved for those with hemodynamic instability, shock, and/or significant right ventricular failure or pulmonary hypertension on echocardiogram.

18. **What are the indications for inferior vena cava interruption (IVC filters)?**
An IVC filter is a barrier that is placed in the IVC by interventional radiologists to prevent clot propagation proximally, thus avoiding a PE. The placement of IVC filters is confined to selected patients with the following indications:
- Contraindications for anticoagulation
- Complications of anticoagulation
- Recurrent VTE despite adequate anticoagulation

Although IVC filters have been proven to prevent PE in patients with the DVT, most nonanticoagulated patients develop postphlebitic syndrome within 2 years.

19. **How long should patients with VTE be treated?**
   After a short course of unfractionated heparin or LMWH, most patients are transitioned to chronic warfarin therapy. The duration of warfarin therapy varies based on the clinical scenario.
   - Patients with the identifiable transient risk factors: 3 months
   - Patients with the first episode of idiopathic VTE: 6–12 months
   - Patients with recurrent idiopathic VTE: lifelong
   - Patients with inherited or acquired thrombophilia in the setting of a DVT or high risk for DVT development: lifelong

KEY POINTS: VENOUS THROMBOEMBOLISM

1. Inpatient mortality from PE in the United States is estimated at 200,000 per year, making it a more common cause of death than breast cancer, AIDS, and liver disease.

2. A negative D-dimer test result nearly rules out significant DVT.

3. Noninvasive testing with a Doppler ultrasound has sensitivity and specificity approaching 95% for diagnosing DVT.

4. The use of LMWH allows most patients with DVT and some patients with documented hemodynamically stable PE to be treated as outpatients.

5. Without prophylaxis, VTE occurs in 10–20% of medical patients and as many as 60–80% of ICU and surgical patients.

6. Chemoprophylaxis should be considered in all patients at high risk for DVT, unless contraindications such as bleeding exist.

20. **What is the prognosis of treated and untreated VTE?**
   Without treatment, the mortality from PE approaches 30%. With timely diagnosis and effective therapy, mortality is reduced to 2–8%. Untreated symptomatic proximal DVT will progress to PE in approximately 50% of cases. In both cases, aggressive treatment aims to limit clot extension, prevent PE, limit the recurrence of DVT, and inhibit the development of the postphlebitic syndrome and pulmonary hypertension.

21. **What is the incidence of VTE in hospitalized patients?**
   The incidence of VTE varies among the different patient groups. Patients with spinal cord injury, hip and knee arthroplasty, hip surgery, and major trauma are at highest risk for VTE. This has to be taken into consideration when choosing the appropriate VTE prophylaxis regimen (Table 57-4).

22. **Can VTE in hospitalized patients be prevented?**
   Most hospitalized patients have multiple risk factors for VTE, but it is impossible to predict which at-risk patients will develop symptomatic VTE. The adverse consequences of VTE include fatal PE, symptomatic DVT and PE, risk of recurrent VTE, chronic postphlebitic syndrome, and cost of treating the clot. Fortunately, thromboprophylaxis is highly efficacious at preventing symptomatic VTE and fatal PE. Cost-effectiveness of prophylaxis has repeatedly been demonstrated. The most favorable approach supported by the best evidence involves the implementation of group-specific prophylaxis routinely for all patients who belong to each major target group.

TABLE 57-4. ABSOLUTE RISK OF VTE IN HOSPITALIZED
PATIENTS

Patient Group	VTE Prevalence (%)
Medical patients	10–20
General surgery	20–40
Major gynecologic surgery	15–40
Major urologic surgery	15–40
Neurosurgery	15–40
Stroke	20–50
Hip or knee arthroplasty, hip fracture	40–60
Major trauma	40–80
Spinal cord injury	60–80
Critical care patients	10–80

23. **List different thromboprophylaxis regimens recommended in common patient groups.**
    - VTE chemoprophylaxis should be used in all critical care patient without a contraindication. Additionally, all hospitalized medical patients with congestive heart failure or acute respiratory disease, or those who are bedridden for >72 hours and have one or more additional risk factors for VTE (i.e., cancer, previous VTE, sepsis, inflammatory bowel disease, or acute neurologic disease) should receive chemoprophylaxis: low-dose unfractionated heparin, 5000 units given subcutaneously three times a day; enoxaparin, 40 mg given subcutaneously each day; or dalteparin, 5000 units given subcutaneously each day.
    - VTE prophylaxis in patients undergoing hip and knee arthroplasty: enoxaparin, 40 mg given subcutaneously each day or 30 mg given subcutaneously twice a day; fondaparinux 2.5 mg given subcutaneously each day; or warfarin, adjusted dose to achieve international normalized ratio of 2.0–3.0.
    - VTE prophylaxis in patients undergoing general surgery, urologic surgery, gynecologic procedures and vascular surgery depends on the extent of the surgical intervention (minor or major) and the presence of additional risk factors for VTE. (See Chapter 77 for more details.)

24. **What is the role of nonchemoprophylaxis in patients at risk for VTE?**
    Nonpharmacologic means of prophylaxis including stockings, sequential compression devices, and ambulation should be considered in patients who have a contraindication for chemoprophylaxis, such as patients with bleeding risks and risk of developing heparin-induced thrombocytopenia. Postsurgical patients who are considered at very high risk for development of VTE should be considered for chemoprophylaxis plus mechanical prophylaxis. Ambulation is recommended in all patients once they can safely ambulate, regardless of whether chemoprophylaxis is used or not.

BIBLIOGRAPHY

1. Agnelli G, Prandoni P, Santamaria MG, et al: Three months versus one year of oral anticoagulation therapy for idiopathic deep venous thrombosis. Warfarin Optimal Duration Italian Trial Investigator. N Engl J Med 345:165–169, 2001.

2. Hirsh J, Guyatt G, Albers GW, et al: The Seventh ACCP Conference on Antithrombotic and Thrombolytic Therapy: Evidence-based guidelines. Chest 126(3 Suppl):1S–173S, 2004.

3. Kearon C, Gent M, Hirsh J, et al: A comparison of three months of anticoagulation with extended anticoagulation for a first episode of idiopathic venous thromboembolism. N Engl J Med 340:901–907, 1999.

4. Konstantinides S, Geibel A, Heusel G, et al: Heparin plus alteplase compared with heparin alone in patients with submassive pulmonary embolism. N Engl J Med 347:1143–1150, 2002.

5. Samama MM, Cohen AT, Darmon JY, et al: A comparison of enoxaparin with placebo for the prevention of venous thromboembolism in acutely ill medical patients. Prophylaxis in Medical Patients with Enoxaparin Study Group. N Engl J Med 341:793–800, 1999.

CHAPTER 58

ANEMIA IN THE HOSPITALIZED PATIENT

Gregory J. Misky, MD

1. **What do hemoglobin and hematocrit measure?**
   - **Hemoglobin:** Hemoglobin is the major pigment in whole blood responsible for carrying oxygen.
   - **Hematocrit:** Hematocrit is the percentage of intact red blood cells (RBCs) occupying a volume of whole blood.

2. **How is *anemia* defined?**
   Anemia is defined as a reduction in the RBC mass in the circulation. In clinical practice, anemia is defined as hemoglobin <13.5 gm/dL or hematocrit <41% in men, and hemoglobin <12.0 gm/dL or hematocrit <36% in women.

3. **Given that hemoglobin and hematocrit represent concentrations, what physiologic variables affect their levels?**
   Altitude and tobacco elevate the hematocrit through hypoxia, which stimulates erythropoietin to produce more RBCs; dehydration increases the hematocrit through loss of plasma volume; and pregnancy produces a lower hematocrit as plasma volume increases out of proportion to RBC mass.

4. **What is the incidence of anemia in hospitalized patients?**
   Anemia is present in up to 45% of inpatients and as many as 95% of patients in the intensive care unit (ICU) within 3 days of admission.

5. **What are the causes of anemia in hospitalized patients?**
   An appropriate cause is found in 65–80%, with anemia of chronic disease (35%) and iron deficiency anemia (15–33%) most common, followed by renal insufficiency and alcohol-induced anemia. No obvious etiology is identified in up to 25% of patients.

6. **What are the physiologic effects of anemia?**
   Patients with anemia may have an increased heart rate, decreased blood pressure, and ultimately impaired delivery of oxygen to vital tissues.

7. **How does a healthy patient compensate for anemia?**
   Healthy patients compensate for anemia by increasing cardiac output, increasing oxygen extraction in peripheral tissue, and shifting the oxygen-hemoglobin dissociation curve. Under normal physiologic conditions, if intravascular volume is maintained and cardiac status is preserved, a healthy patient can effectively deliver oxygen down to a hematocrit of 10%.

8. **What are the symptoms of anemia?**
   Fatigue, weakness, shortness of breath. Symptoms depend on the etiology and acuity of the anemia, as well as a patient's underlying condition. For example, a 42-year-old patient with no medical problems presenting with anemia due to subacute menstrual blood loss is likely to be less symptomatic than an 80-year-old with congestive heart failure, chronic renal insufficiency, and rapid bleeding from a peptic ulcer.

9. **Which conditions are associated with a higher likelihood of morbidity and mortality in an anemic patient?**
    Anemia in patients with chronic renal insufficiency, congestive heart failure, coronary artery disease (CAD), or cancer, as well as certain surgical populations and elderly persons, is associated with worse outcomes.

10. **What is a reticulocyte, and what does the reticulocyte count tell you?**
    An RBC recently released from the bone marrow is termed a *reticulocyte.* A normal reticulocyte count of 1–2% reflects effective RBC production under normal conditions and indicates that approximately 1–2 out of every 100 RBCs are new. However, the normal marrow response is to increase RBC production in the face of anemia. Consequently, as the patient's anemia worsens, the bone marrow response should become more robust such that a reticulocyte count of 1–2% is no longer sufficient. The reticulocyte index (RI) provides a more accurate measure of the bone marrow response to a given anemia.

    $$RI = reticulocytes(percent) \times (patient\ hematocrit/45)$$

    For example, in a patient with a reticulocyte count of 6% and hematocrit of 15%:

    $$RI = 6 \times (15/45) = 2$$

11. **How is the RI useful in classifying a patient with anemia?**
    An RI that does not increase with anemia implies a bone marrow production problem:
    - An **RI ≥ 2.5** reflects a normal response to hemolysis or blood loss
    - An **RI < 2.5** indicates a hypoproliferative state or a maturation defect
    The RBC indices (measured by mean corpuscular volume [MCV]) can then be used to further characterize the anemia.
    - RI < 2.5 and MCV normal = hypoproliferative state
    - RI < 2.5 and MCV is ↑ or ↓ = maturation defect

12. **How is anemia classified?**
    Anemia can be classified functionally or morphologically. Functionally, anemia can be due to a production defect such as bone marrow invasion or impaired RBC maturation (e.g., acute myelogenous leukemia, vitamin B12 deficiency), a destructive process (hemolysis), or blood loss.
    The MCV (a measure of RBC size) helps classify patients morphologically. For example, the MCV helps distinguish microcytic (MCV < 80 fL), normocytic (MCV 80–100 fL), or macrocytic (MCV > 100 fL) causes of anemia (Table 58-1).

TABLE 58-1. MORPHOLOGIC CLASSIFICATION OF ANEMIA BY MCV		
Microcytic MCV < 80 fL	**Normocytic MCV 80–100 fL**	**Macrocytic MCV > 100 fL**
Iron deficiency	Early iron deficiency	Normal variant
Thalassemia	Hemolysis	Liver disease
Anemia of chronic disease	Acute blood loss	Alcoholism
Sideroblastic anemia	Anemia of chronic disease	Myelodysplastic syndromes
Aluminum toxicity	Hypersplenism	Myelophthisis
	G6PD deficiency	Megaloblastic anemia
		Hypothyroidism
G6PD = glucose–6–phosphate dehydrogenase deficiency.		

13. **Name the most common causes of microcytic anemia.**
Iron and dietary deficiencies represent one third of all cases of anemia. Anemia of chronic disease, thalassemia, hemoglobinopathies (e.g., sickle cell), and lead intoxication (in children; now rare in the United States) are less common causes of microcytic anemia.

14. **What laboratory studies are used to confirm a diagnosis of iron deficiency anemia?**
Ferritin represents total body iron stores and is the best screening test. A ferritin level ≤ 30 µg/L has a positive predictive value of 92% for iron deficiency. A ferritin level of >100 µg/L in a nonacutely ill patient virtually excludes the diagnosis. Ferritin is an acute-phase reactant and is artificially elevated in inflammatory states. In such patients, an elevated soluble transferring receptor will be seen. Other useful tests include measurements of iron and iron saturation, which are usually reduced, and transferrin iron-binding capacity (TIBC), which is elevated.

15. **What is the most common cause of iron deficiency anemia?**
Blood loss, primarily occult gastrointestinal (GI) blood loss. Up to two thirds of these patients will have lesions identified, even in the absence of GI-specific symptoms. Peptic ulcer disease and colon cancer are the most frequent causes identified on endoscopy. In premenopausal women, blood loss due to menstruation is a common cause of iron deficiency anemia.

16. **Name the most common causes of normocytic anemia.**
Anemia of chronic disease, chronic renal insufficiency, and bone marrow suppression. In addition, acute blood loss and early iron deficiency are important causes to remember in the differential diagnosis for normocytic anemia.

17. **What are the most common causes of acute blood loss in hospitalized patients?**
Many patients who present to the hospital with anemia have not been bleeding long enough to develop iron deficiency and therefore have a normocytic anemia. The most common cause of acute blood loss anemia is GI tract bleeding. Hematuria, epistaxis, retroperitoneal bleeding (in the setting of recent femoral catheterization), and iatrogenic blood loss (due to frequent draws for laboratory tests) produce less clinically significant blood loss, unless a patient is anticoagulated.

18. **What is anemia of chronic disease?**
Anemia of chronic disease is anemia due to a blunted response to erythropoietin (EPO) and to iron resistance. It is typically associated with chronic inflammatory processes. In 60% of patients, the principal associated diagnosis is a chronic infection (e.g., tuberculosis, abscess), inflammatory (e.g., rheumatoid arthritis) or neoplastic; renal insufficiency is present in over 15%. It presents with a microcytic or normocytic anemia with low iron levels and transferrin iron-binding capacity but high ferritin levels.

19. **How are hemolytic anemias classified?**
Hemolytic anemias are classified by the location of the defect: intracorpuscular or extracorpuscular.
- **Intrinsic defect:** Instability within the RBC structure, usually hereditary. Includes hemoglobin Köln, paroxysmal nocturnal hemoglobinuria, hereditary spherocytosis, thalassemia, and glucose-6-phosphate dehydrogenase deficiency.
- **Extrinsic defect:** Factors outside the RBC structure, usually acquired. Includes trauma (e.g., prosthetic aortic valves), splenomegaly, antibody destruction of RBC membrane

(e.g., autoimmune hemolytic anemia), and microvascular destruction (e.g., disseminated intravascular coagulation).

20. **What are the classic laboratory findings in a patient with hemolytic anemia?**
Reticulocyte count, lactate dehydrogenase level, and indirect bilirubin level are increased; haptoglobin level is decreased. Haptoglobin binds free hemoglobin released from hemolyzed RBCs; a low haptoglobin measurement (i.e., <25 mg/dL) is highly sensitive (83%) and specific (96%) in detecting hemolysis. The peripheral smear can often provide evidence as to the type of hemolytic anemia (Table 58-2).

TABLE 58-2. PERIPHERAL SMEAR FINDINGS IN HEMOLYTIC ANEMIA

Cell Morphology	Description	Disorder
Spherocyte	Spherical, no pale center	Hereditary spherocytosis Immune hemolytic anemia
Target cell	Hypochromic; dark center and periphery with clear ring between	Liver disease Thalassemia
Schistocyte	Fragmented RBC	Microangiopathic destruction (DIC, TTP, HUS)
Spur cell (acanthocyte)	Spiny projections on RBC	Severe liver disease
Howell-Jolly bodies	Spherical blue bodies on/in RBCs (on Wright's stain)	Severe blood loss Severe hemolysis Hyposplenism
Nucleated RBCs	RBCs with nuclei present	Myelophthisic anemia (bone marrow infiltration with tumor, granulomatous disease or fibrosis)

RBC = red blood cell, DIC = disseminated intravascular coagulation, TTP = thrombotic thrombocytopenic purpura, HUS = hemolytic uremic syndrome.

21. **What are the Coombs' studies?**
Coombs' studies are tests that help determine an immune cause of a hemolytic anemia.
- **Direct Coombs' test:** This study measures agglutination that occurs between antibodies specific for either immunoglobulins or complement and a protein present on a patient's RBC. A direct Coombs' test will have a positive result in 98% of patients with an autoimmune hemolytic anemia. Disorders associated with autoimmune hemolytic anemia include viral infections, chronic lymphocytic leukemia, and medications (e.g., penicillin, methyldopa, quinine).
- **Indirect Coombs' test:** This test detects antibodies with anti–immunoglobulin G after serum of a patient is incubated with normal RBCs.

KEY POINTS: ANEMIA IN HOSPITALIZED PATIENTS

1. Recognize that anemia reflects an underlying disease state that must be uncovered.

2. There are frequently multiple causes of anemia in a patient producing a "mixed" anemia. For example, a patient with renal disease may have both anemia of chronic disease and iron deficiency anemia.

3. The ferritin helps distinguish iron deficiency anemia (↓ ferritin) from anemia of chronic disease (↑ ferritin).

4. The most common causes of anemia of chronic disease are chronic infection (e.g., abscess), malignancy (e.g., lymphoma), and inflammatory state (e.g., rheumatoid arthritis).

5. Hemolysis should be suspected in a patient with a rapid decline in hemoglobin and no identifiable bleeding, and it should be diagnosed in those with a high reticulocyte index, high lactate dehydrogenase level, high indirect bilirubin level, and a low haptoglobin level.

6. The decision to treat an anemic patient should be based on physiologic deficiencies rather than an absolute number.

22. **What are the most common causes of macrocytic anemia in the hospital?**
Alcohol abuse is the most common. Liver disease and megaloblastic anemia, a disorder of DNA synthesis of RBC precursors in the bone marrow, also represent a significant proportion. Causes of megaloblastic anemia include folic acid and vitamin B_{12} deficiencies, as well as medications. Hypothyroidism and myelodysplastic syndrome are other etiologies of macrocytic anemia. Myelodysplastic syndrome should be considered in elderly patients, particularly if other cell line abnormalities are seen (e.g., neutropenia, thrombocytopenia and circulating blasts).

23. **What medications are known to cause megaloblastic anemia?**
Hydroxyurea, azathioprine, zidovudine, and methotrexate are the most common inducers of megaloblastic anemia.

24. **Which factors are important in deciding which patients may benefit from RBC transfusion?**
The decision to transfuse should be based on clinical findings of diminished oxygen transport and not a predetermined hematocrit. The use of transfusion to an hematocrit of greater than 30% (hemoglobin of >10 gm/dL) is not evidence based and rarely necessary. Additional considerations for the need to transfuse include the cause of the anemia, the acuity of the anemia (acute bleeding requires more aggressive transfusion), and patient characteristics such as a history of CAD or acute chest pain or hypoxia.

25. **What are the transfusion recommendations in the following populations: CAD, ICU, surgical (vascular and coronary artery bypass graft [CABG], orthopedic), and acute bleeding?**
   - **CAD:** Anemia is a known and significant risk factor; most studies demonstrate transfusion benefit in patients with hematocrit <25%; transfusion for hematocrit between 25–30% is more controversial.

- **ICU:** Up to half of all ICU patients are transfused; little clinical benefit in giving blood until hematocrit <21%. There is potential negative effect of transfusion in the ICU, especially if the patient is less acutely ill or younger (<55 years). An increased number of transfusions correlates with a longer ICU stay and increased mortality.
- **Surgical (vascular and CABG):** Patients have a higher preoperative likelihood of CAD. Low preoperative hemoglobin levels or significant blood loss increases morbidity and mortality rates in these patients, particularly if CAD present. There is threshold and benefit to transfusion when perioperative state involves a hematocrit >25–27%.
- **Orthopedic:** Up to 90% of patients undergoing total joint replacements receive blood despite the fact that 30- and 90-day mortality is not improved if patients with a hematocrit >24% are transfused. A more restrictive transfusion policy (i.e., transfuse to above hematocrit >21%) is reasonable, assuming (1) there are no other comorbid indications such as CAD, and (2) the patient is hemodynamically stable.
- **Acute bleeding:** Because patients bleed blood and not just RBCs, they will lose a proportionate amount of all intravascular components such that the hematocrit (a percentage of RBCs in the blood) will remain unchanged until adequate volume is repleted (diluting the hematocrit to a lower value). In most cases, acutely bleeding patients do not require blood; rather, they need volume (e.g., normal saline) to maintain their blood pressure. However, in major acute hemorrhage, it is often prudent to transfuse both blood (packed RBCs) and volume.

26. What is the downside of transfusion?

The biggest downsides are transfusion reactions, infection, and cost. Transfusion reactions, which can occur in up to 5% of transfused patients, are both immune mediated (i.e., antibody directed) and nonimmune (i.e., volume overload). Immunomodulatory effects of transfused blood are thought to be responsible for diminished cancer survival and increased postoperative infections in patients receiving blood. Viral risks have significantly decreased in recent years, with the combined risk of HIV and hepatitis C < 1 in 2,000,000 units. The cost of a transfusion of packed RBCs is about $150–250 per unit. However, the cost is more significant when the indirect costs of treating transfusion reactions and prolongation of the hospital stay are included.

27. What are the approved indications for EPO?

Erythropoietin stimulates production and differentiation of RBC progenitors at the level of the bone marrow. It is approved in patients with chronic renal insufficiency and chemotherapy-induced anemia. In these patients, the use of EPO is associated with reductions in both mortality and transfusion requirements.

BIBLIOGRAPHY

1. Carson JL: Perioperative blood transfusion and postoperative mortality. JAMA 279:199–205, 1998.
2. Corwin HL: The CRIT Study. Crit Care Med 32:39–49, 2004.
3. Dunne JR: Perioperative anemia: An independent risk factor for infection, mortality, and resource utilization in surgery. J Surg Res 102:237–244, 2002.
4. Guyatt GH, Oxman AD, Ali M, et al: Laboratory diagnosis of iron-deficiency anemia: An overview. J Gen Intern Med 7:145–153, 1992.
5. Hebert PC: A multicenter, randomized, controlled clinical trial of transfusion requirements in critical care. N Engl J Med 340:409–417, 1999.
6. Ioannou GN: Prospective evaluation of a clinical guideline for the diagnosis and management if iron deficiency anemia. Am J Med 113:281–287, 2002.

7. Rao SV: Relationship of blood transfusion and clinical outcomes in patients with acute coronary syndromes. JAMA 292:1555–1562, 2004.

8. Weiss G: Anemia of chronic disease. N Engl J Med 352:1011–1021, 2005.

9. Wu WC: Blood transfusion in elderly patients with acute myocardial infarction. N Engl J Med 345:1230–1236, 2001.

CHAPTER 59

SICKLE CELL DISEASE

Jordan Messler, MD

1. **What is the prevalence of sickle cell disease and trait?**
   Sickle cell is the most common inheritable blood disease and is found in almost every ethnic background. Those from African descents shoulder the majority of the burden in the United States, with 1 in 600 African Americans having sickle cell disease and 8–12% carrying the sickle cell trait.

2. **What are the basic genetics and hereditary pattern of sickle cell development?**
   Normal hemoglobin (Hb), with two alpha chains and two beta chains, is designated hemoglobin A (HbA). Hemoglobin S (HbS) is caused by a single amino acid substitution (valine for glutamic acid) on the hemoglobin beta chain. Hemoglobin C (HbC) results from a substitution of lysine for valine at the sixth position. The heterozygous state (HbAS, sickle cell trait) may cause a slight anemia but does not affect life span; it is thought to be a balanced polymorphism, protective for malaria. The homozygous state, HbSS, manifests as sickle cell disease, an autosomal recessive condition. HbSC phenotypically presents as a milder case of sickle cell disease, and on average, affected patients live 20 years longer than those with HbSS. Other syndromes include hemoglobin S with β-thalassemia. HbSS patients will have elevated levels of HbF, fetal hemoglobin, which is less likely to sickle.

3. **What is the average life expectancy of sickle cell patients (HbSS)?**
   The median life expectancy is 42 years for males and 48 years for females. Risk factors for early death include acute chest syndrome (ACS; the primary cause of death, with a 3% mortality), seizure, elevated white blood cell count (>15,000), low HbF, frequent or prolonged hospitalization, and renal failure.

4. **How does HbS cause abnormalities in blood flow?**
   The amino acid substitution causes the red blood cell (RBC) to form a crescent shape, or sickle (Fig. 59-1). As numerous cells polymerize, strands of hemoglobin develop. These strands reduce RBC deformability and increase occlusion in the smaller blood vessels. These RBCs are more fragile, leading to a hemolytic anemia, and more adherent to each other, increasing blood viscosity.

5. **What events can increase sickling of RBCs?**
   Common triggers include hypoxia, infection, increased physical and psychosocial stress, alcohol, drugs, trauma, and changes in the weather. Other physiologic triggers include acidosis, fever, and dehydration. Often, no clear precipitant is identified.

6. **What are the common complications of sickle cell disease?**
   The complications can be grouped as follows: vaso-occlusive, hemolytic, and infectious.
   - **Vaso-occlusion:** These sometimes involve painful episodes, or acute painful episodes, which are responsible for 90% of emergency department visits and 70% of hospitalizations in sickle cell disease. Other vaso-occlusive complications include strokes, ACS, renal insufficiency, and priapism.

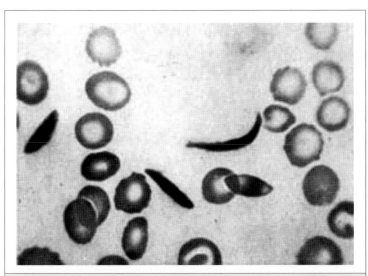

Figure 59-1. Blood smear from the first description of sickle cell disease.

- **Hemolysis:** The chronic hemolysis of sickle cell leads to a mild to moderate anemia and reticulocytosis and frequently causes gallstones.
- **Infection:** The increased risk of infectious complications, such as *Streptococcus pneumoniae* sepsis and osteomyelitis, occurs because of the functional asplenia that develops in most patients at an early age and the resultant susceptibility to encapsulated organisms.

7. **Describe the clinical presentation of an acute painful episode.**
   The usual presentation is symmetric bone pain, most commonly affecting the humerus (38%), tibia (23%), and femur (19%). Recurrent pain episodes tend to be in the same location, and if they are in a new location, alternative diagnoses should be sought. Pain symptoms can range vastly in severity and tend to last from 2 to 7 days.

8. **Describe how to assess the severity of pain.**
   Pain scales, such as the visual analog scale, are useful in gauging initial pain and after the response to treatment in the hospital. (See Chapter 93 for more details). Pain develops chronically in these patients, and objective findings—such as an elevated heart rate—are often absent.

9. **What is the differential diagnosis of bone pain?**
   Additional considerations include avascular necrosis or osteonecrosis, osteomyelitis, septic arthritis, leg ulcers, and rib infarcts. Avascular necrosis occurs in 10% of patients with sickle cell disease and should be considered when the pain is prolonged or described as atypical. Osteomyelitis is usually caused by *Staphylococcus aureus* or *Salmonella* species.

10. **What laboratory abnormalities are commonly seen in pain crises?**
    No laboratory markers are diagnostic of an acute painful episode. A peripheral smear will show sickled cells, and perhaps ovalocytes, target cells, basophilic stippling, or the Howell-Jolly

bodies of asplenia. The white blood cell count is often elevated and the hematocrit is decreased. Except in the case of an aplastic crisis (which has a low reticulocyte count), reticulocytes will be increased from active bone marrow production; hence the mean corpuscular volume will be elevated. Due to ongoing hemolysis, reticulocyte, lactate dehydrogenase, and aspartate aminotransferase levels may be increased.

11. **When should patients be admitted to the hospital for an acute painful episode?**
    Patients should be admitted for inability to tolerate oral medications, poor initial response to intravenous analgesics, signs of infectious complications, acute hypoxia, or anemia requiring transfusion. Patients who report symptoms not typical of their usual pain crises should also be evaluated carefully for admission.

12. **Describe the treatment strategies for pain crisis.**
    Treatment includes reversal of precipitating factors, hydration, appropriate analgesia, adjunctive treatments as described below, blood transfusions (if indicated, see question 17), oxygen supplementation (if patient is hypoxic), and close monitoring. Once the patient is euvolemic, experts generally recommend hypotonic intravenous fluids to avoid the theoretic erythrocyte dehydration that may occur with isotonic or hypertonic fluids. Liberal use of intravenous narcotic pain medications is recommended (see Chapter 93 for more details). Ketorolac (Toradol), given for up to 5 days, is an effective adjunctive therapy and may be used alone in milder crises. Other adjunctive treatments include antiemetics and antihistamines to help combat the nausea and itching often caused by morphine.

KEY POINTS: ACUTE PAINFUL EPISODES OF SICKLE CELL DISEASE

1. Acute painful episodes are the most common vaso-occlusive complication.

2. Pain is subjective; believe the pain.

3. No laboratory markers indicate whether a patient is having a painful crisis.

4. Remember the ABCs of sickle cell treatment: **A**ssess the patient, **B**elieve the pain, rule out **C**omplications, give adequate **D**rugs and **D**istraction, control the **E**nvironment, and give appropriate **F**ollow-up.

13. **Define ACS.**
    The diagnosis of ACS requires a new infiltrate on chest radiograph (not atelectasis), associated with pulmonary or infectious symptoms, such as temperature over 38.5°C, wheezing, shortness of breath, or cough. The most common symptoms in adults are fever (80%), cough (62%), tachypnea (45%), chest pain (44%), dyspnea (41%), arm and leg pain (37%), rib or sternal pain (21%), and reactive airways (13%). Many patients develop ACS while in the hospital, and vigilance is required for an early diagnosis.

14. **What are some of the precipitants of ACS?**
    Rib infarcts, pulmonary emboli (both microvascular and macrovascular), pneumonia, hypoventilation, and fat embolism can all precipitate ACS. Pneumonia accounts for 25% of identifiable causes of ACS, likely to be secondary to an atypical organism such as chlamydia or mycoplasma.

15. **Describe the treatment of ACS.**

Broad antibiotic coverage and judicious use of bronchodilators augment the therapies for acute pain crises outlined earlier. Incentive spirometry reduces the complications of ACS. Transfusions are warranted if the patient's condition is clinically deteriorating. In a rapidly worsening patient, exchange transfusion may have a slight benefit over simple transfusion. Exchange transfusions involve placing a large vascular catheter and removing RBCs to rapidly lower the level of sickle cells. Closer monitoring, such as in an intensive care unit, is appropriate if vital signs are unstable or severe hypoxia develops.

KEY POINTS: ACUTE CHEST SYNDROME

1. ACS is present when a new pulmonary infiltrate appears on chest x-ray concurrent with one of the following: fever, chest pain, or respiratory symptoms.

2. The leading cause of death in patients with sickle cell disease is ACS.

16. **How does the presence of sickle cell disease alter the differential diagnosis for generalized or localized abdominal pain?**

Special considerations include acute cholecystitis, right upper quadrant syndrome, splenic infarct, and priapism. Patients with sickle cell disease have an increased risk of gallstones (30–70% prevalence) as a result of their chronic hemolytic anemia. Many undergo cholecystectomy at an early age. The presentation of right upper quadrant syndrome, or liver sequestration, is similar to that of gallstones, but with greater elevation in liver enzyme levels, jaundice, and a normal ultrasound scan. Splenic sequestration is more common in children, peaking at about 5 years of age, and is diagnosed by the presence of an enlarged spleen and elevated reticulocyte count. By adulthood, the spleen often autoinfarcts.

17. **What are the indications for RBC transfusion in a patient with sickle cell disease?**

See Table 59-1.

TABLE 59-1. INDICATIONS FOR TRANSFUSION IN SICKLE CELL DISEASE	
Definite indications	Acute chest syndrome
	Severe or symptomatic anemia
	Surgery with general anesthesia
	Eye surgery
	Recurrent stroke in children
Possible indications	Complicated obstetric cases
	Severe right upper quadrant syndrome
	Refractory leg ulcers
	Acute, severe priapism
Not indicated	Asymptomatic anemia
	Minor surgery
	Uncomplicated pain crisis

Adapted from Steinberg MH: Management of sickle cell disease. N Engl J Med 340:1021–1030, 1999.

18. **How does hydroxyurea work, and for whom is it indicated?**
    Hydroxyurea increases the levels of HbF, which results in less sickling. It is indicated for patients with a history of stroke, acute chest syndrome, or frequent vaso-occlusive crises (>3 per year). It should be given under the close supervision of a hematologist and is generally started in the outpatient setting. Hydroxyurea use reduces painful crises and hospitalization and improves mortality rates.

19. **What are other discharge considerations?**
    The patient should be counseled to avoid triggers, maintain proper hydration and receive appropriate oral analgesics, and return soon for follow-up. Pneumococcal and influenza vaccines are indicated if not already received. Patients may require pneumococcal revaccination every 7–10 years to maintain antibody levels in the presence of functional asplenia.

WEBSITES

1. The Sickle Cell Information Center: http://www.scinfo.org

2. Sickle Cell Disease Association of America, Inc.: http://www.sicklecelldisease.org

BIBLIOGRAPHY

1. Platt OS, Brambilla DJ, Rosse WF, et al: Mortality in sickle cell disease: Life expectancy and risk factors for early death. N Engl J Med 330:1639–1644, 1994.

2. Steinberg MH: Management of sickle cell disease. N Engl J Med 340:1021–1030, 1999.

3. Steinberg MH, Barton F, Castro O, et al: Effect of hydroxyurea on mortality and morbidity in adult sickle cell anemia: Risks and benefits up to 9 years of treatment. JAMA 289:1645–1651, 2003.

4. Vichinksy EP, Neumayr LD, Earles AN, et al: Causes and outcomes of the acute chest syndrome in sickle cell disease. National Acute Chest Syndrome study Group. N Engl J Med 342:1855–1865, 2000.

CHAPTER 60

THROMBOCYTOPENIA

David Feinbloom, MD, and Joseph Ming Wah Li, MD

1. **Describe platelet production and kinetics.**
   Platelets are produced in the bone marrow by megakaryocytes. This requires healthy bone marrow and stimulation by thrombopoietin, a protein that is produced in the liver in response to a decline in platelet mass. Once formed, platelets survive an average of 8–10 days in the circulation.

2. **How is *thrombocytopenia* defined?**
   The normal platelet count is between 150,000 and 450,000/µL, with *thrombocytopenia* defined as a platelet count of <150,000/µL. However, many healthy persons may have counts lower than this.

3. **At what point do patients develop symptoms from thrombocytopenia?**
   See Table 60-1.

TABLE 60-1. RISK OF BLEEDING DUE TO THROMBOCYTOPENIA	
Platelet Count	**Clinical Risk**
>50,000/µL	Generally asymptomatic
20,000–50,000/µL	Increased risk of posttraumatic or surgical bleeding
5,000–20,000/µL	Serious spontaneous bleeding may occur
<5000/µL	Significant risk of life-threatening bleeding (e.g., intra-cranial hemorrhage)

4. **What are the clinical manifestations of thrombocytopenia?**
   The classic findings are *petechiae*, which are pinpoint hemorrhages into the skin or mucosa. Confluent petechiae form *purpura*, and bleeding into the subcutaneous tissue causes *ecchymosis*.

5. **Name four ways that thrombocytopenia can occur.**
   - Decreased platelet production
   - Peripheral platelet destruction
   - Platelet sequestration
   - Dilutional and pseudothrombocytopenia

6. **Which disease states are associated with decreased platelet production?**
   Bone marrow injury, infiltration, nutritional deficiencies
   - Leukemia, metastatic cancer
   - Aplastic anemia
   - Myeloid metaplasia

- Infections (e.g., tuberculosis, leishmaniasis)
- Chemotherapy
- Radiation
- Vitamin B_{12} or folate deficiency

Megakaryocyte injury or dysfunction
- Viral injury (HIV, measles)
- Alcohol
- Drugs (e.g., thiazides)
- Decreased thrombopoietin levels associated with liver disease
- Amegakaryocytic thrombocytopenia

7. **Which disease states are associated with peripheral platelet destruction?**
   - Immune-mediated platelet destruction
   - Idiopathic thrombocytopenic purpura
   - Posttransfusion purpura
   - Antiphospholipid antibodies
   - Drug-induced thrombocytopenia
   - Mechanical/consumptive platelet destruction
   - Thrombotic thrombocytopenic purpura
   - Hemolytic uremic syndrome
   - Hemolysis, elevated liver enzymes, and low platelet count (HELLP) syndrome
   - Disseminated intravascular coagulation
   - Septicemia
   - Cardiopulmonary bypass
   - Giant cavernous hemangioma

8. **What are the causes of platelet sequestration?**
   At any given time, 30% of circulating platelets are sequestered in the spleen, therefore any disorder that results in splenomegaly may be accompanied by a proportional decline in circulating platelets. Causes of splenomegaly and sequestration include portal hypertension (e.g., cirrhosis, right-sided congestive heart failure), malignancy (e.g., splenic lymphoma), infections (e.g., Epstein-Barr virus, cytomegalovirus, malaria, leishmaniasis), and infiltrative diseases (e.g., Gaucher's, Niemann-Pick, Fabry's diseases).

9. **What is dilutional thrombocytopenia?**
   When a patient has significant blood loss, he or she loses platelets as well. Resuscitation with blood transfusions only replaces the red cells, and the remaining platelets will be diluted in the new blood volume. The result is a true thrombocytopenia that corrects with subsequent increases in platelet production.

10. **What are the causes of pseudothrombocytopenia?**
    As the name implies, pseudothrombocytopenia is not a true thrombocytopenia, and patients are not at increased risk of bleeding. This most commonly occurs when blood specimens are inadequately anticoagulated, resulting in platelet clumping. Additionally, a small number of persons have circulating antibodies that, in the presence of ethylenediamine tetra-acetic acid (EDTA; an anticoagulant used in blood processing), actually cause platelet clumping. In both cases, the resultant platelet clumping is misinterpreted by automated cell counters as white blood cells, thus underestimating the true platelet count.

11. **List the most common causes of thrombocytopenia in hospitalized patients.**
    - Medications: the most common cause (e.g., antibiotics, chemotherapeutic agents, IIb/IIIa inhibitors)

- Infection
- Heparin-induced thrombocytopenia (HIT)
- Disseminated intravascular coagulation
- Dilutional causes (i.e., massive blood transfusion)
- Posttransfusion purpura
- Cardiopulmonary bypass
- Adult respiratory distress syndrome

12. **What are the two kinds of HIT?**
- Non–immune-mediated HIT, or HIT type I, typically occurs 24–48 hours after heparin administration. It is associated with a small decline in the platelet count and resolves without the cessation of heparin therapy.
- Conversely, immune-mediated HIT, or HIT type II, typically occurs between 5–10 days after heparin administration and is associated with a 50% decline in platelet count and an increased risk of thrombosis.

13. **Which of the two types of HIT is more serious?**
Whereas HIT type I is benign, immune-mediated HIT (type II) is associated with a very high risk of venous and arterial thrombosis. The thrombotic diathesis in HIT type II is attributable to the formation of platelet factor 4 (PF4)–heparin complexes, which are able to stimulate an antibody response. The resulting PF4-heparin-antibody complex is able to bind and activate quiescent platelets. If untreated, uncontrolled platelet activation may lead to catastrophic intravascular thrombosis.

14. **When should you suspect immune-mediated HIT?**
First, be vigilant. All patients receiving any heparin should have frequent platelet monitoring—at least every other day. HIT should be expected in any patient who develops an otherwise unexplained decrease in platelets of $\geq$50% from baseline or a venous or arterial thrombotic event occurring 5–10 days after initiation of heparin. Thrombosis may occur in as little as 12 hours in patients who have previously been exposed to heparin.

15. **How is immune-mediated thrombocytopenia confirmed?**
There are presently four assays used to confirm immune-mediated HIT. The most commonly used test is the PF4/heparin enzyme-linked immunosorbent assay, whereas the gold standard remains the functional platelet serotonin release assay. As shown in Table 60-2, all of these tests have reasonably high sensitivity and are therefore useful for excluding the diagnosis of HIT. Unfortunately, their variable specificity would indicate that testing be reserved for patients in whom there is a moderate to high pretest probability of HIT, for example, those with an unexplained drop in platelets or an unexpected thrombotic event.

16. **What is the appropriate approach to the treatment of a patient with suspected HIT?**
Stop the administration of all heparins immediately. This includes unfractionated and low-molecular-weight heparins in the form of drips, flushes, and subcutaneous injections. Patients who develop anti-PF4 antibodies are a high risk for thrombosis and should be prophylactically treated with a direct thrombin inhibitor (DTI) such as argatroban or lepirudin. The DTI should be given until PF4 antibody titers fall, as reflected by the recovery of the platelet count to normal or $\geq$150,000/μL. The management of patients who develop PF4-heparin antibodies, with or without thrombosis, is complicated and should include consultation with a hematologist.

TABLE 60-2. SENSITIVITY AND SPECIFICITY OF ASSAYS FOR DETECTING IMMUNE-MEDIATED HIT ANTIBODIES

Diagnostic Assay	Sensitivity %	Platelet Fall Days 0–4 Specificity %	Platelet Fall Days ≥5 Specificity %
A. Platelet serotonin release assay	90–98	>95	80–97
B. Heparin-induced platelet aggregation assay	90–98	>95	80–97
C. Platelet aggregation test	35–85	>90	82
D. PF4/heparin ELISA	>90	>95	50–93
E. Combination of B or C and D	100	>95	80–97

ELISA = enzyme-linked immunosorbent assay.
Adapted from Warkentin TE, Greinacher A: Heparin-induced thrombocytopenia: recognition, treatment, and prevention: The Seventh ACCP Conference on Antithrombotic and Thrombolytic Therapy. Chest 126:311S–337S, 2004.

KEY POINTS: EVALUATION OF THROMBOCYTOPENIA

1. Immune-mediated HIT is the most serious cause of drug-induced thrombocytopenia, and it must be treated immediately.

2. Medications are the most common cause of thrombocytopenia, and it must be recognized and managed appropriately.

3. Thrombocytopenia may result from decreased production, increased destruction, or splenic sequestration.

4. Clinically relevant bleeding rarely occurs with platelet counts of >20,000/μL.

17. **Is warfarin an acceptable alternative to a DTI in patients with HIT?**
   No. Warfarin therapy should never be started in a patient with suspected HIT because its initial procoagulant effects can lead to acute thrombosis, skin necrosis, limb loss, and even death. Once the patient is established on DTI therapy and the platelet count has returned to normal, the administration of low-dose warfarin can be initiated. However, the DTI must be continued for at least 5 days, with at least 2 days of a therapeutic international normalized ratio.

18. **How much will a platelet transfusion increase the platelet count?**
   A unit of platelet concentrate contains approximately 5000 platelets, and the standard replacement therapy consists of one unit of platelets per 10 kg of body weight. Therefore, after administering 10 units, one should expect an increase in the platelet count of approximately 50,000/μL 1 hour after infusion. However, there is considerable variability in individual responses, which depend on many clinical variables.

19. Outline a mechanistic approach to thrombocytopenia.
See Figure 60-1.

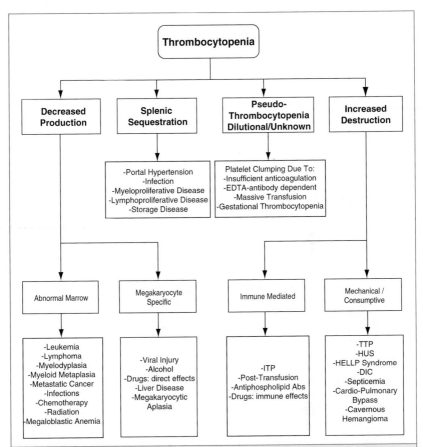

Figure 60-1. A mechanistic approach to thrombocytopenia. EDTA = ethylenediamine tetra-acetic acid, ITP = idiopathic thrombocytopenic purpura, TTP = thrombotic thrombocytopenic purpura, HUS = hemolytic uremic syndrome, HELLP = hemolysis, elevated liver enzymes, and low platelet count, DIC = disseminated intravascular coagulation.

BIBLIOGRAPHY

1. Handin RI: Disorders of the platelet and the vessel wall. In Kasper DL, Braunwald E, et al (eds): Harrison's Principles of Internal Medicine, 16th ed. New York, McGraw-Hill, 2005, pp 673–680.

2. Warkentin TE, Greinacher A: Heparin-induced thrombocytopenia: Recognition, treatment, and prevention. The Seventh ACCP Conference on Antithrombotic and Thrombolytic Therapy. Chest 126:311S–337S, 2004.

CHAPTER 61

ONCOLOGIC EMERGENCIES
Douglas Borg, MD

1. **Which cancers commonly cause hypercalcemia?**

   Hypercalcemia can occur in both solid tumors and leukemia. The most common causes are lung cancer, breast cancer, and multiple myeloma (MM). (See Chapter 46 for more details.)

2. **Why does hypercalcemia occur in patients with cancer?**

   Hypercalcemia is a result of increased bone resorption and release of calcium. There are three major mechanisms involved:

   - **Local osteolysis by metastases:** This is commonly due to breast cancer, MM, and non–small cell lung cancer. Local osteolysis occurs as tumor cells spread to bone. Cytokines, locally produced parathyroid hormone–related protein (PTHrP), and osteoclast-activating factors are involved on a local level at the bone matrix.
   - **PTHrP:** Tumor production of PTHrP, which stimulates PTH receptors, is the most common cause of hypercalcemia in patients with nonmetastatic solid tumors such as squamous cell carcinoma of any type (especially of the lung) and renal cell carcinoma. This also occurs in many patients with non-Hodgkin's lymphoma (NHL). Patients with elevated PTHrP levels usually have a poor prognosis. PTHrP levels can be studied to assess response to treatment. PTH levels are often low or normal in this condition.
   - **Tumor production of calcitriol:** This is a rare cause of hypercalcemia in malignancy but is the cause of most cases related to Hodgkin's disease. It is also seen in adult T-cell lymphomas.

3. **What are the common symptoms of malignant epidural spinal cord compression (ESCC)?**

   - **Pain:** Usually the presenting symptom at the time of diagnosis, pain precedes the diagnosis of ESCC by a number of weeks. The pain is often more severe when the patient is supine, and it is exacerbated by increased intra-abdominal or intrathoracic pressure. Radicular pain is less common than localized pain but, when present, is often bilateral.
   - **Lower extremity weakness:** Found in >50% of patients at the time of diagnosis, lower extremity weakness is associated with hyperactive reflexes, spasticity, and an up-going toe on Babinski's test.
   - **Sensory loss:** Sensory loss is present in approximately 50% of patients at the time of diagnosis. It usually begins in the toes and ascends in a stocking distribution, eventually reaching 1–5 segments below the anatomic level of cord compression.
   - **Bladder dysfunction:** Present in approximately 50% of patients at the time of diagnosis, bladder dysfunction presents as painless urinary retention and is associated with severe weakness and sensory loss in the lower extremities.
   - **Ataxia:** This symptom is present in approximately 4% of patients at time of diagnosis.

4. **What is the incidence of ESCC?**

   ESCC occurs in approximately 5% of patients with cancer. In approximately 20% of cases, ESCC is the initial manifestation of malignancy. Any metastatic tumor can cause ESCC, but prostate, breast, and lung cancer are each responsible for approximately 10–20% of cases. Renal cell cancer, NHL, plasmacytoma, and MM each represent another 5–10% of the total cases of ESCC.

However, the types of tumors that *present* with ESCC as the initial manifestation of cancer differ from those causing ESCC in patients with *known* cancer. In one study, lung cancer, cancer of unknown primary cause, MM, and NHL were responsible for 78% of cases in this group compared with 26% of those with ESCC and known cancer.

Schiff D, O'Neill BP, Suman VJ, et al: Spinal epidural metastasis as the initial manifestation of malignancy: Clinical features and diagnostic approach. Neurology 49:452, 1997.

5. **What are the pathologic mechanisms by which ESCC is thought to occur?**
   In most cases, ESCC is due to hematologic metastasis, but in roughly 10% of cases a paraspinal mass gains access to the epidural space via the neural foramen. This latter mechanism is most common in lymphoma.

6. **Describe the role of radiography in the diagnosis of ESCC.**
   - **Magnetic resonance imaging (MRI):** MRI is the most sensitive and specific imaging modality for localizing malignant epidural lesions. This is important because the discovery of multiple lesions may change the prognosis and management.
   - **Computed tomography (CT) myelography:** This means of imaging is helpful in patients for whom MRI is contraindicated.
   - **CT:** CT scanning alone is rarely indicated because neither the epidural space nor the spinal cord is clearly visualized.
   - **Spinal radiography:** Plain spinal radiographs have abnormal results (i.e., osteolytic lesions, compression fractures) in 85% of cases, but there is an unacceptable rate of false-negative results.
   - **Bone scan:** When a negative bone scan result is combined with a negative plain radiograph result, there is only an approximately 2% risk of ESCC in patients with cancer and spinal symptoms.

Portenoy R, Galer B, Salamon O, et al: Identification of epidural neoplasm: Radiography and bone scintigraphy in the symptomatic and asymptomatic spine. Cancer 64:2207–2213, 1989.

7. **Which factors predict prognosis in patients with malignant ESCC?**
   Ability to ambulate and cancer type are the most useful factors in predicting a patient's prognosis with ESCC. Functional status directly correlates with survival. The average survival time at diagnosis is 6 months, but 50% of ambulatory patients will survive >1 year whereas nonambulatory patients have median survival of 2–4 months. As such, minimizing any delay in diagnosis and consequent loss of function is essential to improve outcomes. Prognosis is better in radiosensitive lesions such as lymphoma, MM, and breast and prostate cancer.

8. **Describe the role of radiation therapy (XRT), corticosteroids, chemotherapy, and surgery in the treatment of ESCC?**
   - **XRT:** XRT is the treatment of choice in ESCC. Goals of therapy are not curative; rather, they are palliative. These goals include pain relief and preservation of neurologic function. XRT alleviates pain in 75% of patients. Patients with radiosensitive tumors and those with the least neurologic deficits tend to do the best with XRT.
   - **Corticosteroids:** For patients with significant neurologic symptoms, steroids are used to minimize further deterioration and to treat pain. Steroids decrease spinal cord edema and improve motor function. Higher doses are typically used in paraplegic or paretic patients.
   - **Chemotherapy:** Unfortunately, the majority of metastatic tumors that cause ESCC are not responsive to chemotherapy. For the occasional tumor that is sensitive, chemotherapy may be used as an adjunctive treatment to XRT and/or surgery.
   - **Surgery:** There is traditionally little role for surgery in this disease, but recent advances suggest that aggressive tumor debulking followed by XRT may allow patients to ambulate longer compared with those who receive XRT alone.

9. **What additional therapy should be considered in patients with ESCC?**
   - **Bisphosphonate:** These medications (e.g., pamidronate) reduce pathologic fractures and alleviate bone pain in patients with breast cancer or MM.
   - **Spine bracing:** For patients with unstable spinal fractures, this can improve mobility.

10. **What is superior vena cava (SVC) syndrome?**
    Obstruction of blood flow in the SVC causes the symptoms and signs of SVC syndrome. A slow, progressive obstruction over a period of months allows for the development of collateral veins. More rapidly occurring obstruction results in less collaterals and more severe symptoms. Dyspnea and head fullness are most common, but other symptoms include facial swelling, cough, arm edema, and cyanosis. Symptoms are often heightened by lying down or bending forward. Physical examination may reveal venous distention in the veins of the neck and chest wall as well as facial edema.

11. **What are the causes of SVC syndrome?**
    Malignancy is responsible for 80–90% of SVC syndrome cases. Of this group, lung cancer and NHL are responsible for 85% of the cases. Thrombosis, commonly associated with central venous catheters, accounts for the remaining 10–20% of the cases of SVC syndrome.

12. **Describe the diagnosis and treatment of SVC syndrome.**
    Since malignancy is the most common cause of SVC syndrome, a majority of patients have abnormal findings on chest radiographs. A widened mediastinum, pleural effusion, and chest masses are the most common findings. A contrast CT scan will demonstrate the degree of obstruction and often the cause of the principal process. A tissue diagnosis is essential because therapy will vary depending on histology. Small cell lung cancer, NHL, and germ cell tumors are usually responsive to chemotherapy. Non–small cell lung cancer is usually treated with chemotherapy with or without concurrent radiation. Data suggest that placement of an endovascular stent should be considered as adjunctive therapy in patients with malignant causes of SVC syndrome. Symptoms usually improve within 24–48 hours of stent placement.

13. **What is tumor lysis syndrome?**
    It is a collection of metabolic abnormalities including decreased urinary output, hyperkalemia, hyperphosphatemia, hypocalcemia, hyperuricemia, uremia, and acute renal failure. If severe enough, renal failure and associated complications such as arrhythmia can be life-threatening.

KEY POINTS: ONCOLOGIC EMERGENCIES

1. Malignancy may induce hypercalcemia via direct metastatic osteolysis, production of PTHrP, or tumor production of vitamin D.

2. Symptoms associated with ESCC include low back pain, lower extremity weakness and sensory loss, bladder dysfunction, and sometimes ataxia.

3. The most important prognostic factors in ESCC are the tumor type and the ability to ambulate at the time of diagnosis.

4. Lung cancer and non-Hodgkin's lymphoma cause most cases of SVC syndrome.

5. CT scan with contrast will often determine the location and degree of obstruction in SVC syndrome as well as the probable underlying tumor type.

6. The tumor lysis syndrome classically presents with hyperkalemia, hyperphosphatemia, hypocalcemia, hyperuricemia, and acute renal failure.

7. The tumor lysis syndrome can often be prevented with alkalinization of the urine, intravenous fluids, and allopurinol.

14. **What causes tumor lysis syndrome?**
    It is usually associated with chemotherapeutic regimens but can also be seen with XRT, corticosteroids, tamoxifen, and monoclonal antibody therapies. It is caused by the rapid release of cellular contents such as potassium and phosphate after the administration of cytotoxic therapy. Additionally, the cellular nucleic acid breakdown products are catabolized to uric acid and other cellular contents that cause direct toxic injury to the renal tubules.

15. **What malignancies are most commonly associated with tumor lysis syndrome?**
    Patients with a large tumor burden and those with a highly proliferative cancer (especially those that are highly responsive to chemotherapy) are at the highest risk to develop the tumor lysis syndrome. Acute lymphocytic leukemia and high-grade NHL are the most commonly associated tumors.

16. **How is tumor lysis syndrome prevented? How is it treated if it develops?**
    Preventative therapy will often reduce the severity or abort tumor lysis syndrome completely. Intravenous fluids given before and continuing for 24–48 hours after chemotherapy are beneficial. Alkalinization of the urine with intravenous bicarbonate and reduction of uric acid before therapy with allopurinol (via inhibition of xanthine oxidase) reduces tubular injury and the incidence of acute renal failure. Rasburicase is a recombinant form of uric acid oxidase that directly breaks down uric acid and can lower the serum uric acid much more quickly than allopurinol. If significant acute renal failure and metabolic abnormalities develop despite these measures, acute hemodialysis should be initiated promptly to prevent irreversible renal damage.

    Pui CH, Relling MV, Lascombes F, et al: Urate oxidase in prevention and treatment of hyperuricemia associated with lymphoid malignancies. Leukemia 11:1813, 1997.

WEBSITE

American Society of Clinical Oncology, Education Book: http://www.asco.org/ac/ 1,1003,_12-002668,00.asp

BIBLIOGRAPHY

1. Biship MR, Cairo MS, Coccia PF: Tumor lysis syndrome. In Abeloff J (ed): Clinical Oncology, 3rd ed. Philadelphia, Elsevier, 2004, pp 987–991.

2. Davidson MB, Thakkar S, Hix JK, et al: Pathophysiology, clinical consequences, and treatment of tumor lysis syndrome. Am J Med 116:546–554, 2004.

3. Gabriel K, Schiff D: Metastatic spinal cord compression by solid tumors. Semin Neurol 24:375–383, 2004.

4. Laskin J, Cmelak AJ, Roberts J, et al: Superior vena cava syndrome. In Abelof J (ed): Clinical Oncology, 3rd edition. Philadelphia, Elsevier, 2004, pp 1047–1059.

5. Patchell R: A randomized trial of direct decompressive surgical resection in the treatment of spinal cord compression caused by metastasis [abstract 2]. Proc Am Soc Clin Oncol 22:1, 2003.

6. Morton Ross AR, Lipton A: Hypercalcemia. In Abeloff J (ed): Clinical Oncology, 3rd ed. Philadelphia, Elsevier, 2004, pp 957–970.

MANAGEMENT OF INPATIENT DIABETES AND HYPERGLYCEMIC SYNDROMES

CHAPTER 62

Sarah Bull, MD, and Eugene S. Chu, MD

1. **How common is hyperglycemia in hospitalized patients?**

   Hyperglycemia is defined as a fasting blood glucose level >100 mg/dL or a random blood glucose level >200 mg/dL. The prevalence of hyperglycemia in hospitalized patients is not well established. Although one study found that almost 40% of hospitalized patients had either a medical history of diabetes, unrecognized diabetes, or hospital-related hyperglycemia, conservative estimates show that 10–25% of hospitalized patients have hyperglycemia. The majority of hyperglycemic patients in the hospital are admitted for complications of chronic hyperglycemia—in particular, vascular diseases such as coronary artery disease, cerebrovascular disease, and peripheral vascular disease. Since hyperglycemia impairs immune function, infection is another common reason for hospitalization. In both cases, hyperglycemia or diabetes is usually a secondary diagnosis, and treatment of these disorders, until recently, has been of secondary importance in the hospital.

2. **What is the impact of diabetes on the hospitalized patient?**

   Diabetes increases the risk of hospitalization by two to four times that of the nondiabetic patient. A medical history of diabetes mellitus is correlated with a 1- to 3-day increase in length of stay. Patients with hospital-related hyperglycemia (high blood sugar levels without a history of diabetes) have a greater length of stay than either diabetic or normoglycemic patients. Finally, hospital-related hyperglycemia has been correlated with an 18-fold increase in hospital mortality compared with normoglycemic patients. Similarly, diabetics have a threefold increased mortality compared with normoglycemic patients.

3. **Describe the glycemic targets for hospitalized patients.**

   For patients in the intensive care unit (ICU), the goal blood glucose level is 80–110 mg/dL. For non-ICU patients, the goal blood glucose level is <110 mg/dL preprandial and <180 mg/dL peak postprandial.

4. **Does achieving tight glycemic control improve hospital outcomes?**

   Tight glycemic control is correlated with a decreased incidence of deep sternal wound infections in patients who undergo cardiac surgery, improvements in functional status in patients who have experienced acute stroke, and reductions in morbidity and mortality in surgical ICU patients and patients experiencing acute coronary syndromes.

5. **Discuss the use of oral diabetic agents in hospitalized patients.**
   - **Sulfonylurea:** These drugs are long-acting medications that are relatively slow to titrate. They also have significant potential for hypoglycemia, especially in persons with erratic food intake such as hospitalized patients.
   - **Metformin:** The use of metformin is associated with lactic acidosis, especially when renal insufficiency, hypoxemia, hypoperfusion, congestive heart failure, or chronic pulmonary diseases are present.
   - **Thiazolidinedione:** These drugs increase intravascular volume and have a slow onset of action; thus, they are relatively ineffective to initiate on an inpatient basis.

Although no significant studies of oral hyperglycemic agents in hospitalized patients have been undertaken, their many limitations make them difficult to use effectively in acutely ill, hospitalized patients.

6. **How is an insulin-deficient patient's daily insulin requirement determined?**
   A patient's daily insulin requirement consists of three different components:
   - **Basal:** Scheduled intermediate- to long-acting insulin to cover basal, endogenous insulin needs.
   - **Bolus:** Scheduled regular or rapid-acting insulin to cover the increased blood glucose associated with meals.
   - **Sliding scale:** Also known as *correctional insulin,* used to supplement scheduled insulin as needed. Correctional insulin is typically dosed before meals and at bedtime. Bedtime doses may be reduced to prevent nocturnal hypoglycemia.

   A patient's total daily insulin requirement may be determined using prehospital insulin requirements or may be estimated as 0.6 units/kg/day. The total daily dosing is divided between basal (40–50%) and bolus (50–60%, divided 10–20% with each meal) doses. For an inpatient who is eating meals, a long-acting insulin such as glargine may be dosed once daily for basal requirements along with a rapid-acting insulin such as lispro or aspart with breakfast, lunch, and dinner. Sliding-scale insulin in the form of regular or rapid-acting insulin would be dosed, as needed, before meals and at bedtime (Table 62-1).

TABLE 62-1. CHARACTERISTICS OF VARIOUS TYPES OF INSULIN

Insulin Type	Time to Onset	Peak Effect	Duration of Action
Lispro (Humalog)	15 minutes	30–90 minutes	3–6 hours
Aspart (NovoLog)	15 minutes	40–50 minutes	3–5 hours
Regular	30–60 minutes	2–4 hours	4–6 hours
NPH	2–4 hours	4–10 hours	14–18 hours
Glargine	60 minutes	None	24 hours

NPH = neutral protamine Hagedorn.

7. **Describe a typical insulin regimen for an insulin-deficient inpatient who is not eating.**
   For an inpatient who is not eating meals, basal requirements could be met with an insulin drip, an intermediate-acting insulin such as neutral protamine Hagedorn (NPH) dosed twice daily, or a long-acting insulin such as glargine dosed once daily. No bolus insulin would be required. Sliding-scale insulin in the form of regular insulin would be dosed every 6 hours or rapid-acting insulin every 4 hours, as needed to control sugars.

8. **What is diabetic ketoacidosis (DKA)?**
   DKA is an acute complication of diabetes mellitus and a common reason for hospitalization in diabetic patients. It can also be the first sign a patient has diabetes. DKA is characterized by hyperglycemia, ketosis, and anion-gap metabolic acidosis.

9. **Discuss the pathogenesis of DKA.**
   DKA develops when there are insufficient levels of insulin in the presence of elevated counter-regulatory hormones (e.g., glucagon, cortisol, catecholamines, and growth hormone).

This leads to an increase in hepatic gluconeogenesis, accelerated lipolysis, and decreased peripheral tissue insulin use. Free fatty acids, released from adipocytes during lipolysis, are oxidized to ketoacids in the liver. These ketoacids are responsible for the anion-gap metabolic acidosis seen in DKA. An osmotic diuresis, resulting from hyperglycemia and glucosuria, causes massive electrolyte and volume depletion.

10. **What are the symptoms and signs of DKA?**
Early symptoms of DKA include polyuria, polydipsia, and polyphagia. As the disease progresses, patients frequently experience abdominal pain, nausea and vomiting, dizziness, and confusion. Physical findings may include Kussmaul's respirations (i.e., rapid, large-volume breathing) and an acetone or "fruity" odor to their breath due to their metabolic acidosis. Patients are often tachycardic and orthostatic due to intravascular volume depletion. Without intervention, metabolic abnormalities can lead to coma, respiratory arrest, or death.

11. **What are the most common precipitating factors for DKA?**
Factors that upset the balance of insulin and counter-regulatory hormones can incite DKA. Infection is the most common precipitating factor, followed closely by inadequate use of insulin. Other factors include alcohol abuse, myocardial infarction, pancreatitis, eating disorders, trauma, hormonal changes (e.g., during pregnancy), and undiagnosed diabetes. Various drugs that affect carbohydrate metabolism, such as corticosteroids, thiazides, and sympathomimetics, may also precipitate DKA.

KEY POINTS: MOST COMMON PRECIPITATING FACTORS FOR DKA

1. Infection

2. Insulin (inadequate dose)

3. Infarction (myocardial)

4. Impregnation (pregnancy)

5. Iatrogenic (corticosteroid administration)

12. **Differentiate hyperglycemic hyperosmotic syndrome (HHS) from DKA.**
HHS, sometimes referred to as *hyperosmolar nonketotic coma,* is less frequent than DKA and is marked by elevated serum osmolality in the absence of ketosis. The pathogenesis of DKA (generally seen in patients with type I diabetes who lack insulin) is better understood than HHS (generally seen in patients with type II diabetes and insulin resistance), yet the underlying mechanisms and precipitating events are essentially the same. The insulin/counter-regulatory imbalance leads to hyperglycemia. The osmotic diuresis caused by the hyperglycemia leads to increased serum osmolality and volume depletion. The presence of even small levels of insulin in HHS patients, although ineffective at lowering glucose levels, inhibits lipolysis and thus ketosis and acidosis. Patients with HHS often have much higher serum glucose levels and more severe volume depletion than patients with DKA, leading to a significantly higher mortality rate (15% versus <5%) (Table 62-2).

13. **What laboratory tests should be performed for patients presenting with DKA or HHS?**
Patients with signs of an acute hyperglycemic crisis should be evaluated urgently with a full chemistry panel to determine blood glucose, creatinine, and electrolyte levels and anion

TABLE 62-2. DIABETIC KETOACIDOSIS AND HYPERGLYCEMIC HYPEROSMOTIC SYNDROME

	DKA	HHS
Plasma glucose (mg/dL)	>250 mg/dL	>600 mg/dL
Ketone formation	Present	Rare
pH	<7.3	Normal
Anion gap	Increased	Normal
Serum bicarbonate	<15 mEq/L	Normal
Average H_2O deficit	6 L	9 L
Serum osmolality	normal	>330 mOsm/kg
Mortality rate	<5%	15%
Presence of comorbidities	Occasional	Frequent
Type of DM	Type I > type II	Type II > type I

DM = diabetes mellitus.

gap; measurement of serum or urine ketones; complete blood count with differential; and arterial blood gas measurement. Additional studies to evaluate for precipitating factors should be guided by the clinical presentation. These may include urinalysis, electrocardiogram, pregnancy test, chest radiograph, blood and urine cultures, and troponin and lipase levels. A hemoglobin A1C measurement may not be useful acutely, but it can help determine the patient's prior range of blood sugar control.

14. **What are the major ketones measured in patients with DKA?**
The anion-gap acidosis seen in DKA is caused by the accumulation of the ketones B-hydroxybutyrate and acetoacetate. Assessment of ketosis is usually performed with a nitroprusside reaction, which provides a semi-quantitative analysis of acetoacetate and acetone levels on urine or serum samples. This assay does not measure B-hydroxybutyrate levels, the major ketoacid in DKA. As DKA resolves and ketogenesis slows, more B-hydroxybutyrate (not measured) is converted back to acetoacetate (measured), which can sometimes result in a paradoxical reemergence of measured ketones.

15. **What are the goals of treatment for a patient with DKA or HHS?**
The therapeutic goals in the treatment of DKA and HHS are similar. They include volume resuscitation, electrolyte repletion, and correction of electrolyte and glucose abnormalities. In DKA, it is important to resolve the ketosis. In both syndromes, serum electrolyte and ketone measurements should initially occur at least every 4 hours. Check the blood glucose level at least every 1–2 hours during intravenous (IV) insulin and dextrose therapy. Alter the laboratory work frequency depending on the patient's clinical status. In general, patients with DKA and HHS are severely volume depleted and require an average of 6 L of isotonic saline over the first 24 hours. At least 1–2 L of normal saline should be given immediately as a bolus followed by continuous IV fluids, the rate of which should be determined by individual patient characteristics and the calculated fluid deficit. The administration of IV fluids should continue until the patient is euvolemic. Changes in clinical status can occur quickly in these patients. Use of a bedside flow sheet is essential to document laboratory results and therapeutic interventions.

16. **Which electrolyte levels are falsely elevated in patients with DKA?**
Both potassium and phosphate levels may be falsely elevated on presentation. Despite total body potassium depletion, hyperkalemia is frequently noted on initial laboratory findings due to dehydration and acidosis. The introduction of insulin will further decrease potassium levels by initiating an intracellular shift. To prevent hypokalemia, potassium replacement should be initiated once the level falls below 5.5 mEq/L, assuming normal renal function. Although there is no definitive evidence supporting the routine repletion of phosphate in DKA, cardiac, respiratory and skeletal muscle weakness may occur at levels <1.0 mg/dL.

17. **Which electrolyte level may be falsely low in patients with DKA or HHS?**
The serum sodium level may be falsely low in patients with significant hyperglycemia. Hyperglycemia raises the serum osmolality and causes free water to leave the *intracellular* space and enter the *intravascular* space, diluting the serum sodium. To account for this effect, assume that for every 100 mg/dL of glucose >100 mg/dL, the serum sodium level will fall by 1.6 mmol/L. For example, a patient with a blood glucose of 800 mg/dL and serum sodium of 120 mmol/L will have a CORRECTED serum sodium of 131.2 mmol/L [120 mmol/L + (1.6 mmol/L × 7) = 131.2 mmol/L]. This is the level of sodium (corrected) one can expect after the blood glucose level corrects to normal.

18. **How should insulin be administered to patients with DKA or HHS?**
IV insulin administration is the most effective route to treat DKA. When given in appropriate doses, insulin reverses gluconeogenesis and lowers serum blood sugar levels by 65–125 mg/dL/h. Once severe hypokalemia is excluded (<3.2 mEq/L) and/or potassium is being repleted, an IV bolus of regular insulin should be given at 0.15 units/kg (usually 10–20 units), followed by a continuous infusion of regular insulin at 0.1 units/kg/h (usually 7–10 units/h). The insulin infusion should be adjusted hourly for an optimal glucose decrease of 100/mg/dL/h until the blood glucose level remains stable within the 70–140 mg/dL range. Since hyperglycemia often resolves before ketosis, dextrose should be added to the IV fluids once the plasma glucose reaches 250 mg/dL so that hypoglycemia does not occur.

19. **How does the treatment of HHS differ from that of DKA?**
Treatment of the two syndromes is essentially the same. With both, the goals are volume resuscitation, electrolyte repletion, and blood glucose correction. Patients with HHS often do not require such high doses of insulin as patients with DKA (since ketosis is not an issue) and should improve significantly with aggressive volume and electrolyte resuscitation.

20. **When should patients be converted from IV insulin to subcutaneous (SC) insulin?**
Patients may be converted to SC insulin once the anion gap has closed and the ketones have cleared. Patients should also be adequately volume resuscitated and able to tolerate oral intake. There should be an overlap in SC insulin initiation and IV insulin therapy, since lack of adequate insulin may result in a recurrence of anion gap acidosis, ketosis, or worsened blood glucose control. IV insulin may be discontinued 30–60 minutes after the first dose of SC insulin has been given.

WEBSITES

1. American Diabetes Association: http://www.Diabetes.org

2. Diabetes Forum: Management of Hyperglycemic Crisis in Patients with Diabetes: http://www.diabetesforum.net

BIBLIOGRAPHY

1. American College of Endocrinology: Position statement on inpatient diabetes and metabolic control. Endocr Pract 10:77–82, 2004.

2. American Diabetes Association: Diagnosis and classification of diabetes mellitus. Diabetes Care 28:S37–S42, 2005.

3. American Diabetes Association: Hyperglycemic crises in diabetes. Diabetes Care 27:S94–S102, 2004.

4. Axelrod DW: Endocrinology. In Zollo AJ (ed): Medical Secrets. Philadelphia, Hanley & Belfus, 1991, pp 37–43.

5. Clement S, Braithwaite SS, Magee MF, et al: Management of diabetes and hyperglycemia in hospitals. Diabetes Care 27:553–591, 2004.

6. Levetan CS, Passaro M, Jablonski K, et al: Unrecognized diabetes among hospitalized patients. Diabetes Care 21:246–249, 1998.

7. Montori VM, Bistrian BR, McMahon MM: Hyperglycemia in acutely ill patients. JAMA 288:2167–2169, 2002.

8. Powers AC: Diabetes mellitus. In Kasper DL, Fauci AS, Longo DL, et al (eds): Harrison's Principles of Internal Medicine, 16th ed. New York, McGraw-Hill, 2005, pp 2152–2180.

CHAPTER 63

ADRENAL INSUFFICIENCY

Jeffrey Carter, MD

1. **What are the defects in primary, secondary, and tertiary adrenal insufficiency (AI)?**

    The hypothalamic-pituitary-adrenal (HPA) axis is responsible for regulation of cortisol synthesis and secretion. The hypothalamus secretes corticotropin-releasing hormone, which in turn stimulates the anterior pituitary gland to secrete adrenocorticotropic hormone (ACTH), which then directly stimulates the adrenal cortex to secrete cortisol.

    - **Primary AI:** In primary AI, or *Addison's disease,* there is destruction of the adrenal cortex. Typically 80–90% of the adrenal glands must be destroyed to develop symptomatic AI.

    - **Secondary AI:** This form of AI results from a complete or relative ACTH deficiency, such that the pituitary is unable to respond to stress by secreting ACTH. The most common cause of ACTH deficiency is administration of exogenous steroids.

    - **Tertiary AI:** Also most commonly caused by exogenous steroid use, tertiary AI involves the failure of the hypothalamus to secrete corticotropin-releasing hormone.

2. **What is the most common cause of AI?**

    Chronic glucocorticoid therapy. Exogenous steroids suppress all aspects of the HPA axis. The degree and duration of suppression are dependent on the duration and doses of steroid therapy. Function typically returns to the hypothalamus first, followed by the pituitary, and then the adrenals. This will initially be demonstrated as inappropriately low ACTH levels for low cortisol levels. As pituitary function recovers, ACTH will rise to a level appropriate for low cortisol. Finally, cortisol levels will normalize. Other drugs that can induce AI are listed in Table 63-1.

TABLE 63-1. DRUGS THAT CAN INDUCE ADRENAL INSUFFICIENCY	
Decrease Cortisol Synthesis	**Increase Cortisol Metabolism**
Corticosteroids*	Rifampin
Etomidate	Barbiturates
Metyrapone	Aminoglutethimide
Ketoconazole	Phenytoin
	Mitotane

*See question 2 for complete mechanism of steroid-induced adrenal insufficiency

3. **Can topical or inhaled steroids cause adrenal suppression?**

    Prolonged, high-potency topical steroid use over a large surface area of skin can suppress the adrenal axis. Suppression can be seen with inhaled steroid doses greater than 0.8 mg (800 µg) per day, although some patients do not experience suppression at even higher doses.

4. **What are the classic signs and symptoms of primary AI?**
   Symptoms tend to be nonspecific and insidious in onset. They include chronic malaise, lassitude, fatigue, generalized weakness, anorexia, weight loss, abdominal pain, hypotension, salt craving, hyperkalemia, hyponatremia, hyperpigmentation, and hypoglycemia.

5. **Describe the patterns of pigmentation associated with Addison's disease.**
   Increased pigmentation is found in sunlight-exposed areas, areas exposed to chronic friction, the palmar creases, areolae, axillae, and perineum. Preexisting pigmentation darkens. The melanotropic activity of ACTH causes melanocytes to increase pigment production.

6. **Why does orthostatic hypotension occur in AI?**
   In primary AI, orthostasis is caused by hypovolemia as a result of mineralocorticoid deficiency. In secondary AI, wherein mineralocorticoid function is intact, the hypotension results from a decreased expression of catecholamine receptors in the vasculature (i.e., lack of vasoconstriction).

KEY POINTS: SIGNS AND SYMPTOMS OF CHRONIC ADRENAL INSUFFICIENCY

1. Fatigue, malaise, and lassitude

2. Weight loss and anorexia

3. Hyperpigmentation

4. Hyponatremia, hyperkalemia, and hypoglycemia

5. Postural hypotension

7. **What is the standard test to confirm AI? What is a normal response?**
   Plasma cortisol testing is complicated by significant diurnal and stress-induced fluctuations. The normal cortisol range is 6–24 μg/dL, with a value < 6 μg/dL or > 24 μg/dL required to definitively rule in or rule out AI. Despite being within the normal range, a normal value may be inappropriately low for the degree of physiologic stress. Consequently, a cosyntropin stimulation (i.e., stress) test is often recommended. A baseline plasma cortisol level is drawn before administration of a 250 μg dose of cosyntropin, with a level > 24 μg/dL effectively ruling out AI. Cortisol levels are measured again at 30 and 60 minutes. A doubling of the plasma cortisol level or an increase to >20 μg/dL are variably defined as normal.

   Grinspoon SK, Miller BM: Clinical review 62: Laboratory assessment of adrenal insufficiency. J Clin Endocrin Metab 79:923–931, 1994.

8. **If the cosyntropin test result is normal, does it rule out secondary AI?**
   No. It does not eliminate the possibility of mild, recent, or subclinical AI. The result of a metyrapone test can be used to distinguish between a healthy subject and one with secondary or tertiary AI. Metyrapone inhibits the final step in the synthesis of cortisol. When given to a healthy subject, ACTH will rise over time, whereas it will not in secondary or tertiary AI.

9. **What is adrenal crisis?**
   Adrenal crisis is defined as hypotension and hemodynamic instability. Whereas many patients will have subnormal responses to an ACTH stimulation test, indicating adrenal suppression, only some will have hemodynamic collapse.

10. **What are the causes of adrenal crisis?**
    Bilateral adrenal hemorrhage, bilateral necrosis secondary to emboli, and sepsis can all induce acute adrenal failure. In patients with a history of AI, the most common cause of adrenal crisis is inadequate replacement or insufficient stress dose steroids in the setting of an acute serious infection, surgical procedure, or trauma. Risk factors and symptoms related to bilateral adrenal hemorrhage are listed in Table 63-2.

TABLE 63-2. BILATERAL ADRENAL HEMORRHAGE: RISK FACTORS AND SYMPTOMS	
Risk Factors	**Symptoms**
Anticoagulation	Hypotension
Acquired coagulopathy	Abdominal pain
Postoperative state	Back/flank pain
Thromboembolic disease	Fever
Trauma	Rigid abdomen
Hypercoagulable state	

11. **Why do patients with AI become hypotensive?**
    Glucocorticoids have a permissive effect on vascular tone, meaning that steroids facilitate vascular response to catecholamines. Failure to respond to such endogenous catecholamines can lead to vasodilation and hypotension.

12. **What is Waterhouse-Friderichsen syndrome?**
    It is bilateral adrenal hemorrhage classically associated with meningococcemia or pseudomonal sepsis. It is associated with vomiting, fever, chills, myalgias, and petechial rash. It is more common in children than in adults.

13. **What are physiologic doses of various steroids?**
    The physiologic dose is the dose that is equivalent to the amount of daily cortisol produced by the adrenal glands. This roughly equates to 25 mg of hydrocortisone, 5 mg of prednisone, 4 mg of triamcinolone, or 0.75 mg of dexamethasone (Table 63-3).

TABLE 63-3. STEROID POTENCY EQUIVALENCY CHART		
Steroid	**Physiologic Dose (mg)**	**Relative Potency**
Hydrocortisone	25	1
Prednisone	5	4
Prednisolone	5	4
Triamcinolone	4	5
Dexamethasone	0.75	~25

14. **At what dose and duration of steroid therapy does the HPA axis become suppressed?**
HPA axis suppression usually requires supra-physiologic doses. Patients receiving the equivalent of ≤5 mg of prednisone are unlikely to be suppressed. Typically, the use of 20 mg of prednisone for 5 days or more is enough to suppress the HPA axis. Mild suppression usually manifests with a normal serum cortisol level but a subnormal response to an ACTH stimulation test, whereas greater suppression will show a low serum cortisol level as well. As a general rule, the greater the dose or the longer the duration of exogenous steroid therapy, the more suppressed the HPA axis will be, and the longer it will take to regain function. Patients chronically taking high doses of steroids, even intermittently, can have HPA axis suppression for up to a year.

15. **Why is dexamethasone the preferred replacement glucocorticoid in adrenal crisis?**
As a synthetic steroid, it does not interfere with the ACTH stimulation test, allowing for empiric treatment before diagnostic testing. Additionally, it has a relatively long half-life (12–24 hours).

16. **Which hospitalized patients should receive stress dose steroids?**
Patients with symptoms of AI or patients receiving chronic steroid therapy who exhibit HPA suppression should receive stress dose steroids in the setting of an acute illness and before surgery. For medical patients at risk of having AI, this can be evaluated with the ACTH stimulation test as outlined in question 7, or it can be treated empirically. Patients on chronic steroids who undergo surgery should receive hydrocortisone 100 mg IV every 8 hours, starting 24 hours before surgery, and 50 mg IV every 8 hours after surgery, in addition to their normal steroid therapy. Patients not taking steroids chronically should receive the previously described therapy with an additional day of hydrocortisone (25 mg IV q8h).

KEY POINTS: SUPPLEMENTAL STEROIDS

1. Any patient who appears cushingoid or has an abnormal response to an ACTH stimulation test should receive supplemental steroids during acute illness or surgery.

2. Any patient taking chronic steroids should continue the usual dose during surgery.

3. For severe stressors, such as major surgery or sepsis, 3 days of replacement glucocorticoid can be given, as hydrocortisone:
   - 100 mg IV q 8h × 24 hours
   - 50 mg IV q 8h × 24 hours
   - 25 mg IV q 8h × 24 hours

17. **Develop a diagnostic algorithm for the work-up of AI.**
See Fig. 63-1.

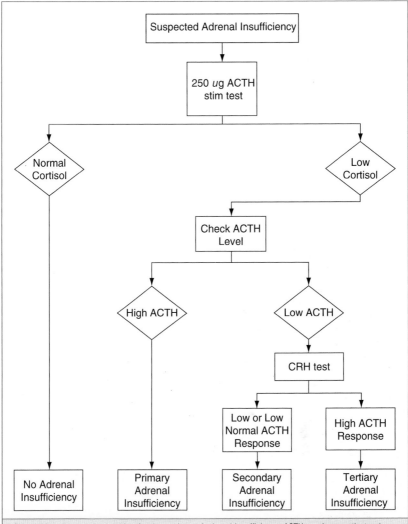

Figure 63-1. Diagnostic algorithm for the work-up of adrenal insufficiency. ACTH = adrenocorticotropic hormone, CRH = corticotropin-releasing hormone.

BIBLIOGRAPHY

1. Axelrod L: Perioperative management of patients treated with glucocorticoids. Endrocrinol Metab Clin North Am 32:367–383, 2003.
2. Coursin DB, Wood KE: Corticosteroid supplementation for adrenal insufficiency. JAMA 287:236–240, 2002.

ACUTE ARTHRITIS

Marina N. Magrey, MD, and Catherine Curley, MD, MS

CHAPTER 64

1. **What is acute arthritis?**

   Acute arthritis is an inflammation of joints characterized by pain, swelling, and increased temperature that develops rapidly within days to a period of less than 6 weeks.

2. **What are the common causes of acute arthritis?**

   The differential diagnosis of acute arthritis is large.

   - **Infectious disease:** Arthritis is often a manifestation of an infectious disease and can be caused by bacteria (e.g., septic arthritis, gonococcal arthritis, infectious endocarditis, Lyme disease), viruses (e.g., parvovirus, rubella, hepatitis B, hepatitis C, HIV), or fungi (e.g., *Candida* species, coccidiomycosis, sporotrichosis, tuberculosis, or nontuberculous mycobacteria).
   - **Genitourinary/gastrointestinal infection:** Reactive arthritis is a form of arthritis involving one or more joints that occurs after genitourinary or gastrointestinal infections. Conjunctivitis or iritis can be seen shortly after the symptoms of urethritis, followed by arthritis typically involving the knees or small joints of the feet, often asymmetric.
   - **Presence of crystals:** Crystal-induced disease causes include gout (urate) and pseudogout (calcium pyrophosphate).
   - **Rheumatoid arthritis and adult Still's disease:** These also present as acute arthritis. Adult Still's disease resembles juvenile rheumatoid arthritis, with patients presenting with high, spiking fevers, arthritis, and an evanescent rash.

   Other causes include systemic vasculitis, systemic lupus erythematosus (SLE), sarcoidosis, malignancy, and familial Mediterranean fever.

KEY POINTS: COMMON CAUSES OF ACUTE ARTHRITIS ✓

1. Infectious arthritis

2. Crystal-induced arthritis

3. Adult Still's disease

4. Reactive arthritis

5. Systemic rheumatic illness

---

3. **What are the most common causes of acute arthritis in hospitalized patients?**

   The most common causes are crystal-induced and septic arthritis.

   Gout is typically a monoarticular arthritis that results from the oversaturation of urate crystals in joint tissue. Patients can present from the community to the hospital with this condition, or it can be seen in patients hospitalized for surgery and trauma, those undergoing chemotherapy for leukemia or lymphoma, and patients with chronic renal failure admitted with an acute illness. Calcium pyrophosphate deposition, known as *pseudogout,* is also commonly seen as a complication of acute illness. Gout and pseudogout can be clinically indistinguishable. Differentiation requires arthrocentesis and evaluation of synovial fluid for crystals. Monosodium urate (gout) crystals appear needle shaped and negatively birefringent under polarized light microscopy. Calcium pyrophosphate (pseudogout) crystals are short, rhomboid, and positively birefringent.

Septic arthritis including non-gonococcal and gonococcal arthritis is another cause of acute arthritis in hospitalized patients. Non-gonococcal, septic arthritis is typically caused by bacteremic seeding of the joint. *Staphylococcus aureus* is the most common pathogen.

4. **What are the seronegative spondyloarthropathies?**
   The seronegative spondyloarthropathies are a group of diseases with some common features: axial spine involvement, asymmetric peripheral joint involvement, and a negative rheumatoid factor (i.e., seronegative). They include entities such as ankylosing spondylitis, reactive arthritis or Reiter syndrome, and inflammatory bowel disease associated arthritis or psoriatic arthritis.

5. **Which viral infections present with arthritis?**
   Parvovirus B19 and rubella cause a self-limited rheumatoid arthritis–like syndrome with morning stiffness and symmetric small joint involvement of the proximal interphalangeal and metacarpal phalangeal joints. Parvovirus B19 arthritis presents acutely and generally resolves within 2 weeks. Arthritis due to rubella can occur up to 1 week before the characteristic rash and typically resolves in 2 weeks. Polyarthritis can precede the symptoms of hepatitis B virus infection. Hepatitis C virus infection can cause a chronic polyarthritis associated with rash and cryoglobulinemia. HIV infection can cause acute and chronic polyarthritis.

6. **How does the pattern of joint involvement aid in diagnosis?**
   Arthritis is characterized by the involvement of one, a few, or many joints (Table 64-1). The various arthritides can present with certain patterns. For example, gout and septic arthritis typically involve a single joint (i.e., monoarticular), whereas rheumatoid arthritis classically involves multiple joints (i.e., polyarticular). In addition, joint involvement can be migratory, symmetric, and additive. Migratory arthritis moves from joint to joint. It is often seen in rheumatic fever, gonococcemia, meningococcemia, viral arthritis, SLE, acute leukemia, and Whipple's disease. Symmetric small-joint synovitis is seen with rheumatoid arthritis, SLE, and viral arthritis.

TABLE 64-1. PATTERNS OF JOINT INVOLVEMENT FOR COMMON CAUSES OF ACUTE ARTHRITIS		
Monoarticular (Single Joint Involved)	**Polyarticular (Multiple Joints Involved)**	**Oligoarticular (2–3 Joints Involved)**
Septic arthritis (non-gonococcal)	Gonococcal arthritis	Inflammatory bowel disease
Gout	RA and Still's disease	Gout
Pseudogout	Rheumatic fever	Rheumatic fever
	Reiter syndrome	Reiter syndrome
	Viral arthritis	
	SLE	

RA = rheumatoid arthritis, SLE = systematic lupus erythematosus.

7. **Which extra-articular manifestations help in diagnosis?**
    Extra-articular manifestations such as fever, rash, skin nodules, and ocular findings are often associated with acute arthropathies and can aid in diagnosis. Table 64-2 lists the extra-articular manifestations and the laboratory values associated with specific types of acute arthritis.

8. **What are Jones criteria for diagnosing acute rheumatic fever?**
    The revised modified Jones criteria for the diagnosis of acute rheumatic fever require the presence of two major criteria, or one major and two minor criteria, supported by evidence of a preceding streptococcal infection (i.e., elevated antistreptolysin O antibody titer, positive pharyngeal culture, or recent scarlet fever).
    - **Major criteria:** Erythema marginatum, carditis, polyarthritis, chorea, and subcutaneous nodules
    - **Minor criteria:** Fever, arthralgias, previous rheumatic carditis, prolonged PR interval on electrocardiography, and elevated inflammatory markers (ESR or CRP)

9. **What is Lofgren's syndrome?**
    The triad of polyarthritis, erythema nodosum, and bilateral hilar adenopathy. Nearly half of such patients have sarcoidosis. Other causes include streptococcal infections, tuberculosis, *Yersinia* infection, leprosy, tularemia, leptospirosis, cat scratch fever, fungal infection (e.g., coccidiomycosis, blastomycosis, histoplasmosis), and viral infection (e.g., infectious mononucleosis).

10. **Which diagnostic laboratory tests are helpful in differentiating the types of arthritis?**
    Standard testing includes complete blood count (CBC) with differential, renal and liver function testing, urinalysis, inflammatory markers including erythrocyte sedimentation rate (ESR) and C-reactive protein (CRP), and tests for antibodies such as rheumatoid factor (RF) and antinuclear antibody (ANA). Derangements of the CBC are common in acute arthritis. The abnormalities can include leukocytosis, thrombocytosis, and cytopenias. In rheumatoid arthritis, anemia is very common, and anemia and other cytopenias can be seen in SLE. Both infectious and crystal-induced arthritis are associated with leukocytosis. Abnormal renal function is typically present only in gout, SLE, and vasculitis. Liver abnormalities are common only in adult Still's disease.

KEY POINTS: LABORATORY EVALUATION OF ACUTE ARTHRITIS

1. CBC

2. Renal function

3. Liver function

4. ESR and CRP

5. RF and ANA

6. Synovial fluid analysis

11. **How useful are ESR and CRP in the evaluation of acute arthritis?**
    Both are nonspecific markers of inflammation. ESR is usually elevated in the presence of an inflammatory process (e.g., infection, malignancy). Elevation of CRP depends on sufficient concentration of inflammatory mediators in the liver, so a normal CRP level does not exclude an inflammatory condition. CRP levels change more rapidly than ESR, making the former a better test for studying disease activity. ESRs can be falsely elevated in common medical conditions such as renal failure, dysproteinemia, occult malignancies, anemia, and infection.

TABLE 64–2. EXTRA-ARTICULAR SYMPTOMS AND LABORATORY ABNORMALITIES IN ACUTE ARTHRITIS

Etiology of Acute Arthritis	Fever	Skin Rash	Subcutaneous Nodules	Eye	ANA Positive	RF Positive	LFT Abnormalities	Renal Insufficiency
Septic	++							
Viral	+	+						
Gout	+		+					+
RA			+	+		+		
Gonococcal	+	+						
Rheumatic fever	++	+	+					
Still's disease	++	++			−	−	+	
Reactive arthritis	+	+		++				
SLE	+	+			+	+		+
Sarcoidosis	+	+		+		+		
Vasculitis	+	+						+

ANA = antinuclear antibodies, RF = rheumatoid factor, LFT = liver function tests, RA = rheumatoid arthritis, SLE = systematic lupus erythematosus, ++ = usually present, + = often present, − = usually not present.

12. **How specific is the RF for rheumatoid arthritis?**

   Unfortunately, RF is not specific for diagnosis of rheumatoid arthritis. However, it tends to be seen only in chronic inflammatory conditions such as viral infections, tuberculosis, subacute bacterial endocarditis, SLE, sarcoidosis, malignancy, and primary biliary cirrhosis.

13. **What are the indications and contraindications for an arthrocentesis?**

   Arthrocentesis, or joint aspiration, should be considered in all patients with acute arthritis. In acute monoarticular arthritis, arthrocentesis is the only way to reliably differentiate crystal-induced arthritis, infectious arthritis, or hemarthrosis. It is also helpful in distinguishing between inflammatory and noninflammatory forms of polyarthritis. Arthrocentesis should not be performed through broken skin or areas of cellulitis. It should be performed with caution in patients who are anticoagulated. The primary complication of arthrocentesis is the introduction of infection into the joint space. This occurs in approximately 1 in 10,000 aspirations.

14. **Which diagnostic tests should be performed on aspirated synovial fluid?**

   The characteristics of the joint fluid can help differentiate the various types of arthritis (Tables 64-3 and 64-4). Most commonly, the fluid is analyzed for cell count, Gram stain, and

TABLE 64-3. CLASSIFICATION OF ARTHRITIS BY JOINT FLUID CHARACTERISTICS

Characteristic	Noninflammatory	Inflammatory	Septic	Hemorrhagic
WBC/mm^3	<2000	2000–100,000	>100,000	<2000
Differential	<25% PMN	>50% PMN	75–95% PMN	>50% PMN
Clarity	Transparent	Variable	Opaque	Opaque/red
Viscosity	High	Variable	Low	N/A

WBC = white blood cell, PMN = polymorphonuclear leukocytes.

TABLE 64-4. COMMON ARTHRITIDES BY FLUID TYPE

Noninflammatory	Inflammatory	Septic	Hemorrhagic
Normal	Seronegative spondyloarthropathies	Non-gonococcal bacterial infection	Trauma
Osteoarthritis	SLE		Coagulopathy
Avascular necrosis	Crystal induced		Tuberculosis
Trauma	RA		
	Lyme		
	Mycobacterial or fungal		
	Viral		
	Sarcoidosis		
	Other connective tissues diseases		
	Gonococcal infection		

SLE = systematic lupus erythematosus, RA = rheumatoid arthritis.

culture. A polarized light microscope will detect crystals. Gross examination of color, clarity, and viscosity should also be performed but often does not add additional information. Measurements of glucose and protein are no longer recommended. Diagnosis of indolent infections (e.g., mycobacterial and fungal arthritis) typically requires synovial tissue biopsy through arthroscopy.

15. **How is disseminated gonococcal infection (DGI) differentiated from other causes of septic arthritis?**
Septic arthritis typically involves only one to two joints. The most common cause is bacteremic seeding of the joint with *S. aureus*. DGI results from gonococcal bacteremia after acute infection, usually genitourinary. Although DGI can present with a septic joint, the more common presentation is the arthritis-dermatitis syndrome with polyarticular, sometimes migratory joint involvement, tenosynovitis of extensor tendons, and a widespread rash consisting of papules and pustules, often hemorrhagic. Joint fluid is typically more inflammatory than other forms of bacterial infections and sterile.

16. **List the common risk factors for septic arthritis.**
Although any bacteremic episodes can result in microbial spread to joints, septic arthritis is seen most frequently in immunosuppressed patients, intravenous drug users, and patients with preexisting joint disease. (See Chapter 56 for more details.)

WEBSITE

Arthritis Foundation: http://www.arthritis.org/

BIBLIOGRAPHY

1. Fye KH: Evaluation of the patient. In Klippel JH (ed): Primer of the Rheumatic Diseases, 12th ed. Atlanta, Arthritis Foundation, 2001, pp 138–144.
2. Gordan DA, Arend WP: Approach to the patient with rheumatic disease. In Goldman L, Ausiello D (eds): Cecil Textbook of Medicine, 22nd ed. Philadelphia, W.B. Sanders, 2004, pp 1623–1627.
3. Ho G Jr, Naides SJ, Sigal LH, et al: Infectious disorders. In Klippel JH (ed): Primer on the Rheumatic Diseases, 12th ed. Atlanta, Arthritis Foundation, 2001, pp 259–283.
4. Pinals RS: Polyarthritis and fever. N Engl J Med 330:769–774, 1994.
5. Reveille JD, Arnett FC, Keat A, et al: Seronegative spondyloarthropathies. In Klippel JH (ed): Primer on the Rheumatic Diseases, 12th ed. Atlanta, Arthritis Foundation, 2001, pp 239–258.
6. Shmerling RH, Delbanco TL, Tosteson AN, Trentham DE: Synovial fluid tests. What should be ordered? JAMA 264:1009–1014, 1990.
7. Terkeltaub RA, Edwards NL: Gout. In Klippel JH (ed): Primer on the Rheumatic Diseases, 12th ed. Atlanta, Arthritis Foundation, 2001, pp 307–324.

CHAPTER 65

VASCULITIS

Alexandra Villa-Forte, MD, MPH, and Brian F. Mandell, MD, PhD

1. **What is vasculitis?**
   The vasculitides are rare diseases characterized by blood vessel inflammation. Vessels of different types, sizes, and locations are affected, resulting in diversity of clinical presentations. Some vasculitic syndromes are associated with characteristic organ inflammation and clinical manifestations. The consequences of blood vessel inflammation are:
   - Stenosis or total vascular occlusion with resultant ischemia
   - Hemorrhage and/or aneurysm formation
   - Various clinical features depending on involved organ system and type of vasculitis

2. **How are the vasculitides classified?**
   The vasculitides are *primary* when there is no known etiology or *secondary* when occurring as a consequence of another primary disorder. The primary vasculitides may be classified according to the size of the predominantly affected vessels and the pattern of clinical involvement (Table 65-1).

TABLE 65-1.   VASCULITIS CLASSIFICATION

Primary Vasculitides

- Large-sized vessel: giant cell arteritis and Takayasu's arteritis
- Medium-sized vessel: polyarteritis nodosa and Kawasaki disease
- Small-sized vessel: Wegener's granulomatosis, Churg-Strauss syndrome, microscopic polyangiitis, Henoch-Schönlein purpura, and cutaneous leukocytoclastic angiitis

Secondary Vasculitides

- Infections: hepatitis B, hepatitis C, HIV, bacterial endocarditis
- Drugs: propylthiouracil, allopurinol, minocycline
- Malignancies: lymphoproliferative and myeloproliferative diseases, carcinomas
- Rheumatologic diseases: systemic lupus erythematosus, rheumatoid arthritis, Sjögren's disease

---

3. **When should the hospitalist suspect a vasculitic syndrome?**
   The vasculitides can be systemic or confined to one organ (e.g., skin, nerve, kidney). Patients may present with a prototypic, specific vasculitic syndrome, unexplained tissue ischemia, or nonspecific features. The concomitant or sequential involvement of multiple organ systems should raise suspicion for a vasculitic syndrome. Glomerulonephritis, purpura, neuropathy, and lung involvement (i.e., infiltrates, nodules, or hemorrhage) more strongly suggest vasculitis. Glomerulonephritis is often asymptomatic. Alveolar hemorrhage need not present with hemoptysis.

4. **What diseases may mimic vasculitis?**
   - Buerger's disease (thromboangiitis obliterans)
   - Occlusive atherosclerosis, cholesterol embolization
   - Thrombotic thrombocytopenic purpura
   - Hypercoagulable syndromes (e.g., antiphospholipid syndrome)
   - Vasospasm
   - Amyloidosis
   - Angiocentric malignancies

5. **What laboratory tests may aid in the diagnosis of vasculitis?**
   Laboratory test results may support the diagnosis, but are not always abnormal. There is no specific test for "vasculitis." Common nonspecific laboratory abnormalities include anemia of chronic disease, leukocytosis, thrombocytosis, and elevated acute phase reactant levels (e.g., erythrocyte sedimentation rate, C-reactive protein). Leukopenia and thrombocytopenia are not typically associated with vasculitis. Eosinophilia associated with manifestations of vasculitis suggests Churg-Strauss syndrome. Examination of fresh urine sediment is mandatory to check for the presence of glomerulonephritis, even if the creatinine value is normal.

   The antineutrophil cytoplasmic antibodies (ANCAs) are useful when Wegener's granulomatosis (WG) or microscopic polyangiitis are clinically suspected. However, ANCA detection is not a screening test for vasculitis. It is not present in all cases of WG or microscopic polyangiitis, and a positive ANCA test result does not mean a confirmed case of "vasculitis." ANCAs may be detected in nonvasculitic diseases (e.g., endocarditis, drug reaction, inflammatory bowel disease).

6. **How can the diagnosis be confirmed?**
   Biopsy or angiography can be used to support a specific clinical diagnosis of vasculitis.
   Biopsy
   - Obtain specimens from accessible and clinically involved sites. Biopsy specimens from asymptomatic sites have very low diagnostic yield and should be avoided.
   - The biopsy site is influenced by the specific suspected diagnosis.
   - Pathologic examination is the definitive diagnostic test, but vessel involvement may be patchy and the pathology may be unrevealing.
   Angiography
   - Angiography is usually performed for suspected large and medium-sized vessel involvement, where biopsy is not feasible.
   - Characteristic but not specific angiographic abnormalities include stenosis or occlusion, and aneurysm formation. Distinction from atherosclerosis may be difficult.

KEY POINTS: DIAGNOSING VASCULITIS

1. Suspect vasculitis in the presence of characteristic clinical patterns or unexplained multisystem or ischemic disease.

2. There are no screening or diagnostic laboratory tests. Examination of fresh urine sediment is mandatory to diagnose glomerulonephritis.

3. Exclude diseases that may mimic vasculitic symptoms and signs.

4. Exclude secondary causes of vasculitis (e.g., infection, malignancy, drug reaction).

7. **How are the vasculitides treated?**
   Treatment is not the same for all the vasculitides. In general, primary vasculitides are initially treated with glucocorticoids. Severe cases and some specific diseases such as WG require a

second immunosuppressive medication in addition to glucocorticoids from the outset. Selected cases of isolated cutaneous leukocytoclastic vasculitis may be treated with other drugs (e.g., colchicine, dapsone) and not glucocorticoids (Table 65-2).

TABLE 65-2. CLINICAL FEATURES AND TREATMENT OF VASCULITIDES

Vasculitis	Clinical Features	Treatment	Comments
Giant cell (temporal) arteritis	Headache, visual loss, jaw claudication, scalp tenderness, polymyalgia rheumatica	GC	Thoracic aortic aneurysm, aortic branch stenoses occur. ESR not always elevated.
Takayasu's arteritis	Visual symptoms, dizziness, headache, pulse abnormalities, extremity claudication	GC	Symptoms and laboratory markers are poor indicators of disease activity
Polyarteritis nodosa	Peripheral neuropathy, mesenteric ischemia, hypertension, renal insufficiency	GC CYC for severe disease	No involvement of lung parenchyma or alveolar vessels No GN
Kawasaki disease	Acute febrile illness, nonsuppurative cervical adenitis, skin and mucous membrane lesions	IV γ-globulin Aspirin	Association with coronary artery aneurysms in ~25% of cases
Wegener's granulomatosis	Upper respiratory tract, lung involvement, GN, skin lesions, eyes, subglottic stenosis	GC + CYC (severe disease) or GC + MTX (mild disease)	High incidence of relapses
Churg-Strauss syndrome	Asthma, pulmonary infiltrates, skin lesions, GN, peripheral neuropathy, coronary disease	GC CYC for severe disease	Striking eosinophilia (CSS)
Microscopic polyangiitis	Pulmonary hemorrhage, GN, peripheral neuropathy, purpura	GC + CYC (severe disease) or GC + MTX (mild disease)	Relapses common

Continued

TABLE 65-2.   CLINICAL FEATURES AND TREATMENT OF VASCULITIDES—CONT'D

Vasculitis	Clinical Features	Treatment	Comments
Henoch-Schönlein purpura	Purpura, bowel involvement, arthralgia or arthritis, GN	Symptomatic treatment or GC	Recovery without therapy more common in children than adults
Essential cryoglobulinemia	Skin lesions, peripheral neuropathy, GN, arthralgias	GC, CYC (severe disease), plasmapheresis	Exclude hepatitis C infection
Cutaneous leukocytoclastic	Skin lesions	Symptomatic treatment, colchicine, dapsone, GC	Exclude systemic vasculitis, infection, drug reaction, and malignancy

GC = glucocorticoids, ESR = erythrocyte sedimentation rate, CYC = cyclophosphamide, GN = glomerulonephritis, IV = intravenous, MTX = methotrexate.

8. **When should cyclophosphamide be considered as a treatment option?**
   Cyclophosphamide is indicated for the treatment of life- or organ-threatening vasculitis, or for vasculitis unlikely to completely respond to corticosteroids alone. General indications include alveolar hemorrhage, progressive glomerulonephritis, neuropathy, cardiac disease, and mesenteric ischemia. Cyclophosphamide treatment ideally should be limited to 3–6 months because of its toxicity, with subsequent transition to methotrexate or azathioprine. Leukopenia is not necessary to achieve disease remission and should be avoided. Severe complications from cyclophosphamide include leukopenia with risk of infection, hemorrhagic cystitis, malignancies (e.g., bladder cancer, myeloproliferative diseases), and sterility.

9. **What infections occur in the immunosuppressed patient that can mimic a flare in vasculitis?**
   - **Bacterial:** Pneumonia, abscesses, and sepsis
   - ***Pneumocystis carinii* pneumonia (PCP)**
   - **Fungal:** Esophagus, skin, lung, and central nervous system
   - **Viral (herpesviruses):** Skin, central and peripheral nervous system, gastrointestinal (cytomegalovirus), and eye
   (See Chapter 53 for more details.)

10. **What prophylaxis should be considered for immunosuppressed patients?**
    - **Osteoporosis:** Calcium and vitamin D for all patients without contraindications; bisphosphonates for selected patients taking corticosteroids.

- ***Pneumocystis carinii* pnemonia (PCP):** Usually indicated for patients treated with a combination of glucocorticoids and a second immunosuppressive medication; sulfamethoxazole/trimethoprim (one double-strength tablet on alternate days), dapsone daily, or monthly inhaled pentamidine. Patients taking methotrexate alone generally do not require prophylaxis.
- **Vaccinations:** Influenza and pneumococcus before initiating immunosuppressive therapy, if possible.
- **PPD:** Before steroid therapy, if possible (prophylactic INH if appropriate).

KEY POINTS: VASCULITIS THERAPY

1. There is a delicate balance between necessary immunosuppression and the risk of serious infections. Cell counts should be checked regularly so that medication doses can be adjusted to avoid leukopenia.

2. PCP prophylaxis is important in significantly immunosuppressed patients.

3. The initial use of cyclophosphamide is useful for severe disease; transition to alternative drug for chronic therapy should be attempted.

4. The need for renal replacement therapy may be transient. If renal failure is acute and due to active vasculitis, therapy should be continued (with doses adjusted for end-stage renal disease).

11. **What is the prognosis for patients with vasculitis?**
    The prognosis depends on the specific disease, the severity of organ damage by the time appropriate therapy is initiated, and the complications of therapy. The need for renal replacement therapy may be transient. If renal failure is acute and due to active vasculitis, therapy should be continued (with doses adjusted for reduced renal function).

WEBSITES

1. Proceedings of the 10th International Vasculitis and ANCA Workshop, April 25–28, 2002: http://www.CCJM.org/TOC/Vasculitis.htm

2. The Johns Hopkins Vasculitis Center: http://vasculitis.med.Jhu.edu

BIBLIOGRAPHY

1. Callen JP: Cutaneous vasculitis: its relationship to systemic disease. In Hoffman GS, Weyand CM (eds): Inflammatory Diseases of Blood Vessels. New York, Marcel Dekker, 2002, pp 529–538.
2. Gabriel SE, O'Fallow WM, Achkar AA, et al: The use of clinical characteristics to predict the results of temporal artery biopsy among patients with suspected giant cell arteritis. J Rheumatol 22:93–96, 1995.
3. Hoffman GS, Specks U: Antineutrophil cytoplasmic antibodies. Arthritis Rheum 41:1521–1537, 1998.
4. Jennette CJ, Falk RJ, Andrassy K, et al: Nomenclature of systemic vasculitides. Proposal of an international consensus conference. Arthritis Rheum 37:187–192, 1994.
5. Langford CA: Management of systemic vasculitis. Best Pract Res Clin Rheumatol 15:281–297, 2001.
6. Masi AT, Hunder GG, Lie JT, et al: The American College of Rheumatology 1990 criteria for the classification of Churg-Strauss syndrome (allergic granulomatosis and angiitis). Arthritis Rheum 33:1094–1100, 1990.

CHAPTER 66

SKIN AND SOFT TISSUE INFECTIONS

Joseph Ming Wah Li, MD

1. **Explain the difference between various types of skin and soft tissue infections.**
   - **Cellulitis:** An infection of the skin and subcutaneous tissue
   - **Erysipelas:** A superficial cellulitis with prominent lymphatic involvement but no involvement of the subcutaneous tissue; in erysipelas, the borders between normal and infected are sharply demarcated, whereas in cellulitis, the borders are indistinct
   - **Impetigo:** An even more superficial cellulitis with a vesiculopustular appearance
   - **Folliculitis:** An infection of hair follicles
   - **Furuncles:** Also known as boils; inflammatory nodules that involve the hair follicles
   - **Carbuncles:** Subcutaneous abscesses that drain purulent discharge via the hair follicles
   - **Hidradenitis suppurativa:** A chronic relapsing inflammatory disease of the apocrine glands that presents as recurrent furunculosis of the axillae and buttocks
   - **Necrotizing fasciitis:** Sometimes referred to as *flesh-eating disease*, involves destruction of the fascial planes
   - **Necrotizing myositis:** Occurs when the necrotic infection involves muscle
   - **Osteomyelitis:** An infection of bone

2. **Name five independent risk factors for cellulitis.**
   - Lymphedema (e.g., after breast surgery for cancer)
   - Wound or trauma at the site of entry (e.g., toe web intertrigo)
   - Venous insufficiency
   - Obesity
   - Leg edema (e.g., after vein harvest for coronary bypass surgery)

3. **List the differential diagnoses for lower extremity cellulitis.**
   The differential diagnosis includes deep and superficial venous thrombosis, contact dermatitis, erythema nodosum, pyoderma gangrenosum, septic arthritis, acute gout, ruptured Baker cyst, postradiation therapy changes, necrotizing fasciitis, anaerobic myonecrosis (gas gangrene), eosinophilic cellulitis (Wells' syndrome), and neutrophilic dermatosis (Sweet's syndrome).

4. **Is it necessary to identify a source of the cellulitis?**
   Although skin trauma is the most common cause, cellulitis can be caused by spread of a local infection (e.g., osteomyelitis) or bacteremic spread from a distant infectious source. Radiographs, needle aspiration, punch biopsies, and blood cultures are not indicated in most cases of cellulitis but should be reserved for cases in which there is suspicion of an alternative cause. Imaging is important if there is concern about foreign bodies or the presence of osteomyelitis. Blood cultures are indicated in all patients with lymphedema because such patients have a higher rate of bacteremia.

5. **Name the most common bacterial pathogens in cellulitis, erysipelas, and impetigo.**
   See Table 66-1.

TABLE 66–1. COMMON BACTERIAL PATHOGENS IN CELLULITIS, ERYSIPELAS, AND IMPETIGO

Cellulitis	Erysipelas	Impetigo
Beta-hemolytic streptococcus: group A, B, and C	Beta-hemolytic streptococcus: mainly group A	Group A streptococcus
Staphylococcus aureus		*Staphylococcus aureus*

6. **Describe the characteristics of patients most commonly affected by group B streptococcal cellulitis.**
   Patients with diabetes mellitus, renal disease, liver disease, or underlying malignancy are at the highest risk.

7. **What is the appropriate empiric antibiotic therapy for uncomplicated cellulitis?**
   - **Parenteral therapy:** Oxacillin, 2 gm given intravenously (IV) every 6 hours *or* cefazolin, 1–2 gm IV every 8 hours
   - **Oral therapy** (for nontoxic patients who can take pills by mouth): Dicloxacillin, 500 mg by mouth (PO) every 6 hours *or* cephalexin, 500 mg PO every 6 hours

8. **Describe appropriate empiric antibiotic therapy for treatment of erysipelas.**
   Group A beta-hemolytic streptococci are responsible the majority of cases.
   - **Parenteral therapy:** Penicillin G, 2 million units IV every 4 hours
   - **Oral therapy** (for nontoxic patients who can take pills by mouth): Penicillin V potassium, 500 mg PO four times/day

9. **Describe the treatment of methicillin-resistant *Staphylococcus aureus* (MRSA) skin infections.**
   Over the past 40 years, MRSA has become endemic in hospitals and is a potential pathogen in the following persons:
   - Patients who reside in a long-term care facility or were recently hospitalized
   - Users of illicit IV drugs
   - Patients who reside in a community with increased rates of MRSA
   Unfortunately, the rate of community-acquired MRSA infections is on the increase. These infections typically involve the skin and are more common in children younger than 2 years old. In high-risk patients or areas where community-acquired MRSA rates are high, clinicians must consider empiric MRSA therapy.
   - **Parenteral therapy:** Vancomycin, 1–2 gm/day IV *or* linezolid, 600 mg IV every 12 hours *or* daptomycin, 4 mg/kg every 24 hours
   - **Oral therapy** (when appropriate to transition from parenteral therapy): Linezolid, 600 mg PO every 12 hours

10. **Why are patients with diabetes at high risk for foot ulcers and infections?**
    Hyperglycemia impairs host immunity, and peripheral vascular disease (PVD) impairs wound healing. Over 60% of patients with diabetic foot ulcers have PVD. Neuropathy, present in more than 80% of diabetic patients with foot ulcers, causes decreased perception of pressure and pain as well as decreased glandular secretions, resulting in dry, cracked skin. All of these factors either promote the formation or inhibit the healing of foot infections in patients with diabetes mellitus.

KEY POINTS: RISK FACTORS FOR DIABETIC FOOT INFECTIONS

1. Hyperglycemia

2. Peripheral vascular disease

3. Neuropathy

11. **Describe the use of the ankle-brachial index (ABI) in patients with diabetic foot ulcers.**

    Persons with diabetes often have associated PVD. The ABI correlates well with arterial occlusive disease. To determine the ABI, use a Doppler probe to measure the systolic blood pressure in the brachial, posterior tibial, and dorsalis pedis arteries. Calculate the ABI by dividing the highest measurement in the lower extremities by the highest brachial measurement. Normal ABI is > 1.0. An ABI < 0.9 is 95% sensitive for detecting PVD. Although many patients with diabetes suffer from microvascular disease in their feet, a low ABI suggests macrovascular disease that may be amenable to surgery.

12. **Describe the physical signs that increase the likelihood of osteomyelitis associated with a diabetic foot ulcer.**

    Osteomyelitis may result from spread of contiguous soft tissue infection; however, the clinical appearance of osteomyelitis may be no different than that of cellulitis with ulcer. The following diabetic patients are at high risk for osteomyelitis:

    ■ Soft tissue infection, especially those over bony prominences, for > 2 weeks
    ■ Larger, deeper ulcers
    ■ Ulcers with exposed bone or bone that can be detected by probing with a sterile, steel probe

    Magnetic resonance imaging is the most sensitive imaging test for diagnosing osteomyelitis, although bone biopsy is the gold standard.

13. **How does the presence of diabetes mellitus affect the treatment of cellulitis associated with a foot ulcer?**

    Foot infections, a major cause of morbidity and mortality in patients with diabetes, may range from superficial localized soft tissue infections to deep ulcerations involving the bone and bloodstream. Organisms obtained from superficial swabs do not necessarily reflect the causative organisms. Whenever possible, deep wound and/or bone culture specimens should be taken and empiric antibiotic therapy started. In addition to beta-hemolytic streptococci and *S. aureus*, coverage should include gram-negative bacilli and anaerobic bacteria.

    ■ **Mild superficial skin infections:** Trimethoprim/sulfamethoxazole double strength (160 mg/ 800 mg) PO twice daily *or* amoxicillin/clavulonate extended release (1000 mg/62.5 mg), two tablets PO twice daily. One to 2 weeks of antibiotics is usually sufficient.

    ■ **Moderate-to-severe soft tissue infections:** Levofloxacin, 500 mg PO daily *or* ciprofloxacin, 750 mg PO twice daily *and* clindamycin, 300 mg PO four times/day. Debridement is often necessary, along with 2–4 weeks of antibiotic therapy.

    ■ **Severe diabetic foot ulcers:** Meropenem, 1 gm IV every 8 hours *or* ertapenem, 1 gm IV daily *or* imipenem, 500 mg IV four times/day *or* piperacillin/tazobactam, 4.5 gm IV three times/day *and* vancomycin, 1 gm IV twice daily *or* linezolid, 600 mg IV every 12 hours. Antibiotic therapy for 4–6 weeks is often recommended for osteomyelitis, but a shorter duration may be sufficient if all infected bone is removed.

14. **What is the difference between periorbital and orbital cellulitis?**
    Periorbital cellulitis involves the eyelid and tissues anterior to the orbital septum. It is important to distinguish periorbital cellulitis from *orbital cellulitis*, which can result in a change in visual acuity, pain with motion of the extraocular muscles, cavernous sinus thrombosis, and occasional blindness.

15. **How does cellulitis on the face affect the choice of empiric antibiotic therapy?**
    Facial cellulitis can result from sinusitis or otitis media, so antibiotic treatment must cover gram-negative pathogens. Before vaccine availability, *Haemophilus influenzae* was a common cause of facial cellulitis. Facial cellulitis in infants may result from pneumococcal bacteremia.

16. **Name the bacterial pathogens associated with cellulitis after water exposure.**
    - **Fresh water:** *Aeromonas hydrophilic*
    - **Salt water:** *Vibrio vulnificus*
    - **Aquacultured fish:** *Streptococcus iniae*
    - **Fish tank exposure:** *Mycobacterium marinum*
    - **Hot tub:** *Pseudomonas aeruginosa*

17. **Name the bacterial pathogens associated with bites.**
    See Table 66-2.

TABLE 66-2.   PRIMARY PATHOGENS IN CELLULITIS AFTER DOG, CAT, AND HUMAN BITES

Dog	Cat	Human
Streptococcus: alpha-, beta-, and gamma-hemolytic species	*Pasteurella multocida*	Streptococcus: alpha- and beta-hemolytic species
Pasteurella multocida, Pasteurella canis		*S. aureus*
S. aureus		Numerous gram-positive and gram-negative organisms
Gram-negative organisms		*Eikenella corrodens*
Erysipelothrix species		
Capnocytophaga canimorsus		

BIBLIOGRAPHY

1. Czachor J: Unusual aspects of bacterial water-borne illnesses. Am Fam Physician 46:797, 1992.
2. Dupuy A, Benchikhi H, Roujeau JC, et al: Risk factors for erysipelas of the leg (cellulitis): Case-control study. BMJ 318:1591, 1999.
3. Eriksson B, Jorup-Ronstrom C, Karkkonen K, et al: Erysipelas: Clinical and bacteriologic spectrum and serological aspects. Clin Infect Dis 23:1091–1098, 1996.
4. Fowkes FG: The measurement of atherosclerotic peripheral arterial disease in epidemiological surveys. Int J Epidemiol 17:248, 1988.
5. Fridkin SK, Hageman JC, Morrison M, et al: Methicillin-resistant *Staphylococcus aureus* disease in three communities. N Engl J Med 352:1436–1438, 2002.
6. Grayson ML, Gibbons GW, Balogh K, et al: Probing to bone in infected pedal Ulcers: A clinical sign of underlying osteomyelitis in diabetic patients. JAMA 273:721, 1995.

7. Karakas M, Baba M, Aksungur VL, et al: Manifestation of cellulites after saphenous vasectomy for coronary bypass surgery. J Eur Acad Dermatol Venereol 16:438, 2002.

8. Lipsky BA, Berendt AR, Deery HG, et al: IDSA Guidelines for the diagnosis and treatment of diabetic foot infections. Clin Infect Dis 39:885–910, 2004.

9. Rasmussen JE: *H. influenzae* cellulites: Case presentation and review of the literature. Br J Dermatol 88:547, 1973.

10. Schrag SJ, Zywicki S, Farley MM, et al: Group B streptococcal disease in the era of intra-partum antibiotic prophylaxis. N Engl J Med 342:15, 2000.

11. Swartz MN: Clinical practice: Cellulitis. N Engl J Med 350:904, 2004.

CHAPTER 67

SKIN ULCERS

Andrew H. Dombro, MD

1. **Which areas are most prone to the development of decubitus ulcers?**
   Decubitus or pressure ulcers can occur in any area overlying a bone that is not well padded with muscle or fat. In decreasing order of frequency, these include the sacrum, ischial tuberosity, greater trochanter, heel, elbow, knee, ankle, and occiput.

2. **What are the physical factors that cause decubitus ulcers?**
   External compression of blood vessels, shear forces, and friction, leading to tissue anoxia and eventually necrosis. This can occur with as little as 12 hours of direct pressure.

3. **What clinical conditions place patients at an increased risk for their occurrence?**
   The Braden scale is often used to assess risk. The main factors are:
   - Altered sensorium, especially with decreased awareness of pain
   - Sensory deficit with decreased pain perception in the affected body region, especially with spinal cord injury
   - Prolonged immobilization
   - Inadequate nursing care
   - Incontinence—urinary or fecal
   - Low blood pressure
   - Poor nutritional status and hypoalbuminemia
   - Presence of a fracture, muscle spasms, or contractures
   - Thin body frame or weight loss
   - Smoking—both higher incidence and slower healing

4. **What other conditions can mimic pressure ulcers?**
   Primary skin infections, such as herpes (especially if immunocompromised) or actinomycosis, burns, skin malignancy, pyoderma gangrenosum, and rectocutaneous fistula (if in perianal area) can mimic decubitus ulcers.

5. **How are decubitus ulcers clinically staged?**
   Per the National Pressure Ulcer Advisory Panel:
   - **Stage I:** Skin is still intact, but there is nonblanching erythema.
   - **Stage II:** This stage involves superficial or partial-thickness necrosis. This may include presence of bullae, dermal necrosis (black in color), and shallow ulcer formation.
   - **Stage III:** Deep necrosis and ulcer formation with full-thickness skin loss are present, extending down to, but not through, the fascia.
   - **Stage IV:** Full-thickness necrosis and ulceration with involvement of muscle and/or bone are characteristics of this stage. Generally, ulcers are quite large and deep with ill-defined borders.

6. **What are the signs and symptoms of secondary infection?**
   Surrounding erythema, purulent exudates, and foul odor (especially if anaerobic) are signs of probable infection. Also, fever, chills, or increasing pain may herald spreading infection, such as cellulitis or osteomyelitis.

7. **What diagnostic studies can be useful if secondary infection is suspected?**
An elevated white blood cell count and/or erythrocyte sedimentation rate is common in secondary infections. Wound cultures (see question 8), blood cultures, skin and bone biopsies, and radiographic imaging may also aid in diagnosis. Remember, ulcer debridement causes a transient bacteremia, so always wait at least 60 minutes to collect blood culture specimens.

8. **Describe the optimal technique for obtaining wound culture specimens.**
Most infections are polymicrobial, and it is very important to differentiate between colonization and infection. The optimal technique involves culture of the deepest portion of a punch biopsy specimen of the ulcer base. Remember to always include anaerobic cultures.

9. **How helpful are bone scans and bone biopsies in the diagnosis of osteomyelitis with advanced ulcers?**
It is often difficult on a bone scan to distinguish osteomyelitis from changes simply associated with chronic pressure sores, so a bone biopsy may be needed to differentiate between the two (See Chapter 56 for more details). Discontinuing antibiotics 24–48 hours before biopsy will increase the diagnostic yield.

KEY POINTS: WARNING SIGNS OF SECONDARY INFECTION OF DECUBITUS ULCERS

1. Surrounding erythema

2. Purulent exudates

3. Foul odor

4. Fever/chills

5. New or increasing pain

10. **What is the overall incidence and impact of decubitus ulcers in hospitalized patients?**
Without appropriate care and prevention, up to 14% of inpatients will develop decubitus ulcers. Most will occur within the first 2 weeks of acute hospitalization. Importantly, patients who develop such ulcers have a fourfold risk of prolonged hospitalization and/or death.

11. **What are the primary measures to help prevent pressure ulcers?**
Frequent patient repositioning—at least every 1 to 2 hours—is the most important preventive measure. Earliest possible mobilization of the patient is crucial, as is frequent inspection of key areas for evidence of skin breakdown. The use of airflow, water-filled or alternating pressure mattresses, foam pads for prone areas, and gentle massage of the areas at risk can help minimize ulcer development. Additional measures include minimizing skin moisture from incontinence, sweating, and wound drainage; cleaning the skin with a mild cleansing agent; and decreasing the head of the bed elevation to ≤30 degrees (reduces shear forces) if clinically appropriate. Finally, it is essential to optimize the patient's nutritional status; some also advocate the use of vitamin C and zinc supplementation.

KEY POINTS: PREVENTION OF DECUBITUS ULCERS

1. Relieve direct pressure to prone areas
2. Reposition patient frequently
3. Mobilize patient early
4. Inspect key areas frequently
5. Keep skin clean and dry

12. Why is it important to prevent secondary infection of an ulcer?
Secondary bacterial infection will not only delay or prevent healing of the ulcer, but it can also cause rapid extension of the ulcer to surrounding and underlying structures. This will often result in cellulitis, osteomyelitis, and/or septicemia. Septicemia carries a very high mortality rate.

13. What is an eschar? Why is it significant?
An eschar is devitalized, necrotic tissue at the base of an ulcer. When present, this increases the propensity to develop secondary infection.

14. How are pressure ulcers treated?
Consultation with a wound care/ostomy nurse is often helpful. In addition to total avoidance of any direct pressure on the ulcer and use of foam pads, treatment is as follows (Table 67-1):

TABLE 67-1. STAGING AND TREATMENT OF PRESSURE ULCERS

	Clinical Appearance	Treatment*
Stage I	Red, nonblanching, intact skin.	Clean with water/gentle soap.
Stage II	Skin loss with open sore/*shallow* ulcer. Bullae and/or necrosis apparent.	Wet-to-dry normal saline dressings and/or hydrotherapy with debridement. Topical silver sulfadiazine with adhesive absorbent bandage (Gelfoam). Hydrocolloid semipermeable dressing (DuoDerm).
Stage III	Full-thickness skin loss with *deep* necrosis and ulcer. No penetration of underlying structures.	Surgical consultation. Will require combination of debridement and skin reconstruction with flaps and/ or grafts. Antibiotics as needed.
Stage IV	Full-thickness necrosis and ulceration involving muscle, bone, tendons, and joints. Large with ill-defined borders.	Same as Stage III, but with the addition of possible bone removal.

*For all, eliminate direct pressure to the area.

- **Stage I/II:** Apply moist sterile gauze, often with topical antibiotics (avoid neomycin; silver sulfadiazine works well) and an adhesive absorbent bandage, such as Gelfoam. If debridement is necessary, use wet-to-dry dressings with normal saline. Consider hydrotherapy as well. Once clean, there are also a variety of hydrogels and hydrocolloid semiocclusive dressings available, such as DuoDerm. To help retain moisture and encourage skin cell growth, these are generally changed every 3–7 days; however, they should be changed immediately if purulent discharge develops.
- **Stage III/IV:** Treatment involves surgical consultation and management. This may include a combination of debridement, bone removal, and skin flaps or grafts.

15. **Are there other treatment options under investigation?**
Yes. They include hyperbaric oxygen, electrotherapy, and topical human growth factors. The last of these has already been approved for the treatment of ulcers in persons with diabetes.

16. **How does the management change if a secondary infection is diagnosed?**
Prolonged antibiotic treatment is necessary, based on culture/sensitivity results, with surgical debridement of necrotic bone if osteomyelitis is present. Antibiotic choice is based on culture results, with some of the most common organisms being *Staphylococcus, Streptococcus* (group B or D), *Proteus, Pseudomonas,* and *Bacteroides* species and *Escherichia coli.* Methicillin-resistant *Staphylococcus aureus* requires treatment with vancomycin, daptomycin, or linezolid. The length of treatment depends in part on the clinical scenario and response but is generally of at least 2–4 weeks duration, and often longer.

17. **How long does it take decubitus ulcers to heal?**
With effective treatment, stage I–II ulcers can heal in 4 weeks or less, whereas stage III–IV ulcers may require 12 weeks or longer.

18. **How do the risk factors, location, and prevention of venous stasis ulcers compare with those of pressure ulcers?**
Unlike pressure ulcers, venous stasis ulcers are generally caused by chronic venous insufficiency. They are often accompanied by varicosities, edema, venous stasis dermatitis, and/or hyperpigmentation. Venous stasis ulcers are associated with advanced age (as are pressure ulcers), but also with obesity, history of leg injury/fracture, and deep venous thrombosis/phlebitis. Venous stasis ulcers most commonly found on the medial, lower aspect of the calf, usually over the malleolus. They can enlarge to involve the entire circumference of the leg. If a patient is morbidly obese, ulcers can also develop in the most dependent parts of the abdominal panniculus. Compression stockings to reduce edema are the most important preventive measure.

KEY POINTS: MAJOR RISK FACTORS FOR VENOUS STASIS ULCERS

1. Advanced age

2. Obesity

3. History of leg injury/fractures

4. Deep venous thrombosis or thrombophlebitis

WEBSITE

National Pressure Ulcer Advisory Panel: http://www.npuap.org

BIBLIOGRAPHY

1. Brem H, Lyder C: Protocol for the successful treatment of pressure ulcers. Am J Surg 188 (1A Suppl):9–17, 2004.

2. Fisher AR, Wells G, Harrison MB: Factors associated with pressure ulcers in adults in acute care hospitals. Adv Skin Wound Care Pract 12:80–90, 2004.

3. Landi F, Aloe L, Russo A, et al: Topical treatment of pressure ulcers with nerve growth factor: A randomized clinical trial. Ann Intern Med 139:635–641, 2003.

4. New PW, Rawicki HB, Bailey MJ: Nontraumatic spinal cord injury rehabilitation: Pressure ulcer patterns, prediction, and impact. Arch Phys Med Rehabil 85:87–93, 2004.

ALLERGIC REACTIONS

Neil Winawer, MD, and Mandakolathur Murali, MD

CHAPTER 68

1. **How common are allergic reactions in hospitalized patients?**
   Although adverse drug events are relatively common among hospitalized patients, <10% of these are caused by allergic or other immunologic mechanisms. Urticaria and pruritus are the most common allergic reactions. More severe cutaneous reactions can occur in as many as 2–3% of hospitalized patients.

2. **What is the mechanism of an allergic reaction?**
   An *allergic reaction* is the immune system's production of immunoglobulin E (IgE) antibody in response to an offending antigen (i.e., allergen). The antibody binds to high-affinity IgE receptors on mast cells and basophils, resulting in sensitization to that antigen. Repeated exposure to the allergen results in cross-linking of mast cell and basophil-bound IgE antibodies, triggering the release of inflammatory mediators (principally histamine) that cause vasodilatation and increased vascular permeability. Examples of allergic (IgE-mediated) reactions include drugs (e.g., penicillin), foods (e.g., peanuts, shellfish), insect stings (e.g., bees, hornets, yellow jackets), latex, parasitic infestations, and aeroallergens (e.g., pollens, spores, dust mites) (Fig. 68-1).

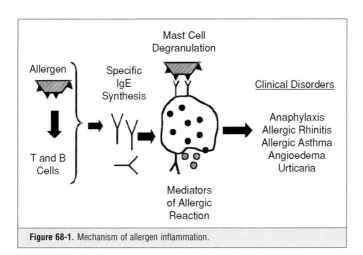

Figure 68-1. Mechanism of allergen inflammation.

3. **Describe the presenting symptoms of an allergic reaction.**
   Patients experiencing mild allergic reactions generally exhibit manifestations on the skin only. These include pruritus, urticaria (i.e., hives), and, in more advanced cases, angioedema. If the allergic reaction is more severe (i.e., larger number of mast cells recruited) then patients may present with bronchoconstriction and hypotension. The most severe form of an allergic reaction

is systemic in nature and is called *anaphylaxis*. It is characterized by acute airway obstruction and circulatory collapse.

KEY POINTS: CHARACTERISTICS OF ALLERGIC REACTIONS

1. Pruritus

2. Urticaria

3. Angioedema

4. **How are allergic reactions treated?**
   - **Mild:** Administer antihistamines (H_1 blockers) and caution patient to avoid the offending allergen.
   - **Moderate:** Administer antihistamines (H_1 blockers), caution patient to avoid the offending allergen, and give systemic steroids and epinephrine (0.3–0.5 mL of 1:1000 epinephrine subcutaneously or intramuscularly).
   - **Anaphylaxis:** Assess/secure airway and evaluate hemodynamics. Begin intravenous fluid resuscitation and administer antihistamines, steroids, supplemental oxygen, and beta-agonists. Where possible, eliminate the offending antigen. Administer epinephrine (0.3–0.5 mL of 1:10,000 epinephrine intravenously every 5–10 minutes as needed or an epinephrine drip at 1.0–10.0 µg/min) if severe bronchospasm, impending airway obstruction, or hemodynamic decompensation is present. In the absence of vascular collapse, administer 0.3 mL of epinephrine 1:1000 by the intramuscular route. Patients receiving beta blockers may not respond to epinephrine and may benefit from intravenous glucagon.

5. **What are the differences between urticaria and angioedema?**
   - **Location:** Urticaria occurs in the dermis (involves superficial vascular plexus), whereas angioedema occurs in the subcutaneous tissue (involves deep vascular plexus).
   - **Urticarial lesions are pruritic and discrete:** In the dermis, where cells are more densely packed, fluid extravasation from the vascular plexus causes a well-circumscribed wheal and flare. Patients often describe intense pruritus given the density of sensory nerve bundles in the skin.
   - **Angioedema can be nonpruritic and is less well defined:** Cell boundaries are less well defined in the subcutaneous tissue, and swelling blends into the neighboring skin. In allergic angioedema, pruritus is common (due to mast cell activation); however, in nonallergic angioedema, pruritus is absent.

6. **Describe severe nonallergic skin reactions that require hospitalization.**
   Stevens-Johnson syndrome (SJS) and toxic epidermal necrolysis (TEN) are bullous and necrolytic reactions (to drugs or infections) that can be life threatening. There is clinical overlap between SJS and TEN. Patients typically present with fever, painful blistering lesions, and mucosal and conjunctival involvement. SJS is characterized by epidermal loss occurring over <10% of body surface area, whereas TEN is characterized by full-thickness epidermal necrosis covering >30% of body surface area. The pathophysiology of the disorders is unknown, and treatment is similar to that of severe thermal burns. This includes aggressive fluid and electrolyte management, supportive therapy (e.g., pain control, nutritional support), and skin care (e.g., paper tapes, whirlpool debridement, antibacterial ointments). Discontinue any

incriminating drugs, and treat infections. The role of intravenous gamma globulin is controversial.

7. **How do anaphylactic and anaphylactoid reactions differ?**
   Patients with anaphylactoid reactions present with signs and symptoms clinically indistinguishable from anaphylaxis. However, the reaction is mediated by mechanisms other than IgE antibody, such as direct mast cell activation, complement activation (e.g., C3a, C5a), and leukotriene-mediated pathways. Since IgE is not involved, anaphylactoid reactions are strictly defined as being nonallergic.

8. **What are the most common anaphylactic and anaphylactoid reactions that occur in the hospital?**
   - **Anaphylactic:** Penicillins/cephalosporins, latex
   - **Anaphylactoid:** Radiocontrast dye, nonsteroidal anti-inflammatory drugs, opiates, anesthetic agents, transfusion reactions

9. **What kinds of conditions or diseases can mimic anaphylactic reactions?**
   Vasovagal reactions, cardiac arrhythmias, bronchoconstriction, and hypoglycemia may be associated with some of the symptoms of anaphylaxis, such as pallor, diaphoresis, hypotension, shortness of breath, and wheezing. Generally, pruritus and urticaria are absent in these conditions. Systemic mastocytosis (a rare disorder characterized by an overabundance of mast cells in the lymphoid tissues) and carcinoid tumors may also present with similar symptoms.

KEY POINTS: MOST COMMON CAUSES OF ALLERGIC AND NONALLERGIC REACTIONS IN THE HOSPITAL

1. Drugs

2. Transfusion reactions

3. Radiocontrast dye

4. Latex

10. **How does the mechanism of hereditary angioedema differ from that seen in allergic reactions? Why is this distinction clinically important?**
    In hereditary angioedema, C1 esterase inhibitor is absent or nonfunctional, resulting in increased C1 (part of the complement cascade) activation. In an acute attack, activated C1 allows the complement cascade to go unopposed, producing the vasoactive peptides, C2 kinin and bradykinin (Fig. 68-2). Unlike allergic reactions, however, mast cells are not involved, and the angioedema is therefore nonpruritic. Thus, standard treatment with antihistamines, steroids, and epinephrine will have little or no effect. Acute episodes are instead managed with supportive care and heat-vaporized C1 esterase inhibitor concentrate. Attenuated androgens such as danazol and stanozolol are effective for prophylaxis.

11. **How is the diagnosis of hereditary angioedema made?**
    In acute attacks, C2 and C4 are consumed, and their levels will be low. Between attacks, the level of C2 is normal but C4 is low because there is always a low level of activated C1 that cleaves C4. Thus, C4 level is a good cost-effective screening test (a normal level excludes hereditary

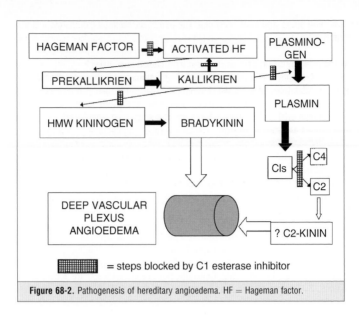

Figure 68-2. Pathogenesis of hereditary angioedema. HF = Hageman factor.

angioedema), and decreased C2 levels reflect the activity of the disease. The measurement of C1 esterase levels is costly and may have pitfalls; thus, it is generally not used in the diagnosis.

12. **What is acquired angioedema?**
    In acquired angioedema, patients produce an antibody against C1 esterase inhibitor that causes the protein to be low or dysfunctional. The result is a presentation that is clinically indistinguishable from hereditary angioedema, with a similar effect on C2 and C4 levels. Acquired angioedema has been documented in patients with lymphoma, plasma cell dyscrasia, systemic lupus erythematous, and rheumatoid arthritis.

13. **What test distinguishes hereditary from acquired angioedema?**
    Although a low C4 level is a good screening test for both hereditary and acquired angioedema, serum C1q levels are low in acquired but normal in hereditary angioedema.

14. **What is the mechanism of angiotensin-converting enzyme (ACE) inhibitor related to cough and angioedema?**
    ACE not only catalyzes angiotensin I to angiotensin II but also breaks down bradykinin, both in tissues and plasma, into inactive peptide fragments. Patients taking ACE inhibitors have elevated levels of bradykinin, which stimulates cough receptors and potentiates angioedema. Other mechanisms exist but are less well understood. For example, angioedema has been described in patients on angiotensin receptor blockers (ARBs), although these drugs do not affect bradykinin levels.

15. **How are ACE-inhibitor cough and angioedema treated?**
    - **ACE-inhibitor cough:** Discontinue course of treatment with ACE inhibitor and follow up in 1–2 weeks. If the cough has resolved, start treatment with an ARB, if clinically indicated. If the cough persists, consider other causes (e.g., postnasal drip, gastroesophageal reflux disease, asthma).

- **ACE-inhibitor angioedema:** This normally occurs in the lips, tongue, uvula, and/or soft palate. Discontinue the use of ACE inhibitor and assess the patient's airway. If mild to moderate edema is present, treat with antihistamines and systemic steroids and follow up in several days; hospitalization is often not required. If the patient has severe edema, continue treatment as above, administer epinephrine, and consider admission to the intensive care unit and elective intubation for airway protection.

16. **Can patients with ACE-inhibitor angioedema be given ARBs?**
    Although there are a few case reports of ARB-induced angioedema in patients with a history of ACE-inhibitor angioedema, it is relatively uncommon. Decisions regarding whether these patients should receive an ARB need to be individualized. First, assess whether there is a strong indication for the ARB (e.g., diabetic nephropathy, heart failure). If so, and if the episode of angioedema was non–life-threatening, then the drug can be instituted with caution.

BIBLIOGRAPHY

1. Kemp SF, Lockey RF: Anaphylaxis: A review of causes and mechanisms. J Allergy Clint Immunol 110:341–348, 2002.

2. Roujeau J, Stern R: Severe adverse cutaneous reactions to drugs. N Engl J Med 331:1272–1285, 1994.

3. Sicherer SH: Advances in anaphylaxis and hypersensitivity reactions to foods, drugs, and insect venom. J Allergy Clin Immunol 111:S829–S834, 2003.

4. Vleeming W, van Amsterdam J, Stricker B, et al: ACE inhibitor-induced angioedema. Drug Safety 18:171–188, 1998.

5. Waytes A, Rosen F, Frank M: Treatment of hereditary angioedema with a vapor-heated C1 inhibitor concentrate. N Engl J Med 334:1630–1634, 1996.

CHAPTER 69

MEDICATION ALLERGY AND DESENSITIZATION

Susan Krekun, MD

1. **What is an adverse drug reaction?**

   Adverse drug reaction refers to all adverse events related to medication administration, whether predictable or unpredictable. Predictable drug reactions are the expected effects of using a drug that can occur in any patient (e.g., side effects, toxicity caused by an overdose, and interactions with other drugs); they are commonly dose dependent. Unpredictable reactions occur in susceptible patients and are usually dose independent. Allergic and pseudoallergic reactions are examples of unpredictable reactions.

2. **Are all adverse reactions to drugs considered drug allergy?**

   Drug allergy is a term reserved for immune-mediated reactions, which occur in a small proportion of patients. The prototypical example of this is β-lactam allergy. Pseudoallergic reactions are unexpected reactions that do not have an immune basis, and thus, are not true allergies, though they can appear clinically identical to allergic reactions. The anaphylactoid reaction seen with radiocontrast media (RCM) is an example. Table 69-1 lists the features of allergic and pseudoallergic reactions.

TABLE 69-1. CHARACTERISTICS OF ALLERGIC AND PSEUDOALLERGIC REACTIONS	
Allergic Reactions	**Pseudoallergic Reactions**
Immune-mediated.	Non–immune-mediated. Typically caused by direct release of mediators from mast cells and basophils.
First exposure is usually uneventful, but reactions may occur several days after drug is started.	Reactions occur immediately upon first exposure and can be severe.
Reactions are not dose dependent and can occur on reexposure to very small doses of drug.	Reactions are usually dose-independent.
Reactions depend on the type of immune response and the target organ involved (e.g., IgE-mediated reactions tend to be anaphylactic with symptoms of urticaria, laryngeal edema, wheezing, and cardiovascular collapse).	Reactions can be characteristic for a given drug but can mimic allergic reaction (e.g., the anaphylactoid reaction seen with radiocontrast media can appear identical to anaphylaxis clinically).
Reactions occur in a small proportion of patients	

3. **Is there a simple classification scheme for the different types of reactions?**
   Immune-mediated drug reactions can be defined using the Gell and Coombs classification (Type 1, IgE mediated; Type 2, cytotoxic; Type 3, immune complex mediated; Type 4, cellular immune mediated). Unfortunately, not all immune-mediated drug reactions fall neatly into these categories because many of the mechanisms are unknown. Drug reactions can also be classified by the organ system affected (e.g., systemic, cutaneous, or visceral).

4. **What is the most common clinical manifestation of drug reaction?**
   Skin manifestations are the most common because the skin is both metabolically and immunologically active. Immune-mediated skin reactions include urticaria, angioedema, contact dermatitis (all of these are common), and exfoliative dermatitis such as Stevens-Johnson syndrome and toxic epidermal necrolysis (less common, but serious).

5. **What drugs most commonly result in allergic reactions in hospitalized patients?**
   Any drug can cause a reaction, but antibiotics, particularly β-lactams or sulfonamides, cause the majority of drug reactions. Other medications that can result in non–immune-mediated reactions that can be mistaken for allergic reactions are aspirin, insulin, chemotherapeutic agents, anticonvulsants, and RCM.

6. **Are there risk factors that predispose patients to allergic reactions to drugs?**
   Table 69-2 lists some of the risk factors for drug hypersensitivity reactions.

7. **What is the appropriate approach to patients with suspected drug allergy?**
   Figure 69-1 shows an algorithm for working up and managing a suspected drug allergy.

8. **How is skin testing done?**
   There are two methods used to test for immediate hypersensitivity: the skin prick test and intradermal testing. In these tests, an allergen solution, starting at 1000-fold dilution, is either pricked into the skin or injected intradermally so a bleb forms. The concentration of allergen

---

TABLE 69-2.   RISK FACTORS FOR DRUG ALLERGY

Patient-Related Factors

Female gender

Infection

HIV infection

Asthma

Systemic lupus erythematosus

Atopy may predispose to more severe reaction

Drug-Related Factors

Exposure to multiple drugs

Frequency of exposure (multiple exposures likely to sensitize)

Molecular structure of drug: large molecules > small molecules

Route of administration: topical > parenteral > oral

Ability to bind to tissue proteins

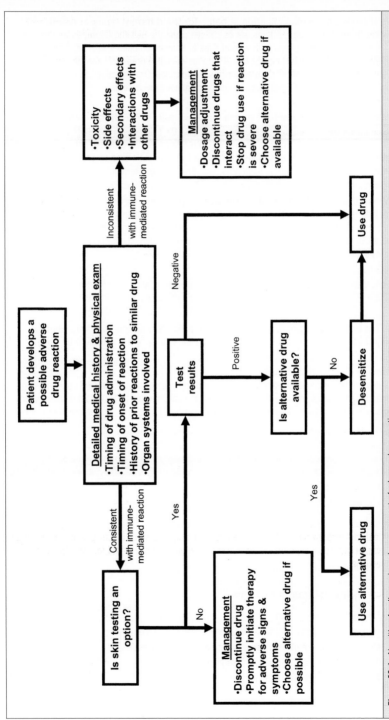

Figure 69-1. Algorithm for diagnosis and management of adverse drug reactions.

progressively increases until the patient has a reaction or until full-strength solution is attained. Readings are taken after 15–20 minutes, with the clinician looking for wheals >3 mm in both testing methods. Drugs with well-defined haptens (like penicillin) can be tested. Of note, medications such as antihistamines and steroids can mask reactions, so these should be discontinued before skin testing is performed.

9. **How safe is skin testing?**
Skin testing is relatively safe. Reactions can resemble the original allergic responses but are usually less intense. Patients can develop systemic symptoms with diffuse pruritus, and sometimes angioedema that can progress to anaphylaxis. Anyone who has had an exfoliative dermatitis or anaphylaxis should not be skin tested with that drug.

10. **Does an allergy to penicillin negate the use of all β-lactams?**
In general, if a patient has a severe reaction to one β-lactam, use of synthetic penicillins (e.g., carbapenems) may be unsafe due to similar chemical structures. Monobactams, like aztreonam, have a different structure and are generally safe to use in penicillin-allergic patients.

11. **Are cephalosporins safe in patients allergic to β-lactams?**
Cephalosporins have a variable degree of cross-reactivity with penicillins because they, too, have a β-lactam ring. Early reports (prior to 1980) noted a cross-reactivity rate of up to 10%, but rates as low as 2% have been reported with the newer generation cephalosporins. Two approaches are reasonable when considering whether to use cephalosporins in penicillin-allergic patients. First, if the history is strongly suggestive of an IgE-mediated reaction to penicillin, then an alternative, non–β-lactam antibiotic should be chosen. The second approach is to perform skin testing on the patient for IgE-mediated allergy to penicillin. If the test result is negative, the patient can receive the cephalosporin. If the test result is positive, and a cephalosporin is necessary, it can be used after desensitization with the cephalosporin has been performed. Of note, there is a cross-reaction between aztreonam and cefepime; so if patients are allergic to one, then the other should be avoided.

12. **Which patients should be considered for desensitization?**
Desensitization is the induction of tolerance to a particular drug to which the patient is allergic. It has been successfully performed with penicillin, cephalosporins, antituberculous agents, vancomycin, sulfonamides, and clindamycin, as well as a few additional drugs. Desensitization should be considered when the offending drug is clearly the best treatment option for a given infection, such as in the case of enterococcal endocarditis (ampicillin or nafcillin) or neurosyphilis (penicillin). However, patients who have had anaphylaxis or exfoliative dermatitis reactions should not be considered for desensitization. It is not useful to attempt desensitization in patients who present with serum sickness, hemolytic anemia, maculopapular rashes, drug fever, or interstitial nephritis because desensitization is mostly useful for IgE-mediated reactions.

13. **How is desensitization performed?**
The procedure should be performed in the intensive care unit or on hospital floors where there is adequate patient monitoring and resuscitation equipment. The initial dose of drug to be used is typically determined by skin testing, in the presence of an allergist. The dose administered is then doubled every 15–30 minutes, either intravenously or orally until the patient manifests a reaction or the therapeutic dose is reached. Patients are closely monitored, watching for vital sign abnormalities and physical manifestations of reaction, such as wheezing. The process may need to be aborted if patients develop severe reactions, such as bronchospasm or hypotension.

Some drugs, such as aspirin and insulin, produce nonallergic reactions in patients. Tolerance to these drugs can also be induced by using a graded-challenge regimen. Although this is technically not desensitization, the concept is similar in that progressively larger doses of the drug are used over days or weeks to induce tolerance.

KEY POINTS: DRUG ALLERGY/DESENSITIZATION

1. True drug allergy occurs in a minority of patients.

2. Drug allergies have some characteristic features that may help distinguish them from non–immune-mediated drug reactions.

3. The skin is the most commonly involved organ in allergic reactions to drugs.

4. Antibiotics, specifically β-lactams and sulfonamides, are the most common inducers of allergic drug reactions in the hospital setting.

5. Patients with true immune-mediated drug allergies should be desensitized when use of the medication is essential.

14. **Are there risks to desensitizing patients?**
    In general, the procedure is safe and effective, but a small number of patients can suffer anaphylactic reactions or, rarely, death. Patients will commonly have mild reactions, such as rash or itching, that can easily be managed without discontinuing the process. The tolerance induced by desensitization lasts as long as the patient receives the drug. After a period of 24 hours, the tolerance disappears and patients will need to be desensitized again before the next drug exposure.

15. **What about patients who need to receive RCM and have previously had anaphylactoid reactions?**
    Patients who have exhibited reactions to RCM do not get desensitized before the next exposure because the reactions are not immune mediated. The use of low-ionic media may lessen the chance of reactions, and patients should be pretreated with steroids (prednisone 50 mg every 6 hours for three doses beginning 18 hours before RCM), diphenhydramine (50 mg orally 1 hour before RCM), and an H_2 blocker (e.g., cimetidine 300 mg orally 1–3 hours before RCM). Some experts also recommend the use of ephedrine, 25 mg orally 1 hour before RCM, but this may be unsafe in patients with a history of cardiac disease or hypertension.

WEBSITE

BIBLIOGRAPHY

1. Anderson JA: Allergic reactions to drugs and biologic agents. JAMA 268:2845–2857, 1992.

2. Executive summary of disease management of drug hypersensitivity: A practice parameter. Joint task force on practice parameters, The American Academy of Allergy, Asthma, and Immunology, and the Joint Council of Allergy, Asthma, and Immunology. Ann Allergy Asthma Immunol 83:665–700, 1999.

3. Gruchalla R: Understanding drug allergies. J Allergy Clin Immunol 105:S637–S644, 2000.

4. Honsinger RW, Green GR: Introduction. In Honsinger RW, Green GR (eds): Handbook of Drug Allergy. Philadelphia, Lippincott, Williams, & Wilkins, 2004, pp xvii–xxvi.

5. Riedl MA, Casillas AM: Adverse drug reactions: Types and treatment options. Am Fam Physician 68:1781–1790, 2003.

5. What are the clinical features of alcohol withdrawal seizures?

Alcohol withdrawal seizures occur in 5-15% of chronic alcoholics. The seizures are generalized tonic-clonic seizures, typically brief, single or occurring in clusters. It is difficult to clearly attribute seizures to alcohol withdrawal ...

XIV. TOXICOLOGY

CHAPTER 70

ALCOHOL WITHDRAWAL

Jeanie Youngwerth, MD

1. **How prevalent is alcohol abuse?**
   Alcohol is the most commonly abused drug in the world. It is used by two thirds of American adults and abused by approximately 10%. Alcohol dependence is present in up to 15–20% of hospitalized patients.

2. **Define *Alcohol Withdrawal Syndrome* (AWS).**
   The criteria listed in the *Diagnostic and Statistical Manual of Mental Disorders,* fourth edition, for AWS include a history of cessation or reduction in heavy and prolonged alcohol use, in addition to two or more of the following: autonomic hyperactivity (e.g., sweating, tachycardia, hypertension, fever), increased hand tremor, insomnia, nausea or vomiting, transient tactile/visual/auditory hallucinations, psychomotor agitation, anxiety, and tonic-clonic seizures.

3. **Who is at risk for developing AWS?**
   Anyone who abruptly stops or reduces intake of heavy or prolonged alcohol use is at risk for developing AWS. A standardized questionnaire, such as the CAGE questionnaire, is recommended to screen for alcohol dependence. The CAGE questionnaire covers the following topics:
   - **Cut down:** Have you ever felt the need to cut down on drinking?
   - **Annoyed:** Have you ever felt annoyed by criticism of your drinking?
   - **Guilty:** Have you ever felt guilty about your drinking?
   - **Eye opener:** Have you ever taken an eye opener (i.e., a drink to help you start the day) in the morning?

   For three or four positive responses, the sensitivity reaches 100% and the specificity 81% for the presence of alcohol dependence.

4. **Name the three major complications of AWS, and outline the time course.**
   Alcohol withdrawal seizures, alcohol hallucinosis, and delirium tremens (DT) are the main complications of AWS. They may occur alone or in any combination with each other. Most alcohol withdrawal seizures occur in the first 24 hours, alcohol hallucinosis in the first 24–72 hours, and DT in the first 72–96 hours (but can be seen as far out as a couple of weeks) (Fig. 70-1).

5. **What are the clinical features of alcohol withdrawal seizures?**
   Alcohol withdrawal seizures occur in 3–33% of chronic alcoholics. The seizures are generalized, tonic-clonic, and usually isolated. Focal seizures or recurrent seizures that are difficult to control are unlikely to be secondary to AWS, and other etiologies should be investigated. A prior history of withdrawal seizures increases a patient's risk for future withdrawal seizures.

6. **What are the clinical features of alcohol hallucinosis?**
   Alcohol hallucinosis occurs in 10–25% of patients hospitalized with AWS. The hallucinations are usually visual (e.g., little pink elephants dancing on the walls, or insects crawling on the ceiling) but can be tactile or auditory. In contrast to DT, wherein patients have confusion or an altered level of consciousness, these patients have a clear sensorium. Alcohol hallucinosis does not predict progression into DT.

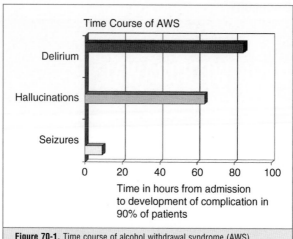

Figure 70-1. Time course of alcohol withdrawal syndrome (AWS) complications.

7. **What are the clinical features of DT?**
DT is the most serious manifestation of AWS and occurs in about 5% of patients hospitalized with AWS. It presents as delirium and extreme autonomic hyperactivity (e.g., agitation, tachycardia, hypertension, fever). The original studies in the 1950s quoted mortality rates as high as 15%; however, more recent data suggests a rate closer to 1–5%. This improvement in outcomes is due to better management and recognition of AWS. Death is usually due to arrhythmias or infections, such as aspiration pneumonia.

8. **What is the Wernicke-Korsakoff syndrome (WKS)?**
Wernicke's encephalopathy (WE) and Korsakoff's psychosis (KP) are long-term sequelae of alcohol abuse but may occur acutely in alcohol withdrawal. These entities are due to thiamine deficiency. WE is characterized by the classic triad of confusion, ataxia, and ophthalmoplegia. The triad is only seen in 10% of cases, with most patients presenting with generalized cognitive impairment. Untreated, WE can progress to KP. KP is a memory disorder consisting of both retrograde and anterograde amnesia. Patients tend to confabulate with KP to fill in the gaps of their disjointed memory. Most experts now consider WKS to be a continuum of one disease state.

9. **What is the mainstay of pharmacologic treatment of AWS?**
Benzodiazepines are the only drugs that have been shown to decrease both the signs and symptoms of AWS and to prevent withdrawal seizures and DT. The commonly used long-acting benzodiazepines in AWS are chlordiazepoxide (Librium), diazepam (Valium), and clorazepate (Tranxene). They undergo oxidative metabolism in the liver producing long-acting active metabolites, which results in their half-lives extending over 100 hours. Lorazepam (Ativan) and oxazepam (Serax) are the most commonly used short-acting benzodiazepines in the treatment of AWS. They undergo glucuronidation in the liver to an inactive form, thereby resulting in a much shorter half-life of around 10–20 hours. No one benzodiazepine has been shown to be more effective than another. In general, the long-acting drugs are preferred but can be associated with oversedation. The short-acting drugs are recommended in elderly patients, those with evidence of hepatic dysfunction, and patients with medical comorbidities that may put them at risk for oversedation and respiratory depression.

KEY POINTS: GOALS OF PHARMACOTHERAPY IN AWS ✓

1. Treat alcohol withdrawal symptoms.

2. Prevent and treat seizures.

3. Prevent and treat DT.

10. **List the three protocol strategies used in AWS.**
    Three methods to treat AWS exist: fixed dose, loading dose, and symptom triggered. There is no evidence demonstrating a benefit of continuous benzodiazepine infusion therapy, and some data supports worse outcomes. However, continuous infusion is commonly used in the intensive care unit for patients who require frequent administration of very high doses of benzodiazepine (Fig. 70-2).

Protocol Strategy	Fixed-Dose Technique	Loading-Dose Technique	Symptom-Triggered Technique
Features	•Classic strategy; original studies only used this technique. •Give drug in scheduled doses, then taper over several days.	•Only used with long-acting benzodiazepines, taking advantage of "self-tapering" effect •Large amounts of drug given up front until symptoms controlled, then discontinue drug.	•Newest strategy; most recent studies use this technique. •Drug is given on a prn basis. •Requires use of a objective scoring system of the severity of AWS, such as the CIWA-Ar scale.
Example Dosing	Chlordiazepoxide 50 mg po q6 hours, then half the dose every 2 days until discontinued.	Diazepam 20 mg po q2 hours until symptoms controlled.	Chlordiazepoxide 50 mg po q4 hours prn CIWA score greater than 8.
Recommendations	Preferred for patients with history of severe AWS, alcohol withdrawal seizures, delirium tremens.	Not commonly used in the inpatient setting, but may be useful in outpatient therapy.	Promising new technique in which lower amouts of drug are used and for a shorter duration of therapy.

Figure 70-2. Protocol strategies for the treatment of alcohol withdrawal syndrome (AWS). prn = as needed, po = by mouth, CIWA-Ar = Clinical Institute Withdrawal Assessment for Alcohol, Revised.

11. **What is the CIWA-Ar scale?**
    The Clinical Institute Withdrawal Assessment for Alcohol revised scale is a 10-item instrument that was developed to objectively measure and quantify alcohol withdrawal severity. Higher scores are predictive of the development of seizures and delirium (Table 70-1).

12. **What adjunctive therapies may be used in AWS?**
    Beta blockers, clonidine, and carbamazepine have been shown to decrease symptoms of AWS; however, they have not been shown to prevent seizures or delirium. Phenothiazines (e.g., haloperidol) also decrease the symptoms of AWS but may lower the seizure threshold. These therapies should only be used as adjuncts to benzodiazepines in managing AWS.

TABLE 70-1. CLINICAL INSTITUTE WITHDRAWAL ASSESSMENT FOR ALCOHOL, REVISED

Symptom Category	Score	Example
Nausea and vomiting	0–7	0 = no nausea or vomiting
		7 = constant nausea, frequent dry heaves and vomiting
Paroxysmal sweats	0–7	0 = no sweats visible
		7 = drenching sweats
Agitation	0–7	0 = normal activity
		7 = thrashes about constantly
Headache	0–7	0 = no headache
		7 = extremely severe headache
Anxiety	0–7	0 = no anxiety
		7 = acute panic state
Tremor	0–7	0 = no tremor
		7 = severe; present with arms not extended
Visual disturbances	0–7	0 = no visual disturbances
		7 = continuous visual hallucinations
Tactile disturbances	0–7	0 = no tactile disturbances
		7 = continuous tactile hallucinations
Auditory disturbances, hallucinations	0–7	0 = no auditory disturbances
		7 = continuous auditory disturbances
Orientation/clouding of sensorium	0–4	0 = oriented and can do serial additions
		4 = disoriented as to person and/or place

Score <8: mild withdrawal symptoms
Score 8–15: moderate withdrawal symptoms
Score >15: severe withdrawal symptoms
Maximum possible score is 67.

13. **What is the role of ethanol in managing AWS?**
The use of ethanol for managing AWS is not recommended. There are no controlled trials demonstrating a benefit of ethanol in managing AWS, and it has not been shown to prevent seizures or DT. Furthermore, no data has evaluated the safety or the relative efficacy of ethanol compared with placebo or benzodiazepines. Ethanol has well-known side effects including neurotoxicity, hepatotoxicity, gastrointestinal toxicity, hematologic toxicity, and respiratory depressant effects.

14. **Is phenytoin effective prophylaxis for alcohol withdrawal seizures?**
No. Phenytoin has not been shown to be effective for prophylaxis of alcohol withdrawal seizures, and its use is not recommended.

15. **What drug is given to prevent and treat WKS?**
Thiamine is used to prevent and treat WKS. The use of parenteral thiamine can potentially reverse WKS if treated promptly.

16. **Why is it important to give thiamine before glucose administration in AWS?**
Glucose is the food of the brain, and thiamine is used as a cofactor in its metabolism. If a glucose load is given without thiamine to a thiamine-deficient patient (e.g., an alcoholic), then a profound thiamine-deficient state can occur, thus precipitating acute Wernicke's encephalopathy.

17. **Name the ingredients of a "yellow bag" or "banana bag."**
A yellow (or banana) bag is the standard nutrients given to a malnourished alcoholic patient. It consists of a one ampule of multivitamin, 100 mg of thiamine, and 1 mg of folate mixed in 1 L of normal saline. These vitamins can also be given orally at the same dose. Treatment doses, route of administration, and duration of therapy are not well documented in the literature. However, there is some evidence that parenteral administration of thiamine is more effective than oral delivery in the prevention and treatment of WKS.

KEY POINTS: PHARMACOTHERAPY IN AWS

1. Benzodiazepines

2. Consider adjunctive therapy with beta blockers, clonidine, carbamazepine, phenothiazines

3. Thiamine

18. **What fluid and electrolyte disturbances are found in AWS?**
Patients experiencing AWS are often dehydrated because of diaphoresis, hyperthermia, and tachypnea from increased sympathetic output and the diuretic effect of alcohol. Hypokalemia, hypomagnesemia, and hypophosphatemia occur as a result of gastrointestinal losses, renal losses, changes in aldosterone levels, and malnutrition. Fluid resuscitation and electrolyte monitoring and repletion are essential.

WEBSITE

American Society of Addiction Medicine: http://www.asam.org

BIBLIOGRAPHY

1. Daeppen JB, Gache P, Landry U, et al: Symptom-triggered vs fixed-schedule doses of benzodiazepine for alcohol withdrawal. Arch Intern Med 162:1117–1121, 2002.

2. Foy A, Kay J, Taylor A: The course of alcohol withdrawal in a general hospital. Q J Med 90:253–261, 1997.

3. Mayo-Smith MF: Pharmacological management of alcohol withdrawal. JAMA 278:144–151, 1997.

4. Mayo-Smith MF, Beecher LH, Fischer TL, et al: Management of alcohol withdrawal delirium. Arch Intern Med 164:1405–1412, 2004.

5. Saitz R, O'Malley SS: Pharmacotherapies for alcohol abuse. Med Clin North Am 81:881–907, 1997.

6. Thomson AD, Cook CCH, Touquet R, Henry JA: The Royal College of Physicians Report on Alcohol: Guidelines for managing Wernicke's encephalopathy in the accident and emergency department. Alcohol Alcoholism 37:513–521, 2002.

CHAPTER 71

APPROACH TO DRUG OVERDOSE

Lisa Shieh, MD, PhD

1. List the most common poison exposures.

Data from poison control centers in 2001 showed exposures were most commonly due to analgesics (10.6%), cleaning substances (9.5%), cosmetics (9.2%), foreign bodies (5.1%), plants (4.7%), sedative-hypnotics and antipsychotics (4.4%), and cough and cold preparations (4.3%).

Litovitz TL, Klein-Schwartz W, Rodgers GC, et al: 2001 annual report of the American Association of Poison Control Centers toxic exposure surveillance system. Am J Emerg Med 20:391–452, 2002.

2. Which exposures are most fatal?

Carbon monoxide poisoning or the ingestion of analgesics, sedative-hypnotics, antipsychotics, antidepressants, street drugs, cardiovascular drugs, or alcohol were most fatal. Analgesics (e.g., acetaminophen, oxycodone, salicylate) accounted for 32% of fatalities due to a pharmaceutical agent.

3. What are the three phases of drug overdose?

- **Preclinical phase:** This phase follows exposure but precedes signs and symptoms. The goal is to reduce or prevent toxicity with early decontamination.
- **Toxic phase:** This is the period from onset to peak clinical/laboratory toxicity. The goal is to shorten the duration and lessen the severity of toxicity with patient stabilization and administration of antidotes.
- **Final phase:** Last is the resolution from peak toxicity to recovery. Management is supportive and guided by clinical status.

4. What should a brief initial screening examination include?

Vital signs, airway assessment, mental status, pupil size, pulse oximetry, core temperature, cardiac monitoring, and electrocardiography (ECG).

5. What are some empiric treatments for a patient with altered mental status and suspected overdose?

Intravenous thiamine for possible Wernicke's encephalopathy and 25 gm of dextrose for hypoglycemia (can be given concurrently). Naloxone (if opiates suspected), or flumazenil (if benzodiazepines suspected). Consider decontamination for certain ingestions (see question 15 for more details).

6. What are the key elements of the history and physical examination?

The patient's history is often unreliable and should be confirmed with family, friends, and outpatient physicians. Examine pill bottles and call pharmacies where prescriptions were filled to obtain a complete medication list. If needle tracks are present, consider street drugs. Correlating signs, symptoms, and laboratory data will help establish a diagnosis. See Table 71-1 for common toxidromes.

7. List the autonomic effects of various ingestions.

- **Physiologic excitation:** Anticholinergics, sympathomimetics, central hallucinogenic agents, drug withdrawal

TABLE 71-1. COMMON TOXIDROMES WITH PRESENTATION AND TREATMENT

Toxidrome	Examples	Vital Signs	Neurologic Signs	Other	Treatment
TCA	Amitriptyline, imipramine, doxepin	Elevated temp, HR, and BP followed by low BP and hypopnea; arrhythmias and conduction disturbances	Confusion, agitation, coma, seizures, myoclonus, choreoathetosis, mydriasis		Activated charcoal, alkalinized serum if arrhythmias/hypotension
Serotonin syndrome	MAOIs, selective serotonin reuptake inhibitors, meperidine, tricyclics	Elevated temp, HR, BP, RR	Confusion, agitation, coma, tremors, myoclonus, hyperreflexia, rigidity, mydriasis	Diaphoresis, flushing, diarrhea	Supportive care, benzodiazepines, cyproheptadine (histamine$_1$-receptor blocker)
Cholinergic	Organophosphate and carbamate insecticides, nicotine, pilocarpine, physostigmine, nerve agents	Low HR, high/low BP, high/low RR	Confusion, coma, weakness, muscle fasciculations, seizures, miosis	Diaphoresis, salivation, urinary and fecal incontinence, diarrhea, emesis, lacrimation, GI cramps, bronchoconstriction	Supportive care and decontamination (oral and skin); atropine and pralidoxime for organophosphate poisoning

Continued

TABLE 71-1. COMMON TOXIDROMES WITH PRESENTATION AND TREATMENT—CONT'D

Toxidrome	Examples	Vital Signs	Neurologic Signs	Other	Treatment
Anticholinergic	Antihistamines, TCA, cyclobenzaprine, antiparkinsonian agents, antispasmodics, atropine, scopolamine, phenothiazines, belladonna alkaloids	High temp, HR, BP, RR	Agitation, delirium, hallucinations, hypervigilance, coma, myoclonus, choreoathetosis, picking behavior, seizures (rare), mydriasis	Dry flushed skin, dry mucous membranes, urinary retention, decreased bowel sounds	Physostigmine for anticholinergic agents
Sedative-hypnotic	Benzodiazepines, barbiturates, alcohols, zolpidem	Low temp, HR, BP, RR	CNS depression, confusion, stupor, coma, hyporeflexia, miosis (usually)		Flumazenil for benzodiazepine, ethanol or fomepizole for ethylene glycol or methanol poisoning (consider dialysis)
Opioid	Heroin, morphine, methadone, oxycodone, hydromorphone, diphenoxylate (Lomotil)	Low temp, HR, BP, RR	CNS depression, confusion, hyporeflexia, pulmonary edema, miosis	Needle marks	Naloxone
Hallucinogenic	PCP, LSD, designer amphetamines (e.g., Ectasy), marijuana, mushrooms	High temp, HR, BP, RR	Hallucinations, perceptual distortions, depersonalization, agitation, nystagmus, mydriasis (usually)		No antidote; treatment is supportive; consider haloperidol or benzodiazepines to calm patients

TABLE 71-1. COMMON TOXIDROMES WITH PRESENTATION AND TREATMENT—CONT'D

Toxidrome	Examples	Vital Signs	Neurologic Signs	Other	Treatment
Sympathomimetic	Cocaine, amphetamines (e.g., crystal methamphetamine), ephedrine, pseudoephedrine, theophylline, caffeine, phenylpropanolamine	High temp, HR, BP, RR, widened pulse pressure	Hyperalert, agitation, hallucinations, paranoia, tremors, hyperreflexia, seizures, mydriasis	Diaphoresis	Supportive treatment of symptoms; diazepam for seizures or agitation, nitroprusside for hypertension, cooling measures for hyperthermia

TCA = tricyclic antidepressant, temp = temperature, HR = heart rate, BP = blood pressure, MAOIs = monoamine oxidase inhibitors, RR = respiratory rate, CNS = central nervous system, PCP = phencyclidine, LSD = lysergic acid diethylamide.

- **Physiologic depression:** Cholinergics, sympatholytics, opiates, sedative hypnotics, alcohol
- **Mixed physiologic effects:** Polydrug overdoses, metabolic poisons (e.g., hypoglycemic agents, salicylates, cyanide), heavy metals (e.g., iron, arsenic, mercury, lead), membrane-active agents (e.g., volatile inhalants, antiarrhythmics, local anesthetics), tricyclic antidepressants
- **Mydriasis (pupil dilation):** Sympathomimetics, anticholinergics, hallucinogens, drug withdrawal, alcohol, nicotine, monoamine oxidase inhibitors, serotonin syndrome
- **Miosis (pupil constriction):** Opioids, sedative-hypnotics, cholinergics, sympatholytics

8. **How can odor help determine an ingestion?**
   Acetone can smell fruity, cyanide like bitter almonds, and arsenic like garlic.

9. **Name some common overdoses that have delayed clinical toxicity.**
   Consider sustained- or enteric-release medications, acetaminophen and salicylates, mushrooms, toxic alcohols, oral hypoglycemic agents, warfarin, fat-soluble organophosphates, ergotamines, and heavy metals.

10. **Discuss the role of laboratory testing in overdoses.**
    Symptomatic patients and those with an unreliable history should undergo urinalysis and measurements of serum electrolytes, blood urea nitrogen (BUN), creatinine, glucose, and acetaminophen and salicylate levels. In more acutely ill patients, also check serum osmolality, ketones, creatinine kinase, liver function tests, amylase, calcium, and magnesium. Women of childbearing age should have a urine pregnancy test. "Toxic" or rapid immunoassay screens commonly detect opiates, benzodiazepines, cocaine metabolites, barbiturates, tricyclics, tetrahydrocannabinol (THC), phencyclidine, salicylates, and acetaminophen. Results are usually available in 1 hour. Comprehensive toxic screening is usually expensive, slow, and unlikely to change management. Exceptions may include methanol, ethylene glycol, digoxin, theophylline, antiepileptics, and lithium.

11. **List common drug-induced electrolyte abnormalities.**
    - **Hyperkalemia:** Alpha agonists, beta blockers, digoxin, fluoride
    - **Hypokalemia:** Beta agonists, diuretics, barium
    - **Hypocalcemia:** Ethylene glycol, oxalate, fluoride
    - **Hyperglycemia:** Beta agonists, calcium channel blockers, acetone, iron
    - **Hypoglycemia:** Beta blockers, insulin, antidiabetic agents, ethanol, salicylates, quinine

12. **How are the anion and osmolal gaps determined? How are they used?**
    - **Anion gap:** The difference between unmeasured anions and cations $[(Na) - (bicarb + Cl)]$. A normal anion gap is three times the serum albumin level or approximately 10–12 in a patient with a normal albumin level.
    - **Osmolal gap:** The difference between the measured and calculated osmolality $[(2 \times Na) + (glucose/18) + (BUN/2.8) + (ethanol/4.3)]$. A normal osmolal gap is approximately 10, with a higher than normal gap indicating more osmoles (measured) than expected (calculated) based on the usually measured osmoles.

    If both the anion and osmolal gap are elevated, consider an alcohol, methanol, or ethylene glycol ingestion. If there is an osmolal gap but no abnormal anion gap, consider isopropyl alcohol poisoning.

13. **Which overdoses can cause an oxygen saturation gap?**
    This gap exists when the oxygen saturation as measured by pulse oximetry is significantly less than the oxygen saturation calculated from arterial blood gas analysis. Overdoses or ingestions that can cause an elevated gap include carbon monoxide, cyanide, and methemoglobin.

KEY POINTS: GENERAL APPROACH TO DRUG POISONING

1. Remember the ABCs (i.e., airway, breathing, circulation).
2. Gather a detailed history of potential and actual exposures.
3. Perform a thorough physical examination for signs of toxidromes.
4. Perform a focused work-up, including urinalysis, ECG, pregnancy screen, and tests of electrolytes, glucose, renal and liver function, and osmolal and anion gaps.
5. Perform rapid "toxic screens" (especially acetaminophen) in severe or unexplained toxicity.
6. Consult regional poison control center at 1-800-222-1222.

14. **When are radiographs useful?**
    Some agents are radiopaque on plain film. The acronym CHIPES may be useful:
    - **C:** Chlorinated hydrocarbons, calcium salts, crack vials
    - **H:** Heavy metals
    - **I:** Iodinated compounds
    - **P:** Psychotropics, packets of drugs
    - **E:** Enteric-coated tablets
    - **S:** Salicylates, sodium salts

15. **When is decontamination indicated, and what methods are available?**
    Some type of gastrointestinal (GI) tract decontamination is routinely recommended early in the management of all patients since the history is often unreliable and it is difficult to predict which patients will benefit. Activated charcoal is the preferred and most effective method if administered within 1 hour of ingestion. The recommended dose of activated charcoal is 1 gm/kg with at least a 10:1 ratio by weight of activated charcoal to intoxicant; the usual single adult dose is 25–100 gm mixed with water and administered as a slurry by mouth or nasogastric tube. Doses >100 gm are not recommended in obtunded patients due to an increased risk of vomiting and aspiration. Some agents (e.g., heavy metals, inorganic ions, lithium, potassium, iron, acids and alkalis, corrosives, hydrocarbons, and alcohols) are not bound by charcoal. Other methods of decontamination include gastric lavage, whole bowel irrigation, cathartics, ipecac, hemodialysis, and hemoperfusion.

16. **Describe the toxicity and basic management of acetaminophen, salicylate, tricyclic antidepressants, benzodiazepine, and opioid overdoses.**
    See Table 71-2 and Fig. 71-1.

17. **What are some useful antidotes for common poisonings?**
    - *Naloxone* (0.4–2 mg IV) and *dextrose* (25 gm as 50 mL of a 50% dextrose solution) are the most common antidotes and should be given routinely to unconscious overdose patients. Consider *flumazenil* 0.2 mg IV every minute to response (up to 3 mg) if benzodiazepine overdose suspected.
    - N-*acetylcysteine* treatment for acetaminophen overdose consists of a 72-hour oral course given as a 140-mg/kg loading dose followed by 17 doses of 70 mg/kg every 4 hours (total dose 1330 mg/kg).
    - *Physostigmine* (1–2 mg IV, slowly) is an antidote for anticholinergic syndrome. Do not use in antidepressant poisoning because of the risk of seizures and bradyarrhythmias.

TABLE 71-2. PRESENTATION AND MANAGEMENT OF COMMON OVERDOSES

Overdose	Presentation/Toxicity	Management
Acetaminophen	Hepatotoxicity, renal tubular necrosis, myocardial damage, pancreatitis	Gastric lavage if within 1 hour of ingestion, activated charcoal mixed with cathartic. Check levels every 4 hours, give N-acetylcysteine if above treatment line on Rumack-Matthew nomogram (see Fig. 71-1).
Salicylates	N/V, tinnitus, fever, diaphoresis, confusion, mixed acid–base disorders (respiratory alkalosis, metabolic acidosis). Toxic > 100 mg/kg Severe > 200 mg/kg Lethal 20–25 gm	Check levels 2 and 6 hours after ingestion. If dermal contact, wash skin. Gastric lavage (regardless of time), activated charcoal with cathartic. Give isotonic fluid with bicarbonate to alkalinize urine to pH > 7.5. Dialyze if decreased mental status, acute renal failure, repeated levels > 100, uncorrectable electrolytes.
Tricyclic antidepressants	High risk if ECG QRS > 0.1 sec, arrhythmias, seizures, altered mental status, respiratory depression, or hypotension. Toxic > 500 ng/mL Life-threatening > 1000 ng/mL Fatal > 5000 ng/mL	Consider intubation, gastric lavage (if <8 hours), activated charcoal with cathartic agent. Alkalinize serum to pH 7.4–7.5 if ECG changes, arrhythmias, or hypotension.
Benzodiazepines	CNS effects (drowsy, slurred speech, ataxia, coma) or anxiety, agitation	Monitor for cardiovascular/respiratory depression. Lavage if < 1 hour from ingestion, give activated charcoal. Flumazenil 0.2 mg IV every minute to response (≤3 mg). Watch for seizures.
Opioids	Classic triad of CNS and respiratory depression, miosis. Findings of miotic pupils, RR < 12 breaths/min and evidence of drug use has a 92% sensitivity of response to naloxone.	ABCs first. Give naloxone (0.4–2.0 mg IV). Can give SC at double the IV dose (if no hypotension). Intubate if respiratory compromise and no response. Check glucose, give thiamine and activated charcoal.

N/V = nausea and vomiting, CNS = central nervous system, IV = intravenous, RR = respiratory rate, ABCs = airway, breathing, circulation, SC = subcutaneous.

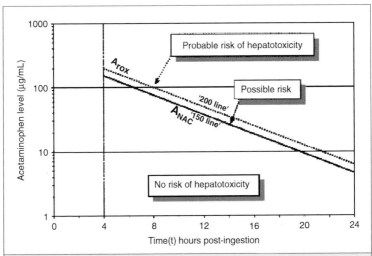

Figure 71-1. Rumack-Matthew nomogram. The lower line of the nomogram (Anac) defines plasma levels 25% below those expected to cause hepatotoxicity; points below this line are not concerning for the development of hepatotoxicity; points between the lower line and upper line (Atox) suggest a possible risk for hepatotoxicity; the upper line (Atox) represents probable risk of hepatotoxicity; points above the upper line are high risk. *N*-acetylcysteine is indicated for any acetaminophen level above the lower line (Anac). (Modified from Rumack BH, Peterson RC, Koch GC, et al: Acetaminophen overdose: 662 cases with oral acetylcysteine therapy. Arch Intern Med 141:380–385, 1981.)

- *Digoxin immune Fab (Digibind)* is an antidote for digoxin poisoning and can rapidly reverse arrhythmias and hyperkalemia. Full response occurs over 20 minutes. For life-threatening overdose, when dose and level are unknown, give 10 vials of Digibind.
- *Atropine* (2–5 mg IV, can double dose until effect) and *pralidoxime* (30 mg/kg IV, slowly) are antidotes for cholinesterase inhibitor toxicity (includes organophosphates and carbamates found in household pesticides). Atropine dries up secretions (mainly pulmonary) and pralidoxime (must be given with atropine) reverses skeletal muscle toxicity.

KEY POINTS: EMPIRIC TREATMENT FOR PATIENTS WITH ALTERED MENTAL STATUS AND SUSPECTED OVERDOSE

1. 100 mg IV thiamine for possible Wernicke's encephalopathy

2. 25 gm dextrose for possible hypoglycemia

3. 0.4–2.0 mg IV naloxone if signs, symptoms, or history are suggestive of opiate intoxication

4. Flumazenil 0.2 mg IV every minute to response (≤3 mg) if benzodiazepine overdose suspected

5. GI tract decontamination with activated charcoal (1 gm/kg)—the earlier the better

18. **What is the role of endotracheal intubation?**
Early airway protection by endotracheal intubation is advisable in a poisoned patient with depressed mental status because of risk of aspiration, especially with GI tract decontamination.

19. **What eight clinical criteria predict a complicated course that could be best managed in the ICU?**
- $PaCO_2 > 45$
- Need for emergency intubation
- Postingestion seizures
- Unresponsiveness to verbal stimuli
- Nonsinus cardiac rhythm
- Second- or third-degree atrioventricular block
- Systolic blood pressure < 80 mmHg
- ECG QRS duration > 0.12 seconds

BIBLIOGRAPHY

1. Brett AS, Rothschild N, Gray R, Perry M: Predicting the clinical course in intentional drug overdose: Implications for use of the intensive care unit. Arch Intern Med 147:133–137, 1987.

2. Chyka PA, Seger D: Position statement: single-dose activated charcoal. American Academy of Clinical Toxicology; European Association of Poisons Centres and Clinical Toxicologists. J Toxicol Clin Toxicol 35:721–742, 1997.

3. Kellermann AL, Fisher SD, LoGerfo JP, et al: Impact of drug screening in suspected overdose. Ann Emerg Med 16:1206–1216, 1987.

4. Kulig K: General approach to poisonings. In Markovchick VJ, Pons PT (eds): Emergency Medicine Secrets, 3rd ed. Philadelphia, Hanley & Belfus, 2002, pp 357–362.

5. Linden CH: General considerations in the evaluation treatment of poisoning. In Rippe JM, Irwin RS, Fink MP, Cerra FB (eds): Intensive Care Medicine. Boston, Little Brown & Company, 1996, p 1455.

6. Olson KR, Pentel PR, Kelley MT: Physical assessment and differential diagnosis of the poisoned patient. Med Toxicol 2:52–81, 1987.

7. Rumack BH, Matthews H: Acetaminophen poisoning and toxicity. Pediatrics 55:871–876, 1975.

8. Savitt DL, Hawkins HH, Roberts JR: The radiopacity of ingested medications. Ann Emerg Med 16:331–339, 1987.

APPROACH TO THE ELDERLY HOSPITALIZED PATIENT

Visalakshi Srinivasan, MD, and Robert M. Palmer, MD, MPH

1. **What is unique about the hospital course of geriatric patients compared with that of younger adults?**
   Patients 65 years and older compose 13% of the American population but account for about 48% of inpatient days of care. Rates of hospitalization are more than twice as great for patients aged 85 years and older compared with patients aged 65–74 years. The oldest patients have longer hospitalizations, higher in-hospital mortality rates, and higher rates of nursing home placement.

2. **What are the hazards of hospitalization for elderly patients?**
   Geriatric patients often suffer functional decline, iatrogenic illness, immobility, and undernutrition while hospitalized.

3. **What is different about history taking in a geriatric patient?**
   It is often necessary to corroborate history from a reliable informant (e.g., family, friend, caregiver, old medical records) because of concerns for the patient's memory. Documentation of baseline function (i.e., basic activities of daily living [BADLs] and instrumental activities of daily living [IADLs]) is essential. The history should also include psychosocial issues such as screening for depression and alcohol abuse, elder abuse, self-neglect (should be suspected with weight loss, noncompliance), noncompliance with medications (should raise suspicion for cognitive impairment, depression), ability to afford medications, and the presence of advance directives.

4. **What are BADLs and IADLs?**
   - **BADLs:** These are the essential elements of self care. Inability to independently perform even one activity may indicate a need for supportive services.
   - **IADLs:** These are associated with independent living in the community and provide a basis for considering the type of services needed in maintaining independence.
   See Table 72-1.

TABLE 72-1. THE BASIC AND INSTRUMENTAL ACTIVITIES OF DAILY LIVING	
BADLs	**IADLs**
Bathing	Using telephone
Dressing/Undressing	Preparing meals
Personal grooming	Housework
Toileting	Taking medicine
Continence	Traveling
Transferring	Shopping
Walking	Managing money
Eating	

5. **Why is functional assessment important in hospitalized elderly persons?**

   Inability to perform BADL predicts mortality, whereas an inability to perform IADLs increases the risk of functional decline. Overall, 25–35% of patients have loss of one or more BADL from admission to discharge (functional decline). This loss of independent functioning during hospitalization is associated with a prolonged hospital stay, greater risk of institutionalization, and higher mortality rates. In preparing a patient for discharge, it is important to determine whether he or she can safely return home to live and, if not, to understand their eligibility for and level of services needed.

6. **How can functional status be determined at the bedside?**

   Observe the patient sit up in bed, transfer out of the bed, walk (with or without assistive device such as a cane, walker, or wheelchair), and eat. Ask about toileting and continence. This assessment of mobility should be done on the day of admission and daily thereafter. If the physician is unable to observe directly, this information can be obtained through discussion with the nursing staff and the physical therapist. Assessment of function is an important factor that influences the disposition of the patient. A patient who resides independently in the community and whose function has declined during the hospitalization may require an assistive device or an alternative site of discharge.

7. **How can gait be assessed quickly at the bedside?**

   The TUG—"Timed Up and Go"—is a test that involves asking a patient to get up from a chair with armrests, walk 10 feet, turn around, and sit down. Performance in 15 seconds or longer is correlated with impairments in BADLs and suggestive that the patient is at risk for falls. Abnormal gait can also be observed during the TUG test.

8. **What steps should you take for a patient who has lost the ability to perform BADLs?**

   Consult physical therapy and occupational therapy personnel early in the hospitalization for patients with impaired performance of BADLs, gait or walking. Physical therapy and occupational therapy consultants often recommend graded bedside exercises (e.g., range of motion, low-impact endurance activities such as walking). Avoid prolonged bed rest and physical restraints and provide assistive devices or aids (e.g., canes, walkers, grab bars) to enhance the patient's independent self-care.

9. **Why is it important to know the patient's living situation before admission?**

   It is important to know whether the patient was at home (house, apartment), in an assisted-living facility, in a skilled nursing facility (SNF), or in a nursing home. This information provides important clues about the patient's prehospital level of functioning and predisposition to certain medical conditions (e.g., colonization with bacteria in nursing home patients). For patients at home, determine whether they live alone, with a spouse, or with another person. Inquiring about personal assistance, especially with regard to performance of ADLs, is essential. Patients living in an assisted-living community may require some assistance with IADLs (e.g., meals, transportation). Patients from a nursing home may require short-term rehabilitation in a skilled nursing facility and are likely to be dependent in most of their ADLs.

KEY POINTS: ASSESSMENT OF GERIATRIC PATIENTS

1. Adverse effects of hospitalization in the elderly include functional decline, iatrogenic illness, immobility, and undernutrition.

2. BADLs are bathing, dressing, toileting, continence, transferring, walking, and eating.

3. The most important predictor of functional decline in medically ill patients is delirium, which is potentially preventable in the hospital.

10. **How is dementia different from depression and delirium?**

Three common causes of decline in an elderly patient are the "three Ds:" dementia, delirium, and depression (Table 72-2).

TABLE 72-2.	THE THREE DS OF COGNITIVE IMPAIRMENT		
Feature	Dementia	Delirium	Depression
Acuity/onset	Insidious (weeks to months)	Acute (hours to days)	Gradual (months to years)
Awareness	Unaffected	Decreased	Clear, but selective
Alertness	Normal	Fluctuates	Normal
Attention	Minimal deficit	Grossly disturbed, easily distractible	Unaffected
Orientation	Impaired as disease progresses	Disoriented	Selective disorientation
Memory	Short-term memory loss, unconcerned about memory deficit	Impaired immediate and short-term memory	May be impaired, concerned about memory deficit
Sleep–wake cycle	Disturbed, day–night reversal	Disturbed, changes hourly	Disturbed, early morning awakening
Progression	Ongoing	Resolves with treatment of underlying precipitating condition	Resolves with treatment

Dementia is a clinical syndrome of at least 6 months of chronic and progressive impairments in two or more domains of cognitive function, such as memory or language in the absence of delirium or a psychiatric or medical illness that can cause cognitive dysfunction. These impairments must interfere with usual and everyday activities. Patients with dementia are usually alert and attentive and do not have fluctuation or altered levels of consciousness as do patients with delirium.

Depression is a clinical condition with an insidious onset of symptoms. Patients usually have a flat affect and disturbances in sleep and appetite.

Delirium is an acute disorder of attention and cognition. Risk factors for hospital-associated delirium in an older patient can be illustrated by the mnemonic DELIRIUM:

- **D:** Dementia
- **E:** Electrolyte disturbances (e.g., hypercalcemia)
- **L:** Low sodium (i.e., hyponatremia)
- **I:** Infection (e.g., urinary tract infection; pneumonia can present as change in mental status)
- **R:** Respiratory failure
- **I:** Injury (e.g., fall, hip fracture, pain)
- **U:** Unfamiliar environment (e.g., sensory deprivation—unavailability of eyeglasses, hearing aids)
- **M:** Metabolic problems (e.g., disturbances of blood sugar, cortisol, thyroid) and medications (e.g., anticholinergics, H_2 blockers, opiates)

11. **Why are depressive symptoms important to recognize?**
    The prevalence of major depression is low among community-dwelling elderly persons but is higher among hospitalized elderly persons, with up to 25–30% having clinical depression. Depressive symptoms are two to four times more common than major depression but are still associated with adverse outcomes during hospitalization. Depressive symptoms are often associated with delayed recovery from an illness, predict functional decline in the hospital, and subsequent mortality. Consequently, early recognition and treatment are warranted.

12. **Describe a rapid method to screen for depression in a hospitalized older patient.**
    The five-item Geriatric Depression Scale is a reliable and effective tool to screen for depression in a cognitively intact patient and requires that the following questions be asked:
    - "Are you basically satisfied with your life?"
    - "Do you often get bored?"
    - "Do you often feel helpless?"
    - "Do you prefer to stay home rather than going out and doing new things?"
    - "Do you feel pretty worthless the way you are now?"

    Positive answers to the depression screening are "no" to the first question and "yes" to the others. The sensitivity and specificity of three positive answers for depression are about 80% and 60%, respectively.

KEY POINTS: GERIATRIC SYNDROMES

1. The most common cause of iatrogenic illness and contributor to delirium in the elderly are adverse drug reactions caused by medications.

2. Complications of malnutrition include impaired wound healing and immunity, predisposition to pressure ulcers and delirium, prolonged hospital stay, delayed functional recovery, and increased mortality.

3. Signs suggestive of depression in the hospitalized elderly include withdrawn appearance, irritability, uncooperativeness, intermittent agitation, and "failure to thrive."

13. **What is protein-energy undernutrition? When should it be suspected?**
    Protein-energy undernutrition is a condition of insufficient energy, protein, or both needed to meet metabolic demands. Suspect undernutrition if:
    - There is a history of significant unintentional weight loss over the preceding 6 months.
    - Physical findings suggest a low body weight (body mass index <19 kg/m^2), loss of subcutaneous fat, muscle wasting, ankle edema, sacral edema, and ascites.
    - The patient has positive biochemical markers (i.e., low levels of hemoglobin, serum albumin level <3.5 gm/dL, low transferrin, low prealbumin, and low cholesterol).

    Deleterious effects of malnutrition include impaired wound healing, predisposition to delirium, pressure ulcers, impaired immunity, prolonged hospital stay, delayed functional recovery, and increased mortality. Serum prealbumin levels are often used to monitor response to nutritional repletion.

14. **What are the causes of malnutrition in a geriatric patient?**
    The mnemonic LOAD can be used to identify these causes:
    - **L:** Low-salt/low-cholesterol diet (e.g., restrictive diets)
    - **O:** Oral factors (e.g., poor dentition, ill-fitting dentures, mucositis, altered taste)
    - **A:** Adverse effects of medications (e.g., anorexigenic drugs—digoxin, metformin)
    - **D:** Depression, dementia, difficulty swallowing, diseases (e.g., hyperthyroidism, hyperparathyroidism, hypoadrenalism)

15. **What are the complications of potentially inappropriate medications (PIMs)?**
    PIMs are drugs whose risks for adverse effects outweigh their benefits at usual or high doses in elderly patients. PIMs can cause the following medical and social effects, illustrated by the mnemonic ABCDEF:
    - **A:** Adverse effects (e.g., drug-drug interaction, drug reaction)
    - **B:** Bedridden (i.e., sleepiness)
    - **C:** Confusion, constipation, cannot urinate (i.e., urinary retention)
    - **D:** Don't take it (i.e., noncompliance)
    - **E:** Empties the wallet (i.e., increasing costs, when less expensive medications are just as efficacious)
    - **F:** Falls (e.g., orthostatic hypotension)

16. **What are some common PIMs used in the hospital?**
    See Table 72-3.

17. **What is a core interdisciplinary health care team, and how can it improve the care of hospitalized geriatric patients?**
    The core interdisciplinary team consists of a patient's nurse, social worker or case manager, and primary attending physician. They collaborate daily in the care of complex patients. The extended interdisciplinary team members include a physical therapist, occupational therapist, dietician, speech pathologist, and home care coordinator. Ongoing collaboration throughout the patient's hospitalization to detect treatable functional impairments (e.g., physical therapy evaluation for patients with generalized weakness, dietary consultation for patients with malnutrition, home care coordinator to help arrange support services on discharge) is important to improve clinical and functional outcomes.

18. **List the common causes of constipation in the elderly patient.**
    Constipation is most often associated with prolonged bed rest, dehydration, a diet low in fiber, and the use of constipating medications (e.g., opioids) (Table 72-4).

19. **What are common causes of urinary incontinence in hospitalized elderly persons?**
    PAMPERS is the mnemonic that describes the common causes of urinary incontinence:
    - **P:** Pee too much (e.g., hyperglycemia)
    - **A:** Acute confusion (e.g., delirium), acute infection (e.g., urinary tract infection), atrophic vaginitis
    - **M:** Medications (e.g., diuretics, anticholinergics)
    - **P:** Psychiatric (e.g., depression)
    - **E:** Enlarged prostate (i.e., overflow incontinence)
    - **R:** Restricted mobility (e.g., physical restraint)
    - **S:** Stool impaction

20. **How can one prevent the occurrence of delirium in hospitalized elderly patients?**
    By identifying high-risk patients (i.e., those with cognitive impairment at baseline, those with serious medical illness), by avoiding immobilization and tethering (e.g., physical restraints, urinary catheter), and by using appropriate orientation techniques (e.g., clocks, calendars, hearing aids, glasses), and limiting stimulation at night (i.e., call bells, bright light, loud talking). Review medications (e.g., restricting the use of long-acting benzodiazepines, H_2 blockers, meperidine, steroids, atropine, and other anticholinergic agents) and encourage family members to visit. (See Chapter 18 for more details.)

TABLE 72-3. LIST OF POTENTIALLY INAPPROPRIATE MEDICATIONS, ADVERSE EFFECTS, AND ALTERNATIVES

Medications That Should Be Avoided	Adverse Effects	Recommendations	Alternatives
Antihistamines Diphenhydramine	Confusion Constipation Falls Oversedation	Avoid use as hypnotic or opioid adjunct. Use lowest effective dose for allergic reactions.	Hypnotics: Zolpidem 5 mg hs Trazodone 50 mg hs
Hydroxyzine	Orthostatic hypotension Urinary retention		Nonsedating antihistamines: Loratadine 10 mg daily Fexofenadine 60 mg daily or b.i.d.
Narcotic analgesics Meperidine Propoxyphene	Confusion Constipation Falls Oversedation Orthostatic hypotension Urinary retention Seizures (metabolite of meperidine)	Use alternative pain medication.	Acetaminophen (equianalgesic to propoxyphene) up to 4 gm/24 hours; add oxycodone 2.5–5 mg q4–6h if needed Morphine: initially low doses (e.g., 1–2 mg q3–4h)
Benzodiazepines Diazepam Chlordiazepoxide	Confusion Falls Sedation	Use shorter-acting agent for anxiety, and for alcohol or benzodiazepine withdrawal. Use low-dose antipsychotic to treat agitation and psychosis.	Anxiety: Lorazepam 0.5–1.0 mg q6h prn Agitation/psychosis: Haloperidol 0.5–2.0 mg b.i.d. or t.i.d. Risperidone 0.5 mg b.i.d. (lower doses daily after symptoms improve)

TABLE 72-3. LIST OF POTENTIALLY INAPPROPRIATE MEDICATIONS, ADVERSE EFFECTS, AND ALTERNATIVES—CONT'D

Medications That Should Be Avoided	Adverse Effects	Recommendations	Alternatives
Tricyclic antidepressants Amitriptiline Imipramine Doxepin	Confusion Constipation Falls Oversedation Orthostatic hypotension Urinary retention	Use fewer anticholinergic agents for neuropathic pain. Use alternative (e.g., SSRI) for depression.	Neuropathic pain: Desipramine 10–20 mg daily Nortriptyline 10–25 mg daily
Histamine₂-receptor blocker Famotidine	Confusion Depression Headache	Reduce usual dose by 50%	Famotidine 10–20 mg daily or 20 mg every other day

hs = at night, b.i.d. = twice a day, prn = as needed, t.i.d. = three times a day, SSRI = selective serotonin reuptake inhibitor.

TABLE 72-4.	CAUSES OF CONSTIPATION: THE SIX MS
Medications	Opiates, anticholinergics, antidepressants, antipsychotics, calcium channel blockers
Mechanical obstruction	Cancer, volvulus, stricture, extrinsic compression, intussusception
Metabolic disorders	Hypercalcemia, hypokalemia, hypophosphatemia, hypomagnesemia, uremia
Many neurologic disorders	Parkinson's disease, multiple sclerosis, spinal cord injury or tumor
Many systemic disorders	Hypothyroidism, diabetes mellitus, congestive heart failure
Miscellaneous	Poor fluid intake, cognitive impairment, immobility

21. **What are some general principles of prescribing medications to older adults?**
Know your patient's medications and medication history. "Start low, go slow," especially when the maintenance dose is unknown. Make adjustments for renal or hepatic impairment. Consider common drug-drug interactions due to hepatic CYP P450 metabolism. Check for orthostatic changes, as this is a common side effect of many medications used to treat older adults. Recognize that any new symptom may be an adverse drug reaction. Consider the occurrence of an adverse effect when behavioral symptoms such as agitation occur. Reevaluate the indications for continued use of all medications. Encourage treatment adherence (i.e., review indications, simplify drug dosing and administration).

22. **What routine preventive measures should be considered on admission in every hospitalized older patient?**
    - **Influenza vaccination:** Status should be determined, and vaccine should be administered to patients who have not received it if they are admitted anytime between October and March, provided they do not have an allergy to eggs.
    - **Pneumococcal vaccination:** This vaccine should also be administered to patients who have never been vaccinated.
    - **Smoking status:** This should be determined, and smoking cessation counseling should be provided as needed.
    - **Abuse and mental status:** Screens for alcohol abuse, depression, dementia, and elder abuse should be completed.

23. **A 65-year-old man is admitted for pneumonia during early winter. He reports having no medical care in 30 years. He responds well to antibiotics and is due to be discharged. What immunizations should he receive on discharge?**
Influenza vaccination, pneumococcal vaccination, and tetanus-diphtheria booster should be administered before discharge. The U.S. Centers for Disease Control and Prevention recommend influenza immunization for those 50 years and older, those with chronic medical conditions or immunosuppression, and all nursing home residents. It is to be administered as early as October provided the patient has no egg allergy. To further protect those who may not mount a protective antibody response, it is also recommended that caregivers for persons at risk also be immunized.

Persons aged 65 or older who were vaccinated with pneumococcal vaccine before age 65 should receive one revaccination 5 years after the initial vaccination. Previously unvaccinated persons should receive one dose at age 65. If an adult has never had a primary series of tetanus, three doses of tetanus toxoid are recommended. Otherwise, a booster dose of tetanus-diphtheria is needed every 10 years.

24. **How do you prevent bowel/bladder dysfunction in hospitalized patients?**
Encourage regular use of toilets/commodes, provide assistance when necessary, and minimize the use of indwelling catheters. Prescribe hyperosmolar laxatives and stool softeners for patients who are bed-bound or on low-fiber diets. Monitor patients for fecal impaction when they are taking medications that affect bowel and bladder functions (e.g., narcotics, anticholinergics, diuretics).

25. **What features identify clinical instability on the day of planned discharge from the hospital?**
New findings of incontinence, chest pain, dyspnea, delirium, tachycardia, hypotension, temperature >38.3°C, or diastolic blood pressure >105 mmHg are suggestive of clinical instability in older patients. Elderly patients who are sent home in an unstable condition have twice the risk of mortality 30 days after hospitalization compared with those whose condition is stable.

Brook RH, Kahn KL, Kosecoff J: Assessing clinical instability at discharge: The clinician's responsibility. JAMA 268:1321–1322, 1992.

KEY POINTS: INTERVENTIONS

1. Iatrogenic illness can be prevented by avoiding PIMs, preventing nosocomial infections, minimizing the use of risky diagnostic procedures, and encouraging mobility.

2. Check for impacted ear wax in a patient who is hard of hearing.

3. Review the "geriatric checklist" on the day of discharge, including a reassessment of performance of ADLs, mobility check, assessment for clinical stability, review of discharge medications, and summary discussion with patient, family, and outpatient provider.

26. **What is the "geriatric checklist" that should be reviewed on the day of planned discharge?**
   - **Reassessing performance of ADLs:** Can the patient transfer, eat and urinate?
   - **Checking mobility:** Is the patient able to walk independently?
   - **Assessing clinical stability**
   - **Reviewing appropriateness of discharge medications**
   - **Family/patient summary conference:** Review the diagnoses, treatment plans, and follow-up medical care.

WEBSITE

Portal of Geriatric Online Education: http://www.pogoe.com

BIBLIOGRAPHY

1. Covinsky KE, Palmer RM, Fortinsky RH, et al: Loss of independence in activities of daily living in older adults hospitalized with medical illnesses: increased vulnerability with age. J Am Geriatr Soc 51:451–458, 2003.

2. Inouye SK: A practical program for preventing delirium in hospitalized elderly patients. Cleve Clin J Med 71:890–896, 2004.

3. Palmer RM, Meldon SW: Acute care. In Hazzard WR, et al (eds): Principles of Geriatric Medicine Gerontology, 5th ed. New York, McGraw-Hill, 2003, pp 157–168.

4. Riedinger JL, Robbins LJ: Prevention of iatrogenic illness. Clin Geriatr Med 14:681–698, 1998.

5. Rinaldi P, Mecocci P, Benedetti C, et al: Validation of the five-item Geriatric Depression Scale in elderly subjects in three different settings. J Am Geriatr Soc 51:694–698, 2003.

APPROACH TO THE PREOPERATIVE EVALUATION

Adrienne L. Bennett, MD, PhD

1. **What determines the perioperative risk, and how does a hospitalist "clear" a patient for surgery?**
   There are three aspects to perioperative risk:
   - Anesthetic risk
   - Surgical/procedural risk
   - Patient risk due to medical comorbidities

   Medical comorbidities (e.g., a patient's underlying coronary artery disease and diabetes) represent the greatest risk for adverse perioperative events. Hospitalists are often asked by surgeons to provide "surgical clearance." Unfortunately, hospitalists cannot deem surgery "safe" since all procedures have inherent risks. Rather, the hospitalist's role is to assess the patient's medical comorbidities and to recommend (and if asked to comanage the patient, to implement) strategies to optimally manage chronic conditions before and after the surgery, thereby improving patient outcomes. It is the surgeon's and the anesthesiologist's duty to take this information back to the patient, making a recommendation based on the urgency and perceived benefit of the procedure. Ultimately, it is the patient's decision as to whether the benefits justify the risks of the overall procedure.

2. **What are the differences between medical consultation and medical comanagement?**
   - **Consultation:** Traditionally, this encompasses the surgeon asking a consultant to evaluate and make recommendations about the management of a particular problem. The role of the consultant is that of an adviser. The consultant should communicate findings (written and through direct discussion for more urgent or critical recommendations) in a timely fashion to the surgeon, who retains overall responsibility for the care of the patient. The consultant should refrain from writing orders for diagnostic or therapeutic interventions unless specifically asked to do so.
   - **Comanagement:** This refers to situations in which the surgeon requests the consultant to evaluate and assume the management for a particular medical problem, including writing orders for appropriate diagnostic tests and therapeutic actions. Hospitalists are frequently asked to comanage patients in the perioperative setting.

3. **What are the risks associated with anesthesia?**
   The risk of perioperative mortality due to the anesthesia itself is quite low (1 death per approximately 250,000 anesthetics administered). The overall risk of anesthetic use is referable to underlying comorbid illnesses. For example, anesthesia-induced hypotension is usually well tolerated unless the patient has a significant premorbid illness such as severe coronary artery disease. The primary risks of anesthesia include hypoventilation, hypoxemia, aspiration, hypotension, arrhythmia, and myocardial depression and ischemia. The decline in anesthesia-related morbidity and mortality is a result of concerted efforts to analyze the causes of adverse events and to introduce clinical guidelines and improve systems to reduce errors (such as the use of pulse oximetry and carbon dioxide detectors to ensure adequate ventilation and oxygenation of patients). All forms of anesthesia carry risks and in particular have effects on cardiovascular physiology. Several studies in selected patient populations have found morbidity

benefits of neuroaxial blockade compared to general anethesia (for example, lower rates of venous thromboembolism in hip fracture patients who undergo operative repair under neuroaxial blockade), although for other patients/procedures no differences have been noted (such as in cardiac outcomes in patients undergoing peripheral vascular surgery). The selection of anesthesia should be determined by the anesthesiologist, taking into account patient preferences.

Rodgers A, Walker N, Schug S, et al: Reduction of postoperative mortality and morbidity with epidural or spinal anaesthesia: Results from overview of randomized trials. BMJ 321:1493, 2000.

4. **What are the risks associated with the surgical procedure?**
   Surgical risk correlates with the physiologic stress response to the surgery, including multiple effects on endocrine and autonomic nervous system functions resulting in alterations in hemodynamics, metabolism, fluid and electrolyte balance, hemostasis, and immune function. The physiologic stress response to surgery is proportional to the magnitude and duration of the surgery. (See Table 74-1 in Chapter 74 for more details.)

5. **What are the key elements of a preoperative evaluation?**
   A thorough history and physical examination focusing on the patient's known medical conditions, any new signs and symptoms, and known risk factors for perioperative morbidity and mortality form the single most important step in determining perioperative risk. A detailed discussion of the pertinent aspects of the preoperative history and physical examination are covered in other chapters and are included in Table 73-1.

TABLE 73-1. FOCUSED PREOPERATIVE HISTORY AND PHYSICAL EXAM	
Component	**Important Aspects for Perioperative Management**
Medical history	Although cardiac and pulmonary illnesses are the most common, they are not the only disease states that can be associated with significant perioperative morbidity and mortality. Diabetes, hypertension, renal insufficiency, chronic liver disease, and cerebrovascular disease—particularly if these conditions are under poor medical control—can lead to major postoperative complications and even death.
Surgical/anesthetic history	Pay special attention to any past adverse events with surgery/anesthesia, particularly past complications (such as reactions to anesthesia, postoperative atrial fibrillation, or congestive heart failure).
Social history	**Tobacco:** $\geq$20 pack-year smoking history is associated with coronary artery disease as well as chronic obstructive pulmonary disease. Although short-term cessation of smoking may be beneficial, 8 weeks of cessation is necessary to significantly reduce the rate of postoperative pulmonary complications.
	Alcohol: Acute alcoholic hepatitis is a contraindication to anesthesia.
	Other drugs: Recreational drug use may have put the patient at risk for HIV and/or viral hepatitis.
	All drugs: Consider the potential for and plan for the management of postoperative withdrawal syndromes (e.g., nicotine patches for heavy smokers, benzodiazepines for chronic alcohol consumers).

TABLE 73-1.	FOCUSED PREOPERATIVE HISTORY AND PHYSICAL EXAM—CONT'D
Component	Important Aspects for Perioperative Management
Family history	Inquire regarding coronary artery disease, bleeding or clotting disorders, and adverse reactions to anesthetics or latex.
Allergies	All adverse reactions to medications should be noted, with particular attention to anesthetics and latex.

6. **How should chronic medications be managed during the perioperative period?**
Obtain a complete list of all medications that the patient takes, including over-the-counter medicines and herbal remedies, with dose, route, and frequency. Most medications can be continued without change throughout the perioperative period. However, several groups of medications do require some management during and after surgery. It is important to reconcile postoperative and discharge medications with preoperative outpatient medications to be sure that any medications that were temporarily suspended are reinitiated, if appropriate (Table 73-2).

TABLE 73-2.	PERIOPERATIVE MEDICATION MANAGEMENT
Medication	Effects and Perioperative Management
Herbal remedies	Several herbal remedies may inhibit clotting (e.g., ginger, gingko) or have hepatotoxic potential (e.g., comfrey, germander) or may affect hemodynamic regulation (ephedra). Others may have unknown potential side effects or drug-anesthetic interactions. Patients should be counseled to discontinue all herbal remedies 2 weeks before elective surgery whenever possible.
Aspirin	Aspirin should be stopped 7–10 days preoperatively based on its irreversible inhibitory effect on platelet function. In the absence of postoperative bleeding, aspirin can be restarted 24 hours after surgery.
Nonsteroidal anti-inflammatory drugs (NSAIDs)	These drugs reversibly inhibit platelet function, and many with short half-lives can be stopped 3 days before surgery. In addition, they inhibit renal prostaglandin synthesis and can induce renal failure in combination with other drugs and hypotension. In the absence of postoperative bleeding, NSAIDs can be restarted 24–48 hours after surgery.
COX-2 inhibitors	These have minimal effect on platelets and can be used in the perioperative period.
Diuretics	Diuretic agents should be withheld on the day of surgery and restarted when the patient is hemodynamically stable postoperatively and can take oral medications.

Continued

TABLE 73-2. PERIOPERATIVE MEDICATION MANAGEMENT—CONT'D

Medication	Effects and Perioperative Management
Inhaled bronchodilators, anticholinergics, steroids, and theophylline	These should be continued throughout the perioperative period.
Cardiac medications	Antianginals and antiarrhythmics, especially beta blockers, should be taken on the day of surgery with a sip of water. The exception may be ACE inhibitors and ARBs, which have been associated with hypotension during induction of anesthesia. Some anesthesiologists prefer to withhold these medications on the day of surgery.
Lipid-lowering agents (statins, niacin and fibric acid derivatives)	These can be continued including on the day of surgery with a sip of water. Recent studies have found a mortality benefit to continuing lipid-lowering agents throughout the perioperative period.
Thyroid replacement	This may be continued but can safely be held for up to 1 week if the patient is NPO postoperatively.
Antithyroid medications	These should be continued, including on the day of surgery.
Oral contraceptives and hormone replacement therapy	Cessation of these drugs is controversial if the woman is of childbearing age. If the patient will receive pharmacologic agents for VTE prophylaxis these agents can be continued perioperatively. In the absence of prophylaxis, these drugs should be discontinued because they increase the risk for thromboembolic complications. To minimize the procoagulant effect, these medicines should be discontinued at least a month before surgery and may be resumed once normal activity levels resume postoperatively.
Antiepileptics and antiparkinson drugs	These drugs should be continued throughout the perioperative period.
Antidepressants including SSRIs, antipsychotics, and benzodiazepines	Administration of these medications should be continued throughout the perioperative period. Care should be taken with monoamine oxidase inhibitors because they can interact with many drugs, including meperidine.
Diabetes medications	See Chapter 76 for more details.

COX-2 = cyclooxygenase-2, ACE = angiotensin-converting enzyme, ARB = angiotensin receptor blocker, NPO = nothing by mouth (i.e., not taking in any food or drink), VTE = venous thromboembolism, SSRI = selective serotonin reuptake inhibitor.

7. **Which patients need stress dose steroids? What dosage is appropriate?**

The use of prednisone ≥20 mg for more than 2 weeks within the past year or chronic use of ≥5 mg of prednisone daily can result in suppression of the hypothalamic-pituitary-adrenal (HPA) axis. However, the dose and duration of steroid use do not correlate in a predictable fashion with HPA suppression. Consequently, a high index of suspicion is required in any patient who has used corticosteroids in the past year and who presents postoperatively with one or more signs and symptoms of adrenal insufficiency. These include fatigue, anorexia, nausea, vomiting, abdominal pain, fever, hypotension, shock, hypoglycemia, and hyponatremia. Rational use of stress dose steroids should parallel the normal physiologic response to surgical stress (Table 73-3).

TABLE 73-3. RECOMMENDATIONS FOR STRESS DOSE STEROIDS

Level of Surgical Stress	Normal Physiologic Response to Surgical Stress	Stress Dose in Patients at Risk for Secondary Adrenal Insufficiency	Postoperative Dosing*
Baseline	~10 mg hydrocortisone/day		
Low (e.g., local/regional anesthetic, procedure <1 hour)	~10 mg hydrocortisone/day	If using chronic steroid therapy, continue the usual dose or give hydrocortisone 25 mg IV × 1 dose given in the OR	Resume usual outpatient dose if patient is using steroids chronically
Intermediate (e.g., orthopedic, urologic procedures)	50 mg hydrocortisone/day, returns to baseline within 24 hours	Hydrocortisone 25 mg IV every 8 hours × 3 doses with first dose given in the OR	Resume usual outpatient dose if patient is using steroids chronically
High (e.g., body cavity operations)	75–150 mg hydrocortisone/day returns to baseline within 2–5 days	Hydrocortisone 50–100 mg IV every 8 hours × 3 doses, with first dose given in the OR	On POD 2, taper to hydrocortisone 25 mg IV every 8 hours × 3 doses, then resume usual outpatient dose

IV = intravenous, OR = operating room, POD = postoperative day.
*Assumes uncomplicated course; complicated course may require higher dose.
Note: Hydrocortisone 10 mg/day = prednisone 2.5 mg/day.

8. **What preoperative screening tests are useful in identifying perioperative risk?**
   There is no evidence that routine screening of asymptomatic surgical patients is helpful in risk stratification or management of perioperative complications. Clinically identifiable medical conditions, recognized during the history and physical examination, are far more likely to result in perioperative adverse events than unrecognized illnesses detected through the use of routine preoperative screening tests. A more cost-effective approach is to determine selected laboratory values that take into consideration findings on the history and physical examination and the type of surgery the patient is undergoing. In general, it is safe to use test results that were performed and were normal within the last 4 months if no change has occurred in the patient's clinical status. Table 73-4 provides evidence-based recommendations for laboratory testing before surgery.

TABLE 73-4. PREOPERATIVE LABORATORY SCREENING	
Test	**Preoperative Indications**
Blood type and screen	Major surgery or anticipated blood loss over 500 ml
Complete blood count	Major surgery or anticipated blood loss over 500 ml, any surgery that requires postoperative anticoagulation, underlying malignancy or myeloproliferative disorder, known bleeding diathesis, prior or ongoing exposure to myelotoxic medications
PT, INR, PTT	Bleeding time, PT, and PTT are not predictive of surgical bleeding. Obtain a PT/INR measurement for patients taking warfarin, those with liver disease or malnutrition, and those with recent/long-term antibiotic use. Obtain PT and PTT measurements for known bleeding diathesis or surgery that requires postoperative anticoagulation.
Electrolytes	Renal disease, diabetes, hypertension, congestive heart failure, medications known to affect electrolytes (e.g., diuretics, digitalis, ACE inhibitor, ARB, corticosteroids)
Blood urea nitrogen and creatinine	Major surgery, cardiac disease, renal disease, diabetes, hypertension, age > 70 years, use of diuretics or other medications known to affect renal function
Glucose and/or glycosylated hemoglobin	Diabetes, obesity, prior corticosteroid use
Liver function tests	Chronic liver disease, history of alcohol abuse
Albumin	Major surgery, liver disease, multiple chronic medical comorbidities, recent major illness, suspected malnutrition, age > 70 years. Correlates with perioperative morbidity and mortality, particularly in the elderly, where albumin serves as a marker of chronic disease and occult protein-energy malnutrition.
Urinalysis	Generally not useful; might consider in diabetics and patients with renal disease

TABLE 73-4.   PREOPERATIVE LABORATORY SCREENING—CONT'D

Test	Preoperative Indications
Chest x-ray	Patients with signs/symptoms of active cardiac or pulmonary disease, or those undergoing intrathoracic surgery
Electrocardiogram	Men > 40 years, women > 50 years, patients with any of the following: coronary artery disease, renal disease, diabetes, hypertension
Medication levels	Digoxin, anticonvulsants, antiarrhythmics

PT = prothrombin time, INR = international normalized ratio, PTT = partial thromboplastin time, ACE = angiotensin-converting enzyme, ARB = angiotensin receptor blocker

KEY POINTS: PERIOPERATIVE RISKS AND THE ROLE OF THE HOSPITALIST

1. The chronic medical illnesses that patients take with them into the operating room put them at the greatest risk of adverse perioperative outcomes.

2. The role of the hospitalist is to assess the risks posed by the patient comorbidities and to recommend strategies to help decrease this risk during the perioperative period, thereby improving clinical outcomes.

9. **How does the serum albumin level predict surgical outcomes?**
Serum albumin levels <3.0 mg/dL correlate with increased perioperative morbidity and mortality. Albumin is a good marker of chronic disease and nutrition. Low levels indicate prolonged illness or protein-malnutrition. If possible, steps should be taken to improve the associated chronic illness or poor nutrition before surgery.

BIBLIOGRAPHY

1. Huddleston JM, Long KH, Naessens JM, et al: Medical and surgical comanagement after elective hip and knee arthroplasty: A randomized, controlled trial. Ann Intern Med 141:28–38, 2004.

2. Shaw M: When is perioperative steroid coverage necessary? Cleve Clin J Med, 69:9–11, 2002.

3. Smetana GW, Macpherson DS: The case against routine preoperative laboratory testing. Med Clin North Am 87:7–40, 2003.

CHAPTER 74

PREOPERATIVE CARDIAC EVALUATION

Neil Winawer, MD, and Steven L. Cohn, MD

1. **What are the goals of preoperative cardiac risk evaluation?**

   Each year, millions of patients undergo noncardiac surgery. A large percentage of these patients have underlying coronary artery disease (CAD) or risk factors for undiagnosed CAD. Cardiac morbidity is the leading cause of death in the perioperative period, making it extremely important to accurately recognize, and subsequently minimize a patient's preoperative cardiac risk. The goals of preoperative cardiac risk evaluation are to:
   - Clinically assess a patient's current medical status
   - Provide a cardiovascular risk profile
   - Decide whether further cardiac testing is indicated before surgery
   - Make recommendations to attempt to reduce the risk of perioperative complications

2. **What historical factors are important in determining perioperative cardiac risk?**

   A history of myocardial infarction (MI), angina, congestive heart failure (CHF), arrhythmias, or valvular heart disease are associated with worse surgical outcome. In the absence of known cardiac disease, risk factors for CAD such as male sex, hypertension, diabetes, dyslipidemia, and tobacco use and age, as well as associated comorbid diseases such as peripheral arterial disease, cerebrovascular disease, chronic renal insufficiency, and chronic obstructive pulmonary disease should be taken into account. Recent angina or dyspnea as well as poor functional status should also be elicited in the preoperative evaluation. Finally, obtaining a list of the patient's current prescribed and over-the-counter medications is essential.

3. **How does the physical examination contribute to cardiac risk assessment?**

   It confirms information obtained in the history and uncovers findings suggestive of cardiovascular disease. The important physical findings include abnormal vital signs, the presence of carotid bruits, elevated jugular venous pressure, murmurs associated with aortic stenosis, gallops (S_3 heart sound), rales or wheezing, edema, and abnormal peripheral pulses.

4. **When is a preoperative electrocardiogram (ECG) indicated?**

   Routine preoperative ECG infrequently alters management. However, the discovery of previously undocumented Q waves or conduction abnormalities should raise concern and may lead to further testing. Guidelines vary, but a preoperative ECG is usually recommended for men older than 40 years and women older than 50 years. An ECG should also be performed in patients with a history or symptoms consistent with cardiac disease, hypertension, diabetes, peripheral vascular disease, pulmonary disease, and those taking certain medications (e.g., diuretics, tricyclic antidepressants) or a history of exposure to chemotherapeutic agents such as doxorubicin.

5. **What is a quick step-wise approach to cardiac risk assessment using the American College of Cardiology/American Heart Association (ACC/AHA) guidelines?**

   The answers to the following questions provide a quick step-wise approach to cardiac risk assessment:
   - How urgent is the need for noncardiac surgery? (Is it *urgent* or *emergent* versus *elective*.)

- Does the patient have a history of previous coronary revascularization including coronary artery bypass graft surgery (CABG) or percutaneous coronary intervention (PCI)?
- When was the most recent coronary evaluation (i.e., stress test or coronary angiography)?
- What clinical predictors does the patient have? (Options are *major, intermediate,* or *minor;* see Table 74-1.)
- What is the patient's functional capacity? (Options are *more than* or *less than 4 metabolic equivalents [METS]*; see Table 74-2.)
- What type of surgical procedure is the patient having? (Is there high, intermediate, or low risk? See Table 74-3.)

See also Fig. 74-1.

TABLE 74-1. ACC CLINICAL PREDICTORS OF INCREASED PERIOPERATIVE CARDIAC RISK (MI, CHF, DEATH)

Major	Intermediate	Minor
Unstable coronary syndromes (MI < 30 days, unstable angina, class III–IV angina)	Mild angina (class I–II)	Advanced age
Decompensated heart failure	Previous MI (>30 days)	Abnormal ECG
Significant arrhythmias	Compensated or prior CHF	Non-sinus rhythm
Severe valvular disease	Diabetes mellitus	Low functional capacity
	Renal insufficiency (creatinine ≥ 2.0)	History of stroke
		Uncontrolled hypertension

TABLE 74-2. MODIFIED DUKE SPECIFIC ACTIVITY STATUS

1 MET:	4 METs:
Take care of self	Climb one flight, go uphill
Eat, dress, toilet	Walk on level ground 4 miles/hour
Walk indoors	Do heavy housework (e.g., scrub floors,
Walk 1–2 blocks (level) at 2–3 miles/hour	move furniture)
Do light work around the house	Do moderate recreational activities
(dust, wash dishes)	Participate in strenuous sports
4 METs	≥10 METs

6. **How do the ACC/AHA and the American College of Physicians (ACP) guidelines differ?**
   The ACC/AHA guidelines are evidence based but use expert opinion in the absence of hard evidence, whereas the ACP guidelines are strictly evidence based, making no recommendation in the absence of conclusive evidence. The ACC/AHA also considers exercise capacity and uses surgery-specific risk. The ACP guidelines do not consider exercise capacity and divide patients' risk into vascular or nonvascular categories. Ultimately, the ACC/AHA tends to over-test while the ACP tends to under-test.

TABLE 74-3.   ACC CARDIAC RISK STRATIFICATION FOR NONCARDIAC SURGICAL PROCEDURES

Level of Risk*	Type of Surgery or Procedure
High risk Cardiac risk >5%	Emergent major operations and aortic and major vascular, peripheral vascular, and prolonged procedures with large fluid shifts or blood loss
Intermediate risk Cardiac risk 1–5%	Carotid endarterectomy, and major head and neck, intraperitoneal, intrathoracic, orthopedic, prostate surgeries
Low risk Cardiac risk <1%	Endoscopic, superficial, cataract, and breast surgeries

*Combined incidence of cardiac death and nonfatal MI.

7. **How does a patient's ability to exercise influence the preoperative assessment?**
Poor exercise capacity, regardless of the cause, correlates with increased risk of postoperative complications. Approximating patients' METs is a useful surrogate of functional status. One MET represents oxygen consumption at rest, approximately 250 mL/min for a 70-kg adult. The ACC/AHA guidelines use the level of >4 METs to represent adequate exercise capacity (see Table 74-2).

8. **Who should undergo noninvasive testing (NIT) preoperatively?**
The ACC/AHA guidelines suggest that testing is indicated if any two of the following are present:
- Intermediate clinical predictors
- Poor functional capacity (<4 METs)
- Procedure with high surgical risk

However, in view of promising results from studies involving prophylactic medical therapy (e.g., beta blockers, alpha agonists, and statins) and the negative findings of a recent prophylactic revascularization study in which no short- or long-term benefit to preoperative CABG or PCI was found, the recommendations for NIT and subsequent revascularization are being reevaluated.

Falls EO, Ward HB, Moritz TE, et al: Coronary artery revascularization before elective major vascular surgery. N Engl J Med 351:2795–2804, 2004.

9. **Which patient group (high, intermediate, or low risk) is likely to benefit from NIT?**
Intermediate-risk patients stand to gain the most benefit from NIT. A negative test result places the patient in a lower-risk group that does not require further testing, whereas a positive test result will lead to an intervention. A positive result in those with a *high pretest* probability only confirms suspicions, whereas a negative test result stands a high chance of being a false negative. Either situation results in proceeding to an interventional procedure. Similarly, an abnormal study in a patient at *low risk* is likely to be a false-positive test result incurring additional risk and cost to intervene. A negative test result in this patient type only confirms the suspected low risk.

10. **Which NIT should be ordered? Is there a "best test"?**
There is no best test. The decision to use a particular test is dependent on individual patient characteristics. Various methods exist to stress and image a patient's heart. Patients can be stressed with exercise or medications. Imaging modalities can add valuable information by

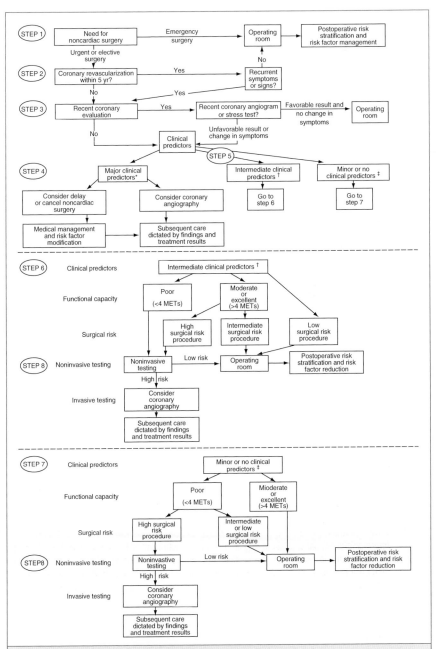

Figure 74-1. ACC/AHA Algorithm for Stepwise Approach to Preoperative Cardiac Assessment. * Major clinical predictors include unstable coronary syndromes, decompensated congestive heart failure, significant arrhythmias, and severe valvular disease. † Intermediate clinical predictors include mild angina pectoris, prior myocardial infarction, and compensated or prior congestive heart failure, diabetes mellitus, renal insufficiency. ‡ Minor clinical predictors include advanced age, abnormal electrocardiogram, rhythm other than sinus, low functional capacity, history of stroke, and uncontrolled systemic hypertension. MET = metabolic equivalent.

allowing visualization of myocardial activity. In general, exercise tests are preferable to pharmacologic (i.e., dobutamine, dipyridamole, adenosine) studies. But many patients are unable to achieve their target heart rates because of poor exercise capacity or disability. Imaging options, including nuclear medicine (e.g., thallium or sestamibi) or echocardiographic modalities appear to be equally efficacious, and use should be dictated by the institutional expertise. Dipyridamole (Persantine) works by causing release of adenosine producing a coronary steal phenomenon with subsequent ischemia in the distribution of stenotic arteries. (See Chapter 26 for more details.)

11. **What types of information do these tests (see question 10) impart?**
    Stress tests provide a patient's exercise capacity (METs), rate pressure product or double product (the peak heart rate multiplied by the peak systolic blood pressure), and ischemic threshold. These tests also demonstrate the presence and extent of ischemia (e.g., symptoms, ECG changes, systolic wall motion abnormalities, and reperfusion abnormalities). This information is useful to the anesthesiologist who will try to maintain the patient's double product below the ischemic threshold in the operating room.

12. **Which patients should be referred for preoperative coronary angiography?**
    Patients with independent criteria for coronary angiography, such as unstable or class III or IV stable angina, regardless of the need for surgery, and those with a strongly positive NIT result (e.g., early ischemia, multiple areas of ischemia) should be considered for coronary angiography. Additionally, patients with three or more intermediate clinical predictors scheduled for high-risk surgery are potential candidates for further intervention.

13. **Does preoperative PCI or CABG result in improved outcome after noncardiac surgery?**
    The only randomized controlled trial to address this issue failed to demonstrate short- or long-term benefit of prophylactic CABG or PCI on the mortality of patients with stable angina scheduled for vascular surgery. Nevertheless, patients who undergo successful bypass surgery have a mortality rate similar to patients without CAD. However, these data do not account for the morbidity and mortality of bypass surgery itself. Since the risk of CABG may equal or exceed the risk of major noncardiac surgery, decisions regarding bypass surgery should not be made solely on the basis of lowering risk. Therefore, the indications for CABG or angioplasty with stenting in the perioperative period remain identical to those in the nonsurgical setting.

    McFalls EO, Ward HB, Moritz TE, et al. Coronary artery revascularization before elective major vascular surgery. N Engl J Med 351:2795–2804, 2004.

14. **A 78-year-old man with stable angina, previous MI, diabetes, and hypertension is scheduled for a cataract extraction. His examination bears unremarkable results, but he can only walk one block slowly due to severe osteoarthritis. Would you recommend an NIT?**
    First do no harm! If the patient's risk of a complication is low, it is difficult to lower that risk much more. Furthermore, all interventions (e.g., PCI) have risks such that the little benefit to be gained from the intervention may be offset by the risk of the procedure itself. Ordering an NIT, which may be reassuring if the result is negative, may only lead to further testing (if the result is positive) that is unlikely to provide benefit due to the overall low risk of the surgical procedure.

15. **At what blood pressure is surgery contraindicated?**
    Like most perioperative decisions, the risk of acute hypertension must be viewed in light of the surgical urgency. In cases of emergent surgery, patients should proceed to the operating room regardless of blood pressure levels. Patients with stage II hypertension (systolic blood pressure >180 mmHg or a diastolic blood pressure >110 mmHg) may be at an increased

risk for MI, stroke, and acute renal failure. Given this, it is reasonable to delay surgery in these patients if the procedure is elective. Patients with mild to moderate hypertension are not at increased risk provided that end-organ complications (e.g., CHF, renal failure) are not present.

16. **How should antiplatelet agents be managed in PCI patients undergoing surgery?**
Antiplatelet agents are usually stopped 7 days before noncardiac surgery to reduce postoperative bleeding. Patients who undergo preoperative balloon angioplasty without stenting can generally proceed to surgery after waiting several days for plaque stabilization. Patients undergoing bare metal stenting, however, are at risk for in-stent thromboses and typically require at least 1 month of dual antiplatelet therapy with aspirin and clopidogrel (to allow for stent endothelialization). Patients receiving drug-eluting stents (which contain antiproliferative agents such as sirolimus or paclitaxel) may require up to 6 months of treatment with aspirin and clopidogrel.

17. **What is the role of prophylactic beta blockers? Who should receive them perioperatively?**
Several observational studies and randomized controlled trials have shown that beta blockers reduce the incidence of perioperative ischemia, MI, and death. Based on these data, beta blockers should be recommended for all high-risk patients undergoing noncardiac surgery. *High-risk patients* are defined as those with intermediate clinical risk predictors who either have poor functional status or are undergoing vascular surgery. Patients who are at intermediate risk may also derive a benefit from beta blockade, particularly if they have a history of hypertension, CAD, diabetes mellitus, stroke, or renal insufficiency. Treatment should be initiated 1–4 weeks before noncardiac surgery with the dose titrated to achieve a resting heart rate of approximately 60 beats/min. However, beneficial effects have been shown with use as little as 24 hours before surgery. Beta blockers should be continued for at least 30 days postoperatively and indefinitely in those with compelling indications (other than just for surgery).

18. **What drugs are acceptable alternatives when beta blockers cannot be used perioperatively?**
A large meta-analysis revealed a statistically significant reduction in mortality and MI in patients treated with alpha agonists (e.g., clonidine) before vascular surgery. Although there are no head-to-head studies, the odds ratios in meta-analyses appear stronger for beta blockers, and based on the available data, it appears best to restrict use of alpha agonists to high-risk patients who have contraindications or intolerance to beta blockers.

19. **Do statins have a benefit in patients undergoing noncardiac surgery?**
Several observational studies and one small randomized controlled trial have shown that use of statins perioperatively was associated with significant cardiac risk reduction in patients undergoing high-risk noncardiac surgery. The beneficial effects of statins in these trials occurred independent of the risk reduction provided by beta blockers. Based on these data, it appears that statins should be continued perioperatively and possibly considered prophylactically in high-risk patients undergoing noncardiac surgery.

20. **What role does invasive monitoring with pulmonary artery catheters play?**
Pulmonary artery catheters are often used in critically ill patients given that physiologic monitoring may help refine treatment and possibly improve outcomes. A recent large randomized controlled trial of high-risk patients found no significant difference in outcomes between patients managed with standard therapy versus patients with a pulmonary artery catheter. Consequently, pulmonary artery catheters should not be used routinely in patients undergoing high-risk surgery.

KEY POINTS: PREOPERATIVE CARDIAC EVALUATION

1. The history and physical examination are the most important elements of the preoperative risk assessment.

2. Risk indices are only tools to assist in clinical decision making; they cannot substitute for good clinical judgment regarding an individual patient's risk.

3. First do no harm. Do not pursue a potentially invasive intervention to "prevent" a complication that is unlikely to occur in low-risk surgery.

4. Patients at intermediate risk are the group most likely to benefit from further cardiac testing.

5. Consider the potential risk of any prophylactic intervention in your risk-benefit analysis.

6. If beta blockers are to be protective, the patient must be adequately beta blocked (resting heart rate < 65 bpm).

21. Who should be monitored with postoperative ECGs or cardiac enzymes?

The ACC/AHA guidelines recommend routine postoperative ECGs in patients with known or suspected CAD who are undergoing high- or intermediate-risk surgical procedures. ECGs should be obtained in the recovery room, daily on the first 2 days after surgery, and whenever there are signs of cardiac dysfunction. Cardiac enzymes should also be measured at 24 hours postoperatively and on either Day 4 or before hospital discharge (whichever comes first) in patients with documented or suspected CAD who are undergoing high-risk surgical procedures.

22. Are patients with aortic stenosis at risk for perioperative complications?

Patients with aortic stenosis are at an increased risk for perioperative complications. As such, consideration of valve replacement should be done before elective surgery in patients with symptomatic aortic stenosis. Asymptomatic patients should have echocardiographic assessment of their valvular and left ventricular function before elective surgery.

BIBLIOGRAPHY

1. American College of Physicians: Guidelines for assessing and managing the perioperative risk from coronary artery disease associated with major noncardiac surgery. Ann Intern Med 127:309–312, 1997. Available at http://www.acponline.org/journals/annals/15aug97/ppcad1.htm.

2. Boersma E, Poldermans D, Bax D, et al: Predictors of cardiac events after major vascular surgery: Role of clinical characteristics, dobutamine echocardiography, and beta-blocker therapy. JAMA 285:1865–1873, 2001.

3. Eagle KA, Berger PB, Calkins H, et al: ACC/AHA guideline update for perioperative cardiovascular evaluation for noncardiac surgery: Executive summary. A report of the American College of Cardiology/American Heart Association Task Force on Practice Guidelines (Committee to Update the 1996 Guidelines on Perioperative Cardiovascular Evaluation for Noncardiac Surgery). J Am Coll Cardiol 39:542–553, 2002.

4. Fleisher LA: Preoperative evaluation of the patient with hypertension. JAMA 287:2043–2046, 2002.

5. Foster ED, Davis KB, Carpenter JA, et al: Risk of noncardiac operation in patients with defined coronary disease: The Coronary Artery Surgery Study (CASS) registry experience. Ann Thorac Surg 41:42–50, 1986.

6. Hlatky MA, Boineau RE, Gigginbotham MB, et al: A brief self-administered questionnaire to determine functional capacity (the Duke Activity Status Index). Am J Cardiol 64:651–654, 1989.

7. Kertai MD, Bountioukos M, Boersma E, et al: Aortic stenosis: An underestimated risk factor for perioperative complications in patients undergoing noncardiac surgery. Am J Med 116:8–13, 2004.

8. Lindenauer PK, Pekow P, Wang K, et al: Lipid-lowering therapy and in-hospital mortality following major noncardiac surgery. JAMA 291:2092–2099, 2004.

9. McFalls EO, Ward HB, Moritz TE, et al: Coronary artery revascularization before elective major vascular surgery. N Engl J Med 351:2795–2804, 2004.

10. Stevens RD, Burri H, Tramer MR: Pharmacologic myocardial protection in patients undergoing noncardiac surgery: A quantitative systematic review. Anesth Analg 97:623–633, 2003.

CHAPTER 75

PREOPERATIVE PULMONARY EVALUATION

Mary H. Pak, MD, and Gerald W. Smetana, MD

1. **Does every patient undergoing surgery require a preoperative pulmonary evaluation?**

   Postoperative pulmonary complications (PPCs) are common and can affect postoperative mortality and morbidity, including an extended hospitalization. Therefore, clinicians should estimate PPC risk for all patients undergoing a preoperative medical assessment.

2. **What are the most clinically important PPCs?**

   Postoperative pneumonia, atelectasis, bronchospasm, exacerbation of chronic obstructive pulmonary disease (COPD), acute respiratory distress syndrome, and respiratory failure.

3. **How common are PPCs?**

   Rates of PPCs are comparable to those of postoperative cardiac complications and are more frequent than thromboembolic complications. Seven percent of all patients undergoing noncardiac surgery develop PPCs. A recent systematic review shows that a PPC occurs in 9% of patients undergoing any abdominal surgery and 25% of patients undergoing upper abdominal surgery. PPCs also increase length of hospital stay.

   Smetana GW, Lawrence VA, Cornell JE: Preoperative pulmonary risk stratification for noncardiothoracic surgery: Systematic review for the American College of Physicians. Ann Intern Med 144:581–595, 2006.

4. **What are the most important patient-related risk factors for PPCs? Do they differ from those for cardiac complications?**

   The most important risk factors are cigarette smoking, COPD, American Society of Anesthesiologists class > 2 (some functional limitation due to effects of systemic disease), poor exercise capacity, abnormal chest examination, and age > 70 years. These differ from the major patient-related risk factors for postoperative cardiac complications, which include coronary artery disease, congestive heart failure, cerebrovascular disease, renal insufficiency, and insulin-treated diabetes mellitus. Thus, it is important to consider separately the risk for cardiac and pulmonary complications during the preoperative medical evaluation. Commonly, a patient may be at high risk for one type of complication but not the other.

5. **Are COPD and asthma risk factors for PPC?**

   COPD increases the risk of PPCs threefold; the risk is greatest for patients with poor exercise capacity, symptoms at rest, or prolonged expiratory phase on chest examination. Despite intuition that suggests otherwise, well-controlled asthma is not a risk factor for PPCs.

6. **Do current smokers have an increased risk for PPCs even if they do not have COPD?**

   Yes! Even among those without chronic lung disease, current (or any time within the previous 2 months) cigarette smoking doubles the risk of PPCs.

7. **Is there an age at which the risk of PPC starts to rise?**

   The risk of PPCs is greater after approximately 60 years old, even for healthy older patients.

8. **What role do obesity, obstructive sleep apnea, and exercise capacity play in determining a patient's risk for PPCs?**
Obesity is not a risk factor for PPCs. For example, even morbidly obese patients undergoing obesity surgery have PPC rates similar to non-obese patients undergoing other abdominal surgeries. Obstructive sleep apnea is a moderate risk factor. The risk is primarily for airway management issues in the postanesthesia care unit (e.g., reintubation, hypercapnia, hypoxia), but obstructive sleep apnea may also increase the risk of traditional PPCs that contribute to morbidity. Good exercise capacity (ability to walk at least four blocks over level ground or climb two flights of stairs) confers a lower risk of PPCs.

9. **How do the site and type of surgery affect the risk of developing PPC?**
Surgical site is the single most predictive factor in assessing risk for PPCs. Proximity of the incision to the diaphragm increases the risk of developing PPCs due to splinting of the abdominal musculature and potential diaphragmatic dysfunction. Abdominal aortic aneurysm surgery carries the highest likelihood of developing PPCs, followed by thoracic and upper abdominal surgeries. Intuitively, laparoscopic surgery should be less likely to result in PPCs compared with open abdominal surgery. The available literature on this point is inconclusive.

10. **Is there a difference in PPC risk between general anesthesia and neuraxial (e.g., spinal, epidural) or regional anesthesia?**
General anesthesia carries a higher risk for PPCs than neuraxial anesthesia. Although neuraxial anesthesia may reduce the risk of PPCs in high-risk patients, in most cases it is best to leave the ultimate choice of anesthetic technique to the anesthesia team.

11. **Does the choice of neuromuscular blockade influence PPC risk?**
Longer-acting neuromuscular blockade agents such as pancuronium increase the risk for PPCs, likely due to residual neuromuscular blockade.

12. **Does emergency surgery increase the risk of PPCs?**
Emergency surgery is second only to surgical site (e.g., abdominal surgery) as a risk factor for the development of PPCs.

13. **Are there indices, similar to the cardiac risk indices, that can help predict the risk of PPCs?**
Yes. There are two well-validated indices: one to predict the risk of postoperative pneumonia and the other to predict the risk of postoperative respiratory failure. These indices are helpful tools to stratify PPC risk (Tables 75-1 and 75-2).

14. **Do preoperative chest radiographs affect preoperative management?**
Less than 1% of routine preoperative chest X-ray (CXR) results are abnormal and change management. The finding of emphysema on CXR will rarely be a surprise because this diagnosis will be apparent by history and physical examination. Obtain a routine CXR for patients older than 50 years of age undergoing major surgery, for patients with known cardiopulmonary disease and for those with symptoms that suggest possible undiagnosed cardiopulmonary disease.

15. **When is preoperative spirometry indicated, and is there a threshold below which surgery poses too much of a risk?**
Preoperative spirometry usually confirms what we already know. It is rare to find significant obstructive or restrictive impairments that are clinically unapparent or silent. Commonly obtained tests include forced expiratory capacity in 1 second (FEV_1) and forced vital capacity (FVC). Although abnormal spirometry (either low FEV_1 or FEV_1/FVC ratio) predicts PPC risks, studies that compare the value of spirometry to the clinical evaluation generally have found

TABLE 75-1. PREOPERATIVE RISK FACTORS FOR POSTOPERATIVE PNEUMONIA OR POSTOPERATIVE RESPIRATORY FAILURE

Preoperative Risk Factor	Postoperative Pneumonia Point Value	Postoperative Respiratory Failure Point Value
Type of surgery		
Abdominal aortic aneurysm	15	27
Thoracic	14	21
Upper abdominal	10	14
Neck	8	11
Neurosurgery	8	14
Vascular	3	14
Age (years)		
≥80	17	6
70–79	13	6
60–69	9	4
50–59	4	—
Functional status		
Totally dependent	10	7
Partially dependent	6	7
History of COPD	5	6
Blood urea nitrogen		
<8 mg/dL	4	—
22–30 mg/dL	2	—
≥30 mg/dL	3	8
Emergency surgery	3	11
Weight loss > 10% in past 6 months	7	—
Albumin (<3 gm/dL)	—	9
General anesthesia	4	—
Impaired sensorium	4	—
History of cerebrovascular accident	4	—
Transfusion > 4 units	3	—
Steroid use for chronic condition	3	—
Current smoker within 1 year	3	—
Alcohol intake > 2 drinks/day in past 2 weeks	2	—

Data from Arozullah AM, Daley J, Henderson WG, Khuri SF: Multifactorial risk index for predicting postoperative respiratory failure in men after major noncardiac surgery. Ann Surg 232:242–253, 2000; and Arozullah AM, Khuri SF, Henderson WG, et al: Development and validation of a multifactorial risk index for predicting postoperative pneumonia after major noncardiac surgery. Ann Intern Med 135:847–857, 2001.

**TABLE 75-2. RISK INDICES FOR PREDICTING POSTOPERATIVE PNEUMONIA
OR POSTOPERATIVE RESPIRATORY FAILURE**

Risk of Pneumonia (Total Point Range)	Risk of Respiratory Failure (Total Point Range)
0.24% (0–15)	0.5% ($\leq$10)
1.19% (16–25)	2.2% (11–19)
4.0% (26–40)	5.0% (20–27)
9.4% (41–55)	11.6% (28–40)
15.8% (>55)	30.5% (>40)

Data from Arozullah AM, Daley J, Henderson WG, Khuri SF: Multifactorial risk index for predicting postoperative respiratory failure in men after major noncardiac surgery. Ann Surg 232:242–253, 2000; and Arozullah AM, Khuri SF, Henderson WG, et al: Development and validation of a multifactorial risk index for predicting postoperative pneumonia after major noncardiac surgery. Ann Intern Med 135:847–857, 2001.

no incremental value from spirometry. Even patients with severely abnormal spirometry (e.g., FEV_1 < 0.5 L) can undergo surgery with an acceptable risk if the indication for surgery is compelling.

16. **Is there any role for preoperative arterial blood gas testing?**
    No. Hypercapnia identifies a high-risk subset of patients, but clinicians can easily identify these patients by virtue of severe obstructive lung disease discovered on history and physical examination. Even when present, hypercapnia is not an absolute contraindication to surgery. Hypoxemia does not increase risk beyond the risk due to the underlying condition, for example, COPD. Do not obtain arterial blood gas measurements as part of the routine preoperative evaluation.

KEY POINTS: PREOPERATIVE PULMONARY EVALUATION

1. All patients undergoing noncardiac surgery need a preoperative pulmonary evaluation, including an assessment of patient-related and procedure-related risk factors.

2. The risk of postoperative pneumonia and respiratory failure can be determined and used to implement a strategy to decrease the risk of postoperative complications.

3. Strategies to decrease the rate of PPCs include deep-breathing exercises, incentive spirometry, continuous positive airway pressure, epidural analgesia, and selective nasogastric decompression.

17. **What other tests help to predict PPC risk?**
    Surprisingly, serum albumin is one of the most important laboratory predictors of PPC risk. A serum albumin level of <3.0 gm/dL confers a three- to fourfold increase in PPC risk; this risk is

equal to the risk of COPD. Measure serum albumin in chronically ill patients preparing for major surgery. An unexpectedly low value should prompt reconsideration of the need for surgery.

18. **What preoperative strategies reduce PPC rates?**
Smoking cessation reduces risk, but only if begun at least 8 weeks before surgery. Teach patients effective lung expansion strategies before surgery. Optimize COPD or asthma to achieve each patient's best baseline status. If a respiratory infection is present, delay the surgery and treat with antibiotics, if appropriate.

19. **What postoperative strategies decrease the risk of PPCs?**
Table 75-3 lists the postoperative maneuvers shown to decrease the PPC risk.

TABLE 75-3. POSTOPERATIVE STRATEGIES TO REDUCE PULMONARY COMPLICATION RATES

Strategy	Comment
Deep breathing exercises	Reduces risk by 50%. Begin teaching before surgery.
Incentive spirometry	Reduces risk by 50%. No advantage to combining with deep breathing exercises.
Continuous positive airway pressure	Use for patients who cannot cooperate with deep breathing or incentive spirometry. Carries a small risk of barotrauma and requires more supervision.
Epidural analgesia	Reduces risk after thoracic, upper abdominal, and aortic surgery.
Selective nasogastric decompression	Selective use of nasogastric decompression after abdominal surgery based on symptoms or distension (as opposed to routine use) reduces PPC rates.

BIBLIOGRAPHY

1. Arozullah AM, Daley J, Henderson WG, Khuri SF: Multifactorial Risk Index for predicting postoperative respiratory failure in men after major noncardiac surgery. Ann Surg 232:242–253, 2000.
2. Arozullah AM, Khuri SF, Henderson WG, et al: Development and validation of a Multifactorial Risk Index for predicting postoperative pneumonia after major noncardiac surgery. Ann Intern Med 135:847–857, 2001.
3. Lawrence VA, Cornell JE, Smetana GW: Strategies to reduce postoperative pulmonary complications after noncardiothoracic surgery: Systematic review for the American College of Physicians. Ann Intern Med 144:596–608, 2006.
4. Smetana GW: Preoperative pulmonary evaluation. N Engl J Med 340:937–944, 1999.
5. Smetana GW, Lawrence VA, Cornell JE: Preoperative pulmonary risk stratification for non-cardiothoracic surgery: Systematic review for the American College of Physicians. Ann Intern Med 144:596–608, 2006.

CHAPTER 76

PERIOPERATIVE MANAGEMENT OF DIABETES

Bindu Sangani, MD, MPH

1. **How common is diabetes mellitus in patients undergoing surgery?**
   As of 2002, 6.3% of the U.S. population had diabetes, with an associated $92 billion in direct medical costs. A third of diabetes cases are untreated or unrecognized before surgery. It is estimated that approximately 25% of persons with diabetes will require surgery at some point. Many undergoing surgery will have preexisting microvascular and macrovascular complications at the time of the surgery.

2. **Describe the pathophysiology and classification of diabetes mellitus.**
   - **Type I:** Patients have an obligate need for insulin due to an underlying insulin deficiency as a result of an autoimmune process. Diabetic ketoacidosis and labile blood sugars are more common in this group, and insulin resistance is less important.
   - **Type II:** Type II includes 95% of persons with diabetes and the hyperglycemia is due to peripheral insulin resistance, hepatic overproduction, relative insulin deficiency, or a combination. These patients may be asymptomatic for years before diagnosis, with half having end-organ compromise at presentation.

3. **Define *Perioperative Hyperglycemia*.**
   Hyperglycemia is defined as a fasting blood sugar level > 126 mg/dL or two or more random blood sugar levels > 200 mg/dL; this finding is very common in hospitalized persons with diabetes.

KEY POINTS: CONSIDERATIONS FOR PRESCRIBING A PERIOPERATIVE DIABETIC REGIMEN

1. Type of diabetes

2. Current diabetic regimen

3. Level of glycemic control

4. Type of surgery

5. Timing of surgery

4. **What are the goals for perioperative glucose control?**
   Fasting glucose levels should ideally be < 110 mg/dL. Glucose levels should be maintained between 80–180 mg/dL at all other times. Levels above 220 mg/dL are strongly associated with worse outcomes.

5. **What factors can worsen perioperative blood sugar control?**
   Surgical stress leads to a release of counter-regulatory hormones such as cortisol, catecholamines, glucagon, and growth hormone, which enhance gluconeogenesis and

glycogenolysis, leading to increased blood glucose levels. Additionally, there is decreased insulin secretion and increased resistance to circulating insulin. Finally, medications such as vasopressors and corticosteroids can worsen glycemic control.

6. **How does poor glycemic control affect postoperative risk of infection and mortality?**

Hyperglycemia is associated with an increased risk for postoperative infection and poor wound healing. Twenty percent of perioperative deaths in patients with diabetes mellitus are due to infection, especially urinary tract and wound infections. Perioperative blood sugars > 220 mg/dL are associated with a nearly threefold higher risk of infection than diabetics with blood sugars maintained below that level. Post–coronary artery bypass graft patients experience higher rates of sternal wound infections and overall mortality when blood sugars rise above 200 mg/dL. Tight control of blood sugars between 80 and 110 mg/dL in critically ill surgical patients (5 or more days in the intensive care unit) leads to a 34% relative reduction in mortality. On the other hand, there was a relative increase in mortality by 30% for each 20 mg/dL rise of blood sugar above 100 mg/dL.

Finney SJ, Zekvaeld C, Elia A, et al: Glucose control and mortality in critically ill patients. JAMA 290:2041–2047, 2003.

Van den Berghe G, Wouters P, Weekers F, et al: Intensive insulin therapy in critically ill patients. N Engl J Med 345:1359–1367, 2001.

7. **How does poor glycemic control affect postoperative wound healing?**

Diabetic patients have a 6–40% chance of developing wound complications after surgery and are five times more susceptible to fungal and bacterial infections. Diabetics have defects in the initial inflammatory response, including decreased phagocytic and chemotactic abilities. Failure of fibroblast growth and collagen synthesis leads to poor tissue strength. Maintaining tight perioperative glycemic control improves the above factors; however, delayed wound healing can still be seen in persons with diabetes, even with noninfected wounds.

8. **How does diabetic autonomic neuropathy affect surgical outcomes?**

Autonomic neuropathy may be associated with hemodynamic lability, particularly orthostatic hypotension, and bradycardia. Gastroparesis may increase the risk of aspiration, and urinary retention may be an issue due to bladder atony.

9. **Which factors must be considered before outlining a perioperative diabetic regimen?**

The type of diabetes, preoperative antidiabetic regimen, recent level of control, and type and timing of surgery all need to be considered. In general, all oral medications and short-acting insulin (e.g., regular insulin, lispro) should be withheld on the day of surgery and restarted when the patient is tolerating oral nutrition. Metformin should be stopped 24–48 hours before surgery and restarted 24–48 hours after the oral nutrition is adequate and it can be ensured that the patient's renal function is normal.

Long-acting insulin, used as basal dosing (e.g., neutral protamine Hagedorn [NPH] or glargine), should be administered as usual the day before surgery. On the day of surgery, one-half to two-thirds of the NPH dose should be given in the morning if the surgery is minor. These patients can be given their evening dose of NPH, assuming the patient is taking adequate oral nutrition. Glargine, which most closely achieves the patient's basal insulin needs, can be given at its usual dose on the day of surgery if the patient is undergoing a minor procedure. Blood sugars should be monitored every 4 hours and covered with sliding-scale regular insulin. Patients whose blood sugars are routinely > 200 mg/dL or those undergoing major surgery should be considered for continuous insulin infusion (Table 76-1).

TABLE 76-1. MANAGEMENT OF DIABETES MEDICATIONS ON DAY OF SURGERY

	Minor Surgery	Major Surgery
DM controlled by diet alone	Monitor glucose perioperatively and treat as needed.	Monitor glucose perioperatively and treat as needed.
DM controlled by oral medications	Withhold medications on morning of surgery until after surgery and patient eating. Consider withholding metformin for 24 hours before surgery.	Withhold medications on morning of surgery. Consider holding metformin for 24 hours before surgery.
DM controlled with short-acting insulin only	Take short-acting insulin as usual the day before surgery. No insulin on morning of surgery. Resume insulin once patient is eating.	Take short-acting insulin as usual the day before surgery. No insulin on morning of surgery. Resume insulin once patient is eating.
DM controlled with basal and short-acting insulin	Take usual dose of short-acting and basal insulin the night before. Take ½ to ¾ dose of basal long-acting insulin on morning of surgery. Use less if patient is NPO past noon meal. Resume bolus insulin once patient is eating.	Take usual dose of short-acting and either full dose or ½ dose of basal insulin the night before, depending on glucose control and timing of surgery. Check blood glucose level on arrival for surgery and treat with IV insulin infusion to maintain glucose in target range.

DM = diabetes mellitus, NPO = nothing by mouth (i.e., taking no food or drink), IV = intravenous.

10. **How should insulin pumps be managed perioperatively?**
Insulin pumps use a basal rate with bolus doses given with meals based on the amount of carbohydrates eaten. Perioperatively, the basal dose should be continued without the bolus doses. Alternatively, the pump can be discontinued in favor of continuous insulin infusion (intravenous drip) or glargine insulin.

11. **Is sliding-scale insulin (SSI) monotherapy sufficient postoperatively?**
SSI should never be used as monotherapy for type I diabetes and is rarely ideal for type II diabetes. SSI treats hyperglycemia but does not prevent it. Its use is associated with poor glycemic control including hypoglycemia and hyperglycemia. In most cases, SSI should only be used as an adjunct to treating hyperglycemia in patients already taking long-acting basal therapy.

12. **Why is NPH insulin given at one half its usual dose whereas glargine is given at full dose?**
Basal insulin, the baseline amount a patient needs, should be given preoperatively while withholding short-acting bolus therapy. NPH, which is shorter acting than glargine, has peak

levels above the basal needs and therefore should be given in half the daily dose. Glargine has a much smoother effect and does not achieve peaks that are so high. Therefore, it can usually be given at its regular dose.

13. **What dose of basal and bolus insulin should be used in hyperglycemic patients who were not treated with insulin before hospitalization?**
Basal insulin doses should start at 0.1–0.3 units/kg and bolus doses at 0.02–0.1 units/kg. NPH 5–10 units given subcutaneously twice daily or glargine 10–15 units given subcutaneously daily are usually good starting doses.

14. **How should basal insulin doses be adjusted?**
Doses should be modified by 10–40% every 12 hours for NPH and every 24 hours for glargine until goal glycemic values are met. For example, a patient started on NPH 10 units twice a day, who consistently has blood sugars > 200 mg/dL, should increase by 1–4 units twice a day.

15. **When should scheduled bolus insulin be used?**
Scheduled short-acting (as opposed to SSI) bolus doses should be given once the patient starts oral nutrition. If glargine is the basal insulin, boluses will be required with each meal. For those using NPH, boluses may only be required for breakfast and dinner, depending on glucose measurements.

16. **How should insulin be dosed in patients receiving total parenteral nutrition (TPN) or tube feeds?**
TPN causes more hyperglycemia than enteral feeds. Consequently, regular insulin is often added to the nutrients in the TPN feeds. For those receiving enteral feeds, a combination of intermediate- and short-acting insulin can be administered. For instance, 70/30 insulin can be given every 8–12 hours with regular insulin coverage as needed. Oral agents alone do not usually provide adequate control.

17. **How often should glucose be monitored perioperatively?**
Patients react to surgery in different ways, and it is difficult to predict how they will react to the perioperative changes in their diabetic regimen. Additionally, hyperglycemia has more obvious and immediate effects perioperatively (e.g., infection). Consequently, more intensive monitoring is required to reduce the risk of hypoglycemia and hyperglycemia. Perioperative monitoring should occur every 4–6 hours. Intraoperative monitoring should be hourly because anesthetized patients may not exhibit signs and symptoms of hypoglycemia. Monitoring frequency can be reduced to pre-meals and bedtime when patients resume an oral diet.

18. **Which type of intravenous fluid should diabetic patients who are fasting for surgery be given?**
Assuming no compelling indication for another type or rate of fluid, patients with type I diabetes should receive one-half normal saline with 5% dextrose added (i.e., D_5 one-half normal saline) at 100 mL/h. Persons with type I diabetes are insulin deficient and therefore need insulin to move glucose into cells. Without a glucose infusion, these patients would not have a substrate to move into the cells and they would be at risk for hypoglycemia. Persons with type II diabetes can receive one-half normal saline at 100 mL/h.

19. **Which laboratory tests are indicated preoperatively in patients with diabetes?**
In addition to more stringent blood sugar monitoring, patients with diabetes should also have their renal function and electrolytes evaluated before surgery. Additionally, they should be assessed for proteinuria because diabetics with abnormal creatinine or proteinuria have an increased risk for postoperative acute renal failure.

KEY POINTS: COMMON PERIOPERATIVE COMPLICATIONS OF DIABETES MELLITUS

1. Wound infection/sepsis

2. Hypotension, cardiac ischemia, myocardial infarction

3. Acute renal insufficiency or failure

4. Stroke

5. Aspiration, urinary retention

6. Foot and pressure ulcers

20. **Is routine preoperative cardiac stress testing indicated?**
   Diabetes is a major risk factor for perioperative cardiovascular events. Diabetics have a two- to four-fold increased risk of cardiovascular complications (e.g., acute myocardial infarction, congestive heart failure, and stroke) and the need for high-risk surgery or an abnormal electrocardiogram further increases this risk. Cardiac stress testing should be considered in diabetics with poor functional status, unexplained dyspnea, or a history of angina or cardiac disease. (See Chapter 74 for more details.)

21. **Should diabetic patients with normal heart rate and blood pressure be started on perioperative beta blockers?**
   Observational and randomized controlled trials have shown that beta blockers attenuate the risk of perioperative ischemia and myocardial infarction. Diabetic patients who have no contraindication to beta-blocker use should be started on a beta blocker preoperatively and the dose titrated to a heart rate of approximately 60 beats/min. There is no clear consensus as to when the first dose should be given, but many suggest as early as possible, allowing enough time to titrate the dose to achieve the desired heart rate. Beta blockers should be continued for 30 days to provide optimal benefit in patients who do not require lifelong therapy.

22. **Should patients with impaired glucose tolerance requiring pharmacologic management of their glucose be discharged on medications?**
   If the patient's glucose normalizes postoperatively, there is no need to discharge them with medications. However, these patients should be monitored for an extended period after discharge to see whether they subsequently develop overt diabetes mellitus.

23. **How can long-term diabetes management be optimized during the hospital stay?**
   If not documented recently, a hemoglobin A1c and lipids should be assessed. Medications should be adjusted as needed to improve glucose and blood pressure control. Smokers should be counseled to quit. Dietary education should be provided, and the need for consistent follow-up and glucose monitoring should be stressed.

WEBSITES

1. American Diabetes Association: http://www.diabetes.org

2. Glycemic control information, April 2005 CME-Today website: http://www.hospitalists.cme-today.com

BIBLIOGRAPHY

1. Coursin DB, Connery LE, Ketzler JT: Perioperative diabetic and hyperglycemic management issues. Crit Care Med 32(No. 4 Suppl):S116–S125, 2004.

2. Hoogwerf BJ: Postoperative management of the diabetic patient. Med Clin North Am 85(Sep):1213–1228, 2001.

3. Schiff RL, Welsh GA: Perioperative evaluation and management of the patient with endocrine dysfunction. Med Clin North Am 87:175–192, 2003.

CHAPTER 77

PERIOPERATIVE VENOUS THROMBOEMBOLISM PROPHYLAXIS AND MANAGEMENT OF LONG-TERM WARFARIN THERAPY

Amir K. Jaffer, MD

1. **How common is venous thromboembolism (VTE) after surgery?**

   VTE is a common complication after surgery and is often silent. Overall, approximately 2 million cases of DVT and 600,000 cases of symptomatic pulmonary embolism occur annually in the United States. According to some estimates, up to one third of the patients with pulmonary embolism will die. It is estimated that about 25% of all the cases of DVT are associated with recent surgery.

2. **What factors determine the prevalence of postoperative VTE?**

   The prevalence of postoperative VTE varies based on the following factors:
   - Patient's risk factors for VTE (Table 77-1)
   - Type of surgery (Table 77-2)
   - Type and amount of prophylaxis

3. **Define and describe Virchow's triad.**

   Virchow's triad includes three underlying predisposing factors for venous thrombosis:
   - Stasis of blood flow (e.g., immobilization)
   - Endothelial injury (e.g., prior DVT)
   - Hypercoagulability (e.g., oral contraceptive therapy)

   Important patient-related risk factors for VTE reflect these underlying pathophysiologic processes and include increasing age, prolonged immobility, malignancy, prior VTE, chronic heart failure, and others listed in Table 77-1. (See Chapter 57 for more details.)

4. **How does surgery increase the risk for developing VTE?**

   During surgery, all three elements of Virchow's triad are present. The supine position coupled with anesthesia leads to stasis. The surgery itself may lead to endothelial injury, and the extent of injury ultimately depends on the type of surgery. For example, trauma to blood vessels occurs more frequently with major joint replacement, such as total knee and total hip arthroplasty, than with gall bladder surgery. Anesthesia also leads to pooling of blood in the extremities with subsequent decreased clearance of the clotting factors, leading to a hypercoagulable state, the final component of Virchow's triad.

5. **What determines the risk of VTE in patients undergoing surgery?**

   During the routine preoperative evaluation, the risk of VTE can be estimated using both patient- and surgery-specific factors. The most recent American College of Chest Physicians (ACCP) guidelines risk-stratify patients based on the type of surgery and also patient-specific risk factors. This allows for four risk categories for postoperative VTE. The corresponding options for prophylaxis in each category are outlined in Table 77-3.

TABLE 77-1. PATIENT-RELATED RISK FACTORS FOR VTE

Strong risk factors (odds ratio, >10)
   Spinal cord injury
Moderate risk factors (odds ratio, 2–9)
   Central venous lines
   Chemotherapy
   Congestive heart failure
   Respiratory failure
   Hormone replacement therapy
   Malignancy
   Oral contraceptive therapy
   Paralytic stroke
   Pregnancy (postpartum state)
   Previous venous thromboembolism
   Thrombophilia
Weak risk factors (odds ratio, <2)
   Bed rest > 3 days
   Immobility due to sitting (e.g., prolonged car or air travel)
   Increasing age
   Obesity
   Pregnancy (antepartum state)
   Varicose veins

Adapted from Anderson FA Jr, Spencer FA: Risk factors for venous thromboembolism. Circulation 107 (23 Suppl 1):I9–I16, 2003.

TABLE 77-2. SURGERY-RELATED RISK FACTORS FOR VTE

	Venographic Prevalence of DVT (%)
Strong risk factors (odds ratio, >10)	
Fracture (hip or leg)	40–60%
Hip or knee replacement	40–60%
Major general surgery	20–40%
Major trauma	40–80%
Moderate risk factors (odds ratio, 2–9)	
Arthroscopic knee surgery	10–20%
Weak risk factors (odds ratio, <2)	
Laparoscopic surgery (e.g., cholecystectomy)	0–10%

TABLE 77-3. VTE PROPHYLAXIS RECOMMENDATIONS ACCORDING TO TYPE OF SURGERY- AND PATIENT-RELATED RISK FACTORS

Level of Risk*	Evidence-based VTE Prophylaxis Options
Low	Early ambulation
Moderate	LDUH q12h or LMWH daily or GCS or IPC
High	LDUH q8h or LMWH or IPC
Highest	LMWH or fondaparinux or warfarin or (IPC/GCS + LDUH q8h or LMWH)[†]

LDUH = low-dose unfractionated heparin, LMWH = low-molecular-weight heparin, GCS = graded compression stockings, IPC = intermittent pneumatic compression device.
*See question 5 for definitions for low, moderate, high, and highest risk.
[†]Recommended LMWH dosing: enoxaparin, 40 mg given subcutaneously daily, or dalteparin, 5000 IU given subcutaneously daily. For total knee procedures consider enoxaparin, 30 mg given subcutaneously every 12 hours, or fondaparinux, 2.5 mg given subcutaneously daily.

- **Low risk:** Patients undergoing minor surgery and younger than 40 years old with no additional risk factors for VTE
- **Moderate risk:** Patients undergoing minor surgery with additional risk factors or major surgery, age 40–60 years, with no additional risk factors
- **High risk:** Patients over the age of 60 years undergoing major surgery without risk factors or major surgery in a patient age 40–60 years with additional risk factors
- **Highest risk:** Patients with multiple risk factors undergoing major surgery, or patients undergoing surgeries with the highest risk: hip or knee arthroplasty, hip fracture surgery, pelvic or abdominal cancer surgery, major trauma surgery, or surgery for spinal cord injury

6. **List some of the available nonpharmacologic options for VTE prevention.**
   - Ambulation is a goal for all patients as soon as possible after surgery.
   - Elastic compression stockings may be used in combination with pharmacologic measures for higher-risk patients but should be used alone only for low-risk patients.
   - Intermittent pneumatic compression devices alone may be effective in high-risk surgical patients but require that they fit properly and be maintained on the patient for approximately 15 h/day to achieve maximal benefit.

   These modalities may be used in those patients who are considered to be at high risk for bleeding after major surgery (e.g., after craniotomy or spine surgery) or used in combination with pharmacologic prophylaxis in the highest-risk patients.

KEY POINTS: POSTOPERATIVE VTE PROPHYLAXIS

1. The prevalence of postoperative VTE is high.

2. Estimate VTE risk by using patient-related risk factors and the type of surgery.

3. VTE risk can be stratified into low-, moderate-, high-, and highest-risk categories.

4. Use the evidence-based prophylaxis recommendations from the ACCP.

7. **What are the available pharmacologic options for VTE prevention?**
   - **Aspirin:** Aspirin inhibits platelet aggregation and is not very effective for prophylaxis against VTE. The ACCP guidelines recommend *against* its use as a single prophylactic agent.
   - **Unfractionated heparin (UFH):** UFH, which inhibits factors II and X, is inexpensive but has a short half-life requiring subcutaneous (SC) dosing two or three times daily for maximal benefit. The anticoagulant effect can be easily reversed with protamine if needed. However, its use carries a significant risk of heparin-induced thrombocytopenia (HIT) (~3% in the postoperative setting).
   - **Warfarin (Coumadin):** This medication inhibits vitamin K–dependent clotting factors II, V, VII, and IX. It is inexpensive and has the advantage of oral administration. However, it requires monitoring with an international normalized ratio (INR), has multiple drug and food interactions, and has a narrow therapeutic index. In addition, it takes approximately 5 days to achieve its maximal anticoagulant effect, and therefore patients are at increased risk for VTE while the INR is subtherapeutic.
   - **Low-molecular-weight heparins (LMWHs):** LMWHs are derived from UFH through a chemical process. They preferentially inhibit factor X more than factor II. They are well absorbed from SC tissue and can be administered once or twice daily. The drugs are renally cleared and cause less HIT compared with UFH. Although they are more expensive, they may be more cost-effective due to less intensive monitoring. Enoxaparin (Lovenox) can be used in renal insufficiency with creatinine clearance of < 30 mL/min (as long as the patient does not have end-stage renal disease on dialysis) by decreasing the recommended dose from 40 mg SC once daily to 30 mg SC once daily.
   - **Fondaparinux (Arixtra):** This is a synthetic pentasaccharide that inhibits factor X, has a long half-life of 18 hours, and is dosed once daily SC. It has a rapid onset of action, but the anticoagulant effect cannot be easily reversed in case of severe bleeding. The drug is cleared by the kidneys and therefore contraindicated in patients with creatinine clearances < 30 mL/min. It does not cause HIT. It is best to start administration of this drug at least 12 hours after surgery, but generally they are begun 18–24 hours after surgery to minimize the risk of bleeding

8. **Outline the surgery-specific VTE prophylaxis recommendations.**
   In addition to Table 77-3, which was developed using both patient-related and surgery-related risk factors by the ACCP, the surgery-specific recommendations for VTE prophylaxis are outlined in Table 77-4.

9. **Which patients need extended prophylaxis after surgery?**
   Certain surgeries confer a high risk for VTE even after discharge from the hospital. Patient groups who benefit from extended prophylaxis include:
   - Patients undergoing abdominal and pelvic cancer surgery, for up to 28 days after surgery
   - Patients undergoing total hip replacement and hip fracture surgery, for up to 35 days after surgery
   Options for extended prophylaxis include LMWHs, fondaparinux, or warfarin.

10. **Do patients undergoing neuroaxial blockade (e.g., spinal and epidural anesthesia) require special attention with regard to perioperative anticoagulation?**
    Spinal hematoma may complicate spinal or epidural anesthesia in patients receiving pharmacologic VTE prophylaxis if special precautions are not exercised. Some important recommendations include:
    - **Placement of epidural catheter:** Withhold prophylactic LMWH for 12 hours and treatment-dose LMWH for 24 hours before placing an epidural catheter. Withhold warfarin for 4–5 days before catheter insertion and ensure INR < 1.5.
    - **Removal of epidural catheter:** Wait 12 hours after a prophylactic dose and wait 2 hours before initiating anticoagulation.

TABLE 77-4. VTE PROPHYLAXIS RECOMMENDATIONS FOR PATIENTS ACCORDING TO TYPE OF SURGERY

Type of Surgery	Type of Prophylaxis*	Duration
Low-risk general surgery	Early mobilization	Until ambulation or discharge
Moderate-risk general surgery	UFH 5000 U SC b.i.d. or LMWH	Until ambulation or discharge
High-risk general surgery	UFH 5000 U SC t.i.d. or LMWH plus IPC or GCS	Until ambulation or discharge, but up to 28 days in major abdominal or pelvic cancer surgery is preferred
Vascular surgery	UFH 5000 U SC b.i.d. or t.i.d. or LMWH	Until ambulation or discharge
Laparoscopic gynecologic surgery > 30 min	UFH 5000 U SC t.i.d. or LMWH plus IPC or GCS	Until ambulation or discharge
Major gynecologic surgery	UFH 5000 U SC t.i.d. or LMWH plus IPC or GCS	Until ambulation or discharge
Urologic surgery other than low-risk	UFH 5000 U SC t.i.d. or LMWH plus IPC or GCS	Until ambulation or discharge
Major joint replacement (e.g., total knee or hip replacement)	LMWH or VKA or fondaparinux†	At least 10 days, and up to 28–35 days for THR is preferred
Hip fracture surgery	Fondaparinux or LMWH or VKA	At least 10 days, and up to 28 days is preferred
Neurosurgery	IPC ± GCS	Until ambulation or discharge
Extracranial	IPC ± GCS	
Intracranial	LMWH or UFH can be added if risk of bleeding is acceptable	

b.i.d. = twice a day, t.i.d. = three times a day, IPC = intermittent pneumatic compression, GCS = graded compression stockings, VKA = vitamin K antagonists (e.g., warfarin), THR = total hip replacement.
*LMWH dosing = enoxaparin, 40 mg SC daily; dalteparin, 5000 IU SC daily; or tinzaparin, 75 IU/kg daily.
†Fondaparinux = 2.5 mg SC daily.
Adapted from Geerts WH, Pineo GF, Heit JA, et al: Prevention of venous thromboembolism: The Seventh ACCP Conference on Antithrombotic and Thrombolytic Therapy. Chest 126(3 Suppl):338S–400S, 2004.

11. **Is warfarin use a problem for patients undergoing an interventional procedure or surgery?**

Periprocedural management of patients who take warfarin is often problematic because of warfarin's long half-life. The drug must be discontinued or the dose adjusted to avoid excessive bleeding, placing patients at risk for recurrent thromboembolism. Therefore, many physicians use "bridging" therapy with short-acting anticoagulants such as UFH or LMWH for patients at moderate or high risk for thromboembolism while the effects of warfarin are wearing off (Table 77-5). A step-by-step protocol to help clinicians perform bridging therapy is outlined in Table 77-6.

TABLE 77-5. THROMBOEMBOLISM RISK STRATIFICATION

High risk: bridging advised

1. Venous or arterial thromboembolism within the preceding 3 months
2. Mechanical heart valve
   - In the mitral position
   - Any position with placement in the preceding 3 months
   - Older valves (e.g., tilting disk, cage ball)
3. History of thromboembolism and known hypercoagulable state
4. Acute intracardiac thrombus
5. Atrial fibrillation
   - With history of stroke, TIA, or systemic embolism
   - Associated with rheumatic valve disease
   - With mechanical valve
   - With multiple risk factors for stroke (e.g., age > 75, HF, DM, HTN)

Moderate risk: bridging on a case-by-case basis

6. Newer mechanical aortic valve (bi-leaflet)
7. Atrial fibrillation with risk factors for stroke
8. Venous thromboembolism within the past 3–6 months

Low risk: bridging not recommended

9. Venous thromboembolism
   - More than 6 months ago
   - Heterozygous factor V Leiden
10. Atrial fibrillation without risk factors

TIA = transient ischemic attack, HF = heart failure, DM = diabetes, HTN = hypertension.
Adapted from Jaffer AK, Brotman DJ, Chukwumerije N: When patients on warfarin need surgery. Cleve Clin J Med 70(11):973–984, 2003.

KEY POINTS: PERIOPERATIVE MANAGEMENT OF LONG-TERM WARFARIN

1. Determine the type of procedure or surgery the patient is having.
2. Determine the patient's risk of thromboembolism if warfarin is stopped.
3. Develop a plan in discussion with the patient, surgeon, and anesthesiologist.
4. Use bridging therapy, if indicated, and provide the patient with written instructions.
5. Follow the patient postoperatively to help guide therapy.

TABLE 77-6. PROTOCOL FOR BRIDGING THERAPY WITH LMWH

Preprocedure Protocol	Postprocedure Protocol
If INR 2–3, stop warfarin 5 days (4 doses) before procedure.	Restart LMWH* approximately 24 hours postprocedure, or consider using a thromboprophylaxis dose of LMWH on postprocedure days 1–3 if patient is at high risk for bleeding.
If INR 3–4.5, stop warfarin 6 days (5 doses) before procedure.	Confer with the surgeon regarding plan to restart anticoagulant therapy.
Start LMWH* 36 hours after last warfarin dose.	Start warfarin at patient's preoperative dose on postoperative day 1.
Give last dose of LMWH 24 hours before procedure.	Check INR daily until patient is discharged and periodically thereafter until INR therapeutic.
Ensure patient is thoroughly educated in self-injection.	Check CBC with platelets at days 3 and 7.
Confer with surgeon and anesthesiologist regarding planned bridging therapy.	Discontinue LMWH when INR is therapeutic for 2 consecutive days.
Check INR on morning of procedure.	

CBC = complete blood cell count.
*Enoxaparin, 1 mg/kg SC every 12 hours, or 1.5 mg/kg SC every 24 hours, or dalteparin, 120 U/kg every 12 hours, or dalteparin, 200 U/kg SC every 24 hours.
Adapted from Jaffer AK, Brotman DJ, Chukwumerije N: When patients on warfarin need surgery. Cleve Clin J Med 70(11):973–984, 2003.

12. **Which surgeries can be performed without discontinuing administration of warfarin?**
Table 77-7 outlines examples of procedures that can be accomplished without stopping warfarin.

13. **How many days before elective surgery should the warfarin be discontinued?**
The goal is to have the preoperative INR < 1.5. White and colleagues showed that for almost all patients with a steady state INR of 2 to 3, the INR falls to below 1.5 within 115 hours (4.8 days) after warfarin is discontinued. Therefore, warfarin should be discontinued 5 days (or held for four doses) before the procedure. If the preoperative target INR range is over 3, the patient is elderly, or both, more time may be required for the INR to drop below 1.5 and therefore patients should be advised to stop taking warfarin 6 days (or held for five doses) before the procedure. If the surgery is emergent (within 12 hours of admission to the hospital) then fresh frozen plasma in addition to intravenous vitamin K (1–2 mg) should be used to lower the INR and to reverse the effects of warfarin. In the case of surgeries occurring >24 hours after admission to the hospital, oral vitamin K (2.5 mg) may be sufficient to reverse the effects of warfarin.

White RH, McKittrick T, Hutchinson R, Twitchell J: Temporary discontinuation of warfarin therapy: Changes in the international normalized ratio. Ann Intern Med 122:40–42, 1995.

TABLE 77-7. EXAMPLES OF PROCEDURES THAT CAN BE PERFORMED WITHOUT STOPPING WARFARIN

Dental
Uncomplicated extractions
Dental hygiene treatment
Periodontal therapy
Gastrointestinal
Upper endoscopy, sigmoidoscopy, or colonoscopy with or without biopsy
Endoscopic retrograde cholangiopancreatography without sphincterotomy
Electroconvulsive therapy
Ophthalmologic
Cataract extractions
Dermatologic
Simple excisions and repairs
Orthopedic
Joint aspiration
Soft tissue injections

WEBSITE

American Society of Regional Anesthesia and Pain Medicine: http://www.asra.com

BIBLIOGRAPHY

1. Bartholomew JR, Begelman SM, Almahameed A: Heparin-induced thrombocytopenia: Principles for early recognition and management. Cleve Clin J Med 72(Suppl 1):S31–S36, 2005.

2. Eikelboom JW, Quinlan DJ, Douketis JD: Extended-duration prophylaxis against venous thromboembolism after total hip or knee replacement: A meta-analysis of the randomized trials. Lancet 358:9–15, 2001.

3. Geerts WH, Pineo GF, Heit JA, et al: Prevention of venous thromboembolism: The Seventh ACCP Conference on Antithrombotic and Thrombolytic Therapy. Chest 126(3 Suppl):338S–400S, 2004.

4. Horlocker TT: Thromboprophylaxis and neuraxial anesthesia. Orthopedics 26(2 Suppl):S243–S249, 2003.

5. Jaffer AK, Brotman DJ, Chukwumerije N: When patients on warfarin need surgery. Cleve Clin J Med 70:973–984, 2003.

6. Turpie AG, Bauer KA, Eriksson BI, Lassen MR: Postoperative fondaparinux versus postoperative enoxaparin for prevention of venous thromboembolism after elective hip-replacement surgery: A randomized double-blind trial. Lancet 359:1721–1726, 2002.

CHAPTER 78

POSTOPERATIVE FEVER

James C. Pile, MD

1. **What is the definition of *fever*?**

   Fever is defined as the regulated elevation of normal body temperature. Based on Wunderlich's work in the 19th century, 37.0°C is commonly cited as "normal" body temperature, although the population mean appears to be slightly lower. A temperature of 38.0°C or higher is a useful, if imperfect, criterion for the diagnosis of fever.

2. **What is the pathophysiology of fever?**

   The body generates fever through a complex set of interactions that remain incompletely understood. Pyrogenic cytokines including interleukin–1 and –6, tumor necrosis factor-α, and interferon-γ are released through a variety of stimuli ranging from infection to trauma, and they operate on temperature regulatory sites in and around the hypothalamus (i.e., the preoptic area). Prostaglandins are then released from the preoptic area, leading to fever mediated by shivering and peripheral vasoconstriction.

3. **How frequent is postoperative fever?**

   Fever in the postoperative period is clearly a common phenomenon. Frequency ranges from 13% to 91%, related in large part to the surgical populations studied as well as the definition of fever. The majority of fever appears in the first 24–48 hours postoperatively and resolves within several days.

4. **What is the most common cause of postoperative fever?**

   An increasing body of evidence supports the idea that most fever results from the release of the pyrogenic cytokines mentioned above as a direct effect of surgical trauma. The extent and type of surgery appears to have a strong correlation with the likelihood of early postoperative fever. For example, an open cholecystectomy conveys a much higher risk of postoperative fever than laparoscopic cholecystectomy. Table 78-1 summarizes the various causes of postoperative fever.

5. **What are the uncommon but not-to-be-missed causes of postoperative fever?**

   - Myocardial infarction
   - Wound myonecrosis
   - Acute adrenal insufficiency
   - Thyroid storm
   - Peritoneal soilage (after intra-abdominal procedures)
   - Stroke
   - Toxic shock syndrome (staphylococcal or streptococcal species)
   - Alcohol withdrawal/delirium tremens

6. **When do surgical site infections (SSIs) typically occur in the postoperative period?**

   The appearance of SSIs is uncommon in the first 2 days after surgery, and the median onset of SSIs is roughly 1 week postoperatively. One important exception to this is wound myonecrosis, which may occur within hours after surgery. This infection, typically caused by either *Clostridium perfringens* or *Streptococcus pyogenes*, is a surgical emergency that requires urgent debridement in addition to antibiotics.

TABLE 78-1. CAUSES OF POSTOPERATIVE FEVER

More Common	Less Common
Direct surgical trauma related	Blood product transfusion reactions
Urinary tract infection	Hematoma
Surgical site infection	Adrenal insufficiency
(including intra-abdominal abscess)	Intravascular device–related infections
Pneumonia	Endocarditis
Clostridium difficile related	Osteomyelitis
Aspiration pneumonitis	Orthopedic hardware–related infections
Venous thromboembolic disease	Acalculous cholecystitis
Gout/pseudogout	Parotitis
Medication induced	Sinusitis
	Wound myonecrosis (group A *Streptococcus, Clostridium perfringens*)
	Blood product–related infections (e.g., cytomegalovirus, West Nile virus)
	Pancreatitis
	Myocardial infarction
	Stroke
	Transplant rejection
	Fat embolism
	Hyperthyroidism ("thyroid storm")
	Alcohol/drug withdrawal syndromes
	Malignancy related
	Malignant hyperthermia

7. **Under which circumstances may postoperative fever be ignored?**
   Although the majority of fevers occurring early in the postoperative period will prove to be benign and self-limited, this cannot be assumed, and the presence of fever after surgery can *never* be safely ignored. Although this applies to fevers appearing in the first 48 hours postoperatively, it is particularly true for fevers appearing on postoperative day 3 or later.

8. **What is the most common cause of fever and diarrhea in the postoperative period?**
   Clostridium difficile colitis is by far the most common culprit in this setting. Hallmarks of *C. difficile* infection include the following:
   - Preceding antibiotic exposure is a common cause; this may be as little as a single prophylactic doses perioperatively.
   - Symptomatic disease may present from 1 day to 1 month after antibiotic exposure.
   - Leukocytosis usually but not always accompanies fever. Those persons with fever and leukocytosis tend to have more severe disease than those who do not.
   - Diarrhea may be absent, and in fact its absence is a risk factor for more severe disease.

9. **Can deep venous thrombosis and pulmonary embolism cause fever?**
   Although a relative paucity of data exists to address this question, an abundance of anecdotal evidence suggests the answer is "yes." In the Prospective Investigation of Pulmonary Embolism Diagnosis (PIOPED) study, 14% of patients with pulmonary embolism and no other discernible

source exhibited fever. Most of these fevers were low grade, although a few patients developed maximum temperatures in excess of 38.8°C.

10. Which drugs are most likely to cause fever in postoperative patients?
Many drugs used in the perioperative period can cause fever, although this is another relatively understudied area. Those agents most strongly linked to fever include antibiotics (especially β-lactams, sulfonamides, and amphotericin B), phenytoin, carbamazepine, and histamine$_2$ blockers. Heparin products (both unfractionated and low molecular weight), although an unusual cause of drug fever, should nonetheless be considered as possible causes given their ubiquitous use in the postoperative setting.

11. Does atelectasis cause fever?
Despite generations of medical students and physicians learning as dogma the "fact" that atelectasis causes most cases of postoperative fever, available data do not support this association. Engoren, for example, demonstrated elegantly that as atelectasis increased shortly after cardiothoracic surgery, fever actually decreased. Attribution of postoperative fevers without another obvious cause to atelectasis resulted, and still results, from a failure to appreciate surgical trauma–mediated release of inflammatory cytokines.

Engoren M: Lack of association between atelectasis and fever. Chest 107:81–84, 1995.

12. Which features of the history should be emphasized in a patient with a postoperative fever?
- Prior history of certain comorbid conditions (e.g., history of crystal arthropathy, atherosclerotic vascular disease)
- Allergies
- Details of the surgery (e.g., operative note, conversation with surgeon)
- All current and recent medications
- Recent administration of blood products
- Cough/sputum production
- Diarrhea
- Location and duration of intravascular catheters

13. Describe the parts of the physical examination that should be emphasized in a patient with postoperative fever.
The examination should begin with a review of the patient's vital signs, including the temperature curve. The cardiovascular examination should evaluate for new murmurs, and the lungs should be assessed for crackles, evidence of consolidation, or dullness. The abdomen should be carefully examined, especially after intra-abdominal surgeries or if *C. difficile* infection is a consideration, joints should be assessed for inflammation, and catheter entry sites should be closely evaluated for inflammatory changes. A careful skin examination is mandatory, with particular attention paid to the operative site.

KEY POINTS: POSTOPERATIVE FEVER

1. Timing of fever in the postoperative period provides a valuable clue to etiology.

2. The majority of postoperative fevers are noninfectious, particularly when the fever occurs in the initial postoperative period.

3. The nature of the surgical procedure dictates consideration of specific causes of postoperative fever.

4. SSIs will frequently mandate a return to the operating theater in addition to antibiotics.

14. **Which laboratory studies should be obtained when evaluating postoperative fever?**

    Laboratory and imaging studies should be ordered judiciously because multiple studies have indicated that their yield is very low when ordered indiscriminately in the setting of postoperative fever. Blood cultures, in particular, are markedly over-ordered in this setting. Febrile patients who appear generally well in the early postoperative period most often do not require any additional studies after a reassuring history and physical examination has been performed. The same principles apply to ordering imaging studies, with the caveat that computed tomography of the abdomen and pelvis should be considered early in the course of the patient who has undergone intra-abdominal surgery.

15. **Should patients with postoperative fever be treated with antibiotics?**

    In general, postoperative patients with fever should not receive antibiotics unless a specific infectious process has been identified. One exception is a toxic-appearing patient; many patients in this condition will require a return to the operating theater in addition to antibiotics.

16. **Identify the pathologic processes that are likely to be encountered in febrile patients after various types of surgery.**

    See Table 78-2.

TABLE 78–2. LIKELY PATHOLOGIC PROCESSES IN FEBRILE PATIENTS AFTER VARIOUS TYPES OF SURGERY

Type of Surgery	Likely Sources of Postoperative Fever
Cardiothoracic	Mediastinitis
	Sternal osteomyelitis
	Endocarditis
Obstetric/gynecologic	Endometritis
	Intra-abdominal/intra-pelvic abscesses
	Suppurative pelvic vein thrombosis (consider especially if fever is prolonged and cryptic)
Intra-abdominal	Intra-abdominal abscesses
	Peritonitis
	Pancreatitis
Orthopedic	Early prosthetic joint infection (especially with *Staphylococcus aureus*)
	Venous thromboembolic disease
Transplant	First several weeks postoperatively: typical bacterial infections predominate
	1–6 months postoperatively: opportunistic infections common
	Noninfectious causes include drug fever, acute rejection episodes

BIBLIOGRAPHY

1. Badillo AT, Sarani B, Evans SRT: Optimizing the use of blood cultures in the febrile postoperative patient. J Am Coll Surg 194:477–487, 2002.
2. Dellinger EP: Approach to the patient with postoperative fever. In Gorbach SL, Bartlett JG, Blacklow NR (eds): Infectious Diseases, 3rd ed. Philadelphia, Lippincott Williams & Wilkins, 2004, pp 817–823.
3. Engoren ME: Lack of association between atelectasis and fever. Chest 107:81–84, 1995.
4. Frank SM, Kluger MJ, Kunkel SL: Elevated setpoint in postoperative patients. Anesthesiology 93:1426–1431, 2000.
5. Mackowiak PA: Concepts of fever. Arch Intern Med 158:1870–1881, 1998.
6. Shaw JA, Chung R: Febrile response after knee and hip arthroplasty. Clin Orthop Rel Res 367:181–189, 1999.

CHAPTER 79

MEDICAL PROBLEMS IN PREGNANCY

Anna Kho, MD, and Noble Maleque, MD

1. **Name the major physiologic changes that occur in pregnancy.**
   See Table 79-1.

TABLE 79-1. PHYSIOLOGIC CHANGES DURING PREGNANCY	
Parameters	**Physiologic Changes**
Systemic vascular resistance	↓
Cardiac output	↑
Blood volume	↑
Red cell volume	↑
Plasma volume	↑
Hematocrit	↓
Tidal volume	↑
Forced vital capacity	No change
Forced expiratory volume in 1 second	No change
Creatinine clearance	↑
Thyroid stimulating hormone	↓ early on, then normalizes later
Free thyroxine	No change

↓ = decreases, ↑ = increases.

2. **What is the most common medical illness complicating pregnancy?**
   Approximately 20–50% of all pregnancies are complicated by hypertension. Hypertension in pregnancy is diagnosed like other types of hypertension, that is, blood pressure ≥ 140/90 mmHg. However, all pregnant women with hypertension should be evaluated for preeclampsia with a complete blood count, blood urea nitrogen and creatinine measurements, liver function tests, and coagulation panel. Four types of hypertensive disorders can complicate pregnancy (Table 79-2).
   - **Type I hypertension:** Also known as *preeclampsia-eclampsia* or *pregnancy-induced hypertension,* type I hypertension refers to new-onset hypertension and proteinuria occurring after 20 weeks of gestation. It complicates 5% of pregnancies and is associated with a defect in placental implantation. Additional clinical features include visual disturbances (e.g., scotomas and scintillations), headaches, epigastric discomfort (due to hepatic edema and capsule swelling), edema of the hands and face, and retinal disease. Patients with preeclampsia may also experience HELLP syndrome (*h*emolysis, *e*levated *l*iver enzymes, and *l*ow *p*latelets), elevated uric acid levels, disseminated intravascular coagulopathy, and renal failure. *Eclampsia* refers to generalized tonic-clonic seizures associated with the preeclamptic state. Primigravida patients and those with twin gestation, diabetes, chronic hypertension, obesity, a personal or family history of preeclampsia, renal disease, and connective tissue

TABLE 79-2. CLASSIFICATION OF HYPERTENSION IN PREGNANCY BY THE AMERICAN COLLEGE OF OBSTETRICS AND GYNECOLOGY

Type	Hypertensive Disorder
I	Preeclampsia/eclampsia
II	Chronic hypertension
III	Preeclampsia superimposed upon chronic hypertension
IV	Gestational hypertension

disease are at the highest risk for developing preeclampsia. Additionally, African-American women are at greater risk for developing this disorder.
- **Type II hypertension:** Type II, or chronic hypertension, is diagnosed when there is a history of hypertension before pregnancy or when repeated blood pressures are ≥ 140/90 mmHg before 20 weeks of gestation.
- **Type III hypertension:** Type III hypertension of pregnancy is the combination of preeclampsia superimposed on chronic hypertension.
- **Type IV hypertension:** Also known as gestational hypertension, type IV hypertension develops during the last month of pregnancy but normalizes postpartum.

3. **At what blood pressure should pregnant women be treated?**
Although pregnant patients with a blood pressure ≥ 140/90 mmHg are considered hypertensive, treatment is not initiated until the blood pressure becomes > 160/110 mmHg. Treating a diastolic blood pressure < 110 mmHg has not been shown to improve fetal or maternal outcomes, and lowering the patient's blood pressure too much may decrease blood flow to the placenta and fetus.

4. **What is the recommended antihypertensive agent used for treating hypertension in pregnancy?**
Methyldopa, labetalol, and hydralazine remain the drugs of choice in treating chronic and gestational hypertension.

5. **What therapies are used to treat preeclampsia?**
Patients with blood pressures ≥ 160/110 mmHg should be treated with intravenous labetalol, hydralazine, or nitroprusside to keep a mean arterial pressure below 126 mmHg. Nitroprusside use is associated with fetal cyanide toxicity, so extended use is not recommended. In addition, seizure prophylaxis with intravenous magnesium sulfate should also be provided. The only cure for patients with preeclampsia or preeclampsia superimposed on chronic hypertension is fetal delivery.

6. **What is the differential diagnosis of shortness of breath in pregnancy?**
The differential diagnosis includes asthma, pneumonia, aspiration, venous thromboembolic disease (VTE), amniotic fluid embolism, congestive heart failure, peripartum cardiomyopathy, valvular heart disease, dyspnea of pregnancy, acute lung injury from tocolytic treatment, and sepsis.

7. **How common is asthma in pregnancy, and how is it managed?**
Asthma affects approximately 4% of all pregnancies and is the most common pulmonary illness seen in pregnancy. About one third of pregnant women with a history of asthma do well during pregnancy, one third remain the same, and one third worsen. Treatment for this disease is similar in pregnancy as in nonpregnant patients, except for a few caveats. First, oxygen saturation should be maintained above 95% to ensure adequate fetal oxygenation. Second,

epinephrine and leukotriene inhibitors should be avoided because the former can cause uterine contractions and the latter has not been used enough to establish its safety. All other standard forms of treatment for asthma can be safely given in pregnancy, including inhaled beta agonists, steroids, and theophylline.

8. **How common is VTE in pregnancy?**
About 1 in 1000–2000 pregnancies is complicated by VTE. It is also the most common cause of non-obstetric mortality in pregnancy. VTE occurs at a similar rate throughout all three trimesters and commonly occurs postpartum. Patients who undergo a cesarean section are twice as likely to develop VTE as those who undergo a vaginal delivery. Therefore, understanding the management and treatment of VTE in pregnancy is especially important.

9. **How should VTE be managed in pregnancy?**
   - **Unfractionated heparin (UFH):** Once VTE has been diagnosed, intravenous UFH should be initiated to achieve a partial thromboplastin time (PTT) of 1.5–2 times the control value. After 5 days of intravenous therapy, adjusted-dose subcutaneous UFH every 12 hours may be started to maintain a PTT of two times the control value. For example, if a patient requires a total of 20,000 units of intravenous UFH per day to achieve a therapeutic PTT, divide this dose in two and administer 10,000 units of subcutaneous UFH every 12 hours. After receiving subcutaneous UFH for 24 hours, check the PTT 6 hours after UFH administration to ensure the PTT is maintained at two times the control value.
   - **Low-molecular-weight heparin (LMWH):** LMWH can also be used in the treatment of VTE in pregnancy. LMWH may be initiated at 1 mg/kg given subcutaneously every 12 hours but should be adjusted to keep the anti-Xa levels between 0.6–1.0 U/mL 4 hours postinjection. There is no consensus on the duration of anticoagulation for VTE in pregnancy, but most experts recommend anticoagulation for 3–6 months. Some experts continue anticoagulation until delivery. Peripartum, stop UFH and LMWH 24 hours before the epidural is placed to minimize the risk of an epidural hematoma. Resume UFH or LMWH postpartum when hemostasis has been established, with plans to convert to warfarin for 4–6 weeks postpartum (due to the high incidence of VTE that occurs postpartum). If LMWH is continued until term, the drug is stopped 24 hours before the epidural is placed to minimize the risk of an epidural hematoma. Therefore, this is best done with a planned date for induction of the pregnancy.

10. **Which medication should be avoided in the treatment of VTE in pregnancy?**
Warfarin crosses the placenta and is teratogenic, causing skeletal malformations, intracerebral hemorrhaging, and mental retardation. However, postpartum, warfarin may be used during breastfeeding since it is not excreted in breast milk.

11. **Which diagnostic tests can be safely obtained in pregnant women?**
Almost all radiologic tests can be safely performed in pregnancy as long as the total amount of radiation exposure is kept below 5 rads (cumulative throughout the entire pregnancy). Above the 5-rad limit, there is a slight increase in the risk of childhood leukemia (about 1 in 2000 versus 1 in 3000 in the general population). However, a few key points must be kept in mind when ordering a radiologic study in pregnancy:
   - Always inform the radiologist of the patient's pregnancy to ensure that the optimal test is ordered to minimize fetal radiation exposure.
   - Although no adverse fetal effects have been reported with the use of intravenous contrast, informing the radiologist of the patient's pregnancy will limit the amount of contrast used during the diagnostic study.
   - Never order a study with the word "radioactive" in its title (such as a radioactive iodine uptake and scan, or radioablation). At 10 weeks gestation, the fetal thyroid begins to trap iodine and exposure to radioactive iodine can cause thyroid ablation and hypothyroidism.

- Avoid all forms of magnetic resonance imaging during the first trimester because its safety has not been well established.

12. **What is the differential diagnosis for proteinuria in pregnancy?**
An often used mnemonic to recall the differential diagnosis of proteinuria is Proteinuria Is **NOT** Very **G**lamorous:
- **P:** Preeclampsia
- **I:** Infection
- **N:** Nephrotic syndrome
- **O:** Orthostatic
- **T:** Transient (7% of cases; benign)
- **V:** Vaginal contaminants (e.g., amniotic fluid, vaginal secretions)
- **G:** Glomerular disease (e.g., glomerulonephritis, polycystic kidney disease)

13. **What are some of the causes of nausea and vomiting in pregnancy?**
Hyperemesis gravidarum, gastrointestinal disorders (e.g., gastroenteritis, hepatitis, pancreatitis), genitourinary tract disorders, diabetes, migraines/headaches, drug toxicity, preeclampsia, HELLP syndrome, and fatty liver of pregnancy.

14. **What is hyperemesis gravidarum?**
Hyperemesis gravidarum presents in the first trimester of pregnancy as intractable vomiting, weight loss of >5% of body weight and ketonuria. Other metabolic derangements include hypokalemia and metabolic alkalosis. Most symptoms of hyperemesis gravidarum resolve spontaneously after the 18th week of pregnancy. Initial treatment involves rehydration, bowel rest, and antiemetics. Early reintroduction of a diet rich in carbohydrates and low in fat is essential.

15. **Name some of the liver diseases commonly seen in pregnancy.**
Pregnant women are susceptible to the same hepatic ailments as nonpregnant women. Additionally, they can suffer from acute fatty liver of pregnancy, intrahepatic cholestasis of pregnancy, and HELLP syndrome. The levels of total bilirubin, alanine aminotransferase, aspartate aminotransferase, prothrombin time, and PTT are useful in differentiating between various causes of pregnancy-induced liver disease. Table 79-3 lists the time course, symptoms, laboratory findings, complications, and management of these various conditions.

16. **What are tocolytic agents?**
Tocolytic agents are used in preterm labor to delay uterine contractions. Commonly used tocolytics include magnesium sulfate and beta-receptor agonists (e.g., terbutaline, ritodrine, albuterol).

KEY POINTS: MEDICAL PROBLEMS IN PREGNANCY

1. Methyldopa is the treatment of choice for hypertension in pregnancy.

2. The only definitive treatment for preeclampsia is fetal delivery.

3. Necessary radiologic studies should not be withheld just because the patient is pregnant. However, the amount of contrast and radiation should be limited and all radioactive studies should be avoided.

4. Abnormal urinalysis should lead to further investigation (bacteriuria or proteinuria).

5. Hyperemesis gravidarum is severe nausea/vomiting in the first trimester that can lead to severe metabolic derangements.

6. Acute fatty liver of pregnancy and HELLP syndrome require urgent delivery of newborn.

TABLE 79-3. COMMON LIVER DISORDERS IN PREGNANCY

	Time Course	Symptoms	Laboratory Tests	Complications	Management
Acute fatty liver of pregnancy	Third trimester	Sudden-onset nausea/ vomiting in 70% RUQ pain 50–80% Flu-like symptoms	Leukocytosis DIC pattern Bilirubin 5–15 mg/dL ALT, AST < 1000 units/L	50% develop preeclampsia Cerebral edema GI bleed Renal failure	Urgent delivery
HELLP syndrome	80% preterm; 20% postterm	Nausea/vomiting RUQ pain One third with headaches	Low platelets Proteinuria Abnormal coagulation studies	Increased incidence of post-partum hemorrhage	Urgent Delivery
Intrahepatic cholestasis of pregnancy	Second or third trimester	Pruritus of hands and feet Jaundice in 10–15%	Increase in conjugated bilirubin (<6 mg/dL) AST, ALT 2–10 × normal PT usually unaffected	Form of preeclampsia	Ursodeoxycholic acid (a bile acid sequestrant)

RUQ = right upper quadrant, DIC = disseminated intravascular coagulopathy, ALT = alanine aminotransferase, AST = aspartate aminotransferase, GI = gastrointestinal, HELLP = hemolysis elevated liver enzymes low platelets, PT = prothrombin time.

17. **What are some adverse effects of the common tocolytic agents?**
Magnesium sulfate can cause flushing, nausea, vomiting, headache, generalized muscle weakness, diplopia, shortness of breath, and, rarely, pulmonary edema. Beta agonists can cause tachycardia (50%) and hyperglycemia. Pulmonary edema is more common if used together with magnesium or with multiple gestations.

18. **What is asymptomatic bacteriuria (ASB)? How should it be managed?**
ASB is diagnosed when urinalysis results are consistent with an infection without symptoms of an infection (i.e., a clean catch urine sample with >10^5 colony forming units of organism). ASB is associated with low birth weight and preterm delivery. *Escherichia coli* is the most common organism (75–90%), and therapy with 7–10 days of antibiotics is required. Nitrofurantoin and ampicillin are safe in pregnancy. Sulfonamides may be used in pregnancy but should be avoided during the third trimester due to an increase risk of kernicterus in newborns. Fluoroquinolones are not safe. Follow up with urine cultures 1–2 weeks after therapy and in each trimester thereafter.

19. **Why is screening for group B streptococci necessary in pregnancy?**
Group B streptococci can lead to various maternal infections and complications such as urinary tract infection, chorioamnionitis, endometritis, wound infection, preterm labor, or premature rupture of the membranes.

20. **Which thyroid disorders are common in pregnancy?**
Up to 1 in 5 pregnant women will have transient subclinical hyperthyroidism due to increased serum human chorionic gonadotropin concentrations. Graves' disease can occur in up to 0.2 % of pregnancies and 5–10% of women develop postpartum thyroiditis.

21. **What medications are safe to use in pregnancy, and which should be avoided?**
See Table 79-4.

TABLE 79-4. MEDICATIONS AND THEIR SAFETY IN PREGNANCY

Medical Issue	Use Justified When Indicated	Not Justified or Contraindicated
Analgesics (including for headache)	*Acetaminophen (A)	NSAIDs (B/C)
	Amitriptyline (B)	Aspirin (D)
	Codeine (C)	Sumatriptan (C)
	Meperidine (C)	Ergotamine (X)
	Morphine (C)	
Antimicrobials	Penicillins (B)	Tetracycline (D)
	Erythromycins (not estolate) (B), azithromycin (B)	Doxycycline (D)
		Clarithromycin (C)
	Cephalosporins (B)	Fluoroquinolones (C)
	Vancomycin (C)	
	Nitrofurantoin (B)	
	Acyclovir (C)	
	AZT (C)	
	Aminoglycosides (D)	
	Rarely justified: Metronidazole (B): okay after first trimester	
	Rarely justified: Trimethoprim (C)	
	Rarely justified: Sulfonamides (C): not close to term	

Continued

TABLE 79-4. MEDICATIONS AND THEIR SAFETY IN PREGNANCY—CONT'D

Medical Issue	Use Justified When Indicated	Not Justified or Contraindicated
Asthma	Beta agonists (all C) Inhaled steroids (all C, except triamcinolone, which is D) Systemic steroids (C) Ipratropium (B) Cromolyn sodium (B) Theophylline (C) Aminophylline (C)	
Depression/anxiety	Amitryptiline (B) Fluoxetine (C)	Lithium (D) Benzodiazepines (D)
Diabetes	Insulin	All oral hypoglycemic agents: glipizide (C), glyburide (B), metformin (B), troglitazone (B)
Diarrhea	Loperamide (B) Diphenoxylate/atropine (C)	
Dyspepsia	*Antacids: Tums, Mylanta Amphogel, Maalox *Sucralfate (B) H₂ blockers: *ranitidine (B), famotidine (B), nizatidine (C), cimetidine (B)	Proton pump inhibitors: omeprazole (B), lansoprazole (C), misoprostol (X)
Hypertension	*Methyldopa (B) *Labetalol (C) Pindolol (B) All other beta blockers (C) Hydralazine (C) Rarely justified: nifedipine (C), clonidine (C), prazosin (C), hydrochlorothiazide (B)	ACE inhibitors (D) Angiotensin II receptor blockers (D)
Laxatives	Bisacodyl (C) Docusate Lactulose (B) Psyllium Sodium biphosphate enema Magnesium hydroxide	

TABLE 79-4.   MEDICATIONS AND THEIR SAFETY IN PREGNANCY—CONT'D

Medical Issue	Use Justified When Indicated	Not Justified or Contraindicated
Nasal congestion	Chlorpheniramine (B), dimenhydrinate (B) *Diphenhydramine (B): avoid in first trimester Pseudoephedrine (C) Nasal steroids (C)	
Nausea	Prochlorperazine (C) Dimenhydrinate (B) Metoclopramide (B)	Ondansetron (B): rarely justified
Seizures	Phenytoin (D) Carbamazepine (C) Phenobarbital (D)	Rarely: valproic acid (D) and gabapentin (C)
Thrombosis	Unfractionated or low-molecular-weight heparin (B)	Warfarin (X)

NSAIDs = nonsteroidal anti-inflammatory drugs, ACE = angiotensin-converting enzyme.
Prescribing in pregnancy should be done only when the risks and benefits to the mother and fetus are carefully weighed.
*Indicates preferred agents; Food Drug and Administration pregnancy safety classes included in parentheses: A = adequate, well-controlled studies in pregnant women have not shown an increased risk of fetal abnormalities, B = animal studies have revealed no evidence of fetal harm; however, there are no adequate and well-controlled studies in pregnant women, or animal studies have shown an adverse effect, but adequate and well-controlled studies in pregnant women have failed to demonstrate fetal risk, C = animal studies have shown an adverse effect and there are no adequate and well-controlled studies in pregnant women, or no animal studies have been conducted and there are no adequate and well-controlled studies in pregnant women, D = studies in pregnant women have demonstrated fetal risk; however, the benefits of therapy may outweigh the potential risk, X = products are contraindicated in women who are or may become pregnant.
Adapted from the Women and Infants' Hospital of Rhode Island: Obstetric Medicine Curriculum for Internal Medicine Residents, 2005.

WEBSITE

1. North American Society of Obstetric Medicine
   http://www.isomnet.org/nasom/home.cfm

BIBLIOGRAPHY

1. Benjaminov F, Heathcote J: Liver disease in pregnancy. Am J Gastroenterol 99:2479–2488, 2004.
2. Lee R, Rosene-Montella K, Barbour L, et al: In Medical Care of the Pregnant Patient. Philadelphia, McNaughton Gunn, 2000, pp xxvi–xxvii, 103–115, 180–208, 387–396, 423–448.
3. Ross D: Overview of thyroid disease in pregnancy, UpToDate, 2005. http://www.utdol.com.
4. Sandhu B, Sanyal A: Pregnancy liver disease. Gastroenterol Clin North Am 32:407–436, 2003.
5. Sibai B: Magnesium sulfate prophylaxis in preeclampsia: Lessons learned from recent trials. Am J Obstet Gynecol 190:1520–1526, 2004.

CHAPTER 80

ADVANCED CARDIAC LIFE SUPPORT

Julius Yang, MD, PhD

1. **Define *cardiac arrest*.**
   Cardiac arrest is defined as the cessation of cardiac mechanical activity confirmed clinically by the absence of a detectable pulse, unresponsiveness, and apnea (or agonal respirations).

2. **Name the three major categories of cardiac arrest.**
   - **Ventricular fibrillation (VF)/pulseless ventricular tachycardia (VT)**
   - **Pulseless electric activity (PEA):** No pulse or evidence of spontaneous circulation despite the presence of an organized cardiac rhythm
   - **Asystole**

3. **What are the outcomes of patients who suffer cardiac arrest in the hospital?**
   Survival after in-hospital cardiopulmonary resuscitation (CPR) is poor. Approximately 30–40% of patients survive 24 hours after the arrest, and only 10–15% survive to hospital discharge. Poor outcomes have been associated with age older than 75 years, unwitnessed arrest, resuscitation efforts lasting longer than 10 minutes, and an initial rhythm that was neither VT nor VF.

4. **What interventions are most critical to an effective resuscitation response?**
   In all cases, the administration of high-quality chest compressions, initiated without delay and continued with minimal interruption, is of primary importance. In cases of VT/VF arrest, early defibrillation improves the likelihood of restoring a perfusing rhythm; it has been estimated that for every minute that defibrillation is delayed, there is an approximately 10% reduction in the likelihood of survival. In cases of PEA/asystolic arrest, prompt recognition and treatment of reversible causes is necessary for successful resuscitation.

5. **Describe the characteristics of "high-quality" chest compressions.**
   - "Push hard, push fast" technique: Compress the sternum 4–5 cm (1.5–2 inches) at a rate of at least 100 compressions/min.
   - Allow complete chest recoil between successive compressions: Within each compression cycle, the time spent pushing down should be roughly equal to the time spent letting up.
   - Minimize interruptions in performance of compressions unless absolutely necessary (e.g., for defibrillation attempt).
   - Rescuers should frequently alternate chest compression duties to avoid decay in the quality of compressions due to provider fatigue.

6. **What are the initial steps in responding to a cardiac arrest victim?**
   If a patient is found to be unresponsive without signs of life (e.g., pulseless, apneic, or with agonal breathing), activate the resuscitation team. Open the airway using a head-tilt/jaw-lift technique, provide two rescue breaths (usually performed with a bag-valve mask when in the hospital), and initiate chest compressions at a rate of 100 compressions/min. Perform compressions alternating with ventilations at a ratio of 30 compressions for every two breaths until a cardiac monitor is available to determine the underlying rhythm. Typically, this is accomplished using the defibrillator unit.

7. **Once basic life support measures have been implemented, what are the next steps if the arrest is due to VT/VF?**

   If the underlying rhythm is VT/VF, continue CPR while charging the unit, then defibrillate with 360 J monophasic or an equivalent biphasic energy level. Immediately after shock delivery, resume chest compressions and ventilations—without rechecking the rhythm. Recharge the defibrillator while performing five cycles of 30:2 compressions and breaths (approximately 2 minutes of CPR), then recheck the cardiac rhythm. If VT/VF persists, repeat shock delivery followed by five more cycles of 30 chest compressions/2 breaths. Consider insertion of an airway adjunct such as endotracheal (ET) tube, laryngeal mask airway, or Combitube; once an invasive airway is established, rescuers should provide 8–10 ventilations/min while chest compressions are continued at 100 per minute—without need to synchronize efforts.

8. **What if VT/VF persists despite chest compressions, ventilation, and attempted defibrillation?**

   Support circulation using either intravenous (IV) epinephrine (1 mg every 3–5 minutes) or IV vasopressin (40 units given once) to replace the first or second dose of epinephrine. Consider antiarrhythmic therapy with IV amiodarone (300 mg, followed by a second dose of 150 mg if needed). To minimize interruptions in the delivery of high-quality CPR, the following sequence has been recommended:

   CPR → rhythm check → CPR(while administering drugs and charging defibrillator) → shock

   Repeat this sequence as needed. CPR should be delivered in uninterrupted spans lasting approximately 2 minutes between rhythm checks and shocks. Note that rhythm checks should be brief, and drug doses should be prepared so that they can be delivered as soon as possible after each rhythm check is completed. Note also that CPR should be continued during the time that the defibrillator is charging and interrupted only prior to "bed clear" instructions preceding actual shock delivery. Pulse checks should be performed if an organized cardiac rhythm is established.

9. **What is an automated external defibrillator (AED)?**

   An AED is a computerized defibrillator device that allows even a responder untrained in advanced cardiac life support (ACLS) to deliver life-saving defibrillation in the setting of VF/VT arrest. Once activated, an AED guides the rescuer, through a series of verbal prompts,
   1. To apply pads to the victim's chest.
   2. To press the "analyze" button. At this point, the AED will automatically analyze the cardiac rhythm for the presence of VF/VT.
   3. If shock is indicated, the device will either automatically charge or guide the responder to press the "charge" button.
   4. Once charged, there will be a verbal prompt to stand clear and press the "shock" button; once pressed, the device will deliver a shock.

   AEDs have been used safely and effectively by lay responders as well as trained professionals responding to victims of cardiac arrest, and studies have found that use of AEDs can improve survival from witnessed out-of-hospital VF arrest.

10. **Once basic life support measures have been implemented, what are the next steps in treating a victim of PEA or asystolic arrest?**

    Support circulation using either IV epinephrine (1 mg every 3–5 minutes) or IV vasopressin (40 units given once) to replace the first or second dose of epinephrine. If bradycardia or asystole is present, consider atropine (1 mg every 3–5 minutes, up to 3 mg). Thoroughly assess for possible causes of PEA/asystolic arrest and promptly treat any reversible causes. A simple mnemonic device for the frequent causes of PEA/asystolic arrest are the 6 Hs and 6 Ts (Table 80-1).

TABLE 80-1. 6 HS AND 6 TS: THE DIFFERENTIAL DIAGNOSIS IN PEA/ASYSTOLIC ARREST

Hypoxia	**T**hrombosis (coronary)
Hypovolemia	**T**hrombosis (pulmonary embolism)
H+/acidosis	**T**amponade (pericardial)
Hyperkalemia or **h**ypokalemia	**T**ension pneumothorax
Hypothermia	**T**oxins (A,B,C,D → TC**A**, **B**eta, **C**a, **D**ig overdose)
Hypoglycemia	**T**rauma

TCA = tricyclic antidepressant, beta = beta blocker, Ca = calcium blocker, Dig = digoxin.

11. **What are the critical medications used in the ACLS response?**
    See Table 80-2.

12. **How does one confirm the appropriate position of an ET tube after an intubation procedure?**
    Listen over the epigastrium. Perform five-point auscultation for breath sounds at the left and right anterior chest, left and right midaxillary line, and over the stomach. Perform secondary confirmation through the use of either commercially available end-tidal CO_2 detector (capnometry) devices or esophageal detector devices.

13. **What are the possible causes of an erroneous reading from an end-tidal CO_2 detector device after attempted tracheal intubation?**
    - **False positive:** A false-positive reading (color change suggests that tube is in the trachea, when in fact it is in the esophagus) can be caused by a distended stomach, recent ingestion of a carbonated beverage, or nonpulmonary sources of CO_2. Esophageal intubation can lead to death if not quickly recognized and corrected.
    - **False negative:** A false-negative reading (lack of appropriate color change even though the tube is correctly placed in the trachea) can result from low blood flow states such as cardiac arrest, in which end-tidal CO_2 production is minimal. This situation may lead to unnecessary removal of a properly placed ET tube if not recognized.

KEY POINTS: ADVANCED CARDIAC LIFE SUPPORT

1. In VF/VT arrest, early defibrillation is crucial. Guidelines state that defibrillation should be provided within 3 minutes of onset for an in-hospital arrest.

2. In the adult, chest compressions should be performed with minimal interruption at 100 compressions per minute, at a compression:ventilation ratio of 30:2 until an advanced airway is secured.

3. Causes of PEA/asystolic arrest can be remembered as the 6 Hs and 6 Ts (see Table 80-1).

4. A misplaced ET tube (e.g., accidental esophageal intubation) is an important and often unrecognized cause of failed resuscitation efforts.

TABLE 80-2. ACLS MEDICATIONS

Condition/Type of Arrest	Medication	Dose	Frequency/Rate	Comments
VF/pulseless VT	Epinephrine	1 mg IV	Every 3–5 min	1:10,000 solution for IV administration
	Vasopressin	40 units IV	May repeat after 10 minutes	
	Amiodarone	300 mg IV initial dose	May repeat with 150 mg IV dose after 3–5 min	Antiarrhythmic of choice in VF/VT arrest
	Lidocaine	1–1.5 mg/kg IV load	Over 1–2 min	
PEA/asystole	Epinephrine	1 mg IV	Every 3–5 min	1:10,000 solution for IV administration
	Atropine	1 mg IV	Every 3–5 min, up to 0.04 mg/kg	
Torsades de pointes	Magnesium	1–2 gm IV		
Hyperkalemia	Calcium chloride	1 gm (1 amp of 10% solution) IV		Administer via central line
	Sodium bicarbonate	1 mEq/kg (1 amp = 50 mEq) IV		
	Insulin with dextrose	10 units IV insulin with 1 amp of D_{50} (25 gm glucose)		
Metabolic acidosis	Sodium bicarbonate	1 mEq/kg (1 amp = 50 mEq) IV	Repeat ½ dose every 10 min as needed	Indications: bicarbonate-responsive acidosis (e.g., DKA), drug overdose (e.g., TCA), prolonged resuscitation with effective ventilation, return of spontaneous circulation after long arrest interval

DKA = diabetic ketoacidosis, TCA = tricyclic antidepressant.

14. **What alternative devices are available to secure an airway when ET intubation is unsuccessful?**

Alternative devices include the laryngeal mask airway and the esophageal-tracheal Combitube. Both offer the significant advantage of allowing blind insertion technique and are associated with a lower risk of malpositioning errors.

15. **Which drugs can be administered through an ET tube?**

Atropine, lidocaine, and epinephrine can be administered via an ET tube. The tracheal dose is 2–2.5 times the IV dose.

WEBSITE

Podrid PJ: Overview of basic and advanced cardiovascular life support. 2005 Up-To-Date Online (v13.2): http://uptodate.com

BIBLIOGRAPHY

1. 2005 American Heart Association Guidelines for Cardiopulmonary Resuscitation and Emergency Cardiovascular Care. Circulation 112(suppl):IV-58–IV-66, 2005.

2. Cummins R (ed): ACLS: Principles and Practice: The Reference Textbook. American Heart Association, Dallas, 2003.

3. Cummins R, Graves J: Clinical results of standard CPR: Prehospital inhospital. In Kaye W, Bircher NG (eds): Cardiopulmonary Resuscitation. New York, Churchill Livingstone, 1989, pp 87–102.

4. DeBard M: Cardiopulmonary resuscitation: Analysis of six years experience and review of the literature. Ann Emerg Med 1:408–416, 1981.

5. In-Hospital Resuscitation: A Statement for Healthcare Professionals from the American Heart Association Emergency Cardiac Care Committee and the Advanced Cardiac Life Support, Basic Life Support, Pediatric Resuscitation, and Program Administration Subcommittees. Circulation 95:2211–2212, 1997.

6. McGrath RB: In-house cardiopulmonary resuscitation: After a quarter of a century. Ann Emerg Med 16:1365–1368, 1987.

7. Recommended Guidelines for Reviewing, Reporting, and Conducting Research on In-Hospital Resuscitation: The In-Hospital "Utstein Style." Circulation 95:2213–2239, 1997.

ECG INTERPRETATION

Amish Ajit Dangodara, MD

1. What is a standard 12-lead electrocardiogram (ECG)?

An ECG is a two-dimensional graph of the heart's electrical voltage plotted against time taken from 12 different standardized vantage points (leads) on the body surface to recreate the three-dimensional representation of the heart's electrical activity. The ECG is plotted on a graph with 1-mm grid lines that has a bold grid line every 5 mm. The standard ECG plots 1 mV/cm (0.1 mV/mm) against 0.4 sec/cm (40 msec/mm) and is denoted by the "standard bar" at the beginning of the ECG tracing. The height of the standard bar *always* equals 1 mV, and its width *always* equals 0.2 sec and is normally 10 mm tall by 5 mm wide (Fig. 81-1, *A*).

2. Where are the leads placed on a standard 12-lead ECG?

The vertical (limb) leads, I, II, III, aVR, aVL, and aVF, are placed on the right arm, left arm, and legs. By changing which of these positions is negative or positive, the direction of the vector can be manipulated (Figs. 81-1, *B* and 81-2). The horizontal leads are V1 through V6. The horizontal leads (chest leads) are placed on the anterior thorax along the fourth intercostal space (Figs. 81-1, *C* and 81-3).

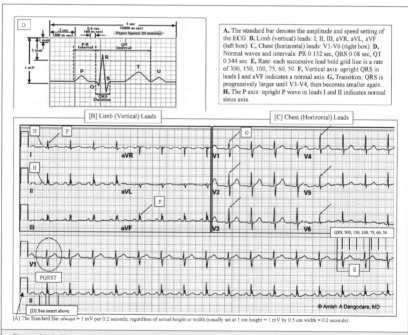

Figure 81-1. The normal 12-lead electrocardiogram.

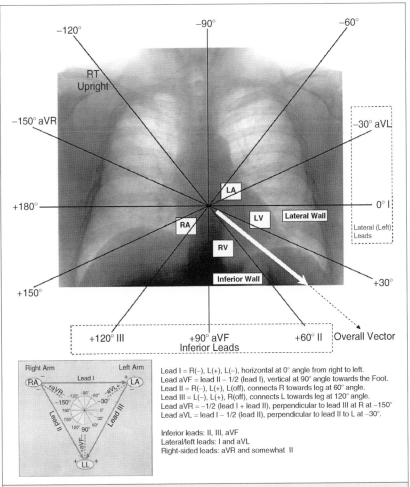

Figure 81-2. The limb (vertical) leads. RA = right atrium, LA = left atrium, RV = right ventricle, LV = left ventricle, R = right arm, L = left arm, F = foot.

3. **Relate the ECG lead positions to the anatomic location of the heart's structures (see Figs. 81-2 and 81-3).**
   - **Inferior leads:** Leads II, III, and aVF correspond to the inferior wall of the heart, the left posterior fascicle (LPF), and the right coronary artery (RCA).
   - **Anterior leads:** Leads V1–V4 correspond to the anterior wall of the heart, the left bundle branch (LBB), and the left anterior descending artery.
   - **Lateral (left) leads:** Leads V5, V6, I, and aVL correspond to the lateral wall of the heart, the left anterior fascicle (LAF), and the left circumflex (LCx) artery.
   - **Septal leads:** Leads V2 and V3 correspond to the septum of the heart, the atrioventricular (AV) node, the bundle of His, and the diagonal (D) branches of the proximal left anterior descending artery.
   - **Posterior leads:** The mirror of V1 and V2 leads correspond to the posterior wall of the heart and the posterior descending artery, a branch of RCA in a right-dominant system.

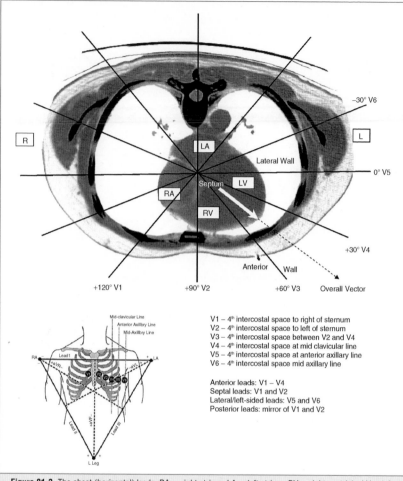

Figure 81-3. The chest (horizontal) leads. RA = right atrium, LA = left atrium, RV = right ventricle, LV = left ventricle.

- **Right-sided leads:** Leads aVR, V1, and V2 correspond to the right atrium (RA), the left atrium (LA), the right ventricle (RV), the right bundle branch (RBB), and the RCA.

4. **How is the electrical activity of the heart's conduction represented on an ECG?**
   Each conduction is represented by a series of waves described as a *PQRS complex,* followed by a T wave that represents electrical repolarization (see Fig. 81-1, *D*):
   - **P wave:** Represents atrial activity and is the first small (usually) upright deflection
   - **PR segment:** The brief horizontal pause after the P wave
   - **Q wave:** The first deflection below the baseline PR segment
   - **R wave:** The first upward deflection above the baseline PR segment after the P wave.
   - **S wave:** The first downward wave below the baseline PR segment after the R wave, which then returns to the baseline; if there is no R wave preceding it, then it is not an S wave but a Q wave

- **QRS complex:** Collectively, the ventricular conduction; may not always contain each of its comprising waves
- **T wave:** Follows the QRS complex after a short pause known as the **ST segment**

KEY POINTS: HEART ANATOMY AND LEAD PLACEMENT ✔

1. Anterior leads (V1–V4): left wall, LBB, left anterior descending artery

2. Septal leads (V2–V3): septum, AV node, bundle of His, D artery, left anterior descending artery

3. Lateral (left-sided) leads (I, aVL, V5–V6): lateral wall, LAF, LCx artery

4. Inferior leads (II, III, aVF): inferior wall, LPF, RCA

5. Right-sided leads (aVR, V1–V2): RA, LA, RV, RBB, RCA

6. Posterior leads (mirror of V1–V2): posterior wall, posterior descending artery

5. **How does the normal electrical vector move through the heart?**
   The overall vector of the heart's electrical activity normally points downward and outward through the apex of the heart (see Figs. 81-2 and 81-3). The heart's electrical activity originates in the sinoatrial (SA) node in the RA, moves anteriorly, then circles posteriorly to the LA (Fig. 81-4). This is represented by the P wave. The electrical activity then travels inferiorly to the AV node and down the bundle of His through the septum of the heart (see Fig. 81-4). Delays in

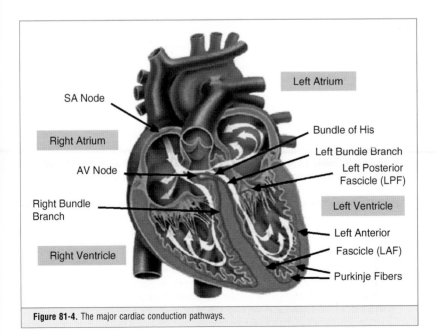

Figure 81-4. The major cardiac conduction pathways.

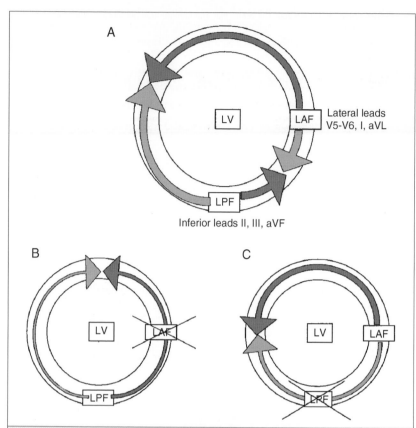

Figure 81-5. Fascicular blocks. **A,** Normal conduction of left anterior fascicle (LAF) and left posterior fascicle (LPF). **B,** LAF block. Small Q waves in lateral leads (LAF) and deep S waves (vector moving away) in inferior leads. **C,** LPF block. Small Q waves in inferior leads (LPF) and deep S waves (vector moving away) in lateral leads. LV = left ventricle.

conduction here are seen as AV blocks. It then splits down the RBB to the RV and the LBB to the left ventricle (LV). Delays in conduction here are seen as bundle blocks. The LBB splits further into the left anterior fascicle (LAF) and LPF. Delays in conduction here are seen as fascicular blocks. Finally, the electrical activity travels through the Purkinje fibers to depolarize the myocardial cells of the ventricles in a circular fashion, moving both clockwise and counterclockwise from the end of the terminal fascicles (Fig. 81-5, *A*). The QRS complex represents ventricular conduction. Abnormal conduction here is seen as a Q wave. The myocardial cells then "recharge." The repolarization is represented by the T wave.

6. **How do you measure the rate on the ECG?**
   Rate can be measured in terms of atrial rate (P wave) or ventricular rate (QRS complex) by counting either the number of P waves or QRS complexes, respectively, per unit of time (usually 1 minute). The normal sinus rate is 60–100 beats/min. Fifteen centimeters (30 bold grid lines) equals 6 sec, so the number of P waves or QRS complexes within 15 cm multiplied by 10 (60 sec) equals the rate per minute. Another method uses the bold grid lines. Start by identifying

a QRS complex aligned with a bold grid line on the ECG tracing, and count each successive bold grid line (5 mm or 0.2 sec) until the next QRS complex. Each successive bold grid line is a rate of 300, 150, 100, 75, 60, and 50. The rate can be estimated at somewhere between the two bold grid lines on either side of the next QRS complex (see Fig. 81-1, *E*).

7. **What is the normal axis of the heart?**
   The normal vertical axis of the heart is between −30 and +90 degrees on the vertical plane. The normal horizontal axis (transition) of the heart is between −30 and +90 degrees on the horizontal plane (Figs. 81-1, *F* and *G*, 81-2, 81-3, and 81-6). The term *axis* refers to the vertical axis, whereas the term *transition* refers to the horizontal axis (see Fig. 81-1, *G*). If the vertical axis is less than −30 degrees, then there is left axis deviation (LAD). If the vertical axis is greater than +90 degrees, then there is right axis deviation (RAD). The horizontal axis in the chest leads can have early, normal, or late transition.

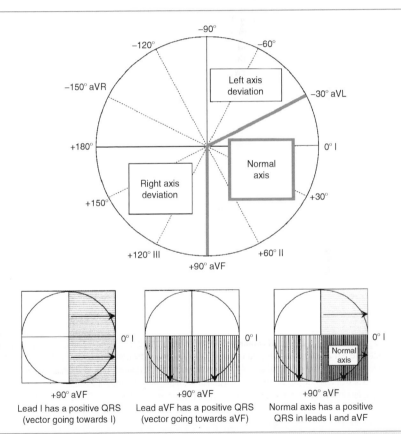

Figure 81-6. How to determine the axis. By looking at the direction of the QRS complexes in leads I and aVF, the axis can be narrowed to one of the four intersecting quadrants above. Then identify the most isoelectric limb lead (QRS is almost equally positive and negative). The axis is perpendicular (i.e., 90 degrees) to this lead in the direction of the intersecting quadrant. In Fig. 81-1, for example, the most isoelectric limb lead is aVL, and the lead perpendicular to it is lead II. Because the intersecting quadrant is normal (0–90 degrees), the axis is heading in the direction of this quadrant and lead II in this quadrant is +60 degrees, which would be the estimated vertical axis.

8. **How do you measure the axis of the heart?**
   A normal axis should result in an upward QRS complex (large R wave) in leads I (0 degrees) and aVF (+90 degrees) since the normal axis is between these two leads (see Figs. 81-1, *F*, and 81-6). The overall vector of electrical activity points down and left at approximately 45 degrees (see Fig. 81-2).

9. **What is the normal PR interval?**
   The normal PR interval is 0.12–0.21 (easy to remember as "12–21") sec (3–5 mm) and is measured from the start of the P wave to the start of the QRS complex (see Fig. 81-1, *D*). A prolonged PR interval indicates an AV nodal block.

10. **What is the normal QRS duration?**
    The normal QRS duration is 0.08–0.12 sec (2–3 mm) and is measured from the start of the QRS complex to the J point, or the end of the QRS complex (see Fig. 81-1, *D*). A prolonged QRS duration indicates a bundle branch block.

11. **What is the normal QT interval, and how is it measured?**
    The normal QT interval is measured from the start of the QRS complex to the end of the T wave (see Fig. 81-1, *D*). It represents the duration of electrical activation and recovery of the myocardial cells of the ventricles. When the QT interval is corrected for the heart rate, it is known as the *corrected QT interval* (QTc) (Fig. 81-7), which is based on a heart rate of 60 beats/min. The normal QTc is usually 0.300–0.460 sec (see Fig. 81-7). The QTc can be calculated by the measured QT divided by the square root of the R-to-R interval in seconds:

    $$QTc = QT \ sec/\sqrt{(\text{R-R seconds})}$$

    A normal QTc can be estimated by determining whether the QT interval is less than half of the R-R interval:

    $$normal \ QTc = < \tfrac{1}{2} \ \text{R-R interval}$$

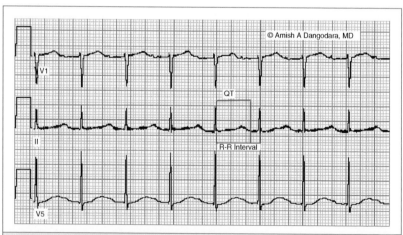

Figure 81-7. The corrected QT interval (QTc). The QTc can be estimated by measuring the R-R interval. The normal QTc should be less than one half of the R-R interval. In this case, the QTc is abnormally prolonged since it is greater than half of the R-R interval.

12. **What is the significance of the P wave? Where is it best seen?**

   The P wave represents atrial electrical activity (Fig. 81-8). An upright P wave in leads I and II indicates a normal P (sinus) axis (see Fig. 81-1, *H*). All of the inferior leads, II, III, and aVF, should have an upright P wave because the vector moves from the atria downward to the AV node toward those leads. All of the left-sided leads, I, aVL, and V4–V6, should have an upright P wave because the vector curves left from the RA to the LA toward those leads. The P wave is seen best in leads II and V1 because these leads are closest to the atria (see Figs. 81-2 and 81-3).

13. **What is the Q wave? When is it significant? What does it signify?**

   The Q wave is the first downward deflection after the P wave and preceding the upright R wave and is usually not present. When significant, it indicates infarcted or dead myocardium. The Q wave is significant if its depth is greater than one third of the height of the QRS complex or >0.04 sec (1 mm) in duration (Fig. 81-9; also see Fig. 81-17). The Q wave is significant if it appears in two or more anatomically contiguous leads. The presence of the Q wave may be normal and insignificant if neither of the above criteria is met.

14. **What does the QRS complex signify? How should it be analyzed?**

   The QRS complex signifies ventricular conduction that originates below the level of the AV node. It is not necessary for each of its comprising waves to be present. The R wave is larger in leads that are closer to the ventricular conduction since the ventricular vector is moving toward that lead. The R wave is really composed of two different R waves buried within each other—one from each ventricle—but appears as one wave since both ventricles normally conduct simultaneously. If there is a delay in conduction between the two ventricles, then the R wave may appear widened, or there may be two distinct R waves known as an R and R′ wave. The S wave is deeper in leads that are further from the ventricular conduction since the ventricular vector is moving away further from that lead. The normal ventricular vector points downward

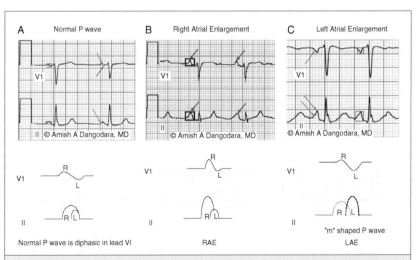

Figure 81-8. The normal P wave **(A)** and atrial enlargement **(B and C)**. The P wave represents the combination of right and left atrial activity. The right atrium normally conducts first, followed by the left atrium. Enlargement of either chamber leads to greater prominence of the corresponding P wave and alters the overall appearance of the P wave such that the amplitude is >0.2 mV (>2 mm height) or the duration is >0.12 sec (>3 mm width). In lead V1, the P wave is normally diphasic, but in right atrial enlargement only the upright portion may predominate and obscure the downward portion; whereas in left atrial enlargement, only the downward portion may predominate and obscure the upright portion. Biatrial enlargement has features of both right atrial enlargement (RAE) **(B)** and left atrial enlargement (LAE) **(C)** where the diphasic P wave in V1 has a larger amplitude than normal.

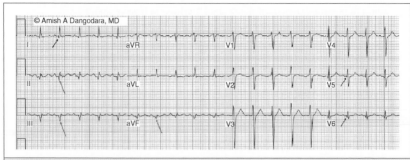

Figure 81-9. Significant Q Waves. Significant Q waves are >1 mm wide (>0.04 sec) or have a depth of greater than one third of the total QRS height and must occur in at least two or more anatomically contiguous leads. In this case, they are present in all three of the inferior leads, II, III, and aVF (*leftward arrows*). Not all of these criteria need to be met at once for Q waves to be significant, but if none of these criteria is met, then the Q wave is probably normal. On this ECG, there are also small Q waves in the lateral leads, I, V5, and V6 (*rightward arrows*), which are not >1 mm wide and are not greater than one third of the total QRS complex height, but do occur in more than two anatomically contiguous leads. Small Q waves in the lateral leads can be seen in left anterior fascicular block (Fig. 81-23); however, there are no deep S waves in the inferior leads, so this is not left anterior fascicular block. Therefore, the small lateral Q waves are actually significant, especially when viewed in the context of the significant Q waves in the inferior leads. This ECG represents an old inferolateral myocardial infarction, most likely due to an occlusion of the right coronary artery with a right dominant system (see question 4).

and outward through the apex of the heart at approximately 45 degrees in the horizontal and vertical planes (see Figs. 81-2 and 81-3).

15. **What is the J point? What does the ST segment signify?**
The J point is the terminal end of the QRS wave and signals the beginning of the ST segment. The ST segment starts at the end of the QRS complex and ends at the onset of the T wave. It is usually horizontal and signifies the duration that the ventricular myocardium remains in a depolarized state. The ST segment can be described as depressed, normal, or elevated, referring to its position in comparison to the PR segment baseline. The ST segment can be described as downsloping, flattened, or upsloping as it progresses from the J point to the onset of the T wave (Fig. 81-10). The first part of the normal ST segment is usually at the same baseline level as the PR segment, although it may feature a slight upsloping or downsloping.

If the J point is elevated and the ST segment quickly returns to the baseline level of the PR segment, this is known as *J-point elevation*, which is a normal variation. A short, mildly elevated, flat or mildly upsloping ST segment with J-point elevation may indicate *early repolarization*, especially if the following T-wave morphology is normal. The QRS may have a tiny terminal upward deflection that can be mistaken for an R′ wave but is actually highly characteristic of early repolarization (Fig. 81-11).

16. **What does the T wave signify? What is its normal morphology?**
The T wave signifies ventricular repolarization and is normally symmetrically rounded (see Fig. 81-1). The T wave is usually upright in leads I and V2–V6. The T wave is usually inverted in aVR and may also be inverted in lead V1. The T wave is usually oriented in the same direction as the overall QRS complex in the remaining limb leads, II, III, aVL, and aVF.

17. **What is a U wave? What does it signify?**
A U wave is a small symmetrically rounded wave that follows the T wave after the TU segment and has the same orientation as the accompanying T wave (see Fig. 81-1, *D*). It may represent electrical activity generated by the "M" cells in the mid-myocardial portion of the LV. The U wave is normally absent and disappears at fast heart rates because it merges with the following

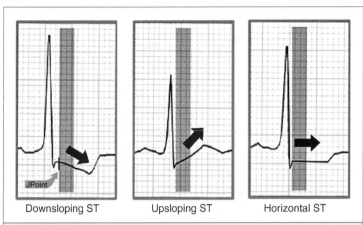

Figure 81-10. ST-segment depression. The J point occurs at the end of the QRS complex. The ST segment begins at the J point and extends to a user-defined interval.

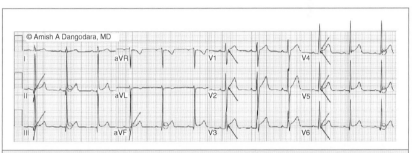

Figure 81-11. J-point elevation and early repolarization. The J point is denoted by the *upright arrows* and is elevated in most leads. The small "blip" at the very end of the QRS complex *(ovals and downward arrows)* is sometimes mistaken for an R' wave but is actually very characteristic of early repolarization. It is typically followed by an upsloping or flat ST segment and normal T wave. These findings together are seen in early repolarization, which is a normal variation. Therefore, in this case, the ST elevation and J-point elevation are *not* suggestive of changes seen with myocardial infarction or ischemia.

P wave. The U wave can be seen with significant bradycardia or QTc prolongation. The U wave is most commonly associated with hypokalemia (Fig. 81-12).

18. **What is an artificial pacer spike?**
    An artificial pacer spike is the electrical activity generated by an artificial electronic pacemaker and appears as a perfectly vertical line (Fig. 81-13). If the pacer spike precedes the P wave, then this is an atrial pacemaker. If the pacer spike precedes the QRS complex, then this is a ventricular pacemaker. Dual-chamber pacing is indicated by a pacer spike that precedes both the P wave and the QRS complex.

19. **What are the various pacemaker rates in normal adults?**
    Normally, the SA node initiates the electrical pacing of the heart, but other lesser pacemakers can take over if the SA node is diseased or fails to activate electrical impulses. The lesser pacemakers include ectopic atrial, junctional, or ventricular pacemakers (Fig. 81-14). Sinus

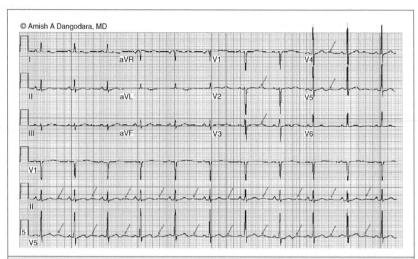

Figure 81-12. Hypokalemia. There is a U wave following the T wave *(arrows)*, which is characteristic of hypokalemia.

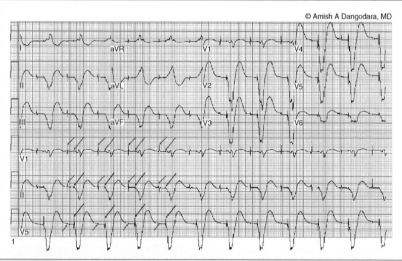

Figure 81-13. Dual-chamber AV sequential pacemaker. The perfectly vertical lines *(small arrows)* indicate the artificial signal for atrial contraction from the implanted artificial electronic pacemaker. The inverted P wave triggered by this impulse is only seen in lead V1 on this ECG. The perfectly vertical lines *(larger arrows)* preceding each QRS complex indicate the artificial signal for ventricular contraction from the implanted artificial electronic pacemaker. Note that the QRS complex has an abnormal wide appearance similar to a natural cardiac ventricular pacemaker (see Fig. 81-14, *C*) because the signal originates in the ventricle.

tachycardias are usually 100–150 beats/min. Paroxysmal atrial, junctional, and ventricular tachycardias are usually 150–250 beats/min. Atrial and ventricular flutter rates are usually 250–350 beats/min. Atrial and ventricular fibrillation rates are usually >350 beats/min (Table 81-1).

20. **What does an abnormal axis signify?**
    An abnormal axis means that the overall cardiac vector has shifted either as a result of cardiac injury, asymmetric hypertrophy, or an alteration of the anatomic position of the heart (see Fig. 81-6).

21. **What is LAD? What does it signify?**
    LAD results in an upright QRS in lead I and a downward QRS in lead aVF (Figs. 81-2 and 81-15). LAD can be seen with left ventricular hypertrophy (LVH) and pathology that can lead to LVH such as hypertension, aortic valve stenosis or regurgitation, mitral valve regurgitation, atrial septal defect, or idiopathic hypertrophic cardiomyopathy. LAD can be seen when pathology of the anterior conduction pathways preferentially shifts conduction to the left, such as in left anterior fascicular block (LAFB). LAD also results from artificial pacing with an implanted electronic pacemaker.

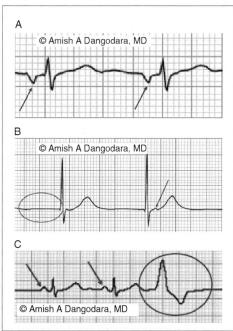

Figure 81-14. The cardiac pacemakers. The QRS complex tends to be wider as the origination of the pacemaker is lower (ventricular versus atrial). The P wave is only present in pacemakers originating in the atria or traveling retrograde to the atria, which does not occur in pacemakers of ventricular origin. It may be helpful to look at multiple leads to identify the P wave. **A,** Ectopic atrial pacemaker. The P wave is present but inverted. The QRS is narrow complex. Normal atrial rates are 60–100 beats/min. **B,** Junctional pacemaker. The P wave is absent in first beat *(oval)* and retrograde in next beat *(arrow)*. The QRS is narrow complex. Normal junctional rates are 40–60 beats/min. **C,** Ventricular pacemaker. The first two beats are sinus with a normal P wave *(arrows)* and the next beat has an absent P wave *(oval)*. The QRS is wide complex and usually associated with T-wave abnormalities. Normal ventricular rates are 20–40 beats/min.

TABLE 81-1.	PACEMAKER RATES BY CARDIAC CELL TYPE			
Pacemaker	Normal	Bradycardia	P Wave	QRS Complex
Atrial (SA)	60–100 beats/min	<60 beats/min	Present	Narrow
Junctional (AV)	40–60 beats/min	<40 beats/min	Retrograde or absent	Narrow
Ventricular	20–40 beats/min	<20 beats/min	Absent	Wide

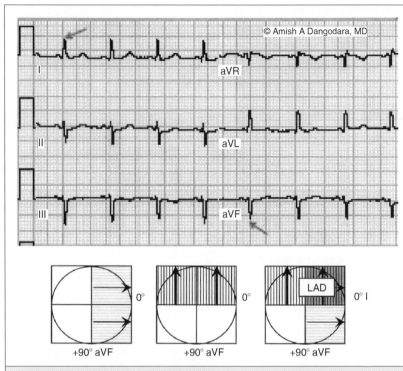

Figure 81-15. Left axis deviation (LAD). QRS is positive in (toward) lead I (0 degrees) and negative in (away from) lead aVF (+90 degrees). This means that the axis is in the intersecting quadrant, somewhere between −90 degrees and 0 degrees. The most isoelectric lead is lead II, which runs from −120 degrees toward +60 degrees (see Fig. 81-6). The lead perpendicular (90 degrees) to lead II is lead aVL (see Fig. 81-6), which is −30 degrees in the intersecting quadrant. Therefore, the vertical axis is initially estimated at −30 degrees. Even though lead II is the most isoelectric, it has a more negative component than a positive one, which means that the axis is pointing slightly away from lead II and is closer to −120 degrees. Therefore, the true axis is slightly negative of the initially estimated axis of −30 degrees, or approximately −50 degrees. This represents LAD because the axis is less than −30 degrees.

22. **What is RAD, and what does it signify?**

    RAD results in a downward QRS in lead I and an upright QRS in lead aVF (Figs. 81-2 and 81-16). RAD can be normal in tall, thin people whose hearts are anatomically shifted vertically or to the right. RAD can be seen with right ventricular hypertrophy (RVH) and pathology that can lead to RVH such as chronic lung disease, pulmonary hypertension, pulmonary embolism, atrial septal defect, ventricular septal defect, or mitral valve stenosis. RAD can be seen when pathology of the left-sided conduction pathways preferentially shifts conduction to the right, such as with left posterior fascicular block (LPFB).

23. **What does an abnormal transition (horizontal axis) of the heart signify?**

    An abnormal transition means that the overall cardiac vector has shifted either as a result of cardiac injury, asymmetric hypertrophy, impedance of electrical forces, or alteration in the normal anatomic position of the heart (see Figs. 81-1, G, and 81-3).

    Early transition can be due to RVH or posterior myocardial infarction. Myocardial injury to the lateral wall is distinguished from early transition by the sudden loss of R wave in leads V5–V6, even though the R wave peaks normally by V4. In early transition, the R wave peaks by V2 then

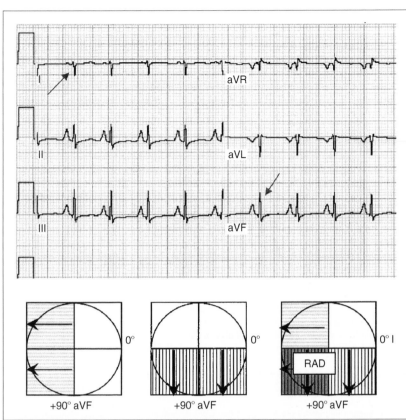

Figure 81-16. Right axis deviation (RAD). QRS is negative in (away from) lead I (0 degrees) and positive in (toward) lead aVF (+90 degrees). This means that the axis is in the intersecting quadrant, somewhere between +90 degrees and +180 degrees. The most isoelectric lead is lead aVR, which runs from +30 degrees toward −150 degrees (see Fig. 81-6). The lead perpendicular (90 degrees) to lead aVR is lead III (see Fig. 81-6), which is +120 degrees in the intersecting quadrant. Therefore, the vertical axis is initially estimated at +120 degrees. Because aVR is almost exactly isoelectric, the true axis is approximately +120 degrees.

becomes gradually smaller by V6. Therefore, lateral wall infarction will result in poor R-wave progression but not in early transition. Impedance to electrical activity in the chest leads (V1–V6) can result in hypovoltage, or poor R-wave progression.

Late transition can be due to LVH or enlargement of the left ventricular chamber without hypertrophy of the wall. This contrasts with poor R-wave progression seen with myocardial injury of the anteroseptal wall, which will result in small or absent R waves in V1–V2, which overlie the septum, but normal R waves in V3–V6, which overlie the anterolateral wall (Fig. 81-17). This is distinguished from late transition by the sudden appearance of a normal sized R wave in V3 that peaks by lead V4 and becomes smaller in leads V5–V6. In late transition, the R wave peaks in leads V5–V6.

24. **What is the significance of an abnormal PR segment?**
    ■ **Shortened PR interval:** A shortened PR interval of <0.12 sec can be seen in pericarditis or early depolarization such as Wolff-Parkinson-White (WPW) syndrome. It can also be seen in

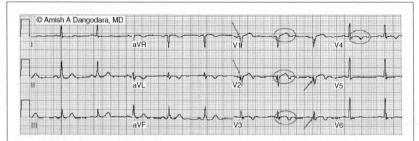

Figure 81-17. Anteroseptal myocardial infarction. The R waves are small or nearly absent in the septal leads *(downward arrows)*, showing abnormal transition or poor R wave progression. There are small Q waves in leads V2 and V3 *(upward arrows)*. Even though the Q waves are small and narrow in leads V2–V3, they are still considered "significant" because they are in two anatomically contiguous leads in association with other findings consistent with myocardial infarction. There are associated abnormal asymmetric, biphasic, or inverted T waves in leads V1–V4 consistent with infarction or ischemia. This constellation of findings represents anteroseptal myocardial infarction, likely due to an occlusion of the left anterior descending artery.

high junctional beats, where the conduction originates high in the bundle of His and is transmitted retrograde to the atria. Low junctional beats may result in a retrograde P wave *after* the QRS (see Fig. 81-14, *B*).

- **Depression of the PR segment:** A delayed PR interval (relative to the TP segment) can be seen in pericarditis. A delayed PR interval suggests a delay in conduction from the AV node to ventricular conduction, which may be due to medications that affect the AV node (e.g., beta blockers) or due to a diseased AV nodal pathway.
- **Prolonged PR interval:** A prolonged PR interval of >0.21 sec is associated with AV heart blocks.

25. **What are the various types of AV nodal heart blocks?**
    - **First-degree AV block:** A fixed PR interval of >0.21 sec associated with each QRS complex (Fig. 81-18).
    - **Second-degree AV block:** Seen in two types, known as Mobitz I (or Wenckebach) and Mobitz II. *Mobitz I* second-degree block is a progressively lengthening PR interval associated with each successive QRS complex until the QRS complex no longer conducts (a dropped beat), after which the cycle of progressive lengthening may start again (Fig. 81-19, *A*). In a *Mobitz II* second-degree AV block, the PR interval does not progressively lengthen with each successive QRS complex, but the QRS complex occasionally does not conduct (a dropped beat). The other PR intervals may be normal or prolonged at a fixed interval (Fig. 81-19, *B*).

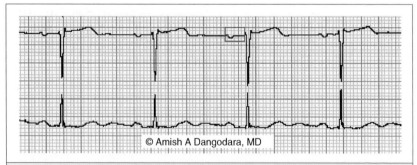

Figure 81-18. First-degree AV block results in a prolonged PR interval. The normal PR interval is 0.12–0.21 msec. In this case, it is approximately 0.24 msec and remains constant with each successive conduction.

- **Third-degree AV block:** Also known as *complete heart block* or *AV dissociation*, there is no correlation of atrial conduction with ventricular conduction. The atria are pacing but not being transmitted through the AV node, so an "escape" pacemaker below the atria assumes control of ventricular pacing, usually at a slower rate than the atrial pacemaker. The P wave occasionally appears to correlate with QRS conduction, but this is usually by coincidental timing of the atrial pacemaker aligning with the timing of the ventricular pacemaker. The atrial rate is usually regular and the ventricular rate can be regular or variable, but the atria and ventricles are pacing independent of each other, each one with its own rate (Fig. 81-20).

KEY POINTS: AV BLOCKS ✔

1. First-degree AV block: fixed PR interval prolonged > 0.21 msec with each conduction

2. Second-degree AV block, Mobitz type I (Wenckebach): increasing PR interval prolongation with each conduction, dropped QRS

3. Second-degree AV block, Mobitz type II: fixed PR with occasional dropped QRS

4. Third-degree AV block (AV dissociation): fixed P-P rate, variably slower R-R rate independent of P-P rate

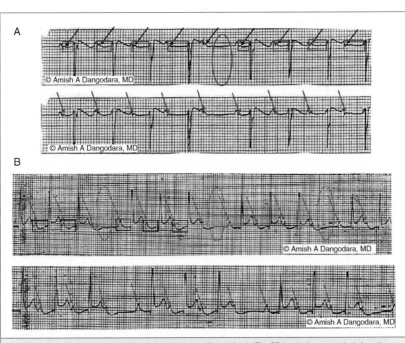

Figure 81-19. Second-degree AV block. **A,** Mobitz I or Wenckebach. The PR interval progressively lengthens *(boxes)* until there is a dropped beat *(oval)*. The P waves are marked by the arrows. **B,** Mobitz II. The PR interval does not lengthen *(boxes)*, but the QRS drops *(ovals)*. Again, the P waves are marked by the arrows.

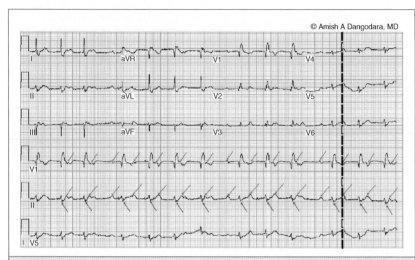

© Amish A Dangodara, MD

Figure 81-20. Third-degree AV block is also known as *AV dissociation* or *complete heart block*. The atria pace at a normal rate *(downward arrows)* but fail to transmit a signal to the ventricles. Therefore, a lower pacemaker, in this case, a junctional pacemaker *(upward arrows)*, which is narrow complex (see Fig. 81-14, *B*), takes over and usually paces at a slower rate than the atrial pacemaker. Since any vertical line on the ECG tracing *(dashed line)* represents the same point in time across all leads, the P wave can be identified in one lead (in this case, it is easy to find in lead V1) and traced vertically to other leads where it may be more difficult to find.

26. **What is the significance of an abnormal QRS duration?**
    - **Bundle branch block:** A widened QRS duration of >0.12 sec signifies a delay in electrical conduction from the AV node to the Purkinje fibers, or a bundle branch block (see Fig. 81-4). Because there is a block, or delay, in the conduction of one of the bundle branches, the ventricles do not depolarize simultaneously. This results in a widened QRS complex or a QRS with a second delayed overlapping R wave, giving the appearance of an R wave followed by a second R wave known as an R′ wave.
    - **Right bundle branch block (RBBB):** An RBBB is seen best in the right-sided leads (V1–V2, aVR), which overlie the RV. The RSR′ pattern is not as noticeable in the left-sided leads (V4–V6, I, aVL) since these leads are further from the right bundle. The negative vector of the left leads represents right-sided electrical forces, so the S wave is wide in the left leads (Fig. 81-21).
    - **Left bundle branch block (LBBB):** An LBBB is seen best in the left-sided leads (V4–V6, I, aVL), which overlie the LV. The R wave in V1 is usually very small or absent. The RSR′ pattern is not noticeable in the right-sided leads (V1–V2, aVR) since these leads are farther from the left bundle. The negative vector of the right leads represents left-sided electrical forces, so the S wave is wide in the right leads (Fig. 81-22).
    - **Incomplete bundle branch block (IRBBB or ILBBB):** An IRBBB or ILBBB has the same appearance as a bundle branch block, either right or left, but the QRS duration is only mildly delayed at the upper limit of normal at 0.10–0.12 sec.

27. **What is a hemiblock?**
    A hemiblock is a block of one of the left bundle fascicles (fascicular block) with a normal QRS duration of 0.08–0.12 sec and increased QRS voltage in the vertical leads (see Fig. 81-4). Normally, the electrical activity moves in both clockwise and counterclockwise directions around the ventricle from the terminal point of each fascicle (see Fig. 81-5, *A*). When one of the fascicles

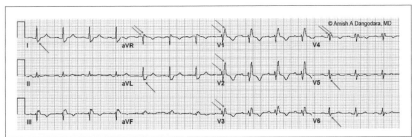

Figure 81-21. Right bundle branch block. The right-sided leads, aVR, V1, and V2, reveal an obvious delay in the right and left ventricular conduction with an RSR′ pattern *(downward arrows)*. The S wave in the left-sided leads, I, aVL, and V5–V6, represents electrical forces moving away from the left leads, or toward the right *(upward arrows)*. This is why the left-sided leads have a widened (delayed) S wave in right bundle branch block.

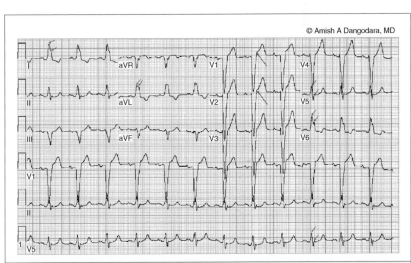

Figure 81-22. Left bundle branch block. The left-sided leads, I, aVL, and V5–V6, reveal an obvious delay in the right and left ventricular conduction with an RSR′ pattern *(downward arrows)*. The S wave in the right-sided leads, aVR, and V1–V2, represents electrical forces moving away from the right leads, or toward the left. This is why the right-sided leads have a widened S wave in left bundle branch block. There is also usually an elevation of the J point in leads V1–V3 *(upward arrows)*.

is blocked, the electrical vector moves predominantly *away* from the location of the remaining *active* fascicle since there is no electrical activity from the blocked fascicle to counter its forces. This results in a deep S wave (moving *away* from) in the leads representing the *active* fascicle. A fascicular block also results in very small Q waves in the leads representing the blocked fascicle, since Q waves indicate absence of electrical activity.

Therefore, an LAFB has small insignificant Q waves in the lateral leads (i.e., I, aVL, V6), since the LAF is located in the lateral wall. It also results in deep S waves in the inferior leads (i.e., II, III, aVF), representing the residual electrical activity of the LPF, which is located in the inferior wall. This is usually associated with left axis deviation (LAD) (Fig. 81-23).

An LPFB has small insignificant Q waves in the inferior leads (i.e., II, III, aVF) because the LPF is located in the inferior wall. It also results in deep S waves in the lateral leads (i.e., I, aVL, V6), representing the residual electrical activity of the LAF, which is located in the lateral wall. This is usually associated with right axis deviation (RAD), but there is no evidence of RVH (Fig. 81-24).

28. **What are bifascicular and trifascicular blocks?**
The RBB, LAF, and LPF constitute the three major electrical pathways. Since a block of both the LAF and the LPF essentially constitutes an LBBB, this does *not* qualify as a bifascicular block. Since a

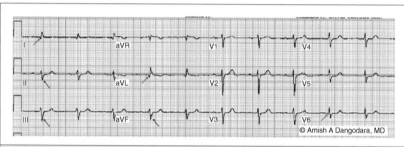

Figure 81-23. Left anterior fascicular (LAF) block. LAF block is a block in the conduction of the LAF, which is located in the lateral wall. This results in very small insignificant Q waves in the lateral leads, I, aVL, and V5–V6 *(rightward arrows)* since the lateral LAF is not conducting. The residual electrical activity is conducted through the inferior left posterior fascicle. The electrical activity moves quickly away from the initial direction that it was generated around the ventricle (see Fig. 81-5, *B*). This is why the negative vector (moving away), represented by the S wave, is more prominent in the inferior leads, II, III, and aVF *(leftward arrows)*.

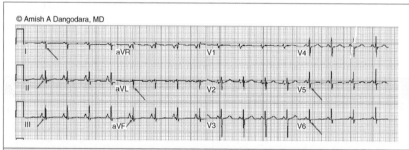

© Amish A Dangodara, MD

Figure 81-24. Left posterior fascicular (LPF) block. LPF block is a delay in conduction of the LPF, which is located in the inferior wall. This results in very small insignificant Q waves in the inferior leads, II, III, and aVF *(rightward arrows)*, since the inferior LPF is not conducting. The residual electrical activity is conducted through the lateral left anterior fascicle. The electrical activity moves quickly away from the initial direction that it was generated around the ventricle (see Fig. 81-5, *C*). This is why the negative vector (moving away), represented by the S wave, is more prominent in the lateral leads, I, aVL, and V5–V6 *(leftward arrows)*.

complete RBBB and a complete LBBB essentially constitutes a block of all three major electrical pathways, this is a complete heart block or third-degree AV block. Any other combination of two "blocks" of the three major electrical pathways constitutes a *bifascicular block* (Fig. 81-25). Any other combination of three blocks, including first- or second-degree AV nodal blocks, constitutes a *trifascicular block*, which is usually an indication for a pacemaker. Examples include IRBBB + LAFB (or LPFB) + first- or second-degree AV block; RBBB + LAFB (or LPFB) + first- or second-degree AV block; or IRBBB + LBBB (or ILBBB) + first- or second-degree AV block.

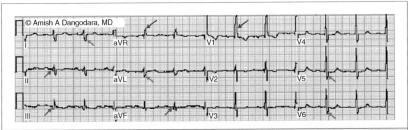

© Amish A Dangodara, MD

Figure 81-25. Bifascicular block. Bifascicular block due to right bundle branch block (RBBB) (see Fig. 81-21) and left posterior fascicular block (LPFB) (see Fig. 81-24). The RSR′ pattern of the RBBB is best seen in the right-sided leads aVR and V1 (*downward arrows*). The small Q waves of the LPFB are seen in the inferior leads, II, III, and aVF (*upward rightward arrows*). The deep S waves of the LPFB are seen in the lateral leads, I, aVL, and V5–V6 (*upward leftward arrows*). These same left-sided leads also have widening of the S wave due to the RBBB.

29. **What are the causes of an abnormal QTc interval?**
    Abnormal QTc intervals are usually due to drug toxicity or electrolyte disturbances, but they can also be found in patients with artificial electronic pacemakers or neuromuscular cardiomyopathies. Antiarrhythmics such as quinidine, procainamide, disopyramide, flecainide, amiodarone, or sotalol can cause QTc prolongation, which can lead to a potentially lethal type of ventricular fibrillation known as *torsades de pointes*. Neuropsychiatric drug toxicity due to phenothiazines, tricyclic antidepressants, and phenytoin can cause QTc prolongation. Drug-to-drug interactions with any of the above medications in safe doses can occur with theophylline; aminophylline; antihistamines such as cimetidine or terfenadine; promotility agents such as cisapride, promethazine, or prochlorperazine; and azole antifungals such as ketoconazole. These interactions can lead to QTc prolongation. Electrolyte disturbances such as hypokalemia, hypocalcemia, or hypermagnesemia can also result in QTc prolongation. Hypercalcemia causes shortening of the QTc, usually without any other harmful arrhythmias. *Digitalis toxicity* causes a shortened QTc and can lead to premature atrial contractions, AV blocks, or tachycardias with AV dissociation.

KEY POINTS: ABNORMAL INTERVALS

1. The PR interval (normal = 0.12–0.21 sec, or 3–5 mm) may be prolonged by AV blocks and certain drugs; it may be shortened by WPW syndrome, pericarditis, or junctional block.

2. The QRS interval (normal = 0.08–0.12 sec, or 2–3 mm) may be prolonged by bundle branch blocks.

3. The QTc interval (normal = <½ R-R interval, or 0.30–0.46 sec) may be prolonged by certain drugs, electrolytes, and pacers; it may be shortened by digitalis and hypercalcemia.

30. **What are the signs of atrial enlargement?**

Atrial enlargement results in an enlarged P wave that is >0.2 mV (>2 mm height) or >0.12 sec (>3 mm) in duration (see Fig. 81-8).

- **Right atrial enlargement (RAE):** RAE results in an enlarged P wave (> 2 × 3 mm) in lead II and a predominantly upright P wave in lead V1 (see Fig. 81-8, *B*). Any condition that causes increased volume or resistance to blood flow out of the right atrium can result in RAE, such as tricuspid stenosis, moderate to severe tricuspid regurgitation, pulmonic stenosis, pulmonary hypertension, pulmonary embolism, atrial septal defect, or ventricular septal defect resulting in left-to-right shunting. RAE predisposes the development of atrial arrhythmias because it anatomically distorts the SA node.

- **Left atrial enlargement (LAE):** LAE results in an enlarged P wave (> 2 × 3 mm) with a notched (dicrotic) *M* or triangle-shaped P wave in lead II and a predominantly downward P wave in lead V1 (see Fig. 81-8, *C*). Predisposing conditions include mitral stenosis or regurgitation, aortic stenosis or regurgitation, LVH, or left ventricular failure resulting in left-sided congestive heart failure. Biatrial enlargement fulfills criteria for both RAE and LAE, resulting in a large P wave in lead II and a large diphasic P wave in lead V1.

31. **What does "loss of R wave" signify?**

A small or absent R wave in leads that are expected to have a prominent R wave may be due to myocardial injury or impedance to conduction caused by anatomic variations. Impedance of electrical activity in the chest leads (V1–V6) can result in hypovoltage due to obesity, large breasts, hyperinflated emphysematous lungs, or pericardial effusion. Small or absent R waves in leads V1–V2 may indicate septal infarction (see Fig. 81-17), signifying an occlusion of the left anterior descending or the proximal diagonal artery branches. Similar changes in leads V1–V4 may indicate anterior wall infarction. This signifies an occlusion of the left anterior descending artery distal to the branch of the LCx artery. Small or absent R waves in leads V5–V6 may indicate lateral wall infarction, signifying occlusion of the LCx artery with a normal left anterior descending artery. Loss of R wave may be accompanied by a Q wave, indicating late myocardial injury or death, or it may be accompanied by ST segment and T wave abnormalities in the absence of Q waves, indicating ischemic injury or "non–Q wave infarction" (Fig. 81-26).

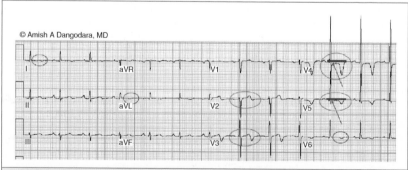

© Amish A Dangodara, MD

Figure 81-26. Anterolateral ischemia. There is poor R wave progression in leads V1–V2. The J point is denoted by the arrows in leads V4 and V5. It signals the end of the QRS complex and the beginning of the ST segment. There is J-point and horizontal ST-segment depression in leads V4 and V5. There are upsloping ST-segment elevations in leads V2 and V3. There are abnormal deep symmetric T-wave inversions in leads V3–V6 and flattened T waves in leads I, aVL, and V6. This constellation of findings is consistent with anterolateral ischemia and corresponds to an occlusion of the *proximal* left anterior descending artery, which results in ischemic changes of its distal branches, including the diagonal branches (causing septal ischemia) and the left circumflex artery branch (causing lateral ischemia).

32. **What are the signs of RVH?**

Increased amplitude of the R wave in the right-sided leads, aVR, and V1–V2; RAD; or early transition may be present in RVH (Fig. 81-27). RAD can be the earliest and most subtle sign of RVH, but RAD can also be caused by conditions other than RVH. Increased amplitude results in early transition, or a larger than expected R wave in lead V1 and V2, which are closest to the RV. This is associated with deep S waves in leads V5–V6, which have deep negative deflections since the rightward vector is moving away from these left-sided leads. If the sum of the R wave in lead V1 and the S wave in lead V5 or V6 is >11 mm (>1.1 mV), RVH is present. A prominent R wave in aVR and RAD can also be seen with associated asymmetric T-wave inversions in the right-sided leads due to right ventricular strain. These findings are the most severe signs of RVH.

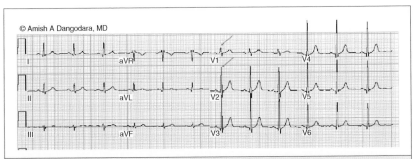

© Amish A Dangodara, MD

Figure 81-27. Right ventricular hypertrophy (RVH). The R wave in V1 and V2 (right-sided leads) is larger than expected *(arrows)*, indicating early transition due to prominent right-sided electrical forces. These findings are characteristic of RVH.

33. **What are the signs of LVH?**

Increased amplitude of the R wave in the left-sided leads, I, aVL, and V4–V6; LAD; or late transition may be present in LVH (Fig. 81-28). An R wave in lead aVL >11 mm (>1.1 mV) indicates LVH. LVH results in deep S waves in leads V1 and V2, the right-sided leads, which have a deep negative deflection since the leftward vector is moving away from these leads. There is late transition since the R wave peaks in leads V5–V6, which are closest to the LV. Therefore, if the sum of the S wave in lead V1 or V2 and the R wave in lead V5 or V6 is >35 mm (>3.5 mV), LVH is present. An R wave in V4, V5, or V6 of >25 mm (>2.5 mV) is a minor criterion for LVH. Associated asymmetric T-wave inversions may indicate a hypertrophic strain pattern (Fig. 81-29, *B*; Table 81-2).

34. **What do abnormalities of the ST segment signify?**

- **ST depression of >1 mm (>0.1 mV):** This generally signifies myocardial ischemia, especially if it is in two or more anatomically contiguous leads and associated with T-wave abnormalities (see Fig. 81-26).
- **ST depression:** ST depression with a rounded upsloping ST segment that merges with the T wave is a sign of digitalis effect, sometimes referred to as the "Dali sign" (Fig. 81-30).
- **ST elevation of >1 mm (>0.1 mV):** This elevation generally signifies acute myocardial infarction if it is in two or more anatomically contiguous leads and associated with T-wave abnormalities (Fig. 81-31). Upsloping and flattened ST elevations are usually easy to identify. However, downsloping ST elevations may blend in with the QRS complex and the following T wave, giving the false appearance of QRS widening, and can be difficult to identify.
- **Diffuse ST elevation:** This elevation in every lead is seen in pericarditis and is usually associated with a shortened and depressed PR segment. There may also be associated T-wave abnormalities.

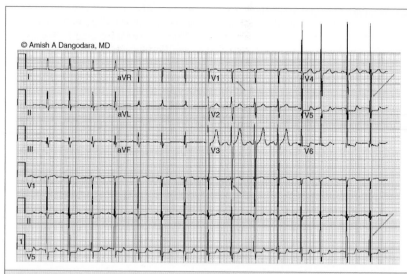

Figure 81-28. Left ventricular hypertrophy. There is a large R wave *(downward arrow)* in the left leads (V5 and V6) and a deep S wave *(upward arrow)* in the right leads (V1 and V2). The downward S wave in the right leads represents the vector moving away from the right leads, or toward the left leads. The sum of the R wave in the left leads plus the S wave in the right leads is > 35 mm. Additionally, the R wave is > 25 mm in either leads V4, V5, or V6. The aVL criteria of an R wave > 11 mm is not present on this ECG.

- **Persistent ST elevation:** ST elevation present for >6 weeks in anatomically contiguous leads is seen in aneurysmal dilation of the ventricle.

35. **What do abnormalities of T-wave morphology signify?**
    Abnormalities of the T wave are nonspecific and may represent anything from normal variation due to differences in anatomy to electrolyte disturbances, drug effects, and cardiac or neurologic ischemia or infarction (see Fig. 81-29). Symmetric inversions of the T wave, especially if they occur in leads in which the T wave is supposed to be inverted, are normal.
    - Small symmetric inversions of the T wave in leads that are supposed to have an upright T wave may signify ischemia or drug effects (see Fig. 81-29, *F*).
    - An asymmetrically inverted T wave with a gradual and long downward component and a rapid upward component is usually associated with a hypertrophic ventricular strain pattern, especially if criteria for RVH or LVH are met (see Fig. 81-29, *B*). This can sometimes also be seen with ischemia, especially if there are no associated criteria for ventricular hypertrophy. An upsloping ST segment can blend with the onset of the T wave to give the false appearance of asymmetric T-wave inversions when the T wave is actually symmetric and due to ischemia. These types of T waves are also seen with beats of ventricular origin, in which there is no preceding P wave or with artificially paced ventricular beats that are preceded by a pacer spike (see Figs. 81-13 and 81-14, *C*).
    - An asymmetric upright T wave that has a gradual initial component and a rapid terminal component is usually associated with bundle branch blocks, especially if there are criteria for RBBB or LBBB. T waves with similar morphology are *inverted* in the right-sided leads, aVR, and V1–V2 in RBBB and *inverted* in the left-sided leads, I, aVL, V5–V6 in LBBB (see Fig. 81-29, *C*). The presence of bundle branch blocks makes it difficult to interpret ischemic changes.

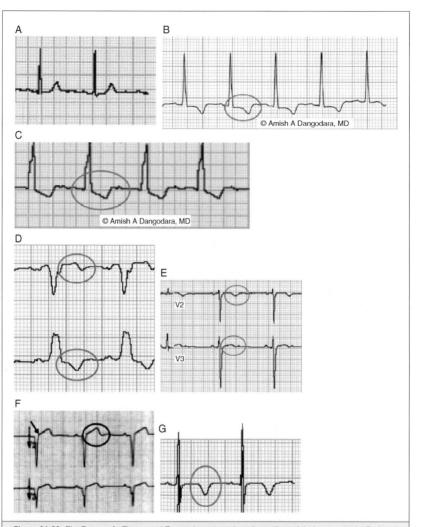

Figure 81-29. The T wave. **A,** The normal T wave is symmetric and usually upright in most leads. **B,** An asymmetrically inverted T wave with a shallow downward component *(oval)* and a rapid upward component is usually associated with a hypertrophic ventricular strain pattern, especially if criteria for right or left ventricular hypertrophy are met. **C,** Right bundle branch block (RBBB) and **D,** left bundle branch block (LBBB). An asymmetric upright or inverted T wave that has a gradual initial component due to an upsloping or downsloping ST segment blending in with the T wave and a rapid terminal component is usually associated with bundle branch blocks, especially if criteria for RBBB or LBBB are met. **E,** Nonspecific T wave changes with an abnormally inverted T wave in V2 and a flattened T wave in V3 may represent ischemia, electrolyte problems, medication effects, or many other nonspecific problems, or it may be a normal variant. **F,** Asymmetric biphasic T wave with J point and upsloping ST-segment elevation seen in acute myocardial infarction. The arrow points to the J-point and upsloping ST-segment elevation. **G,** Symmetric T-wave inversion *(oval)* in ischemia.

TABLE 81-2. VENTRICULAR HYPERTROPHY

	Major Criteria	Minor Criteria
RVH	Large R wave in V1 or V2 or deep S wave in V5 or V6 or R V1 + S V5 or V6 = >11mm	RAD Large R in aVR with RAD
RVH with strain pattern	T wave inversions in aVR, V1, V2	
LVH	S V1 or V2 + R V5 or V6 = >35 mm or R aVL = > 11mm	LAD R V4,V5, or V6 = > 25mm
LVH with strain pattern	T-wave inversions V1–V6, I, aVL	

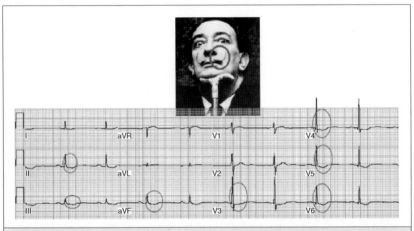

Figure 81-30. Digitalis effect, or the "Dali sign." The effect of the drug digitalis results in smooth, rounded, usually depressed ST segments, similar to the shape of the mustache of the famous eccentric artist Salvador Dali. On this ECG, the T waves are somewhat flattened or blend into the ST segment and become difficult to distinguish from the ST segment.

- T-wave flattening is a nonspecific finding that may be seen with ischemia, drug effects causing QTc prolongation, hypokalemia, obesity, pancreatitis, renal failure, and many other medical conditions that can effect fluid and electrolyte balance (see Fig. 81-12, *D*). Hypokalemia is usually associated with the presence of a U wave (see Fig. 81-2).
- Large, symmetric, peaked T waves with normal orientation are seen with hyperkalemia (Fig. 81-32).
- Deep, symmetric T-wave inversions indicate myocardial or cerebral ischemia, especially if these changes appear in two or more anatomically contiguous leads (see Fig. 81-26). ST elevation in almost every lead is more consistent with pericarditis (Fig. 81-33).
- Potentially ischemic-appearing T-wave changes are much more likely to be ischemic if there are associated ischemic abnormalities of the ST segment or if significant Q waves are present. Ischemic-appearing T wave changes can also be seen with ventricular aneurysms, cardiomyopathy, or neuromuscular cardiac diseases such as muscular dystrophy.

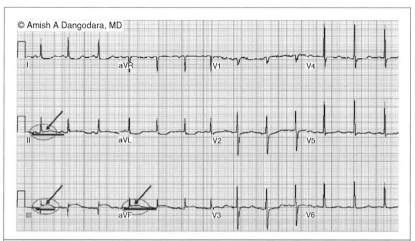

Figure 81-31. Acute inferior wall myocardial infarction. There is flat, horizontal ST-segment elevation of >1 mm above the baseline in the inferior leads II, III, and aVF *(arrows)*. This represents an acute inferior wall infarction in the distribution of the right coronary artery (see question 3).

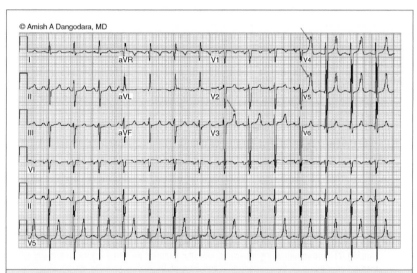

Figure 81-32. Hyperkalemia. Hyperkalemia results in tall, peaked, symmetric T waves that have a normal upright or inverted orientation for the respective lead (see question 16). The peaked effect may not be readily evident in all leads but is usually best seen in the chest leads, V1–V6. The arrows point to the peaked T-waves.

36. **What pattern of ECG changes is unique to myocardial infarction?**
    Myocardial infarction can be divided into ST-segment elevation myocardial infarction (STEMI) or non-STEMI. STEMI is associated with ST-segment elevations in the acute or subacute phase (see Fig. 81-31) and significant Q waves in the late phase (see Fig. 81-9), involving anatomically contiguous leads. This represents transmural infarction of the full thickness of the ventricle.

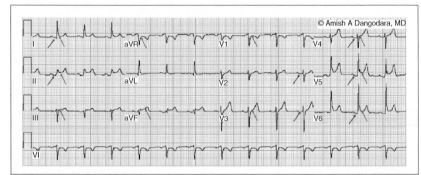

Figure 81-33. Pericarditis. There is ST elevation in almost every lead (leftward arrows pointed at the elevated J point). In the right-sided leads, aVR and V1, the leads are opposite to the overall vector, so the J point and ST segment are depressed instead of elevated, with associated T-wave inversion in these leads. If these findings were isolated to just one or two segments of the heart, then they may be due to acute myocardial infarction. Because the ST-segment elevation is diffuse, involving every wall, the findings are more consistent with pericarditis. Other findings in pericarditis include depression of the PR segment and shortening of the PR interval. On this ECG, the PR segment is depressed below the baseline *(rightward arrows)*, but the PR interval is not shortened.

Non-STEMI may be associated with ST-segment depressions from ischemia in the acute phase (see Fig. 81-26) and/or T-wave abnormalities, both in the acute and late phases (see Fig. 81-29, *G*), involving anatomically contiguous leads. Because Q waves do not develop in the late phase, this is sometimes referred to as "non–Q wave" myocardial infarction. This represents nontransmural infarction or partial-thickness injury to the ventricle.

37. **What pattern of ECG changes is unique to WPW syndrome?**
    The presence of a preexcitation wave of the QRS, or delta wave (Fig. 81-34), is most characteristic of WPW and can be seen with a sinus rhythm or reentry tachycardia. There may also be a shortened PR interval.

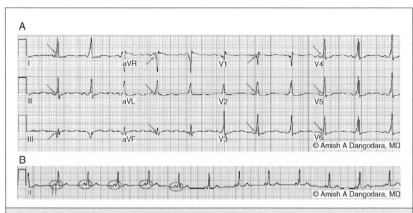

Figure 81-34. Wolff-Parkinson-White syndrome (WPW). WPW is a preexcitation, reentry supraventricular tachycardia due to either a right- or left-sided accessory bypass tract. **A,** It is characterized by a preexcitation wave *(arrows)*, or delta *(triangle)* wave, at the onset of the QRS complex. **B,** There may also be a shortened PR interval *(oval)* due to the preexcitation of WPW.

38. **What pattern of ECG changes is consistent with pulmonary disease?**

    Pulmonary disease pattern on an ECG reveals signs of right ventricular strain from pulmonary hypertension or chronic pulmonary diseases, including chronic obstructive lung disease, obstructive sleep apnea, and pulmonary embolism. These findings include early transition, RAD (see Fig. 81-16), RVH (see Fig. 81-27), RAE (see Fig. 81-8, *B*), or RBBB (see Fig. 81-21).

39. **What pattern of ECG changes is unique to pulmonary embolism?**

    Pulmonary embolism is associated with a unique set of ECG findings that occur in <15% of cases of pulmonary embolism. These specific but insensitive findings result in a deep S wave in lead I, a Q wave in lead III, and inverted T wave in lead III (S1Q3T3). The more common but less specific findings are those of a pulmonary disease pattern.

40. **How should the rhythm be evaluated?**

    Evaluate the rate, axis, intervals, waves and complexes, and the relationship of the P wave to the QRS complex to evaluate the rhythm. Arrhythmias are divided into supraventricular (narrow complex) and ventricular (wide complex) classifications. Arrhythmias are defined by the source of the underlying pacemaker as sinus, atrial, junctional, supraventricular, ventricular, or asystole (see Fig. 81-14). The rate can also define the arrhythmia as bradycardia, tachycardia, flutter, or fibrillation, depending on the underlying pacemaker. Arrhythmias are defined by the mechanism of the abnormal beat as AV nodal blocks, escape beats, reentry tachycardias, unifocal, multifocal, wandering, or paroxysmal. Arrhythmias are also defined by the frequency of the abnormal beat as pauses, premature, nonsustained, or sustained based on the origin of the abnormal pacemaker. The pattern of the abnormal beat in relation to the underlying rhythm can define the arrhythmia as a pattern of *bigeminy* (one abnormal beat per baseline beat) or *trigeminy* (one abnormal beat per two baseline beats, or vice versa). (See Chapters 32 and 33 for further details.)

BIBLIOGRAPHY

1. Dubin D: Rapid Interpretation of EKG's, ed 6. Tampa: Cover Publishing, 2000.
2. Wagner GS: Marriott's Practical Electrocardiography. Philadephia: Lippincott Williams & Wilkins, 2001.

CHAPTER 82

CHEST X-RAY INTERPRETATION

Sunil Kripalani, MD, MSc

1. **What are the first things to look at when viewing a chest radiograph?**
   Before looking for abnormalities, confirm you have the correct radiograph by reviewing the patient's name, medical record number, and date. Describe the type of film, its penetration, the patient positioning, and the degree of inspiration.

2. **Describe the advantages and disadvantages of portable radiographs.**
   Although portable radiographs may be more convenient, they are often inadequate for assessing the thorax due to inadequate inspiration and the single view provided. Structures near the mediastinum, lung bases, lung apices, and retrocardiac area (basically, the whole thorax!) are poorly seen.

3. **Describe the differences in technique between portable radiographs and posterior-anterior (PA) radiographs.**
   PA radiographs are taken with the patient standing, arms abducted, with the x-ray plate against the anterior chest wall and the machine behind the patient. This position promotes maximum inspiration of the chest and minimizes enlargement of the heart shadow as it is projected by x-rays (traveling posterior to anterior) onto the nearby film. Portable radiographs are usually taken when the patient is lying on a stretcher, arms adducted, with the plate against the patient's back. The film is shot anterior to posterior, so the heart (which is anterior in the chest) appears larger when projected onto the x-ray plate. Clues that a particular radiograph may be portable include an absent gastric bubble (air only rises to create the bubble when the patient is standing), horizontal orientation (the viewed radiograph is wider than it is tall), arms are adducted (confined by the bed rails), monitor leads are visible, and the recumbent patient often takes a poor inspiration.

4. **How is film penetration assessed?**
   Intervertebral disk spaces should be slightly visible through the heart shadow on the frontal view. In an underpenetrated film, the spaces are not visible, and the radiograph appears white overall. In an overpenetrated film, the radiograph looks dark, and subtle structures are not seen.

5. **Name several different ways to position the patient for a chest radiograph.**
   The patient's position may be upright, supine, decubitus (i.e., lying on the side), or lordotic (i.e., leaning back). In a properly positioned, nonrotated, upright radiograph, the vertebral spines will lie exactly between the heads of the clavicles. Decubitus radiographs are useful for assessment of pleural effusions. Lordotic radiographs provide a better view of the apices.

6. **What features indicate an adequate degree of inspiration for the radiograph?**
   Count ribs. On a PA radiograph, the right hemidiaphragm should be at or below the 5th anterior or 10th posterior intercostal space.

7. **On a normal frontal view of the chest, what structures compose the central (cardiac) shadow?**
   On the patient's right side are the right brachiocephalic artery and vein, ascending aorta and superior vena cava, right atrium, and inferior vena cava. The structures composing the left side

of the shadow are the left brachiocephalic artery and vein, aortic knob, pulmonary trunk, left atrial appendage, and left ventricle (Fig. 82-1).

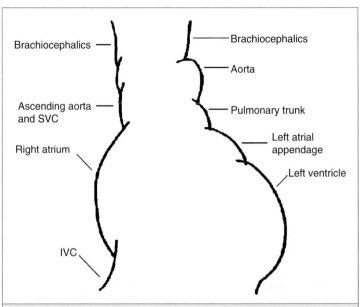

Figure 82-1. Structures comprising the central shadow. IVC = inferior vena cava; SVC = superior vena cava.

KEY POINTS: WHY PORTABLE CHEST RADIOGRAPHS ARE USUALLY INADEQUATE FOR ASSESSING THORACIC PATHOLOGY

1. They provide only a single view.

2. The degree of patient inspiration is often poor.

3. The heart appears enlarged due to the anterior-posterior technique.

4. Structures near the mediastinum, lung bases, lung apices, and retrocardiac area are poorly seen.

8. **On a normal lateral view of the chest, what structures compose the cardiac shadow?**
The right ventricle is located anteriorly. The posterior aspect of the shadow includes the aorta and left atrium.

9. **Where are the lobes of each lung located?**
The right lung comprises the upper, middle, and lower lobes, which are separated by the horizontal and oblique fissures. The left lung has only upper and lower lobes, separated by the

oblique fissure; the lingula is part of the upper lobe. The right middle lobe and lingula are located anteriorly. The lower lobes extend posteriorly behind them (Fig. 82-2).

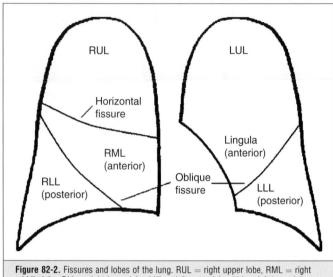

Figure 82-2. Fissures and lobes of the lung. RUL = right upper lobe, RML = right middle lobe, RLL = right lower lobe, LUL = left upper lobe, LLL = left lower lobe.

10. **Apart from the cardiac shadow, what structures are normally asymmetric on a chest radiograph?**
    - There are more vascular markings in the lower than in the upper lungs.
    - The left hilum is slightly (<3 cm) higher than the right.
    - The left dome of the diaphragm is slightly (1 intercostal space) lower than the right.

11. **Describe a systematic approach for reading chest radiographs.**
    After confirming administrative data and assessing the radiograph's quality, describe the patient's general features (e.g., body size, sex) and the location of foreign objects (e.g., intravenous lines, tubes, monitor leads). Then progress from the soft tissues to the lung fields. Immediately focusing on the lungs may result in other findings being overlooked. After searching for abnormalities, look for absent structures (e.g., missing parenchymal markings that may indicate a pneumothorax), as well as findings associated with the abnormalities detected. For example, if the radiograph shows a lung nodule, go back and look for associated adenopathy, lobar collapse, effusion, etc. The phrase, "Stop and be careful. His lungs appear abnormal," helps organize this systematic approach (Table 82-1).

12. **What is the silhouette sign?**
    The silhouette sign helps localize pulmonary infiltrates. When adjacent objects have similar density, their borders blend together. For example, an infiltrate that appears in the lower half of the right lung field on frontal view is located in the right middle lobe if it is confluent with the right heart border, and in the right lower lobe if it is confluent with the diaphragm.

TABLE 82-1. STOP AND BE CAREFUL, HIS LUNGS APPEAR ABNORMAL	
Mnemonic Clue	**Structures to Examine**
Soft tissues	Neck, axillae, breasts, chest wall
Abdomen	Liver, stomach, colon, spleen, aorta
Bones	Spine, shoulder girdle, sternum, ribs
Central shadow	Trachea, great vessels, heart border
Hila	Pulmonary vessels, bronchi, lymph nodes
Lungs	Pleura, diaphragm, fissures, lung parenchyma
Absent structures	Absent parenchyma or vascular markings, volume loss
Abnormalities	Look for associated abnormalities

13. **What is the difference in appearance between alveolar and interstitial processes?**
   - **Alveolar:** Small (5–10 mm), fluffy, coalescent; air bronchograms
   - **Interstitial:** Nodular type (2–3 mm multiple discrete nodules), reticular type (thin 1–2 mm well-defined linear densities), or reticulonodular

14. **What are air bronchograms?**
   Highlighting of bronchioles when surrounding alveoli are filled. They are seen in pneumonia, radiation pneumonitis, bronchoalveolar cancer, lymphoma, pulmonary edema, and other alveolar processes.

15. **What are signs of volume loss?**
   Volume loss is usually caused by lobar collapse or fibrosis. Radiographic findings include an elevated hemidiaphragm, mediastinal shift, narrowed intercostal spaces, compensatory emphysema of the contralateral lung or remaining lobes, displaced hilum, and displaced interlobar septa bounding the affected lobe.

16. **What are Kerley's B lines?**
   Kerley's B lines are septal lines (2–3 cm marks perpendicular to the lateral chest wall) in the lung periphery. They are seen in pulmonary edema, interstitial pneumonitis, and lymphatic obstruction (e.g., lymphangitic carcinomatosis).

17. **What is the significance of air under the diaphragm?**
   This usually signifies free air in the abdomen, which rises to the level of the diaphragm in an upright patient. It may be caused by an intestinal perforation and should be considered a surgical emergency.

18. **Describe the classic radiographic appearance of common diseases.**
   See Table 82-2.

19. **Name several conditions that can cause localized or widespread pulmonary infiltrates.**
   - **Localized:** Pneumonia, infarction, contusion, edema, postradiation changes, lung cancer, lymphoma
   - **Widespread:** Edema, pneumonia, hemorrhage, adult respiratory distress syndrome, lung cancer, hematogenous metastasis, lymphoma, sarcoid, eosinophilic pneumonia

TABLE 82-2.   CLASSIC RADIOGRAPHIC APPEARANCE OF COMMON DISEASES

Disease	Radiographic Appearance
Adult respiratory distress syndrome	Diffuse infiltrates, normal-sized heart, no pleural effusion
Aortic dissection	Mediastinal widening
Emphysema	Hyperinflated, hyperlucent lung fields; flat diaphragms; avascular zones; small, vertical-appearing heart
Lung abscess	Thick-walled cavity, air-fluid level
Lung cancer	Nodule or large mass; may have multiple lesions, adenopathy, or effusion
Pericardial effusion	Enlarged "water bottle" heart shadow
Pneumonia (lobar)	Consolidation that respects fissures, air bronchograms; silhouette sign against adjacent structures
Pneumonia (atypical)	Diffuse alveolar and interstitial infiltrates
Pneumothorax	Sharp line of collapsed pleura, no vascular markings peripherally
Pulmonary edema	Bilateral, soft, fluffy, coalescing infiltrates; interstitial markings; cephalization of vasculature; Kerley's lines; may have pleural effusion or fluid in fissures
Pulmonary embolism	May be normal; classic triad (i.e., basal infiltrate, elevated hemidiaphragm, blunting of costophrenic angle); subsegmental atelectasis; Hampton's hump (i.e., pleural-based, wedge-shaped consolidation); Westermark's sign (i.e., wedge-shaped absence of vascular markings)
Tuberculosis	Upper lobe cavity superimposed on infiltrate

20. **What is the differential diagnosis for hyperlucency?**
    - **Unilateral**
        - □ *Structural:* Poor technique, rotation, scoliosis
        - □ *Chest wall:* Mastectomy, atrophy or absence of pectoralis muscle
        - □ *Lung:* Compensatory emphysema, obstructive emphysema, unilateral bullae, pulmonary embolism (PE), pneumothorax
    - **Bilateral**
        - □ *With overexpanded lungs:* Emphysema, asthma, tracheal/laryngeal/bilateral bronchial stenosis;
        - □ *With normal/small lungs:* Pulmonary hypertension, multiple PE, pulmonary artery stenosis

KEY POINTS: CLASSIC RADIOGRAPHIC APPEARANCE OF LOBAR PNEUMONIA

1. Dense consolidation that respects the lung fissures

2. Air bronchograms (highlighting of bronchioles when surrounding alveoli are filled)

3. Silhouette sign (confluence of borders with adjacent structures)

21. **Name common processes that can cause hilar enlargement.**
    Lung cancer, lymphoma, tuberculosis, sarcoidosis, perihilar pneumonia, fungal infection, pulmonary artery aneurysm, PE, pulmonary hypertension, hypersensitivity pneumonitis, silicosis, and berylliosis.

22. **What processes typically cause infiltrates in the upper lung fields?**
    Tuberculosis, radiotherapy, sarcoidosis, chronic hypersensitivity pneumonitis, histoplasmosis, silicosis, progressive massive fibrosis, ankylosing spondylitis, cystic fibrosis, and eosinophilic pneumonia.

23. **What are some of the noninfectious causes of fever with pulmonary opacification?**
    Pulmonary hemorrhage, Goodpasture's disease, Wegener's granulomatosis, systemic lupus erythematosus, idiopathic pulmonary hemosiderosis, allergic bronchopulmonary aspergillosis, eosinophilic pneumonia, eosinophilic granuloma, hypereosinophilic syndrome, bronchoalveolar cancer, lymphoma, pulmonary infarct, adult respiratory distress syndrome, bronchiolitis obliterans-organizing pneumonia, aspiration of gastric contents, drugs, radiation pneumonitis, pulmonary alveolar proteinosis, sarcoid, toxic gas inhalation, and fibrosing alveolitis.

24. **What conditions can cause lung nodules?**
    - **Solitary:** Lung cancer, metastatic cancer, tuberculosis, histoplasmosis, hydatid cyst, carcinoid, hamartoma, pneumonia, bronchogenic cyst, sequestration, teratoma, pulmonary infarct, hematoma, arteriovenous malformation
    - **Multiple:** Metastatic cancer, abscesses, coccidiomycosis, histoplasmosis, hydatid cysts, Wegener's granulomatosis, rheumatoid nodule, Caplan's syndrome, progressive massive fibrosis, arteriovenous malformation

25. **How can the location of a mediastinal mass guide the differential diagnosis?**
    - **Anterior:** Thymoma, teratoma, retrosternal thyroid, aortic aneurysm, lymphoma, sternal tumor, pericardial fat pad, Morgagni's hernia, diaphragmatic hump, pericardial cyst
    - **Middle:** Lymphoma, metastatic lymph node enlargement, granulomatous disease, bronchogenic cyst, mediastinal vessel aneurysm, bronchial cancer
    - **Posterior:** Neurogenic tumor, esophageal achalasia, hiatal hernia, extramedullary hematopoiesis, abscess, lymphoma, Bochdalek's hernia, aorta (e.g., dilated, ruptured, tortuous), anterior thoracic meningocele

26. **What conditions can cause cavitary lesions?**
    - **Abscesses:** *Staphylococcus aureus*, *Klebsiella* species, tuberculosis, aspiration, coccidiomycosis, *Cryptococcus* species
    - **Cancer:** Squamous, metastasis, Hodgkin's lymphoma
    - **Granulomas:** Wegener's, rheumatoid, sarcoid, progressive massive fibrosis
    - **Other:** Septic emboli/infarction, cystic bronchiectasis, bronchogenic cyst, sequestrated lung, hematoma, traumatic lung cyst

27. **What is the differential diagnosis of pleural effusion (with otherwise normal chest radiograph)?**
    Primary tuberculosis, viruses, mycoplasma, lung cancer, metastasis, mesothelioma, lymphoma, systemic lupus erythematosus, rheumatoid, pancreatitis, subphrenic abscess, post-thoracic/abdominal surgery, Meig's syndrome, nephrotic syndrome, congestive heart failure, cirrhosis, hypothyroidism, PE, closed chest trauma, and asbestosis.

28. **What causes elevation of the diaphragm?**
    Bilateral elevation is seen with poor inspiratory effort, obesity, ascites, pregnancy, pneumomediastinum, restrictive lung disease, and bilateral basal pulmonary collapse. Unilateral

elevation can be caused by phrenic nerve palsy, unilateral pulmonary collapse, pulmonary infarct, pleural disease, splinting of the diaphragm, hemiplegia, eventration of the diaphragm, gaseous distention of the stomach or splenic flexure, hepatomegaly, splenomegaly, abdominal mass, scoliosis, and decubitus positioning (dependent side has raised diaphragm). It is important to rule out subpulmonic effusion or abscess.

BIBLIOGRAPHY

1. Carpenter W: Basic chest x-ray review. Available at http://rad.usuhs.mil/rad/chest_review/index.html
2. Chandrasekhar AJ: Chest x-ray atlas. Available at http://www.meddean.luc.edu/lumen/meded/medicine/pulmonar/cxr/atlas/cxratlas_f.htm
3. Fanta CH: Harvard Medical School Radiology for Second-Year Students. Available at http://brighamrad.harvard.edu/education/online/clerk_2/read.html
4. Jaffe CC, Lynch PJ: Introduction to cardiothoracic imaging. Yale Center for Advanced Instructional Media. Available at http://info.med.yale.edu/intmed/cardio/imaging/
5. Ritter B: Basics of chest x-ray interpretation. A programmed study. Available at http://nps.freeservers.com/chestxra.htm

CHAPTER 83

LUMBAR PUNCTURE

Alex Carbo, MD, and Craig Gordon, MD

1. **What is a lumbar puncture? When is it indicated?**

   A lumbar puncture is the insertion of a hollow needle between lumbar vertebrae to withdraw cerebrospinal fluid (CSF) for diagnostic or therapeutic purposes. It is most commonly used in the evaluation of altered mental status or to aid in the diagnosis of suspected meningitis, encephalitis, subarachnoid hemorrhage, central nervous system (CNS) vasculitis, or normal pressure hydrocephalus.

2. **How does one identify the proper anatomic interspace to insert the spinal needle?**

   A lumbar puncture should typically be performed at the L3–L4 or L4–L5 interspace, below the conus medullaris. Locate the posterior superior iliac spines and draw a horizontal line to determine the location of the L3–L4 interspace. The patient can be positioned in either a lateral decubitus position or seated upright, but only the lateral decubitus position yields an accurate result for CSF opening pressure.

3. **Describe how to perform a lumbar puncture.**

   After proper anatomic location is selected, first sterilize and drape the area and administer local anesthesia. Place the needle in the selected intervertebral space in the midline of the back with the open bevel pointing towards a lateral flank. Advance the needle, while firmly holding the stylet in place, at a 30-degree angle cephalad aiming toward the umbilicus. There may be a "popping" sensation as the needle passes through the ligamentum flavum. Otherwise, you may have to remove the stylet periodically to see whether CSF is draining. Never advance the spinal needle without the stylet in place. If the tip of the needle encounters bone, retract the needle and redirect at a slightly different angle. Once CSF is freely flowing, attach the stopcock and manometer to the needle to measure the opening pressure. Opening pressure done in a seated patient will result in an inaccurate reading. Collect fluid for analysis in four tubes. Replace the stylet before attempting to remove the needle.

4. **Under what circumstances should neuroimaging be performed before lumbar puncture?**

   Patients with altered level of consciousness, immunocompromised state (e.g., AIDS, use of immunosuppressants), age older than 60 years, papilledema, or focal neurologic deficits are at an increased risk of having a CNS mass lesion and subsequent increased risk of herniation. These patients require CNS imaging before a lumbar puncture. In the absence of these predictors, the rate of significant CNS herniation is minimal.

   Hasbun R, Abrahams J, Jekel J, Quagliarello VJ: Computed tomography of the head before lumbar puncture in adults with suspected meningitis. N Engl J Med 345:1727–1733, 2001.

5. **Are there coagulation or platelet values at which lumbar puncture is contraindicated?**

   There are no studies reported in the literature that describe a cutoff value for international normalized ratio or platelet count. However, clinical judgment should prevail, and significant coagulopathy should be corrected before lumbar puncture.

6. **What are the potential complications of a lumbar puncture?**
   The most common complication is post–lumbar puncture headache, which complicates up to 30% of lumbar punctures. Use of a small-bore needle (24-gauge or smaller) reduces this rate. The volume of fluid removed and operator experience have no effect (Table 83-1).

TABLE 83-1. COMPLICATIONS OF LUMBAR PUNCTURE	
Common Complications	**Uncommon Complications**
Post–lumbar puncture headache	Tonsillar herniation
Back pain at site of needle insertion	Ascending subarachnoid hemorrhage
Local self-limited hemorrhage	Spinal cord/nerve root injury
	Infection

7. **What are the treatment options for post–lumbar puncture headache?**
   This type of headache is hypothesized to be related to persistent CSF leak through the dural puncture site. The initial management is aggressive pain relief with acetaminophen or nonsteroidal anti-inflammatory drugs but often requires opiate analgesia. If these measures are ineffective, 500 mg of intravenous caffeine results in a 75% rate of headache relief (versus 15% in control subjects). If this is not effective, an epidural blood patch (instilling autologous blood into the epidural space at the site of the lumbar puncture) is a relatively safe procedure that is extremely effective (95%). Blood patches seal the dural puncture site and prevent further leak of CSF. There is no data to support the use of bed rest or intravenous fluids in the management of post–lumbar puncture headache.

KEY POINTS: LUMBAR PUNCTURE

1. Lumbar puncture is indicated in the evaluation of altered mental status or to aid in the diagnosis of suspected meningitis, encephalitis, subarachnoid hemorrhage, CNS vasculitis, or normal pressure hydrocephalus.

2. During a lumbar puncture, the patient may be positioned in either the lateral decubitus position or seated upright, but only the lateral decubitus position yields an accurate result for CSF opening pressure.

3. Potential complications of lumbar puncture include post–lumbar puncture headache, back pain at site of needle insertion, local self-limited hemorrhage, tonsillar herniation, ascending subarachnoid hemorrhage, spinal cord/nerve root injury, and infection.

8. **What are the different tests that can be sent to aid the evaluation of cerebrospinal fluid?**
   The presence of red blood cells (RBCs) in the CSF may indicate subarachnoid hemorrhage. In this situation, one would expect either the same or increasing numbers of RBCs in tube 4 as are present in tube 1. More commonly, the presence of RBCs is due to trauma caused by the lumbar puncture. Under this scenario, the number of RBCs decreases from tube 1 (more) to tube 4 (less) (Table 83-2).

TABLE 83-2. ANALYSIS OF CSF AFTER LUMBAR PUNCTURE*	
Tube Number	Test
1	Cell count and differential
2	Total protein
	Glucose
3	Gram's stain
	Bacterial culture
4	Cell count and differential

*A wide variety of additional tests may be indicated, depending on the specific clinical circumstance.

BIBLIOGRAPHY

1. Chen H, Sonnenday C, Lillemoe K: Neurosurgical procedures. In Manual of Common Bedside Surgical Procedures, 2nd ed. Philadelphia, Lippincott Williams & Wilkins, 2000, pp 180–186.

2. Hasbun R, Abrahams J, Jekel J, Quagliarello VJ: Computed tomography of the head before lumbar puncture in adults with suspected meningitis. N Engl J Med 345:1727–1733, 2001.

CHAPTER 84

THORACENTESIS

Vaishali Singh, MD, MPH, MBA

1. **What is a thoracentesis? When is it indicated?**

   Thoracentesis is the removal of fluid from the pleural space for diagnostic or therapeutic purposes. Diagnostic thoracentesis is performed to help establish the cause of a pleural effusion. Therapeutic thoracentesis is performed to relieve respiratory difficulties caused by large pleural effusions or to introduce sclerosing (pleurodesis) or antineoplastic agents into the pleural space to treat recurrent pleural effusions and malignancy, respectively.

2. **What are the contraindications to thoracentesis?**

   The contraindications for thoracentesis include coagulopathy, local chest wall infection, an uncooperative patient, hemodynamic instability, severe cough or hiccups, and major respiratory impairment with the contralateral lung. Relative contraindications include mechanical ventilation and acute coronary syndrome.

3. **Describe the preparations for a thoracentesis.**

   Inform the patient of the risks and benefits associated with a thoracentesis, and obtain his or her written consent to undergo the procedure. Equipment needed for the procedure includes thoracentesis needle, catheter device with three-way stopcock and vacuum collection system, gauze, sterile drape and gloves, Betadine, 1% lidocaine, specimen test tubes, 22G and 25G injection needles, and syringes to aspirate fluid (20–60 ml syringes are acceptable, depending on the amount of fluid to be withdrawn). Most hospitals have a kit that provides all the necessary equipment in one convenient package.

4. **How is a thoracentesis performed?**

   Thoracentesis is generally performed with the patient sitting upright and leaning slightly forward with his or her arms supported in front of the body (Fig. 84-1). Localize the optimal site to tap by physical examination (dullness to percussion of the chest wall). Chest x-ray, computed tomography scan, and ultrasound are helpful imaging tools that can be used to localize fluid. If the effusion is free flowing, select a site that is 1–2 intercostal spaces below the fluid level and above the diaphragm between the midscapular and posterior axillary line. Using sterile technique, clean the skin with Betadine and drape the patient. At the superior border of the rib, use a 25G or smaller needle to inject local anesthetic (usually 1% lidocaine) and create a small wheal beneath the skin (Fig. 84-2). Avoid the lower border of the upper rib, which contains the neurovascular bundle. Using a 22G (1.5-inch) needle with intermittent aspiration, infiltrate the anesthetic agent into the subcutaneous tissue along the superior aspect of the rib, the periosteum, and finally the parietal pleura. Advance the needle slowly in this fashion until a slight give is felt. Once pleural fluid is aspirated, remove the needle and insert the thoracentesis needle to a similar depth. For diagnostic taps, attach the thoracentesis needle to a 20–60 ml syringe to aspirate pleural fluid. For therapeutic taps, connect the thoracentesis needle to a larger syringe or vacuum container system. Be cautious never to expose the open end of the anesthesia or thoracentesis needle to air while in the pleural space.

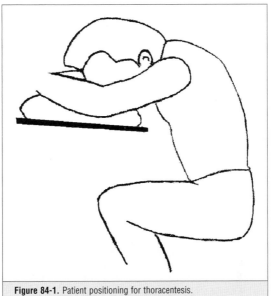

Figure 84-1. Patient positioning for thoracentesis.

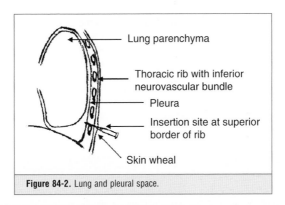

Lung parenchyma

Thoracic rib with inferior neurovascular bundle

Pleura

Insertion site at superior border of rib

Skin wheal

Figure 84-2. Lung and pleural space.

5. **Describe the use of ultrasound in thoracentesis.**
   Ultrasound is used to evaluate or guide aspiration of pleural fluid by marking the fluid level site at which the thoracentesis should be performed. It also permits the identification of free versus loculated effusions. Ultrasound-guided thoracentesis offers safety advantages in patients receiving mechanical ventilation and those with small effusions or potentially misleading physical examination or radiograph findings.

6. **How much fluid can safely be removed with thoracentesis?**
   Removal of more than 1L of pleural fluid may increase the chance for reexpansion pulmonary edema, although this is thought to be a generally uncommon complication. Reexpansion pulmonary edema is thought to result from the reinflation of the lung after a prolonged period of collapse.

7. **What can you tell from the appearance and smell of pleural fluid aspirate?**
   Transudative pleural effusions generally appear pale or straw colored. Grossly bloody effusions may result from trauma (including traumatic thoracentesis), neoplasm, esophageal rupture, pulmonary embolus with infarction, or cardiothoracic surgery. Parapneumonic effusions can appear serosanguinous. A milky effusion suggests trauma to the thoracic duct (e.g., chylous effusion) or chronic inflammation (e.g., tuberculosis, connective tissue disease). Gross pus or a putrid smell suggests purulent infection or empyema. Fluid that smells like urine or ammonia may suggest urinothorax, which can be verified by demonstrating that the pleural creatinine level is higher than the serum creatinine level.

8. **What are the different tests that can be ordered to aid the evaluation of pleural fluid?**
   Pleural fluid is routinely withdrawn for cell count with differential, cytology, Gram's stain, fungal and bacterial cultures, acid-fast bacilli stain, lactate dehydrogenase, glucose, protein, creatinine, amylase, lipids, and pH. A spun hematocrit test of grossly bloody pleural fluid assists in the diagnosis of hemothorax, in which the hematocrit level of the pleural fluid is >50% of the peripheral hematocrit level. (See Chapter 24 for more details.)

9. **What if a patient starts coughing during the thoracentesis?**
   Patient coughing has been associated with large-volume thoracentesis and increases the risk of pneumothorax during the procedure. The tip of the needle may be touching the pleura. Try to either withdraw the needle slightly to avoid injury to the lung and/or discontinue removal of fluid until the coughing stops. Ask the patient to take shallow breaths during the procedure if possible.

10. **When the catheter is in, can I introduce air into the pleural space?**
    Yes, airflow from the atmosphere can enter the pleural space via the catheter or needle. This most often occurs as the syringe is removed from a needle or catheter, and it can be avoided by placing the operator's gloved finger over the open area until the connection is made.

11. **What are complications of thoracentesis?**
    Potential complications of thoracentesis include pain at puncture site, pneumothorax, cough, shortness of breath, vasovagal reaction, introduction of infection, hemothorax, reexpansion pulmonary edema, and liver or splenic laceration.

KEY POINTS: THORACENTESIS

1. Thoracentesis is the removal of fluid from the pleural space for diagnostic or therapeutic purposes.

2. Contraindications to thoracentesis include coagulopathy, uncooperative patient, and major respiratory impairment of the contralateral lung.

3. Common complications from thoracentesis are pain at puncture site, pneumothorax, cough, vasovagal reaction, bleeding, and introduction of infection.

4. When performing thoracentesis, be sure to prepare all needed equipment and obtain written consent from the patient before starting the procedure.

5. Obtain a post-thoracentesis chest x-ray if pneumothorax is suspected clinically or when air is aspirated during the procedure.

12. **Do all patients undergoing diagnostic thoracentesis require a routine chest x-ray after the procedure for identification of a pneumothorax?**

In a study of 174 hospitalized patients undergoing diagnostic thoracentesis for a pleural effusion, a subgroup was identified in whom the risk for pneumothorax was low enough (approximately 1%) to justify the avoidance of about 60% of chest radiographs obtained after the procedure. The characteristics of the patients were clinical stability, no prior chest irradiation, only one pass attempted without the aspiration of air, and no other indication of pneumothorax.

BIBLIOGRAPHY

1. Colice GL, Jeffrey RB: Practical management of pleural effusions. Post Grad Med 105:67–70, 73–77, 1999.

2. Collins TR, Sahn SA: Thoracocentesis: Clinical value, complications, technical problems, and patient experience. Chest 91:817–822, 1987.

3. Doyle JJ, Hnatiuk OW, Torrington KG, et al: Necessity of routine chest roentgenography after thoracentesis. Ann Intern Med 124:816–820, 1996.

4. Gomella LG: Thoracentesis. Clinician's Pocket Reference, 7th ed. Norwalk, CT, Appleton & Lange, 1993, pp 257–259.

5. Jones PW, Moyers P, Rogers JT, et al: Ultrasound guided thoracentesis: Is it a safer method? Chest 123:418–423, 2003.

6. Light RW: Useful tests on the pleural fluid in the management of patients with pleural effusions. Curr Opin Pulm Med 5:245–249, 1999.

7. Villena V, Lopez-Encuentra A, Garcia-Lujan R, et al: Clinical implications of appearance of pleural fluid at thoracentesis. Chest 125:156–159, 2004.

CHAPTER 85

PARACENTESIS

Craig Gordon, MD, and Alex Carbo, MD

1. **What is an abdominal paracentesis? When is it indicated?**

   A paracentesis is the removal of fluid from the abdominal cavity by use of a hollow needle. It is useful for determining the etiology of new-onset ascites or ascites of unknown etiology, diagnosis of spontaneous bacterial peritonitis in a patient with ascites and change in clinical status (e.g., fever, nausea, abdominal pain, confusion), and treatment of symptomatic large-volume ascites.

2. **Describe the best anatomic location to insert the paracentesis needle.**

   Patients should be placed in the supine position. The right or left lower quadrants should be selected to avoid injury to the liver or spleen. Insert the needle lateral to the rectus abdominus muscle to reduce the risk of a rectal sheath hematoma. Avoid inserting the needle near a surgical scar because this can increase the risk of bowel perforation. Some recommend a medial approach through the relatively avascular linea alba, but this should be undertaken only in patients with large amounts of ascites and dullness to percussion in this region.

3. **Describe how to perform a paracentesis.**

   After selecting an appropriate site for needle insertion, sterilize and drape the area and administer local anesthesia. Use a small-bore finder needle (22G to 25G) to locate the ascitic fluid. After identifying the presence of ascites, insert and advance the larger-bore paracentesis needle while aspirating with a syringe. Remember not to use the larger-bore paracentesis needle until fluid is aspirated with the smaller needle. Once fluid is freely flowing into the syringe, retract the needle and, if the kit allows, leave only the catheter in place to withdraw fluid into vacuum bottles. When switching bottles, use the stopcock to clamp the tubing to stop the flow of fluid into the vacuum container. When the procedure is completed, remove the catheter and apply pressure for a few minutes before covering with a bandage.

4. **When is the use of an ultrasound advisable?**

   Common indications for ultrasound are to identify and sample loculated ascitic fluid, or to safely obtain fluid in patients with bowel obstruction or during pregnancy. There are no data available to support the use of ultrasound to "mark" fluid that will be sampled at a later time.

5. **Are there coagulation or platelet values at which paracentesis is contraindicated?**

   There is no absolute cutoff for coagulopathy or platelet dysfunction in the performance of a paracentesis. One study found no increased rate of hemorrhagic complications (hemoglobin decrease of 2 mg/dL) in patients with an international normalized ratio (INR) as high as 3.8, a partial thromboplastin time as high as 63 seconds, or platelet counts as low as 50,000/μL.

   McVay PA, Toy PT: Lack of increased bleeding after paracentesis and thoracentesis in patients with mild coagulation abnormalities. Transfusion 31: 164–171, 1991

6. **How can the potential complications of paracentesis be minimized?**

   - **Hemorrhage:** Consider platelet transfusion for a platelet count < 50,000 and fresh frozen plasma for elevated INR.

- **Perforation of bowel:** Ensure patient does not have bowel obstruction. Do not insert needle through a surgical scar.
- **Hypotension or other hemodynamic compromise:** Administer albumin (see question 7) for large-volume paracentesis (>5 L).
- **Persistent leakage of ascites:** Use the "z-tracking" technique of inserting the needle at an oblique angle through retracted skin. After the procedure, allow the skin to return to normal position to tamponade any direct tract that may have formed.
- **Liver or spleen laceration:** Do not insert the needle into the right or left upper quadrants. Ensure there is no organomegaly at the site of needle insertion.
- **Bladder laceration:** Ask the patient to void completely or place a urinary catheter before paracentesis.

See Table 85-1.

TABLE 85-1. MAJOR COMPLICATIONS OF PARACENTESIS	
Type of Complication	**Rate Quoted in Literature**
Persistent leakage of ascites	0.3–6.8%
Hypotension	2.7%
Hemorrhage/hematoma	1.4–2.2%
Perforation of bowel	0.3–0.8%
Liver or spleen injury	Unknown
Bladder perforation	Unknown

7. **What are the appropriate indications for the use of albumin?**
   In patients with ascites from portal hypertension who are undergoing large-volume paracentesis (>5 L), those who receive albumin (6–10 gm/L of ascites removed) have statistically lower rates of renal insufficiency, hypotension, and hyponatremia compared with those who do not receive albumin.

   Gines P, Tito L, Arroyo V, et al: Randomized comparative study of therapeutic paracentesis with and without intravenous albumin in cirrhosis. Gastroenterology 94: 1493–1502, 1988

KEY POINTS: PARACENTESIS

1. Paracentesis is the removal of fluid from the abdominal cavity for diagnostic or therapeutic purposes.

2. Paracentesis is indicated in patients with new or worsening ascites, those with symptoms consistent with spontaneous bacterial peritonitis, or as a treatment for patients with a large volume of ascites.

3. Potential complications include pain at puncture site, bleeding, bowel perforation, liver, bladder and spleen laceration, hypotension, and persistent leakage of ascitic fluid.

4. Albumin should be given to most patients from whom more than 5 L are removed to avoid hypotension and acute renal failure.

8. **How much ascites fluid can I safely remove?**
   There is no predefined limit to the removal of ascites fluid. However, the risks of hypotension and acute renal failure increase if >5 L are removed without the use of albumin. Most clinicians feel comfortable removing up to 10 L in what is called *total paracentesis*, as long as albumin is administered.

9. **What are the different tests that can be ordered to aid the evaluation of ascitic fluid?**
   See Table 85-2. See Chapter 40 for more details.

TABLE 85-2. ANALYSIS OF ASCITIC FLUID AFTER PARACENTESIS	
Tests Required for Nearly All Patients	**Tests for Specific Clinical Circumstances**
Cell count and differential	LDH
Albumin (to calculate SAAG)	Glucose
Total protein	Cytology
Gram's stain	AFB smear and culture
Bacterial culture	Fungal culture
	Others*

LDH = lactate dehydrogenase, SAAG = serum to ascites albumin gradient, AFB = acid-fast bacillus.
*A wide variety of additional tests may be indicated depending on the specific clinical circumstance.

BIBLIOGRAPHY

1. Gines P, Cardenas A, Arroyo V, Rodes J: Management of cirrhosis and ascites. N Engl J Med 350:1646–1654, 2004.
2. Runyon BA: Current concepts: care of patients with ascites. N Engl J Med 330:337–342, 1994.
3. Runyon BA: Paracentesis of ascitic fluid: A safe procedure. Arch Intern Med 146:2259–2261, 1986.

CHAPTER 86

VASCULAR ACCESS

Benjamin A. Hohmuth, MD

1. **Describe and contrast some common types of vascular access catheters.**
   See Table 86-1.

2. **Define *central venous access*.**
   Central venous access is access to the superior or inferior vena cava via a vascular catheter.

3. **List some typical indications for central venous access.**
   Common indications include administration of vasoactive medications (e.g., norepinephrine, Neo-Synephrine) or hyperosmolar solutions (e.g., total parenteral nutrition); hemodynamic monitoring (e.g., central venous pressure); transvenous cardiac pacing; rapid resuscitation with crystalloid and blood products; hemodialysis; and inability to secure peripheral access.

4. **What are the common sites and approaches for placement of a central venous catheter (CVC)?**
   - **Subclavian (SC) vein** (Fig. 86-1): Enter at the soft spot in the chest wall just inferior and lateral to where the convexity of the clavicle changes and the clavicular head of the sternocleidomastoid inserts. With your free hand, place your index finger in the sternal notch and your thumb on the clavicle. The needle should be aimed toward the sternal notch and directed just below the clavicle, hugging its posterior surface. The needle bevel should be facing upward. If the attempt is unsuccessful, subsequent attempts should be redirected slightly more cephalad.
   - **Internal jugular (IJ) vein** (Fig. 86-1): The point of entry is at the apex of the triangle formed by the two heads of the sternocleidomastoid muscle and the clavicle. The needle should be at an angle approximately 45 degrees to the coronal plane and aiming toward the ipsilateral nipple with the needle bevel facing upward. Use your free hand to palpate the carotid artery (which lies just medial to the IJ vein) as you advance the needle. If the first pass is unsuccessful, subsequent attempts should be directed slightly more medial.
   - **Femoral vein** (Fig. 86-2): The femoral artery should be palpated with the index and middle fingers of one hand while the other hand holds the needle. The skin should be entered at a 45 degree angle approximately 1 cm medial to the artery and just below the inguinal ligament (which runs from the pubic symphysis to the anterior superior iliac spine), with the needle bevel facing upward.

5. **What is the appropriate position of the patient for placement of a CVC?**
   For both SC and IJ attempts, the patient should be in 10–25 degrees of Trendelenburg with the head rotated 45 degrees away from the side of entry. Placing a rolled towel between the shoulder blades and parallel to the spine is helpful for the SC approach. For a femoral approach, the patient should be supine without flexion at the hips.

6. **What is appropriate sterile technique for placement of a CVC?**
   The use of sterile gloves, sterile gown, sterile drape, cap, mask, and local skin preparation with chlorhexidine solution, which is superior to iodine-based solutions for skin antisepsis, are associated with a reduction in CVC infections.

TABLE 86-1. OVERVIEW OF THE DIFFERENT TYPES OF VASCULAR ACCESS CATHETERS

Type of Catheter	Site of Entry	Utility	Duration*	Pros	Cons
Nontunneled CVC	Subclavian, internal jugular, or femoral vein	Central venous access	Days to weeks	Easy bedside insertion and removal	Highest rates of bloodstream infections
Tunneled CVC	Catheter is tunneled under the skin for several centimeters between where it enters the skin and where it enters the vein	Central venous access	Months to years	Lower rates of bloodstream infections compared with nontunneled catheters	More invasive than nontunneled catheter and generally placed in the operating room by a surgeon or interventional radiologist
Totally implantable CVC	In addition to tunneling the catheter, the access port remains subcutaneous and is accessed percutaneously with a needle	Central venous access	Months to years	Lowest rates of bloodstream infections of all the CVCs	More invasive placement and removal
Peripherally inserted CVC	Entry at basilic, cephalic, or brachial veins but with catheter tip terminating in superior vena cava	Central venous access	Weeks to months	Lower rates of bloodstream infections than nontunneled catheters and least invasive of the CVCs	Although rates of infection are lower than other CVCs, they remain higher than peripheral venous catheters

TABLE 86-1. OVERVIEW OF THE DIFFERENT TYPES OF VASCULAR ACCESS CATHETERS—CONT'D

Type of Catheter	Site of Entry	Utility	Duration*	Pros	Cons
Midline catheter	Basilic or cephalic vein	Peripheral venous access	Days to weeks	Less phlebitis than short peripheral venous catheters and can be left in for >96 hours	A few reports of anaphylactoid reactions to certain catheters
Peripheral venous catheter	Hand or arm veins	Peripheral venous access	Should be changed every 72–96 hours to minimize incidence of phlebitis and infection	Easy and least invasive	Potential for phlebitis and need for frequent replacement
Peripheral arterial catheter	Usually in the radial artery but femoral, brachial, and axillary arteries are also used	Peripheral arterial access	Days to weeks	Allows for continuous blood pressure monitoring and arterial blood sampling	Potential for ischemic complications in addition to low risk of bloodstream infections

*All catheters should be removed if a complication arises (e.g., infection).
CVC = central venous catheter.

7. **What is a finder needle?**
A finder, or seeker needle, is a 22G needle used to locate the vein before passing the much larger introducer needle alongside it.

8. **How do you know when you have successfully entered the venous system?**
Gentle traction on the plunger should be applied while advancing the needle. The sudden return of dark, nonpulsatile blood suggests successful entry into the venous system. Apply traction on the plunger while withdrawing after an unsuccessful pass because you may enter the vein on the way out. Bright red, pulsatile return suggests arterial blood. Sometimes it is difficult to determine whether you are in a vein or artery simply by looking at the blood (especially in patients with hypoxemia). Passing an 18G single-lumen catheter does not require a dilator and can be used to transduce a pressure and check blood gases, which may help clarify the placement before using a dilator and passing a larger catheter.

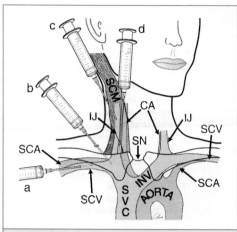

Figure 86-1. Sites of needle entry for central venous catheterization using (a) infraclavicular subclavian approach, (b) supraclavicular subclavian approach, (c) posterior internal jugular approach, and (d) middle internal jugular approach. CA = carotid artery, IJ = internal jugular vein, INV = innominate vein, SCA = subclavian artery, SCM = sternocleidomastoid muscle, SCV = subclavian vein, SN = suprasternal notch, SVC = superior vena cava. (From Kruse JA, Fink MP, Carlson RW [eds]: Saunders Manual of Critical Care. Philadelphia, W.B. Saunders, 2003, p 684.)

9. **How many attempts are too many?**
After two unsuccessful needle passes, there is an increased risk of complications, and changing sites and/or getting help from a more experienced operator is appropriate.

Mansfield PF, Hohn DC, Fornage BD, et al: Complications and failures of subclavian-vein catheterization. N Engl J Med 331:1735–1738, 1994.

10. **What is the Seldinger technique?**
The Seldinger technique involves insertion of a catheter over a wire. After the vein is located with the introducer needle, the syringe is taken off of the needle, which is held in place in the vein. A wire is then passed through the needle into the central vein, and the needle is taken out while leaving the wire in place. Once the needle is out, a slight cut is made in the skin at the entry point with a scalpel and a dilator is passed over the wire to enlarge the passage. The dilator is then removed and the desired catheter is passed over the wire. The wire is then removed, leaving the catheter in the vein. Keep hold of the wire during all steps of the above procedure to avoid migration of the wire out of the desired location. Losing the wire in the patient's venous system is a rare but dangerous complication.

11. **When and why should a chest radiograph be ordered?**
After placement of any central line other than a femoral line. This is to confirm correct placement and to rule out pneumothorax. The catheter tip should be >2 cm past an imaginary line joining the lower surfaces of the clavicles and should not cross the midline.

12. **What is an air embolism? How is it recognized and treated?**

An air embolism is a rare complication of CVC placement and removal. If there is communication between the central veins and the atmosphere during inspiration, the negative intrathoracic pressure can suck air into the veins, resulting in acute cardiopulmonary decompensation. When the diagnosis is suspected, the patient should be placed on 100% supplemental oxygen with the left side down in Trendelenburg position to attempt to trap the air in the right atrium. Attempts to aspirate the air should be made via the catheter.

13. **List some common complications of CVCs relative to their site.**

The femoral vein site has been shown in some studies to have significantly higher rates of thrombotic and infectious complications than the SC site. The infectious risk at the IJ site is likely more similar to the SC site than the femoral site. Although the numbers in Table 86-2 vary

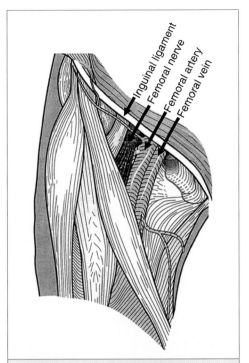

Figure 86-2. Anatomic relationships of femoral vein, femoral artery, femoral nerve, inguinal ligament, and adjacent muscles of the upper anterior thigh. (From Kruse JA, Fink MP, Carlson RW [eds]: Saunders Manual of Critical Care. Philadelphia, WB Saunders, 2003, p 689.)

between studies, as many as one in five femoral catheters will be complicated by an infection.

TABLE 86-2. COMPLICATION OF FEMORAL VERSUS SUBCLAVIAN NONTUNNELED CENTRAL VENOUS CATHETERS

Complication	Femoral Site	Subclavian Site
Overall infection	19.8%	4.5%
Sepsis	4.4%	1.5%
Thrombotic	21.5%	1.9%
Major mechanical*	1.4%	2.8%

Major mechanical complications were defined as those requiring a therapeutic procedure (e.g., pneumothorax requiring a chest tube or bleeding requiring transfusion).
Adapted from Merrer J, De Jonghe B, Golliot F, et al: Complications of central venous catheterization in critically ill patients. JAMA 2001 286:700–707, 2001.

14. **Is there a preferred site of central venous access?**
The SC vein is the preferred site due to lower rates of infectious complications relative to the femoral vein and IJ vein catheters. A common exception to this is in patients who will need long-term vascular access (e.g., patients receiving hemodialysis), a situation in which the SC vein should be avoided due to increased risk of stenosis. The right IJ and left SC vein sites offer the most favorable courses to the right ventricle if passing a pulmonary artery catheter or a transvenous pacer is anticipated.

15. **When might a femoral approach be preferred?**
If a patient is unstable and emergent access is needed, a femoral approach offers quick access that does not interfere with cardiopulmonary resuscitation or intubation. A femoral site is also easier to compress if urgent central access is needed in someone at high risk for bleeding (e.g., coagulopathy). In patients in whom a neck hematoma or pneumothorax would be devastating (e.g., patients with very tenuous pulmonary status), a femoral vein catheter may be preferable.

16. **Is coagulopathy a contraindication to attempting central venous access?**
In the absence of renal failure or thrombocytopenia, patients with modestly elevated prothrombin time and/or partial thromboplastin time values are probably not at increased risk for bleeding complications due to central line placement performed by or supervised by an experienced operator.

   Doerfler ME, Kaufman B, Goldenberg AS: Central venous catheter placement in patients with disorders of hemostasis. Chest 110:185–188, 1996.

17. **What is an introducer catheter?**
Most percutaneously inserted CVCs have 1–5 lumens, each of which is fairly narrow (e.g., 18G). An introducer catheter is a single-lumen catheter with a very large internal diameter that can be used for rapid infusion and can accept another catheter passed through it such as a pulmonary artery catheter or a transvenous cardiac pacer.

18. **How is catheter size measured?**
Either by French size or by the gauge system. A higher French number means a greater-diameter catheter, whereas a higher gauge number means a smaller-diameter catheter. There is no easy conversion between the two metrics. Often a French size is given to describe the external diameter of a multilumen catheter, whereas gauge is used to describe the various lumens within.

19. **Which is better for rapid infusion—a central line or large-bore peripheral lines?**
The flow rate in a catheter is determined by its length (inversely related) and its radius (directly related to the fourth power). Doubling a catheter's length will decrease flow by half. Doubling a catheter's internal radius will increase flow 16-fold. Because central catheters are generally 3–4 times longer than peripheral catheters, large-bore (14G to 18G) peripheral access is more effective for rapid infusion.

20. **What is the Allen test? How is it performed? How useful is it?**
The Allen test verifies effective ulnar arterial blood supply of the hand in case cannulation of the radial artery leads to compromised radial blood flow. Locate the radial and ulnar pulses. Occlude both the radial and ulnar arteries with digital pressure and have the patient make a tight fist to drain the blood from the hand. Have the patient open the hand, which should appear blanched, and then release the pressure on the ulnar artery. Rubor should return to the hand within 5–10 sec. The clinical utility of this test remains unclear because a positive test result does not reliably predict ischemic complications of radial artery cannulation and a negative test result does not rule out the development of ischemic complications.

KEY POINTS: CENTRAL VENOUS CATHETERS

1. The SC site is preferred in most circumstances.

2. Infectious complications are highest at the femoral site.

3. Appropriate sterile technique decreases the risk of infection.

4. Peripherally inserted CVCs are less invasive and have lower rates of bloodstream infections than nontunneled CVCs.

21. **What are the indications for arterial catheterization?**
    Continuous blood pressure measurement (e.g., patient in shock) and frequent arterial blood sampling (e.g., patient on a mechanical ventilator) are the most common indications.

22. **How is an arterial line placed?**
    A radial arterial line can be placed the same way a peripheral venous catheter is placed, using an angiocatheter in a direct over-the-needle approach and then securing the catheter with sutures. An alternative approach is to use the Seldinger technique described previously. The hand is generally taped to a small arm board with a roll of gauze behind the wrist to maintain some mild dorsiflexion (Fig. 86-3).

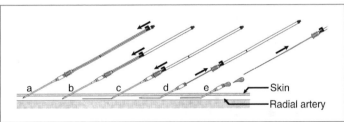

Figure 86-3. Percutaneous cannulation of the radial artery by a modified Seldinger technique using a catheter-over-needle device with integral guidewire. (a) A tab is used to advance the guidewire into the needle after the artery is punctured. (b) The tip of the guidewire is at the level of the needle orifice once the tab reaches the marker. (c) The guidewire is advanced into the artery. (d) The catheter is advanced over the needle and the guidewire into the artery. (e) The needle and guidewire are removed. (From Kruse JA, Fink MP, Carlson RW [eds]: Saunders Manual of Critical Care. Philadelphia, WB Saunders, 2003, p 688.)

BIBLIOGRAPHY

1. Centers for Disease Control and Prevention: Guidelines for the Prevention of Intravascular Catheter-Related Infections. MMWR 51(no. RR–10):[1–29], 2002.

2. Latto IP, Ng WS, Jones PL, Jenkins BJ: Percutaneous Central Venous and Arterial Catheterisation, 3rd ed. Philadelphia, WB Saunders2000.

3. Marino P: In The ICU Book, 2nd ed. Baltimore, MD, Williams & Wilkins, 1998, pp 53–93.

4. McGee DC, Gould MK: Preventing complications of central venous catheterization. N Engl J Med 348:1122–1133, 2003.

5. Merrer J, De Jonghe B, Golliot F, et al: Complications of central venous catheterization in critically ill patients. JAMA 286:700–707, 2001.

6. Peters PC, Tisnado J, Mauro MA: Venous Catheters A Practical Manual. New York, Thieme Medical Publishers, Inc, 2003.

CHAPTER 87

PALLIATIVE CARE ASSESSMENT

Stephanie Grossman, MD, and Melissa Mahoney, MD

1. **What is palliative care?**

   Palliative care is an interdisciplinary approach to relieving suffering and improving the quality of life for patients with a life-threatening or terminal illness. This includes malignant as well as nonmalignant diseases. Expert control of pain and other symptoms, whether they are physical, psychological, social, or spiritual, is integrated with other appropriate medical treatments. It is often referred to as *whole person care.*

2. **Why should we practice palliative care?**

   Traditionally, modern medicine has been focused exclusively on curing illness and prolonging life. As medicine has advanced and our population has aged, physicians find themselves caring for many patients with chronic and terminal illness. This "chronic" or "terminal" phase can last weeks to months as in certain types of incurable cancer, or months to years as in nonmalignant chronic diseases. Palliative care seeks to address the physical, social, and psychological ramifications of a patient's disease by providing effective communication, goals of care, symptom management, and spiritual, psychological, and bereavement support. The overall goal is to relieve suffering and improve quality of life.

3. **Which nonmalignant chronic diseases may benefit from palliative care?**

   Patients with any debilitating chronic disease may benefit, especially those with congestive heart failure, chronic obstructive pulmonary disease, dementia, stroke, amyotrophic lateral sclerosis, or acquired immune deficiency syndrome.

4. **When should palliative care start? Does it prohibit management of acute medical issues?**

   Traditionally, palliative care was deemed necessary only after curative therapy failed. However, when patients are living with a chronic or terminal illness, palliative care can be introduced at any stage of illness. Ideally, it should begin as soon as the diagnosis of a life-threatening illness is confirmed, and it should be integrated with acute care management (Fig. 87-1).

5. **When is consulting a palliative care expert helpful?**

   Ideally, all physicians would be expert in providing palliative care. Realistically, most physicians have not received adequate training. In these instances, consulting with an expert is essential. A palliative care consult team can help with establishing goals of care, conflict resolution, symptom management, and withdrawal of life-prolonging interventions, such as mechanical ventilation, dialysis, or artificial nutrition and hydration. A palliative care consult is also time intensive. A busy clinician may not have the time or resources to provide appropriate care, even if he or she has the appropriate skills.

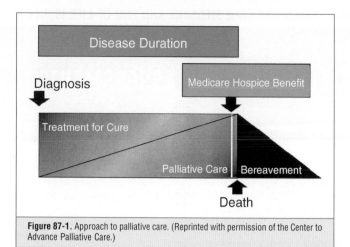

Figure 87-1. Approach to palliative care. (Reprinted with permission of the Center to Advance Palliative Care.)

KEY POINTS: PALLIATIVE CARE CONSULTATION

1. Useful for a variety of chronic, debilitating diseases.

2. May assist with symptom management and addressing goals of care at any time in the course of the illness.

3. Use should not be limited only to the last few days of life.

6. **Name key members of the palliative care team.**
The core palliative care team usually consists of a physician, nurse, social worker, and chaplain. An extended team may include pain management specialists, a psychiatrist or psychologist, a member of the ethics committee, a clinical pharmacist, a nutritionist, a physical and occupational therapist, member of the administration, and a lay volunteer from the community.

7. **What is the physician's role in the palliative care team?**
The physician works with the core team to identify the goals of care for the patient and family, perform the initial and subsequent assessment and plan, provide expertise in palliation of common symptoms of the terminal illness, build relationships among the interdisciplinary care team, teach health care professionals and lay public about principles of palliative care, and participate in research protocols as appropriate.

8. **What is a quality of life questionnaire, and how is it beneficial?**
Improving patients' quality of life is the main goal of palliative care. Several quality of life instruments have been developed and validated in palliative care, and there are a series of questionnaires that cover physical, psychological, and social aspects of life. Diagnostically, the questionnaires can uncover uncontrolled symptoms such as pain, which is the most reliable predictor of poor quality of life. Therapeutically, the process of completing the questionnaires can help patients reflect on issues related to their illness, living, and dying. The quality of life questionnaires currently available are most useful in research and may not be suited for use in daily clinical practice.

9. **Name 10 common symptoms that should be considered in a palliative care assessment.**
   Fatigue, pain, anxiety, depression, anorexia, nausea, constipation/bowel obstruction, dyspnea, delirium, and dysphagia should all be addressed.

10. **What is "total pain"?**
    Total pain is the combination of the following four types of pain: physical, emotional or psychic, social or interpersonal, and spiritual or existential. Each type of pain can exist and interact with the others, resulting in increased overall suffering. Palliative care teams must therefore assess and treat each type of pain to relieve suffering.

KEY POINTS: TOTAL PAIN

1. Involves the following four types of pain: physical, emotional or psychic, social or interpersonal, and spiritual or existential.

2. Each type of pain can exist and interact with the others, resulting in increased overall suffering.

11. **What are some barriers to assessment of these symptoms?**
    Denial, misconceptions about pain medication (e.g., narcotic addiction), and issues related to culture, religion, gender, or finances.

12. **How can physicians prognosticate outcomes for chronic illnesses?**
    The National Hospice and Palliative Care Organization has developed consensus guidelines for identifying patients with non-cancer diagnoses who are likely to have a life expectancy of 6 months or less if the illness were to run its normal course. More research is needed to establish their accuracy and validity. Other prognostic scales include the Karnofsky Performance Scale (KPS), which is more oriented toward hospitalization based on functional status. (See Chapter 89 for more details.) The Palliative Care Performance Scale is similar to KPS but also includes nutritional limitations and mental status deterioration and may be a better predictor of hospice length of stay. It is important to communicate to patients using ranges of time (i.e., days to weeks, weeks to several months) rather than specific amounts of time.

13. **Where do the majority of people want to die, and where do they currently die?**
    In the United States, 90% of patients wish to die at home. Currently, however, among American adults dying of nontraumatic causes, 23.4% of deaths take place at home, 23.2% in nursing homes, 49.5% in hospitals, and 3.9% in other locations.

    Facts on dying 2004: Policy relevant data on care at the end of life. USA and State Statistics. Brown University Center for Gerontology and Health Care Research. Available at http://www.chcr.brown.edu/dying/USASTATISTICS.HTM.

14. **Name several distressing symptoms at the time of death, and describe methods of alleviation.**
    Common physical signs in the terminal phase include pain, dyspnea, a "death rattle," anxiety, and delirium. Pain may be treated with opioids delivered through a non-oral route (e.g., subcutaneous, sublingual, intravenous). Dyspnea can be alleviated with morphine or analgesic equivalent. A death rattle (i.e., gurgling or rattling sound sometimes made in the throat of a dying person) is treated with a scopolamine gel or patch; sublingual hyoscyamine; nebulizer

solution consisting of atropine, morphine, and dexamethasone; or atropine and furosemide. Benzodiazepines such as lorazepam and alprazolam are effective in the treatment of anxiety. Delirium may be managed with haloperidol, methotrimeprazine, chlorpromazine, or midazolam. (See Chapter 94 for more details.)

15. **Describe the steps for withdrawing ventilatory support.**
    1. Decision and documentation
       a. Document goals of care; discuss them with all team members.
       b. Establish date and time for the removal of mechanical ventilation.
       c. Encourage family members to initiate cultural rituals/ceremonies in preparation for death.
       d. Discontinue tests and treatments that do not meet the goals of care.
       e. Confirm/document do-not-resuscitate order.
    2. Preparation for removal of mechanical ventilation
       a. Discontinue artificial fluids and feeding.
       b. Provide counseling to family members and determine whether they wish to be present at the time of death.
       c. Discuss organ donation with the family, if appropriate.
       d. Contact a respiratory therapist to assist with the procedure.
       e. Administer premedication to ensure comfort (benzodiazepines and opioids).
       f. Remove restraints and other medical devices.
       g. Have suction equipment and towels available.
       h. Write an order to discontinue the ventilator.
    3. Removal of mechanical ventilation
       a. Silence ventilator alarms.
       b. Remove mechanical ventilation.
       c. Monitor the patient for signs of discomfort, and treat accordingly.
    4. Follow-up
       a. Invite family members into the room.
       b. When the patient dies, allow the family time to say good-bye.
       c. Debrief staff; provide support.
       d. Initiate the family bereavement plan.

    Adapted from Marr L, Weissman D: Withdrawal of ventilatory support from the dying adult patient. J Support Oncol 2:283–288, 2004.

WEBSITES

1. American Academy of Hospice and Palliative Medicine
   http://www.aahpm.org

2. Center to Advance Palliative Care
   http://www.capc.org

3. The Education in Palliative and End-of-life Care (EPEC) Project
   http://www.epec.net

4. End of Life/Palliative Education Resource Center
   http://www.eperc.mcw.edu

5. Harvard Medical School's Program in Palliative Care Education and Practice
   http://www.hms.harvard.edu/cdi/pallcare

6. National Hospice and Palliative Care Organization
   http://www.nhpco.org

BIBLIOGRAPHY

1. Head B, Ritchie CS, Smoot TM: Prognostication in hospice care: Can the Palliative Performance Scale help? J Palliat Med 8:492–502, 2005.

2. Kassa S, Loge J: Quality of life in palliative medicine: Principles practice. In Doyle D, Hanks G, Cherny N, et al (eds): Oxford Textbook of Palliative Care, 3rd ed. Oxford, Oxford University Press, 2004, pp 195–210.

3. Story P: UNIPAC Book Series: Hospice/Palliative Care Training for Physicians: A Self-Study Program, 2nd ed. New York, Mary Ann Liebert, 2003.

CHAPTER 88

ESTABLISHING GOALS OF CARE

Ruben O. Halperin, MD, MPH

1. **Why, and in which patients, is it important to establish goals of care?**

   Goals of care should be established for all patients, especially those with advanced or terminal diseases, whose limited options often involve tradeoffs between function, longevity, and comfort. Patients may have different desires regarding cure versus palliation, and not everyone will want the most aggressive therapies, especially when there are significant risks and morbidity involved. Others may not be good candidates for certain treatments. Patients with similar disease processes may have very different goals of care, and these goals may change over time. Discussions about goals of care should ideally include the patient, physician, family, and any other members of the health care team. (See Chapter 90.)

2. **In patients with advanced or terminal illnesses, what are the three most common, but often contradictory goals of care?**

   - **Prolongation of life:** Patients whose main interest is prolongation of life may be willing to initiate treatments with significant risks and discomfort for any possible increase in life expectancy.
   - **Maintenance of function:** Some patients might forego treatments that could potentially extend their lives if the treatment involves significant threats to their functional status, such as amputation or high-risk surgery.
   - **Maximization of comfort:** Patients who primarily wish to remain symptom free and comfortable might forego potentially life-prolonging therapies that involve discomfort (e.g., chemotherapy or surgery) or impair function (e.g., amputation).

3. **How is quality of life defined and measured?**

   Quality of life is defined as how one's physical, emotional, and social well-being are affected by a medical condition and its treatment. Quality of life is subjective and should be assessed by the patient, not the physician or a family member. Most instruments include up to seven aspects of quality of life: physical well-being, functional well-being, emotional well-being, family well-being, social functioning, treatment satisfaction, and sexuality/intimacy.

4. **What is an advance directive? What are some of the specific instruments that can constitute an advance directive?**

   Advance directives are specific written documents created by a patient to express his or her wishes. They guide decision making during times when the patient may be incapable of verbalizing those desires. Specific instruments include the following:

   - **Health care proxy (also known as *durable power of attorney for health care*):** Formally names a surrogate decision-maker.
   - **Living will:** Provides a general sense of the patient's wishes in case of terminal illness. It can be modified to include specific wishes regarding interventions such as cardiopulmonary resuscitation, ventilators, and tube feedings. Living wills are generally vague and only apply to a patient recognized to be in the terminal stages of illness. They may not be considered applicable in settings of severe, but not necessarily life-threatening, illness.
   - **Instructional directive:** Serves as a more specific form of the living will that addresses use of various interventions in four different scenarios: coma with virtually no chance for recovery,

coma with a small chance of recovery to an impaired state, advanced dementia with a terminal illness, and advanced dementia. One limitation is that these documents do not discuss goals and thus do not distinguish between indefinite and short-term use of an intervention, such as a ventilator for a severe but reversible pneumonia.

- **Combined directive:** Combines a living will, a values history, and an instructional directive in an attempt to get a much broader picture of a person's wishes with regard to multiple different scenarios. The Five Wishes, which specifies the following, is an example of such a document:
  1. Which person you want to make health care decisions for you when you can't make them
  2. The kind of medical treatment you want and don't want
  3. How comfortable you want to be
  4. How you want people to treat you
  5. What you want your loved ones to know

KEY POINTS: ESTABLISHING GOALS OF CARE

1. Establishing patients' goals for care is an essential step in creating a treatment plan for all patients, especially critically or terminally ill patients for whom treatment choices may require tradeoffs.

2. Discussing end-of-life preferences with a patient is an ongoing process that ideally should begin well before a patient is faced with a terminal illness.

3. All patients should be encouraged to establish documentation of their end-of-life preferences. These should be updated by each patient as his or her physical condition changes over time.

5. **What are the principles of autonomy and beneficence?**
   - **Autonomy:** This is the right to make choices about one's life, including choosing among different therapeutic options and the right to refuse treatment.
   - **Beneficence:** This is the principle that medical professionals have an obligation to help further the patient's legitimate interest. This can often come into conflict with the principle of autonomy. A physician may feel that prolongation of life is achievable and in the best interest of a patient, but that patient may refuse life-prolonging therapy. In cases where there is a conflict, there is a consensus in the United States that the principle of autonomy takes precedent.

6. **What are nonmaleficence and nonabandonment?**
   - **Nonmaleficence:** This is the principle of not inflicting harm. This precludes physicians from offering treatments that they reasonably believe have the potential for more harm than benefit. This gives physicians the right to refuse to participate in practices or to refuse treatments that they consider harmful.
   - **Nonabandonment:** Another ethical principle, this may come into conflict with nonmaleficence. Although physicians are obliged to not participate in practices believed harmful, they also are morally obligated to not abandon a patient. Physicians must try to explain the issues involved, and if the patient insists on pursuing the questioned practices, it is appropriate to help the patient find another physician.

7. **How have patient and physician roles changed in the decision-making process?**
   - **Paternalism:** A generation ago, society believed in medical paternalism—physicians making decisions without significant patient input. This practice assumed that the physician would act in the patient's best interest, per the concepts of beneficence and nonmaleficence.
   - **Patient autonomy:** In the mid 1980s, patient autonomy began to replace paternalism. The role of the physician became to impartially discuss the treatment options and let the patient or his or her surrogate make a decision based on the risks and benefits of each treatment.
   - **Enhanced autonomy:** In recent years there has been a move toward enhanced autonomy, in which patients and physicians partner to make the choices. Patients may differ in what style they prefer.

8. **How much information is required for decision making or consent to be considered truly informed?**
   Three legal standards are available. The *professional community standard* involves providing as much information as would other physicians in the community. Under the *reasonable person standard*, the appropriate amount of information is what would be desired by an individual free of mental and physical illness and who has no conflict of interest. The *subjective standard* allows the physician to use experience and judgment to decide what information is required.

KEY POINTS: DECISION MAKING

1. Decision making is a partnership between the physician and the patient and/or the patient's surrogates.

2. The decision to withhold or withdraw care will be made easier if the patient's goals are established, documented, and understood by all parties involved in the patient's care.

9. **What are common reasons for withholding or withdrawing particular treatments?**
   Treatments may be withheld or withdrawn if the burdens (e.g., pain, suffering, or loss of function) are felt to outweigh the potential benefits, if the treatment is ineffective, or if the treatment is unlikely to meet a patient's goals.

10. **Is withholding care ethically different than withdrawing care that has already been initiated?**
   Ethically, these concepts are similar. It is important to establish the goals of a particular treatment before initiation. If it later becomes clear to the patient, the physician, or the patient's surrogate that the therapy is not meeting established goals, then withdrawing the treatment is completely appropriate and ethical. For example, a patient who does not wish to be on prolonged life support may develop a severe respiratory illness and agree to a short period of mechanical ventilation while he or she attempts to recover from that illness. If after a defined time no progress has been made, then the therapy can be reevaluated and withdrawn.

WEBSITE

Aging with Dignity: Five Wishes:
http://www.agingwithdignity.org

BIBLIOGRAPHY

1. Bergner M: Quality of life, health status, and clinical research. Med Care 27(3 Suppl):S148–S156, 1989.
2. Danis M, Garrett J, Harris R, Patrick DL: Stability of choices about life-sustaining treatments. Ann Intern Med 120:567–573, 1994.
3. Gillick MR: Advance care planning. N Engl J Med 350:7–8, 2004.
4. Lynn J: Conflicts of interest in medical decision-making. J Am Geriatr Soc 36:945–950, 1988.
5. Rosenfeld K, Wenger N, Kagawa-Singer M: End-of-life decision-making: A qualitative study of elderly individuals. J Gen Intern Med 15:620–625, 2000.
6. Tierney WM, Dexter PR, Gramelspacher GP, et al: The effect of discussions about advance directives on patients' satisfaction with primary care. J Gen Intern Med 16:32–40, 2001.

CHAPTER 89

ESTABLISHING CODE STATUS

Ben Keidan, MD

1. **When should discussions about advance directives and code status take place?**
   Whenever a patient's goals of care are uncertain or might be expected to change. Ideally, all patients will have begun this discussion with their primary care physician, making this topic familiar to them. A brief discussion is crucial in every hospitalized patient. More detailed discussions are essential when patients are medically unstable or have had acute changes in their status.

2. **What information is important to know before this discussion?**
   Knowing the prognosis and goals of care for each individual patient will allow the provider to place the conversation in the larger context of meeting the goals of care.

3. **Should we provide prognostic estimates? Are there methods that physicians can use to be more accurate when estimating prognosis?**
   Studies confirm that the majority of patients want to know a realistic, individualized prognosis, which often has significant implications for treatment decisions. Physicians tend to avoid prognostication, but when they do provide such information they tend to overestimate survival by a factor of 2. The Karnofsky Performance Status (KPS) is a useful tool to assist in estimating an accurate prognosis. A KPS < 50 suggests a life expectancy of < 8 weeks (Table 89-1).

   Hagerty RG, Butow PN, Ellis PM, et al: Communicating with realism and hope: Incurable cancer patients' views on the disclosure of prognosis. J Clin Oncol 23:1278–1288, 2005.

4. **What percentage of patients who suffer cardiopulmonary arrest in the hospital survive to hospital discharge?**
   Hospitalized patients generally suffer an arrest as a complication of a severe illness. Overall, approximately 10–15% survive, though many are neurologically impaired. Among patients with

TABLE 89-1.	KARNOFSKY PERFORMANCE SCALE
100	Normal, no complaints, no evidence of disease
90	Able to carry on normal activity: minor symptoms of disease
80	Normal activity with effort: some symptoms of disease
70	Cares for self: unable to carry on normal activity or active work
60	Requires occasional assistance but is able to care for needs
50	Requires considerable assistance and frequent medical care
40	Disabled: requires special care and assistance
30	Severely disabled: hospitalization is indicated, death not imminent
20	Very sick, hospitalization necessary: active treatment necessary
10	Moribund, fatal processes progressing rapidly
0	Dead

systemic *noncardiac* disease, the likelihood of survival to hospital discharge is significantly lower (< 1%).

Ebel MH, Becker LA, Barry HC, Hagen M: Survival after in-hospital cardiopulmonary resuscitation: A meta-analysis. J Gen Intern Med 12:805–816 1998.

5. **How should I initiate discussions about code status?**
In a routine hospitalization with low risk of cardiopulmonary arrest, a brief discussion at the time of admission is appropriate. For example:

We are admitting you to the hospital for treatment of pneumonia. I expect you will do well and be home soon; however, it is important for me to know your wishes in the unlikely event of a rapid change in your status. If you were to die despite all of our efforts, would you want us to perform heroic measures to try to bring you back to life?

In patients with severe acute or chronic medical conditions, a brief assessment of previous code discussions is essential, followed by a more complete discussion going through the steps listed in the Key Points.

Weissman D: Fast Fact and Concepts #23: DNR Orders in the Hospital—Part 1. (October 2000). End-of-Life/Palliative Education Resource Center. Available at: http://www.eperc.mcw.edu.

KEY POINTS: DISCUSSING CODE STATUS

1. Establish an appropriate setting. Sit down in a comfortable setting with appropriate family members present, if the patient desires.

2. Ask the patient and family what they understand. For example, "What do you understand about your illness? What have the doctors told you so far?"

3. Find out what they expect and what their wishes are. For example, "What are your goals/expectations/concerns for the future?" If the patient's expectations are unrealistic, this is the time to educate and clarify. It is often necessary to search for realistic goals.

4. Discuss a DNR order, including situations when it would apply.

5. Respond to emotions (e.g., with silence or reassurance, by offering a tissue or a hand, by expressing empathy). For example, "I wish things were different."

6. Establish, document, and implement the plan.

6. **How should I describe cardiopulmonary resuscitation (CPR)?**
The key is to start general (e.g., heroic measures) and work toward specifics (e.g., CPR, defibrillation, ventilation) later in the conversation if they arise. It is generally best to avoid mechanical descriptions of CPR unless asked to elaborate, instead focusing on the patients' goals.

7. **Is it appropriate to make a recommendation?**
Yes; once the goals of care have been established, a physician should make a recommendation that is consistent with the patient's goals. For example:

We have agreed that your goals are to be comfortable and to spend as much time at home as possible. Given your wishes, if you were to die despite all of our current efforts, I do not recommend the use of artificial or heroic measures to bring you back to life.

A clear, respectful recommendation has the potential to spare patients and their family feelings of guilt that they "did not do everything possible" or "just let her die." There is no need to discuss every specific circumstance, nor is it necessary to ask patients and families to go through a checklist detailing their wishes if you understand the patients' goals of care.

8. **How can I discuss code status without destroying a patient's hope?**
   By focusing on what can be done and anticipating worst-case scenarios. For example:
   I will do everything to try to improve your current condition. I am hoping for the best. At the same time, we should prepare for the worst.

9. **Why should you avoid the phrase, "Do you want everything done?"**
   This implies that you are currently holding back on effective treatments. It is also difficult for patients and families to say no to such a leading question.

10. **Is there any role for "slow codes" or "chemical codes"?**
    No. There is no role for resuscitation outside of standard CPR and advanced cardiac life support procedures. These situations generally arise when there is conflict regarding CPR decisions and signal the need for continued communication among the medical team, patient, and family. Performing CPR with less than standard procedures undermines communication and trust.

11. **What do palliative care experts do differently when they discuss do-not-resuscitate (DNR) orders?**
    Experts spend twice as much time (15 minutes), are less verbally dominant (i.e., they listen better), give less specific information, focus on psychosocial and lifestyle discussions, and engage more in partnership building.

    Roter DL, Larson S, Fischer GS, et al: Experts practice what they preach: A descriptive study of best and normative practices in end-of-life discussion. Arch Intern Med 160:3477–3485, 2000.

12. **Is there anything I can do once we have established that a patient has a DNR order?**
    Yes. DNR status has no bearing on other aspects of care. It does not preclude curative therapies when they are available or palliative care when cure is not possible. When goals of care are comfort, offering outstanding palliative care (e.g., pain and symptom management, attending to the spiritual and psychosocial needs of the patient and caregivers) and continued emphasis on nonabandonment of patients and families is essential.

WEBSITES

1. Education in Palliative Care and End-of-Life Care Project:
   http://epec.net

2. End-of-Life/Palliative Education Resource Center:
   http://www.eperc.mcw.edu

BIBLIOGRAPHY

1. Back AL, Arnold RM, Quill TE: Hope for the best, and prepare for the worst. Ann Intern Med 138:439–443, 2003.
2. Quill TE, Arnold RM, Platt F: "I wish things were different": Expressing wishes in response to loss, futility, and unrealistic hopes. Ann Intern Med 135:551–555, 2001.
3. Von Gunten C: Discussing do-not-resuscitate status. J Clin Oncol 19:1576–1581, 2001.
4. Weissman D: Fast Fact and Concepts #24: DNR Orders in the Hospital Setting—Part 2. October, 2000. End-of-Life Physician Education Resource Center. Available at http://www.eperc.mcw.edu.

CHAPTER 90

ETHICAL AND LEGAL ISSUES AT THE END OF LIFE

Barbara Cleary, MD

Note: This chapter is not intended to substitute for legal counsel with respect to individual cases. Many laws and regulations vary in different jurisdictions. All decisions about end-of-life issues should be made with the appropriate legal and ethics consultations, as needed.

1. **Who decides about treatment options at the end of life?**
   The patient and his or her physicians as well as other members of the health care team should discuss the possible benefits and risks of treatment options. Ultimately, the patient makes the decision. This is the ethical principal of patient autonomy. If a patient lacks capacity, a surrogate decision maker makes the decision.

2. **Can patients decline life-sustaining treatment or choose to withdraw treatment?**
   In 1990, the U.S. Supreme Court established that patients have a constitutional right to refuse medical treatment (including nutrition and hydration), even when such treatment is life sustaining.

3. **Can a surrogate decision maker decline or withdraw life-sustaining treatment on an incapacitated patient's behalf?**
   Some states accept surrogate decisions made in the patient's best interest, although states may require "clear and convincing evidence" that this was the patient's wish. Living wills or advance directives that address the medical situation constitute "clear and convincing evidence."

4. **What is the difference between competence and capacity?**
   Competence and *capacity* are both terms that describe the ability to understand one's medical choices and make informed decisions about one's health care. The word *capacity* tends to be used in the medical arena, whereas *competency* tends to be used more in a legal context. An attending physician makes this initial determination, although a psychiatry consultation may be useful as well. If it is unclear whether a patient lacks the capacity to make a certain decision, then a judge may be needed to make the legal determination.

5. **Who makes the medical decisions when a patient lacks the capacity to do so?**
   The decision maker may be someone with durable power of attorney, a proxy, or a court-appointed guardian. In an emergency, one must proceed with treatment until a decision maker is identified. If an incapacitated patient disagrees with the surrogate decision maker, or if interested persons cannot decide on a proxy, the court must appoint a guardian for medical decisions after determining a patient is incompetent (Fig. 90-1).

6. **What is medical futility?**
   No consensus definition of *futility* exists in the medical profession. Opinions about futility are often based on values from life experience and religious and cultural backgrounds. Futility may be described as physiologic, quantitative, or qualitative.
   - **Physiologic futility:** The desired physiologic effect cannot be achieved with the proposed treatment (e.g., using a diuretic to treat cancer).

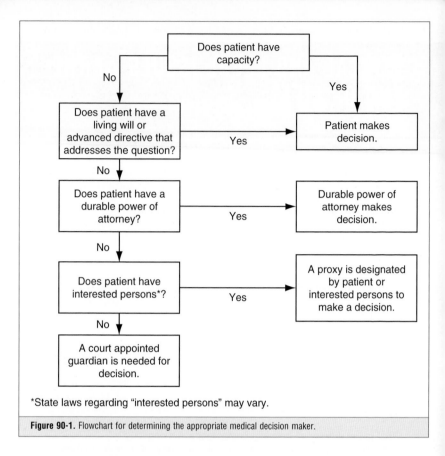

Figure 90-1. Flowchart for determining the appropriate medical decision maker.

- **Quantitative futility:** Experience and studies predict failure of an intervention to provide a benefit to a patient (e.g., aggressive resuscitation for end stage pulmonary fibrosis).
- **Qualitative futility:** The potential effect of the treatment is not worthwhile.

7. **What are some examples of differing values surrounding futility?**
   Treatment that prolongs dying might seem futile to a physician but worthwhile to a patient with a specific goal, such as living long enough to say good-bye to family. Someone who believes that life is the ultimate goal, rather than quality of life, will likely believe any potential treatment is worthwhile. Many studies show that physicians frequently rate a patient's quality of life lower than the patient does. Many patients choose life-prolonging treatments despite chronic or terminal illnesses based on their perceived quality of life.

8. **Can futility be defined in terms of medical resource allocation?**
   No. These are two separate issues. Decisions about futility involve a judgment about appropriate care rather than how best to allocate limited resources.

9. **Who decides whether a potential treatment is worthwhile?**
   Ideally, the physician, patient, and family come to the same consensus. But when they do not, the patient or his or her surrogate has autonomy to accept or decline potential treatments. Ethics consults may be useful to ensure communication and help define goals of care.

10. **Are physicians required to provide treatment they feel is futile when family or patients request the treatment?**
Many hospitals have policies on how to approach ethical dilemmas about futility, but when no consensus is reached between family members and care teams, most hospitals defer to patient or surrogate requests for treatment or arrange transfers to teams or hospitals willing to provide the requested treatments. Withholding treatment is a complex issue, and conflicts are best managed with the assistance of an ethics committee.

11. **What are cultural sensitivity and cultural competence?**
   - **Cultural sensitivity:** This is an understanding and acceptance that different values and beliefs exist based on one's culture.
   - **Cultural competence:** This involves possessing knowledge about the beliefs and values of those from different cultures. It is important to recognize your own values and beliefs and understand that they may not be the same as your patient's. Caregivers should familiarize themselves with commonly held cultural and religious beliefs but not assume that all patients from similar cultures embrace the same values. Trained interpreters and clergy should be available and used to help facilitate patient care.

12. **What are some common themes that occur at the end of life?**
   - **Religious beliefs:** Some religions hold that suffering is redemptive and should be endured. Patients with these beliefs are more likely to request aggressive treatment until death. Most religions hold that "extraordinary" treatment is not required at the end of life; however, they may differ on what is considered "ordinary" versus "extraordinary" treatment. Clergy can help to facilitate discussions with families, patients, and caregivers about this.
   - **Truth telling:** Many cultures and religions do not endorse disclosing medical diagnoses and treatment options to patients. Rather, information should only be shared with family members. It is important to ask patients whether they want to hear the details of their diagnoses, or if they prefer this information be given to family. With a patient's consent, it is both legal and ethical to discuss information with the family. This should be documented in the chart.
   - **Trust:** Some patients believe that medical professionals will not provide needed treatments because the patient lacks funds or because of cultural differences. This mistrust may lead patients to request aggressive treatment until death.

KEY POINTS: FUTILITY

1. Medical futility has no agreed-upon definition.

2. Personal experience and values shape the way physicians identify "futile" cases.

3. To date, the legal system has supported decisions to preserve life in "futile" cases.

4. Many hospitals have policies on how to approach conflicts about futility.

13. **What is the difference between treatment and care?**
   - **Treatment:** This implies therapy aimed at curing disease or prolonging life.
   - **Care:** This implies therapy aimed at providing comfort or palliation to patients. The term *withdrawal of care* imparts a feeling that the patient is abandoned by his or her caregivers. When withdrawing life-sustaining or curative treatments, it should be stressed that care aimed at palliation will continue.

14. **Is it legal to provide escalating doses of pain medication to relieve pain even if death is anticipated as a result of the narcotic dose?**
   This is both legal and ethical care if the goal of treatment is to relieve pain or suffering. This ethical concept, called *double effect,* allows that what would be morally wrong if caused intentionally is ethical if foreseen but unintended.

15. **How does this differ from euthanasia and physician-assisted suicide?**
   - *Euthanasia* refers to the deliberate ending of a person's life with or without that person's request, usually to end suffering. Euthanasia is not legal in the United States.
   - *Physician-assisted suicide* refers to providing a patient with a method to end his or her own life, usually a prescription for a large dose of narcotic or barbiturate. In 1997 the U.S. Supreme Court ruled that there is no constitutional right to physician-assisted suicide. Oregon has legalized physician-assisted suicide; however, many states have subsequently criminalized the practice.

WEBSITES

1. American Society of Law, Medicine, & Ethics
   http://www.aslme.org

2. Bioethics.net
   http://www.bioethics.net

BIBLIOGRAPHY

1. Anderson J, Brescia F, Davis RS, et al: Health Care Ethics Consortium of Georgia 1997 Task Force on Futility Report.
2. Batlle JC: Legal status of physician-assisted suicide. JAMA 289:2279–2281, 2003.
3. Cohen CB: Religious, spiritual, ideological perspectives on ethics at the end of life. In Doka KJ, Jennings B, Corr CA (eds): Living with Grief: Ethical Dilemmas at the End of Life. Hospice Foundation of America, 2005, pp 19–40.
4. Crawley LM, Marshall PA, Lo B, et al: Strategies for culturally effective end-of-life care. Ann Intern Med 136:673–679, 2002.
5. Jonsen AR, Siegler M, Winslade WJ: Clinical Ethics: A Practical Approach to Ethical Decisions in Clinical Medicine, 5th ed. New York, McGraw-Hill, 2002, pp 25–30, 41–66, 69–73, 83–86, 95–101, 105–114, 134–146.
6. Lo B, Ruston D, Kates LW, et al: Discussing religious and spiritual issues at the end of life: A practical guide for physicians. JAMA 287:749–754, 2002.
7. Meisel A, Jennings B: Ethics, end-of-life care, the law: Overview. In Doka KJ, Jennings B, Corr CA (eds): Living with Grief: Ethical Dilemmas at the End of Life. Hospice Foundation of America, 2005, pp 63–79.
8. Meisel A, Snyder L, Quill T: Seven legal barriers to end-of-life care: Myths, realities, and grains of truth. JAMA 248:2495–2501, 2000.
9. Tiano N, Beyer E: Cultural religious views on non-beneficial treatment. In Doka KJ, Jennings B, Corr CA (eds): Living with Grief: Ethical Dilemmas at the End of Life. Hospice Foundation of America, 2005, pp 41–62.

CHAPTER 91

BREAKING BAD NEWS: AN ART BEYOND SCIENCE

Jeffrey L. Greenwald, MD, and Barry S. Greenwald, PhD

1. **What constitutes "bad news"?**

   Bad news is hard to define, but most of us think we know it when we hear it. "Your tumor is inoperable." "I'm afraid we won't be able to restore your sight." "The pills are no longer sufficient for your diabetes, so we'll need to consider starting you on insulin." Bad news has been defined as "situations where there is either a feeling of no hope, a threat to a person's mental or physical well-being, a risk of upsetting an established lifestyle, or where a message is given which conveys to an individual fewer choices in his or her life." Remember, bad news is subjective. Something you might consider devastating may not be received that way by a patient. Alternatively, information you consider minor may trigger a greater reaction than you anticipate.

   Bor R, Miller R, Goldman E, Scher I: The meaning of bad news in HIV disease: Counseling about dreaded issues revisited. Cousel Psychol Q 6:69–80, 1993.

2. **How do I know whether a patient is ready to hear bad news? How can I prepare him or her?**

   People are never really ready to hear bad news. There is always some degree of shock and surprise. However, most patients have some awareness that something out of the ordinary is taking place. Patients vary enormously in what they want to know, how much they want to be involved in decision making, and their willingness to give control over to their doctor. The better you know your patient, the more able you are to discuss his or her wishes openly and modulate your approach to the patient's readiness to hear the news. Watch your patient's face. Make eye contact. Patients, even the most open ones, can "close down" in an instant.

3. **What do I need to do to prepare myself to give bad news to a patient?**

   Take a moment to think about the message you wish to convey and how you believe the patient will want to hear it. Try to find a location that minimizes distractions and is comfortable. Always have tissues and water handy for the patient and family. Remember to use simple language, avoid jargon, and be cognizant of cultural barriers and expectations. If you have introduced the possibility of bad news previously, try to use similar wording. If you are not an expert on the issue, try to familiarize yourself with the basic information but be prepared to say that you do not have all the answers and that you will assist in obtaining them where possible.

4. **How long does breaking bad news take?**

   Breaking bad news is a process. You do not need to complete the discussion in one sitting. Allocate sufficient time to initiate the conversation and engage the patient and family in discussion. At a minimum, you should leave yourself 15 minutes, though these discussions can take more than an hour. Inform the patient that you will return later to answer further questions. Try not to rush. Patients and family members can sense it, and it may make them feel like you no longer want to care for them.

5. **Who should be present when I break the news to the patient?**

   Some patients prefer to receive the news alone, whereas others prefer to have a friend or family member around. If you can anticipate when the news will be delivered (e.g., you know when the

HIV test results will return from the laboratory), you may wish to ask the patient whether he or she prefers to have someone there when the results return. If you think it is appropriate and helpful, you might also include a senior clinician, a nurse, a member of the clergy, or a mental health specialist. Often including the patient's primary care physician (PCP) is useful, especially if the PCP has a longstanding relationship with the patient. You must decide what situation will make the patient, family, and you most comfortable.

6. **How do I begin the conversation?**
If you have news to share, especially if the patient expects that news is coming, avoid small talk and get right to it. Offering a warning shot like, "I am afraid I have some bad news," or, "I have something serious to share with you," is often a helpful way to begin. Then, proceeding slowly, break the news down into small chunks. Patients rarely want or can handle all the news with all the associated options, implications, and decisions that may be required immediately. Take it step-wise, allowing the patient to ask questions and drive the conversation. Remember, patients often absorb little after the initial shock of the news. Repetition during the conversation and subsequently is useful and should be expected.

7. **What if there is no hope of fixing the problem?**
Maintaining hope, even if based on a long shot, is important, especially initially. If there really is no reasonable or even slim hope of "fixing" the problem, remember that fixing problems is only one aspect of care. You must convey that the focus of care will now shift toward controlling the patient's symptoms, maintaining his or her independence, and, most importantly, preserving the patient's dignity. Beginning to explore the patient's wishes regarding desired care, therapies, and interventions is important so you can tailor your plans to the patient's goals.

8. **What other messages are important for the patient to hear?**
When there are no longer curative treatments to suggest, physicians sometimes feel they have nothing further to offer. It is critical to reassure patients that you will not abandon them and that you will continue to care for them and offer palliative therapies to make them comfortable, keep them functional, and preserve their dignity. Your body language can also help to convey this message. Sit near the patient; if possible, do not stand over him or her. A gentle touch on the patient's hand, arm, or shoulder can be calming to some patients, helping them realize they are not alone.

9. **What if they cry, yell, or do not respond at all?**
It is difficult to deal with a patient's intense emotions or absolute silence. Common physician reactions are, "How do I stop this?" "Why can't I fix this?" or "How do I get as far away from this as possible?" The patient who dissolves in tears needs to cry. The patient who fights back his or her emotions may be trying desperately to remain in control. The silent patient, stunned by the news or not able to absorb what has been said, is doing the best he or she can to cope. These reactions need to be respected. The best response is to sit quietly with the patient and allow the feelings to take their course.

10. **Will I ever get used to giving bad news?**
No matter how many times you deliver bad news, there is no getting used to it. We are trained to heal, and when that training no longer suffices, we face the human condition of helplessness that none of us enjoy. Bad news forces the physician to come to terms with his or her limits. It can drive us behind a wall of supposed professionalism that disallows feelings, defining everything as "just a part of the job." Any and all of these reactions are costly. Nonetheless, when done well, the physician may feel satisfied that he or she has had a positive impact on the life transition the patient is facing. Sharing this experience with colleagues is helpful also. Just plain talk, including the feelings, frustrations, and doubts, can be restorative.

KEY POINTS: AN APPROACH TO BREAKING BAD NEWS

1. Think about what you want to say and how you want to say it before you begin the conversation with the patient.

2. When you begin the conversation, get to the news quickly. Consider a warning shot like "I'm afraid I have some serious news."

3. Tailor your discussion of the bad news to the level of readiness and reactions of the patient. Never assume how patients will react to your news.

4. Leave yourself plenty of time to have the conversation. It cannot be rushed.

5. Make sure your patient understands that you will continue to care for him or her irrespective of the course of his or her illness.

11. What do I do when it is over?

It is important to do two things after such a conversation with a patient. First, it is often helpful to request feedback and observations about how the discussion went from someone who was present so you may learn from the experience. Although there is no one right way to break bad news, you will certainly learn from the experience, and feedback will assist along the way. The second important step is to document your discussion in the chart so that other physicians will know exactly what information has been given to the patient and where you believe the patient is in the process of understanding the information.

WEBSITES

1. Beyond Breaking Bad News: Helping Patients Who Suffer
   http://www.studentbmj.com/back_issues/0300/education/65.html

2. Breaking Bad News
   http://www.breakingbadnews.co.uk/

3. A Framework for Breaking Bad News
   http://www.skillscascade.com/badnews.htm

BIBLIOGRAPHY

1. Farber NJ, Urban SY, Collier VU, et al: The good news about giving bad news to patients. J Gen Int Med 17:914–921, 2002.
2. Ptacek JT, Eberhardt TL: Breaking bad news: A review of the literature. JAMA 276:496–502, 1996.

CHAPTER 92

HOSPICE

Solomon Liao, MD

1. **What is hospice?**

   Hospice is not a physical place but rather a model of care that addresses the physical, emotional, social, and existential needs of the whole person and the family. To achieve this comprehensive care, an interdisciplinary team approach is essential.

KEY POINTS: COMMON MYTHS ABOUT HOSPICE

1. Hospice is a place.

2. Patients must have prognosis of 6 months or less to be eligible for hospice.

3. Patients must have a DNR order to be eligible for hospice.

4. Hospice chaplains try to push religion.

5. Going onto hospice means "giving up all hope."

6. Patients cannot have chemotherapy, radiation treatments, blood transfusions, or surgery while on hospice.

7. Hospice patients cannot come back to the emergency department or hospital.

---

2. **How is hospice different from palliative care?**

   Hospice care is a type of palliative care but limited to the final stage of life. Like palliative care, patients do not have to give up curative options, especially if not related to the terminal condition (e.g., providing antibiotics for cellulitis in a cancer patient is a form of a curative therapy not aimed at the underlying terminal diagnosis). However, unlike palliative care, in hospice, patients and families do have to put comfort care as the primary goal of care. (See Chapter 87.)

3. **Who is eligible for hospice?**

   Anyone with a limited prognosis (generally considered 1 year or less) or life-threatening illness is eligible for hospice. Although most hospices use standard guidelines developed by the National Hospice and Palliative Care Organization for determining prognosis and eligibility, studies have shown that these guidelines are no more accurate than a clinician's judgment. By Medicare regulations, the ultimate judgment of prognosis is the physician's overall clinical evaluation. Patients are not required to have a do-not-resuscitate (DNR) order, nor must they have a tissue diagnosis of cancer to be eligible for hospice (Table 92-1). They must, however, have a designated caregiver, and the patient and family must accept a palliative approach to care.

4. **What does hospice provide?**

   Hospice provides all the palliative therapies that are related to the end-stage illness. These therapies include professional services, medications, and durable medical equipment, such as oxygen, a

TABLE 92-1. TYPICAL PROFILE OF NON-CANCER HOSPICE PATIENTS

General system decline

- Elderly patient not clearly dying of one diagnosis or organ problem but clearly declining significantly. Also called multiorgan failure, multisystems failure, failure to thrive, general debility, or terminal debility.

Dementia

- Recurrent aspiration pneumonia
- Weight loss
- Lethargic delirium

Heart failure

- Accelerated hospitalization: increasing frequency or shortening duration between hospitalizations
- Refractory symptoms despite maximal therapy
- Severe functional impairment

Chronic obstructive pulmonary disease

- Accelerated hospitalization
- Unable to eat, losing weight (e.g., pulmonary cachexia)
- Needs or uses nebulizers and inhalers more frequently than every 4 hours

Acquired immunodeficiency syndrome

- Increasing infections or development of drug-resistant infections
- Progressive multifocal leukoencephalopathy
- Malignancy
- Failed or unable to take highly active antiretroviral therapy

Amyotrophic lateral sclerosis

- Requiring respiratory support
- Declined or failed artificial nutrition

hospital bed, and bedside commode. Hospice services can include antibiotics, artificial hydration/nutrition, blood transfusions, chemotherapy, radiation, and surgery (as long as the goal is palliative and not curative, and if no other options are available to relieve the symptom). Home hospice provides emergency services 24 hours a day and 7 days a week. This includes on-call nurses, social workers, and chaplains who are available to come to the house as necessary. Hospice is required to provide bereavement follow-up for the family for a minimum of 13 months.

5. **What doesn't hospice cover?**
   Hospice does not cover custodial or "non-skilled" needs, such as cooking and cleaning. Non-skilled needs are those things that can be done by a family member and do not require a licensed health professional. Hospice also will not cover preexisting or non–terminal-related conditions, such as diabetes or hypertension. Additionally, they will not cover experimental trials or interventions that have a curative or preventive intent. Some palliative treatments may extend life or prevent complications of diseases and are allowed as long as the primary goal of care is palliative and not curative.

6. **What are the different levels of hospice care?**
   Most (80%) of hospice care is done at home under *routine* care. Routine care provides visits by an interdisciplinary team (Table 92-2), generally 2–3 times a week. For patients and families

---

TABLE 92-2.   MEMBERS OF THE INTERDISCIPLINARY HOSPICE TEAM AND THEIR ROLES

- **Medical director:** Supervises medical care, signs certification, assists primary care physician
- **Nurse:** The case manager in most hospices, interacts most commonly with the patient and family (typically visits 1–3 times a week)
- **Social worker:** Psychosocial assessment and intervention (typically visits 1–2 times a month)
- **Chaplain:** Coordinates spiritual and existential care (typically visits once a month)
- **Bereavement coordinator:** Assesses risk of family for complicated grief and coordinates or provides bereavement services
- **Home health aide (bath aide):** Provides baths and massages
- **Volunteer coordinator:** Supervises and coordinates volunteers

---

requiring more intensive attention (at least daily visits), either *continuous* care or *general inpatient* (GIP) care can be instituted. *Respite* care provides custodial nursing home placement for up to 5 days at a time, allowing overwhelmed caregivers a break.

7. **What are the advantages of continuous and GIP care?**
   Continuous care provides around-the-clock skilled care at home (usually by a licensed nurse), allowing the patient to stay at home. GIP care covers the cost of admission to a nursing home, inpatient hospice unit, or a palliative care bed in a hospital, including room and board. Actively dying patients (with a prognosis of < 2 weeks) requiring intensive monitoring often opt for GIP. Use of GIP can shorten the length of hospital stay for these patients.

8. **What if the patient lives past 6 months on hospice?**
   The traditional 6-month marker should no longer be used. Although the initial physician certification for hospice patients still uses this mark on the paperwork, in practice there is nothing special about this time marker in the current recertification process. As long as the patient's condition continues to decline, they can be recertified almost indefinitely. Recertification occurs at the first 90 days, the second 90 days, and then every 60 days thereafter. In other words, there is no penalty for the patient, family, hospice, or physician if the patient lives past the 6-month point.

9. **Can a patient be discharged from hospice?**
   Patients can be discharged from hospice if their condition stabilizes (i.e., if they are no longer declining), if they are admitted to an acute care hospital for nonpalliative reasons, or if the hospice can no longer provide care (e.g., the patient moves out of the coverage area or the environment is unsafe for staff visits). Patients or family can also choose to disenroll from hospice at any time—most commonly because they want to seek life-prolonging measures. Patients can return to hospice status, assuming they still qualify, as many times as they wish without penalty.

10. **Who pays for hospice?**
    Most hospice care in the United States is paid through Medicare. The rest is provided through Medicaid or private insurance. Nonprofit hospice agencies will often provide hospice care to patients who lack insurance and are unable to pay. Hospice care is therefore completely free for most patients and families. Medicare and Medicaid pay a rate nationally of approximately $120 a

day directly to the hospice with no deductible for the patient. Private insurers may use different payment structures, such as capping the total cost at a fixed amount (e.g., $10,000), paying for each unit of service (e.g., each nursing visit) as they do for home health, or requiring the patient to pay a deductible.

WEBSITES

1. American Academy of Hospice and Palliative Medicine
   http://www.aahpm.org

2. End of Life/Palliative Education Resource Center
   http://www.eperc.mcw.edu

3. National Hospice and Palliative Care Organization
   http://www.nhpco.org

BIBLIOGRAPHY

1. Herbst L: Hospice care at the end of life. Clin Geriatr Med 20:753–765, vii, 2004.
2. Perron V, Schonwetter R: Hospice and palliative care programs. Prim Care 28:427–440, 2001.

CHAPTER 93

PAIN MANAGEMENT IN THE HOSPITALIZED PATIENT

Bradley Flansbaum, DO, MPH

1. What is pain? Why is pain management important?

Pain is a subjective complaint without reliable objective measures. Two commonly used definitions are:

- An unpleasant sensory and emotional experience associated with actual or potential tissue damage.
- Whatever the experiencing person says it is, existing whenever he or she says it does.

Pain in both the community and hospital setting is *very* common. It is distressing to patients, affects psychological well-being, and detracts from their quality of life. Additionally, lost productivity and overuse of health care services exert a huge economic toll. Poorly managed pain in a hospitalized patient may also lead to increased length of stay and adverse medical outcomes such as an increased risk of deep venous thrombosis and pneumonia.

2. Do physicians underdiagnose pain?

Yes. Pain management has less value as a bona fide discipline within the medical community. As trainees, students and residents are infrequently "rewarded" for diagnosing pain and have limited positive mentoring experiences. It is also unlikely that recognizable complications will result from disregarding pain complaints.

3. Do physicians undertreat pain?

Even when diagnosed, physicians inadequately medicate patients experiencing pain. In many studies, physicians fail to relieve pain in up to half of patients experiencing generalized pain. The magnitude of cancer pain is often underappreciated, contributing to unnecessary end-of-life suffering. Patients often report severe pain early in their hospital stay, but physicians may be fearful of dispensing narcotics because of increasing federal and state regulations or concerns about narcotic adverse effects. Some have called this "opiophobia."

4. What are key factors in assessing pain?

Predicting patients at high risk for pain, such as persons with sickle cell anemia, is a straightforward task. However, selecting patients at low risk for pain is difficult, and thus, a broad-based, nonselective approach to screening is prudent. Behavioral and physiologic signs and symptoms are *not* accurate guides for assessing pain. A patient's self-report is the most reliable indicator of pain.

KEY POINTS: PAIN

1. Chronic and acute pain are common, and awareness of the problem among physicians is poor.

2. Inattention to and neglect of pain are the largest barrier to its appropriate treatment.

3. Mandates to assess and treat pain are common, and physicians will need to improve their pain management skills.

5. **When is it necessary to assess pain? How is this done?**
   Pain assessment is necessary in all hospitalized patients. Recognized as "the fifth vital sign," pain assessment has been mandated in U.S. hospitals since 2001. The use of numeric or visual tools assists physicians in translating the pain experience of patients. The reliability of these instruments is contingent on patient education, language, cognition, and culture and is at times imperfect.
   - **Numeric scale:** Patients rate pain based on a 0–10 self-report scale.
   - **Visual analog scale:** The patient points to a place on a short horizontal line, with the left and right boundaries of the line representing the extreme absence or presence of pain.
   - **FACES Pain Scale:** Faces portraying emotional states, smiling to tearful, move from left to right (Fig. 93-1). The patient chooses the face that best represents his or her condition.

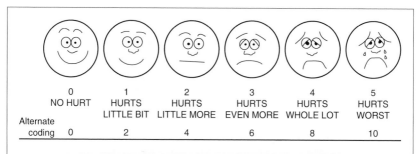

	0 NO HURT	1 HURTS LITTLE BIT	2 HURTS LITTLE MORE	3 HURTS EVEN MORE	4 HURTS WHOLE LOT	5 HURTS WORST
Alternate coding	0	2	4	6	8	10

Figure 93-1. Wong-Baker FACES Pain Rating Scale. (From Hockenberry MJ, Wilson D, Winkelstein ML: Wong's Essentials of Pediatric Nursing, 7th ed. St. Louis, Mosby, 2005, p 1259, with permission.)

6. **How is mild, moderate, and severe pain characterized?**
   Both the visual analog and FACES pain scale have a 0–10 numeric dimension to represent mild (0–3) moderate (4–7), and severe pain (8–10). *The goal for pain treatment is a pain rating <3.*

7. **What is the World Health Organization (WHO) analgesic ladder?**
   The WHO designed a progressive three-step approach to the treatment of pain (Fig. 93-2). Although the algorithm was intended for use in patients with cancer, it is applicable to any person with pain.

KEY POINTS: PATIENT ASSESSMENT

1. A patient's self-report is the most reliable indicator to assess pain.

2. All hospitalized patients require documentation of pain assessment action.

3. Measuring severity of pain is important and will assist in the choice of an appropriate therapy.

8. **List appropriate medications to treat mild, moderate, and severe pain.**
   - **Mild:** Nonopioid analgesics are the treatment of choice (e.g., nonsteroidal anti-inflammatory drugs [NSAIDs], acetaminophen, and aspirin).
   - **Moderate:** Less potent narcotics (e.g., codeine, hydrocodone) are recommended, or stronger ones (e.g., morphine) in lower doses combined with nonopioid analgesics.

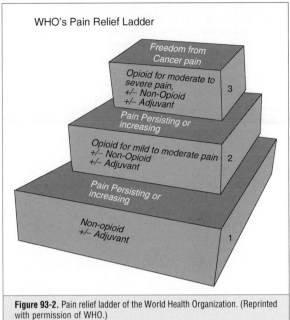

Figure 93-2. Pain relief ladder of the World Health Organization. (Reprinted with permission of WHO.)

- **Severe:** More potent narcotics such as morphine, hydromorphone, and oxycodone are appropriate.

9. **What are adjuvant drugs, and how are they used?**
   Adjuvant drugs, including antiepileptics, antidepressants, and corticosteroids, have primary indications other than pain management. However, they are helpful in the setting of subacute or chronic pain, have narcotic-sparing effects, and are particularly useful for treatment of neuropathic pain (see question 26).

10. **What narcotics are best for everyday practice?**
    There are many products on the market, and few are "better" than the rest. It is important to become knowledgeable about the most common drugs and learn their properties. Table 93-1 lists the drugs frequently encountered in the hospital setting.

11. **Do all narcotics behave similarly?**
    No. Commonly used narcotics such as hydrocodone and codeine have "ceiling effects." A dose is reached beyond which additional side effects, but not pain relief, occur. Narcotics like morphine and hydromorphone have no such properties, so dose escalation should continue until pain relief is achieved, barring adverse effects.

12. **Which pain medications are not ideal for routine use?**
    Narcotic agonist/antagonist medications such as butorphanol and pentazocine are problematic in patients using narcotics chronically and may cause opioid withdrawal. Given its toxicity and multiple drug interactions, meperidine use should be avoided. Additionally, its touted clinical advantage (mainly, its lack of spasmodic effect on the biliary tree) is unfounded. Methadone's unpredictable kinetics and potential stigmatization, and the difficulty in obtaining prescriptions for this drug make this a second-line choice that is not ideal for acute pain.

TABLE 93-1. ANALGESIC EQUIVALENTS OF COMMONLY USED NARCOTICS

Generic Name	Sample Trade Name	Oral Dosing Interval	Equivalent Oral Doses (mg)	Equivalent Intravenous Doses (mg)†	Other Available Routes of Administration
Codeine/acetaminophen	Tylenol #3 (30 mg codeine)	q4h	200*	N/A	PO
Hydrocodone/acetaminophen	Vicodin (5 mg hydrocodone)	q4–6h	30*	N/A	PO
Oxycodone/acetaminophen	Percocet	q4–6h	20*	N/A	PO
Oxycodone, controlled-release	OxyIR	q4–6h	20		
	OxyContin	q12h	60		
Morphine, controlled-release	MSIR	q4h	30	10	Rectal, subcutaneous, epidural, intrathecal, sublingual
	MS Contin	q12h	90		
Hydromorphone	Dilaudid	q4–6h	7.5	1.5	Rectal, subcutaneous, epidural, intrathecal
Fentanyl	Duragesic (transdermal)	N/A	N/A	100 μg	Transdermal, epidural, intrathecal, oral transmucosal

PO = by mouth.
*Excluding acetaminophen.
†See question 14.

13. **List the various routes of administration available for analgesics.**
    Opioid analgesics in their various forms are available for virtually every route of administration—oral, rectal, subcutaneous, intramuscular, intravenous, topical, intranasal, and intraspinal.

14. **What narcotics are best for parenteral use?**
    Morphine and hydromorphone. Both are available for subcutaneous or intravenous administration. Avoid intramuscular use because absorption is unpredictable and painful. The potency ratio of morphine to hydromorphone is 6:1. Usual subcutaneous starting doses are 5–10 mg every 3–4 hours and 1–2 mg every 3–4 hours, respectively. Intravenous administration can be given continuously or via bolus.

15. **Describe the approach to initiating an analgesic regimen for a hospitalized patient.**
    Assess the degree of pain using a pain scale, and begin nonopioid therapy for mild to moderate pain and opioids for moderate to severe pain. For opioids, start with a scheduled short-acting formulation using around-the-clock dosing. Oral dosing is preferred, but the patient's condition or need for immediate relief may require the use of a subcutaneous or intravenous route. Simultaneously, make available breakthrough doses of medication to cover recurrent pain between regular administrations of drugs (typically 50% of the fixed short-acting dose). An order for a person with severe pain might look as follows: (1) morphine sulfate, 10 mg given orally every 4 hours, plus (2) morphine sulfate, 5 mg given orally every 2 hours as needed for breakthrough pain. Reassess pain every few hours and increase fixed dose based on pain scale findings or frequent need for breakthrough medication.

KEY POINTS: PAIN MANAGEMENT

1. The primary treatment consideration is always patient comfort, with the dose of narcotic being secondary.

2. No best narcotic exists. Route and response dictate the ideal drug for the patient.

3. Morphine is versatile, very effective, and inexpensive—become comfortable with its use.

16. **What is the difference between analgesics administered in fixed-dose versus breakthrough fashion?**
    Pain intensity sometimes fluctuates and requires additional treatment above regularly prescribed doses. Patients need breakthrough or "rescue" medication in the event pain increases. Both forms of dosing should always be available simultaneously, especially when pain is acute.

17. **When is long-acting medication necessary?**
    Long-acting or controlled-release medication is the preferred therapy for patients with unremitting pain. Morphine and oxycodone are available in long-acting oral formulations. Fentanyl is available in a transdermal patch that requires a change once every 3 days. After adequate pain control is achieved with short-acting and breakthrough medication, tally the total used in a 24-hour period and convert to a long-acting formulation. For example, if a patient used 60 mg of fixed-dose morphine and 5 mg of breakthrough over 24 hours, converting to morphine 30 mg every 12 hours, controlled-release would be appropriate. Always continue breakthrough medication with long-acting formulations. A good general rule is that the breakthrough dose should be 10–20% of the 24-hour dose every 2 hours. In the case of a patient receiving long-acting morphine, 30 mg taken orally every 12 hours, an appropriate breakthrough dose would be morphine sulfate 10 mg every 2 hours as needed.

18. **What are the pitfalls of treating patients with pain medications on an "ask-only" (PRN) basis?**

Treating patients in a fixed-dose fashion ensures they will receive analgesia at prescribed intervals. Ask-only dosing allows patients to receive analgesia only when they request it. It is problematic in patients who cannot make their needs known or who have not consented to this approach of treatment. Such patients are unable to maintain adequate blood levels of medication and may suffer needlessly. Ask-only dosing should only be used in persons with mild pain or for those who receive appropriate education.

19. **What options are available if the initial response to treatment is suboptimal?**

Continue to increase the current dose of narcotic based on breakthrough and pain scale needs, monitoring for adverse effects. Schedule a nonopioid therapy such as an NSAID or acetaminophen. These work synergistically with narcotics and enhance their analgesic effects. Switch medications using equianalgesic doses of another narcotic (see Table 93-1), since patients may respond more favorably to another drug. There is incomplete cross-tolerance among narcotics, so it is best to reduce the dose by 25–50% of the equivalent dose when switching.

20. **What is a patient-controlled analgesia (PCA) pump?**

PCA is a form of analgesia that uses an automated pump to administer narcotics in response to patient demand. The pump settings, such as the maximum individual and hourly doses, are set in advance by the physician. PCA pumps are helpful in the setting of severe pain when patient narcotic needs are difficult to predict. When pain is controlled, transition the patient to oral medications.

21. **How does management of chronic pain differ from that of acute pain?**

The management philosophy is similar: use long-acting medications continuously and provide short-acting rescue medication for pain exacerbations. Ideal regimens may take 1–2 months to titrate. Use of adjuvant medications such as antidepressants or antiepileptic drugs is common. Issues such as tolerance, opioid rotation, and use of less common narcotics such as methadone and levorphanol are more commonplace. Patients with long-term pain needs are best referred to a pain specialist.

KEY POINTS: PAIN IN HOSPITALIZED PATIENTS

1. Only use PRN drug dosing when the pain is mild and the patient is educated and consents to this treatment.

2. Long-acting narcotics are not appropriate for the initial treatment of acute pain.

3. Continue to titrate narcotics until pain is relieved or an adverse effect appears.

4. Administering narcotics in a fixed-dose and breakthrough fashion is always the preferred method to manage moderate to severe pain.

5. There is incomplete cross-tolerance between narcotics. Reduce doses of narcotics when switching therapy.

22. **When narcotics are no longer necessary, can they be abruptly discontinued?**

No. Dependence may develop, and narcotics must be decreased slowly over time to avoid opiate withdrawal.

23. **List common adverse effects often associated with analgesics.**
   - **Urinary retention:** This occurs especially in men with prostatic hypertrophy
   - **Sedation:** Tolerance develops rapidly.
   - **Constipation:** The only adverse effect that will not diminish with time. Always anticipate and routinely use cathartics.
   - **Itching and hives:** Respond to antihistamines.
   - **Nausea and vomiting:** Begin antiemetics.
   - **Delirium:** Elderly particularly susceptible, stop or decrease dose.
   - **Respiratory depression secondary to narcotics:** This is rare in patients with pain. Pain is a potent stimulus to breathe.

24. **Is parenteral administration of narcotics better than the oral route?**
   In severe pain, the onset of action and peak effects of subcutaneous or intravenous administration make these routes preferable. Once pain is controlled, however, convert to oral dosing as soon as convenient. It is a misconception among patients and health providers that shots are "better." These routes are equivalent once a steady state is reached.

25. **Should patients with acute abdominal pain receive analgesics?**
   Despite classic teaching that pain control will mask important changes in status, withholding analgesia in patients with acute abdominal pain is not necessary. Randomized controlled trials examining this question are numerous, and the use of narcotics in this situation does not adversely affect outcomes.

26. **What is neuropathic pain? How is it treated?**
   Pain is an appropriate response to noxious stimuli. However, when a nerve injury occurs, it processes signals in an aberrant fashion and can lead to pain without a precipitant—that is, neuropathic pain. Diabetes mellitus is the most common cause of neuropathy. Neuropathic pain responds variably to antiepileptic drugs, tricyclic antidepressants, and narcotics, often leading to patient and physician frustration.

27. **Characterize the differences between the following terms as they relate to narcotic use: physical dependence, addiction, pseudoaddiction, and tolerance.**
   - **Physical dependence:** The appearance of an abstinence syndrome with abrupt cessation or diminution of chronic narcotic intake.
   - **Addiction:** A negative behavioral pattern of drug use for reasons other than pain control.
   - **Pseudoaddiction:** Drug-seeking behavior that seems similar to addiction but is due to unrelieved pain. Aberrant behavior disappears with treatment.
   - **Tolerance:** The need for increased dosage of a drug over time to produce the same level of analgesia, assuming no worsening of pain.

WEBSITE

Pain: Current Understanding of Assessment, Management, and Treatments. National Pharmaceutical Council
http://www.npcnow.org/

BIBLIOGRAPHY

1. ACP Observer: Pain Management for the Internist, December, 2004, pp 1–12.
2. Ballantyne JC, Mao J: Opioid therapy for chronic pain. N Engl J Med 349:1943–1953, 2003.
3. Whelan CT, Jin L, Meltzer D: Pain and satisfaction with pain control in hospitalized medical patients: No such thing as low risk. Arch Intern Med 164:175–180, 2004.

MANAGEMENT OF COMMON PHYSICAL AND PSYCHOLOGICAL SYMPTOMS

Jeanie Youngwerth, MD, and Daniel Johnson, MD

1. **Why is it important to be aware of and treat symptoms at the end of life?**
   Terminal illness is associated with significant disability and suffering. Aggressive care focused on symptom management can improve functional ability and quality of life. In addition to pain, other distressing symptoms such as nausea and vomiting, constipation, dyspnea, agitation and delirium, and depression are common in patients with advanced and terminal illness. For example, patients with advanced cancer have high rates of nausea (75%), constipation (50–95%), dyspnea (18–79% in the last week of life), delirium (15–85%), and depression (25–53%).

2. **Describe a general approach to managing symptoms in a patient with advanced illness.**
   When assessing symptoms in a patient with advanced illness, it is important to understand the patient's goals and identify expectations for treatment. When consistent with patient goals, treat reversible causes and use symptomatic therapies to relieve symptom distress (Fig. 94-1).

3. **What are common causes of nausea and vomiting in a patient with advanced illness?**
   Common causes of nausea and vomiting in advanced illness include medications, constipation, obstruction, tumor, uremia, infection, metabolic abnormalities, and increased intracranial pressure. When choosing symptomatic treatment, target therapies based on the four pathophysiologic mechanisms that mediate nausea and vomiting (Table 94-1).

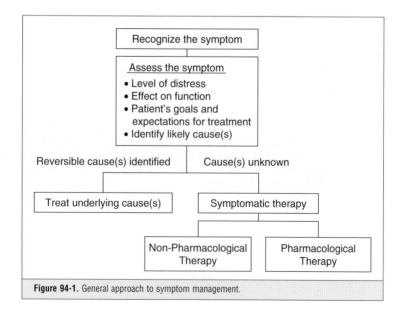

Figure 94-1. General approach to symptom management.

TABLE 94-1. COMMON CAUSES OF NAUSEA AND VOMITING IN ADVANCED ILLNESS

Mechanism	Causes	Primary Neurotransmitters and Mediators	Pharmacologic Treatments
Cerebral cortex	Increased intracranial pressure	? Pressure receptors	Corticosteroids (e.g., dexamethasone)
	Psychosocial factors (e.g., pain, anxiety, memories, odors)	Learned responses	Benzodiazepines (e.g., lorazepam)
Chemoreceptor trigger zone	Chemically induced factors (e.g., drugs, electrolyte abnormalities)	Dopamine	Dopamine blockers (e.g., haloperidol, chlorpromazine, prochlorperazine)
	Infections (cytokine-mediated)		
Vestibular apparatus	Motion or positional factors	Acetylcholine	Anticholinergic agents (e.g., scopolamine)
	Local tumors	Histamine	Antihistamines (e.g., hydroxyzine, diphenhydramine)
GI tract	Irritation of the GI tract (e.g., mucositis, gastritis, organ distention, constipation, bowel obstruction)	Acetylcholine Serotonin	Anticholinergic agents (e.g., promethazine, scopolamine) Serotonin blockers (e.g., ondansetron, metoclopromide)

GI = gastrointestinal.

4. **What nonpharmacologic interventions can be used to treat nausea and vomiting?**
   Review the patient's medication list for potential culprits that can be stopped (e.g., opioids, digitalis, iron, chemotherapeutic agents, NSAIDs). Utilize small, frequent meals with bland food, and consider using distraction, visualization, and/or relaxation techniques. Control the patient's pain or other symptoms, as this may exacerbate nausea and vomiting. Attend to concomitant social, psychological, and spiritual problems.

5. **Which medications are most effective in managing nausea and vomiting?**
   Select an antiemetic based on the likely underlying pathophysiologic mechanism. This approach will optimize therapy by targeting key receptors while minimizing unnecessary adverse effects (see Table 94-1).

6. **How should a patient with refractory nausea and vomiting be managed?**
   Reevaluate the patient's condition and identify potentially reversible causes. Maximize the dose of the selected antiemetic agent before adding a second agent. When choosing a second agent,

use an antiemetic from a different class. Use combinations of drugs targeting multiple mechanisms (e.g., diphenhydramine, dexamethasone, and metoclopramide). Although expensive, ondansetron is frequently effective in the treatment of severe nausea.

7. **What are common causes of constipation in patients with terminal illnesses?**
   - **Medications:** Opioids, anticholinergics, iron, antihypertensives
   - **Metabolic abnormalities:** Hypercalcemia, hypothyroidism
   - **Gastrointestinal factors:** Bowel obstruction, anal fissures, hemorrhoids, tumor
   - **Neurologic conditions:** Nerve or spinal cord compression, visceral neuropathy
   - **Environmental factors:** Inactivity, poor food and fluid intake, poorly accessible toilet facilities
   - **Psychological conditions:** Depression, anxiety, confusion

8. **How can constipation be prevented?**
   Opioids are one of the most common causes of constipation in terminally ill patients. Provide scheduled stimulant laxatives (e.g., senna or bisacodyl) with or without a stool softener in patients taking scheduled or frequent opioids. Fiber can potentially worsen constipation in opioid-dependent, sedentary patients with poor oral intake. When possible, encourage oral hydration and regular activity.

9. **What nonpharmacologic interventions can be used to manage constipation?**
   Minimize or stop the administration of constipating medications. Establish a regular bowel routine that takes advantage of the gastrocolic reflex that occurs after eating. Toilet facilities should be easily accessible. When consistent with patient goals, encourage fluid intake and activity.

10. **Name the seven major categories of laxatives and their mechanism of action.**
    See Table 94-2.

TABLE 94-2. MAJOR CATEGORIES OF LAXATIVES AND MECHANISMS OF ACTION		
Laxative Category	**Mechanism**	**Medications**
Bulk-forming	Increase stool bulk by absorbing water	Methylcellulose
	Decrease colon transit time	Psyllium
Surfactant	Enhance fat dissolution in water	Docusate
	Increase water content	
Osmotic	Increase water retention of stool	Lactulose
	Increase peristalsis	Sorbitol
		Milk of magnesia
Stimulant	Irritate the bowel	Senna
	Increase peristalsis	Bisacodyl
Prokinetic	Stimulate the mesenteric plexus	Metoclopramide
	Increase peristalsis	
Lubricant	Lubricate stool	Glycerin suppositories
	Irritate the bowel	Mineral oil
	Increase peristalsis	
Large-volume enemas	Increase water content of stool	Warm water enemas
	Distend/irritate the colon	Soap suds enemas
	Increase peristalsis	

11. **How should a patient with refractory constipation be managed?**
Reevaluate the patient's condition and identify potentially reversible causes. For patients taking opioids, titrate maintenance stimulants (e.g., senna or bisacodyl) to achieve a bowel movement every 1–3 days. The dose of the selected laxative should be maximized before additional agents are added. When adding a second agent, consider choosing an osmotic agent (e.g., sorbitol, lactulose, or magnesium citrate). For patients with impaction or hard stool in the rectal vault, use lubricant agents and large-volume enemas to soften stool before manual disimpaction. When possible, use nonopioid and adjuvant analgesics to minimize opioid-induced constipation.

12. **What are common causes of dyspnea in the palliative care patient?**
Dyspnea is the sensation of breathlessness. The "BREATH AIR" mnemonic can be helpful in identifying common causes of or contributing factors to breathlessness.
  - **B:** Bronchospasm (chronic obstructive pulmonary disease, asthma)
  - **R:** Rales (pneumonia)
  - **E:** Effusion (pleural or pericardial), edema (congestive heart failure, end-stage renal disease), embolism (pulmonary embolism)
  - **A:** Anemia, acidosis, ascites
  - **T:** Thick secretions
  - **H:** Hypoxia, hypercapnia
  - **A:** Anxiety
  - **I:** Interpersonal issues (family, financial, legal)
  - **R:** Religion/spiritual concerns

13. **What nonpharmacologic interventions are useful in managing dyspnea?**
When consistent with patient goals, identify and treat reversible causes. Optimize the environment by humidifying the air, using fans, cooling the ambient temperature, and eliminating respiratory irritants. Patient comfort should be optimized by means of positioning and managing anxiety by using breathing and relaxation techniques. Avoid excess fluid intake, especially in patients with congestive heart failure and end-stage renal disease.

14. **Does oxygen provide relief for patients with dyspnea?**
Oxygen can provide relief of dyspnea in many patients with advanced illness. Recognize, however, that many patients with dyspnea are not hypoxic and that measurements of hypoxia, hypoxemia, or respiratory rate do *not* correlate with the sensation of dyspnea. Cool air moving across the face may provide the same level of relief as oxygen. Oxygen delivered via nasal cannula is typically tolerated better than oxygen via masks and interferes less with communication and oral intake.

15. **Which medications are most effective for treating dyspnea?**
Opioids are the drugs of choice for the symptomatic treatment of dyspnea. Less evidence supports the use of benzodiazepines for dyspnea. Anxiety from breathlessness may respond better to opioid therapy than to benzodiazepines.

16. **Does treating dyspnea with opioids lead to premature death?**
There is no evidence that opioids, when used appropriately to treat dyspnea, lead to premature death. Opioids can relieve dyspnea in most patients without significant effect on their respiratory rate or oxygenation. In opioid-naïve patients with severe lung disease (e.g., advanced chronic obstructive pulmonary disease), "start low and go slow" when titrating opioids for dyspnea. Try to avoid using combinations of sedating drugs (e.g., opioids with benzodiazepines) to minimize the risk for respiratory depression.

17. **How should a patient with refractory dyspnea be approached?**
Reevaluate the patient and identify potentially reversible causes. Corticosteroids (e.g., dexamethasone) may be helpful as a nonspecific adjunctive therapy. Low doses of chlorpromazine or promethazine may augment the positive effects of opioids on breathlessness. For patients experiencing unacceptable adverse effects from higher opioid doses, consider rotation to an alternative opioid or deliver the selected opioid via nebulization.

18. **What are common causes of agitation and delirium in a patient near the end of life?**
- **Medications:** Number-one cause in the hospital setting (e.g., analgesics, anticholinergics, histamine blockers, sedative-hypnotics)
- **Pain or other concurrent symptoms**
- **Environmental factors:** Unfamiliar environment, excessive stimuli
- **Metabolic abnormalities:** Hypercalcemia, uremia, hyponatremia, hypernatremia
- **Physiologic factors:** Hypoxia, hypercarbia, dehydration, constipation, urinary retention, infection

19. **Which nonpharmacologic interventions are useful in managing agitation and delirium?**
Identify and treat reversible causes, if consistent with the patient's goals. Discontinue all nonessential medications. Create a calm and supportive environment, with frequent reorientation using clocks and diurnal light variations. Avoid sleep deprivation or other disruptions in the sleep cycle. Optimize impaired vision or hearing when possible.

20. **What medications are most effective for managing agitation and delirium?**
If sedation is desired, use neuroleptics (e.g., haloperidol or chlorpromazine) as first-line agents. Although more costly, the atypical neuroleptics (e.g., risperidone, olanzapine, or quetiapine) are also effective. For patients who require long-term therapy for confusion and agitation, the atypical agents reduce the risk for extrapyramidal adverse effects. However, the atypical neuroleptics may increase mortality in the elderly. Use benzodiazepines with caution because these drugs are commonly associated with "paradoxical agitation," especially in the elderly.

21. **How should the patient with refractory agitation and delirium be treated?**
Reevaluate the patient's condition and identify potentially reversible causes. Maximize the dose of the chosen neuroleptic agent before adding additional medications. Consider rotating the neuroleptic to a more sedating neuroleptic/atypical neuroleptic or adding a benzodiazepine. If opioid toxicity is suspected, then consider opioid rotation. "Palliative sedation" with propofol, phenobarbital, or thiopental is used in extreme cases, where all other efforts have failed to bring relief from symptom distress.

22. **What factors commonly contribute to depression in a patient receiving palliative care?**
- **Psychological:** Spiritual pain, lack of social support, progressive physical impairment, loss of independence, feelings of burden on family
- **Physiologic:** Pain and other concurrent symptoms, cancer
- **Medications:** Chemotherapy, corticosteroids, interferon

23. **Name the factors that reliably predict depression in patients with advanced illness.**
Reliable predictors of depression in advanced illness are feelings of hopelessness, helplessness, worthlessness, loss of self-esteem, and suicidal ideation. Somatic symptoms (e.g., anorexia,

fatigue, insomnia) are less predictive given the high prevalence of these symptoms in patients with terminal illness. The simple question, "Are you depressed?" is a sensitive and specific screen for depression in advanced illness.

KEY POINTS: MANAGEMENT OF COMMON PHYSICAL AND PSYCHOLOGICAL SYMPTOMS ✔

1. An assessment of a symptom in advanced illness is not limited to simply looking for causes but needs to elicit the patient's concerns and level of distress, the effect on function, and the patient's goals and expectations for treatment.

2. Target medication therapy based on the common physiologic pathways and receptors that mediate nausea and vomiting.

3. Scheduled opioids require scheduled bowel stimulants. Fiber, fluids, and stool softeners are not enough!

4. Trust the patient's report of breathlessness. Measurements of hypoxia, hypoxemia, and respiratory rate do *not* consistently correlate with the sensation of dyspnea.

5. Common somatic complaints, such as insomnia, fatigue, and changes in appetite, do *not* accurately predict clinical depression in patients with advanced illness.

24. **Which nonpharmacologic interventions may be helpful in managing end-of-life depression?**
Cognitive and behavioral therapies, including relaxation therapy and meditation, can be helpful in managing end-of-life depression. These techniques can be used in conjunction with psychotherapy, which may involve individual and/or group counseling.

25. **Which medications are most effective for treating depression in advanced illness?**
Selective serotonin reuptake inhibitors (SSRIs) are often effective for depression in advanced illness. However, because the antidepressant effects of SSRIs may not be achieved for 4–6 weeks, consider starting a psychostimulant (e.g., methylphenidate) for patients needing more immediate relief (24–48 hours). Tricyclic antidepressants may be useful in patients with neuropathic pain and depression, although these drugs are usually less well tolerated due to their prominent anticholinergic adverse effects.

26. **How should a terminally ill patient with refractory depression be approached?**
Reevaluate the patient's condition and identify potentially reversible causes. For patients already taking an SSRI, consider adding methylphenidate. Incorporate an interdisciplinary team approach to address the physical, psychological, social, spiritual, and emotional needs of the patient. Consult a psychiatrist in cases of patients with refractory depression or suicidal ideation.

WEBSITE

1. End of Life/Palliative Education Resource Center—Fast Facts
http://www.eperc.mcw.edu

BIBLIOGRAPHY

1. Centeno C, Sanz A, Bruera E: Delirium in advanced cancer patients. Palliat Med 18:184–194, 2004.
2. EPEC Participant's Handbook, EPEC Project. The Robert Wood Johnson Foundation, Modules 6 and 10, 1999.
3. Klaschik E, Nauck F, Ostagathe C: Constipation—modern laxative therapy. Support Care Cancer 11:679–685, 2003.
4. Kvale PA, Simoff M, Prakash UBS: Palliative care. Chest 123:2845–3115, 2003.
5. Lipman AG, Jackson KC, Tyler LS: In Evidence Based Symptom Control in Palliative Care. Binghamton, NY, Pharmaceutical Products Press, 2000, pp 47–89, 109–127, 163–181.
6. Rao A, Cohen HJ: Symptom management in the elderly cancer patient: Fatigue, pain and depression. J Natl Cancer Inst Monogr 32:150–157, 2004.
7. Storey P, Knight CF: In UNIPAC Four: Management of Selected Non-pain Symptoms in the Terminally Ill, 2nd ed. Glenview, IL, Mary Ann Liebert, Inc., 2003, pp 29–52.

INDEX

Page numbers in **boldface type** indicate complete chapters.